Second Edition

Medical TERMINOLOGY

FOR HEALTH CAREERS

Alice G. Ettinger, RN, MSN, CPNP

Division of Pediatric Hematology-Oncology
Saint Peter's University Hospital
New Brunswick, New Jersey

Pamala F. Burch

Ozarks Technical Community College
Springfield, Missouri

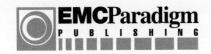

EMCParadigm
PUBLISHING

Senior Developmental Editor	Sonja Brown
Project Editor	James Patterson, RN
Developmental Editor	Barbara Cox, PhD
Cover and Text Designer	Leslie Anderson
Illustrator	Electronic Illustrators Group
Desktop Production	John Valo
Copy Editor	Ann Warren
Proofreader	Joy McComb
Indexer	Nancy Fulton

Photo credits appear on page I-14.

Reviewers—The authors and publisher wish to thank the following instructors and healthcare professionals for their valuable suggestions during the development of this book.

First Edition:
- H. JEFFREY TURNER, Ivy Tech State College, Muncie, IN
- P.J. MILLSPAUGH, Dallas County Community College, Dallas, TX
- WANDA WILSON, North Hennepin Community College, Brooklyn Park, MN
- PAT MCLANE, Henry Ford Community College, Dearborn Heights, MI
- BARBARA TINKER, Allentown Business School, Allentown, PA
- HELEN LITTRELL, Medical Transcriptionist, Klamath Falls, OR

Second Edition:
- WAYNE BECKER, MA, (ret.), Normandale Community College, Bloomington, MN

Publishing Team—Robert Cassel, Publisher; Janice Johnson, Vice President, Marketing; Lori Landwer, Marketing Manager; Shelley Clubb, Electronic Design and Production Manager.

Text: ISBN 0-7638-2273-6
Text + Encore CD: ISBN 0-7638-2270-1

Trademarks
Some of the pharmaceutical product names used in this book have been used for identification purposes only and may be trademarks or registered trademarks of their respective manufacturers.

© 2007, 1999 by Paradigm Publishing Inc.
Published by **EMC**Paradigm
875 Montreal Way
St. Paul, MN 55102
(800) 535-6865
E-mail: educate@emcp.com
Web site: www.emcp.com

Printed in the United States of America
10 9 8 7 6 5 4 3 2 1

Contents

Chapter 9: The Special Senses: Vision, Hearing, Smell, Taste, and Touch — 339

Chapter 10: The Respiratory System — 383

Chapter 11: The Cardiovascular System — 419

Chapter 12: The Gastrointestinal System — 461

Preface

This text has been written for students who are preparing for a variety of professional and paraprofessional careers in the medical field, including the areas of direct patient care and support services. It integrates the anatomy, physiology, and pathology information for each body system with exercises and activities designed to assist students in building a foundation of medical terminology.

Building on the Success of the First Edition

In planning the second edition of this text, we have worked to retain the key features that have made this a popular and highly successful tool for students learning the language of healthcare, including:

- chapter content structure that follows the order and focus of a medical visit
- special focus on wellness and illness vocabulary related to the developmental changes from infancy to maturity
- set of stimulating exercises after each of the three sections of concepts and related terms
- integration of language instruction with realistic medical scenarios and documents
- full-color, easily comprehensible illustrations

New Elements to Enhance Student Achievement

This edition has new elements to make the text even more inviting and accessible for today's student.

Students want to tackle the essential content as quickly as possible, so we have reduced the four introductory chapters from the first edition to two chapters that teach the foundations of word structure and the whole-body terms common to all medical specialties.

Students enjoy working with a variety of learning media, including electronic tools. Available with the second edition is an easy-to-use multimedia CD offering an array of rich content that includes stimulating, varied exercises for every chapter plus audio term pronunciations and related full-color images, chapter quizzes, and an end-of-book exam. Test scores are reported by e-mail to both the student and the instructor.

Responses to Instructor Feedback

Instructors have asked us to create fewer exercises of the type that require individual student answers and thus demand more time to evaluate. In response, we have revised the intrachapter exercises so that students can check all of their own work against the definitive answers provided in Appendix A. Each chapter's Performance Assessment includes activities of varying difficulty and type. Students who successfully complete them will have mastered the chapter content. To add a little fun to the learning experience, we have incorporated a crossword puzzle.

Full Complement of Product Components

A complete set of ancillaries is available with the text, including:

Encore Multimedia CD	0-7638-2276-0
Printed Instructor's Guide and CD	0-7638-2274-4
Flash Cards	0-7638-2275-2
Test Generator and Item Bank	0-7638-2277-9
Internet Resource Center	www.emcp.com
Class Connections (WebCT and Blackboard)	(Contact your sales representative.)

Comments and Questions

We hope this text adds to the pleasure of learning about the fascinating language of medicine, and we welcome your comments about how we can improve the instruction in future editions. You may contact us via this e-mail address: educate@emcp.com. Please visit the company's Web site at www.emcp.com to see the full array of high-quality products for schools and colleges.

Dedication

To my husband, Larry, who also is my work partner as Clinical Professor of Pediatrics, Drexel College of Medicine and Chief of the Division of Pediatric Hematology-Oncology at Saint Peter's University Hospital, New Brunswick, NJ, for his support and patience as well as his professional expertise and assistance. And to all of my patients and their families who taught me everything I know.

—A.G.E.

To my daughter, Stephanie Burch, without whose assistance I could not have completed this project.

—P.F.B.

To the Student

This text represents the first step in a journey of learning. It teaches the skills to help you understand and use medical language immediately and presents the foundation for continuing to learn new words throughout your career. Even though the subject matter may seem quite difficult and perhaps even overwhelming at times, remember that you can have fun with the language as you learn. Experiment with words—try combining prefixes, roots, and suffixes to create new words that make sense. You will find this activity both creative and enjoyable, and you will add to your knowledge about the medical language in the process. If you are not using the flash cards available with the text, consider making your own. Flash cards have a long history as a successful memorization tool. Another important learning aid is the Glossary of terms on the multimedia Encore CD that is available with the book. The Glossary offers audio pronunciations of the major terms in the text (from the tables marked with a CD icon) and displays a related illustration, if available, to help you understand the term and remember its meaning.

You may find it helpful to spend some time becoming familiar with the text before beginning your study. Chapters 1 and 2 introduce the concepts of word formation. You will learn how prefixes, word roots, and suffixes are combined in various ways to create common medical terms. Knowing these typical combinations will help you analyze and understand the new terms presented with each body system in Chapters 3-16. The body systems chapters contain three major sections that follow the order of a typical medical visit. The first section, "Examining the Patient," deals with anatomy and physiology, or the body structures and functions of a particular system, for example, the respiratory system. The second section, "Assessing Patient Health," focuses on the common illnesses and conditions associated with the three major life stages. The third section, "Diagnosing and Treating Problems," presents the key procedures and treatments related to the system. This section correlates to the part of the medical visit in which the doctor or another health professional tells the patient what's wrong and prescribes medicines, procedures, or surgery, if necessary. Major combining forms are presented at the beginning of the chapter. A table of key terms and six exercises follow each of the three content sections. You can check your work by looking up the answers in Appendix A. At the end of the chapter is a Performance Assessment that tests your mastery of the key terms and how to use them in the medical workplace.

As you progress through this text, you will find that your medical vocabulary is expanding significantly, and learning will become easier, even fun. In a few short weeks, you will have a foundation of skills and knowledge that are vital to a successful career in your chosen profession. You will be speaking the language of healthcare.

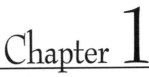

Chapter 1

The Language of Healthcare

Learning Outcomes

Students will be able to:

- Describe the parts of words used to create medical terms.
- Analyze medical terms to determine meaning.
- Give the meanings of a beginning set of roots, combining forms, suffixes, and prefixes.
- Form the plural and adjective forms of medical terms.
- Name the referents of abbreviations; list abbreviations for various medical phrases.

Medical terminology is a language in itself. If you understand from the beginning that you are learning a new language, you will be better prepared to use an effective approach and attitude to learning a huge body of terms. This chapter will begin your mastery of this language by familiarizing you with the parts of words that combine to create medical terms. Rather than setting out to memorize thousands of words and phrases, you will analyze medical terms and begin to build a vocabulary of word parts. You will also learn various medical abbreviations, as well as how to form plural and adjectival forms.

Learning the meanings of basic medical word parts will provide important tools and shortcuts for mastering this language of medicine, but the process of mastering medical terminology still requires significant amounts of memorization. You will need to practice and review persistently and patiently. Use every tool provided by this text, the Encore CD that accompanies it, and your instructor to facilitate your learning. Once you have mastered a core vocabulary of word parts, you will be well on your way to understanding and using the language of health professionals.

THE ORIGINS OF OUR MEDICAL LANGUAGE

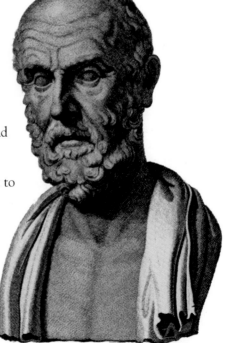

We owe most of the development of early medical language to the ancient Greeks and Romans. Hippocrates (460–370 BC), the Greek physician recognized as the "Father of Western Medicine," was among the first to study anatomy, physiology, and disease processes. Prior to his work, myths and superstition dominated teachings about healing and the human body. Hippocrates and other early Greek anatomists dissected cadavers and attempted to treat disease in living humans. They named body structures using terms familiar to them. For

Code of Medical Ethics

In addition to medicine, Hippocrates studied philosophy and ethics. His work in these areas spurred him to write the oath of ethical conduct that became the standard for Greek and Roman physicians. The Hippocratic Oath is the basis for today's code of medical ethics. Although this ancient oath is no longer followed by all institutions, its basic premises are still very much a part of modern medicine.

Hippocratic Oath

I swear by Apollo, the physician, and Aesculapius, and Health and Allheal, and all the gods and goddesses, that I will keep this oath and stipulation to reckon him who taught me this art equally dear to me as my parents, to share my substance with him and relieve his necessities if required; to regard his offspring as on the same footing with my own brothers, and to teach them this art if they should wish to learn it, without fee or stipulation, and that by precept, lecture, and every other mode of instruction, I will impart a knowledge of the art to my own sons and to those of my teachers, and to disciples bound by a stipulation and oath, according to the law of medicine, but to none other.

I will follow that method of treatment, which according to my ability and judgement, I consider for the benefit of my patients, and abstain from whatever is deleterious and mischievous. I will give no deadly medicine to anyone if asked, nor suggest any such counsel; furthermore, I will not give to a woman an instrument to produce abortion.

With purity and holiness, I will pass my life and practice my art. I will not cut a person who is suffering with a stone, but will leave this to be done by practitioners of this work. Into whatever houses I enter I will go into them for the benefit of the sick and will abstain from every voluntary act of mischief and corruption; and further from the seduction of females or males, bond or free.

Whatever, in connection with my professional practice, or not in connection with it, I may see or hear in the lives of men which ought not to be spoken abroad, I will not divulge, as reckoning that all such should be kept secret.

While I continue to keep this oath unviolated, may it be granted to me to enjoy life and the practice of the art, respected by all men at all times, but should I trespass and violate this oath, may the reverse be my lot.

example, they thought of the thyroid gland as shaped like a shield and named it with the Greek word for shield, *thyreos*. The eardrum looked to them like a tambourine, and they named it accordingly, with the Greek word *tympanon*, which is the source for our term tympanic membrane.

During the Roman Empire, Latin became the dominant language, and many new anatomy terms used Latin words. For example, the term bowel (intestine) originated from the Latin *botulus*, meaning sausage. In ancient times as now, sections of animal intestines were used as sausage casings.

Over subsequent centuries, German, French, and English researchers and physicians tended to dominate medicine in the Western world and gave names based in those languages to new discoveries about the body, diseases, and therapies. For example, the old English *drogge* gave us the word drug; French terms yielded fontanel (the soft spot in an infant's skull) and tourniquet (a band pressed against an artery to stop the bleeding); and Trendelenburg position (a position of patients for treatment of shock) is named after the German physician who first used it. The result is a medical language that is 90 percent Greek and Latin in origin, with influences of several other cultures.

UNDERSTANDING THE STRUCTURE OF MEDICAL TERMS

Most medical terms are composed of word parts—prefix, root or the combining form of a root, and suffix. The parts combine to form a complete term that conveys a specific idea. For example, the word parts *intra* (a prefix meaning inside), *muscul* (a root meaning muscle), and *ar* (a suffix meaning pertaining to) combine to form the word intramuscular, which means "pertaining to the inside of a muscle."

A **root** is just what its name implies: the word part that forms the basis or "root" of a term's meaning. Sometimes a combining vowel is added to the root to connect it to a suffix or another root. When a root has a combining vowel attached to it, we call it the **combining form** of the root. Combining forms often make a word easier to pronounce. A **prefix** is a word part that comes before the root or combining form and adds to or changes the meaning of the root. A **suffix** is a word part that follows the root and adds to or changes the meaning of the root. Consider the medical term **pathology**. It is constructed from the combining form (*patho*) of the root *path* (meaning disease) plus the suffix *-logy* (meaning study of). The resulting word, *pathology*, means the study of disease. Using the same combining form *patho* with the suffix *-logist*, which means "one who specializes in the study or treatment of," results in the word term *pathologist*, which is the name for the physician who specializes in the study of diseases. Notice that using the pure root for these words yields words that would be more difficult to pronounce—pathlogy or pathlogist.

ROOTS AND COMBINING FORMS

Most medical terms are formed by joining a *root* or a *combining form* with a *suffix*. The next two sections address the identification and use of roots and combining forms.

Roots

Each body system has a set of roots. For example, many terms used to describe the cardiovascular system (the heart and blood vessels) derive from the roots *cardi-* (heart) and *angi-* (vessel). Many terms relating to the respiratory system (the lungs and airways) use the roots *pneum-* (air or lung), *pulmon-* (lung), or *bronch-* (airway).

Learning Medical Terminology

Today's medical dictionaries contain more than a hundred thousand entries. Fortunately, learning to use medical language correctly does not require you to memorize every word in the dictionary. Approach the study of medical terminology with the idea of dividing the work into smaller, more manageable tasks:

- Memorize the meanings and spellings of common prefixes and suffixes.
- Learn the most commonly used terms that apply when discussing the whole body, since you will encounter these terms with each of the body systems.
- Memorize the roots and combining forms associated with each body system.
- Learn the ways different word parts are combined into the major terms associated with each body system.
- Apply the standard rules for spelling the plural forms of nouns and memorize the unusual plural spellings.
- Listen to the pronunciation of medical terms and practice saying them correctly.

And many words related to the nervous system (the brain, spinal cord, and nerves) are formed from roots *neur-* (nerve) or *cerebr-* (brain).

Table 1.1 lists some roots and meanings related to the body systems. (Details on many more roots related to specific body systems will be addressed in subsequent chapters.) *Sometimes two or three roots have the same meaning.* You will use one root word in some contexts, and a different root word in other contexts. When we have two or more roots with the same meaning, they are *not* interchangeable. You do not get to pick which root you wish to use for which meaning. Certain roots make specific words. Why do we have more than one root with the same meaning? Because medical terminology grew in several places at once. The most common example is the existence of a Latin root and a Greek root for the same meaning. For the meaning "kidney," for example, we have the Latin root *ren*, as in *renal*, and the Greek root *nephr*, as in *epinephrine*. Growing familiarity with medical terminology will help you learn which root to use. You will learn some things by exposure to the correct form. Concentrate on learning the roots in Tables 1.1 and 1.2, and notice which root fits each body system.

Table 1.1

Roots Associated with Specific Body Systems

Root	Meaning	Example
cardi-	heart	cardiac
gastr-	stomach	gastric
hemat-	blood	hematic
muscul-	muscles	muscular
nephr-	kidneys (from Greek)	nephron
nerv-	nerve (from Old English)	nervous
neur-	nerve (from Greek)	neuron
ren-	kidneys (from Latin)	renal
skelet-	skeleton (bones)	skeletal
ur-	urine	urine
vascul-	(blood) vessels	vascular

Not all roots are associated with a specific body system. Some roots are used more broadly and can be applied to any body system. For example, the roots in Table 1.2 can be combined with prefixes, suffixes, and combining vowels to produce terms that describe something (adjectives, adverbs) or name something (nouns). These roots are often used in terms that describe *conditions* or *diagnoses*.

Table 1.2

Common Roots Used With Various Body Systems

Root	Meaning	Example
abdomin-	abdomen	abdominal
bacter-	bacteria	bacteremia
bas-	base	basal
carcin-	cancer	carcinoma
cephal-	head	cephalic
corp-	body	corpus
cost-	ribs	intercostal
electr-	electric	electrolyte
fibrin-	fiber	fibrinous
lip-	fat	lipids
necr-	death	necrotic
sarc-	tissue	sarcoma
thromb-	clot	thrombin
viscero-	organs	visceromegaly

Use the exercise below to practice your knowledge of roots and their meanings.

Matching Roots and Meanings   Exercise 1

Read the root word carefully, paying attention to its spelling, and match the root with its meaning. Write the letter of the meaning beside the root. Remember that more than one root can have the same meaning.

Root	Letter of the meaning	Meaning
1. nephr	c	a. fiber
2. necr	f	b. ribs
3. fibrin	a	c. kidneys
4. thromb	g	d. fats
5. cost	b	e. cancer
6. carcin	e	f. death
7. sarc	h	g. clot
8. cephal	i	h. tissue
9. lip	d	i. head
10. hemat	j	j. blood

Combining Forms

Adding a *connecting* or *combining vowel* to a root word creates a word part called a *combining form*. As described before, connecting vowels make medical terms easier to spell and pronounce, but they can also connect a root with another root when more than one root is used to form a term. For example, in the word *musculoskeletal*, the root *muscul* adds the connecting vowel *o* to make the combining form *muscul/o* so that the two roots (*muscul* and *skelet*) can be combined. In addition, a combining vowel may be used to join a root word and a suffix. The most commonly used combining vowel is *o*; the second most common is *i*.

Sometimes a root is used with a suffix to form a word, and sometimes the combining form of that same root is used with a suffix to form a word. Whether a root is used or its combining form is used depends on the suffix, its spelling, and the meaning it conveys. For example, a root meaning head is *cephal*. A combining form for *cephal* is *cephal/o*. The root (*cephal*) plus suffix (*ic*) gives us the word *cephalic*; the combining form (*cephalo*) plus another root (*pelv*) plus suffix (*ic*) gives us *cephalopelvic*; and the combining form *electr/o* plus prefix (*en*) plus combining form (*cephal/o*) plus suffix (*graph*) gives us *electroencephalograph*.

Study the way combining forms and suffixes are joined in the following examples, and then work on memorizing the combining forms shown in Table 1.3. Note that when combining forms are shown, a slash separates the root and the connecting vowel, as in *carcin/o*, which is the root *carcin* plus connecting vowel *o*.

> **Example: abdominocentesis (*abdomin/o* + -*centesis*)**
> *abdomin/o* = combining form for abdomen
> -*centesis* = puncture for withdrawal of fluid
> Abdominocentesis is the puncture of the abdomen for withdrawal of fluid.

> **Example: cardiogram (*cardi/o* + -*gram*)**
> *cardi/o* = combining form for heart
> -*gram* = record
> A cardiogram is a record of the activity of the heart.

Table 1.3

Common Combining Forms Related to Diseases and Conditions

Combining form	Meaning	Example
bacteri/o	bacteria	bacteriology
carcin/o	cancer	carcinogenic
fibrin/o	fiber	fibrinolysis
necr/o	death	necrosis
onc/o	tumor	oncology
thromb/o	clot	thrombosis
path/o	disease	pathology

Tables 1.4 and 1.5 contain additional combining forms related to anatomy and colors, respectively.

Why learn combining forms about colors? We use them in many areas of medicine. Dermatologists apply them to skin lesions, cytologists use them to discuss various cell types, and all physicians use them to describe various conditions.

Table 1.4

Common Combining Forms Related to Anatomy

Combining form	Meaning	Example
abdomin/o	abdomen	abdominothoracic
angi/o	vessel	angiography
cardi/o	heart	cardiologist
cephal/o	head	cephalopathy
cyst/o	sac or cyst containing fluid (also urinary bladder)	cystogram
cyt/o	cell	cytology
enter/o	intestines	enteritis
gynec/o	woman; female	gynecologist
hem/o	blood	hemolysis
hemat/o	blood	hematology
hepat/o	liver	hepatology
lip/o	fat	lipodystrophy
mamm/o	breast	mammography
nephr/o	kidney	nephrotomy
pelv/io	basin; pelvis	pelviotomy
sarc/o	flesh	sarcophagic
trache/o	trachea	tracheotomy
uter/o	uterus	uteroscopy

Table 1.5

Combining Forms Describing Colors

Combining form	Meaning	Example
cyan/o	blue	cyanosis
erythr/o	red	erythrocytosis, erythroderma
leuk/o	white	leukocyte
melan/o	black	melanocyte
xanth/o	yellow	xanthochromia

Note that the roots for the color purple are the Greek "purpur" (from which we get the words purpure, purpura, purpurate, and purpurin) and the Old English "purpul" (from which we get purple and empurple). These roots do not have a combining form.

Identify Combining Forms

Exercise 2

Read each sentence and circle the medical term that contains the combining form(s). Write the definition of the combining form in the blank. If the term has more than one combining form, write the definition for each of them.

1. Linda sees the gynecologist once a year. _female Dr._

2. The lab test revealed that the child had leukocytosis. _high white blood cell count_

3. A tracheostomy was necessary to allow the patient to breathe. _open trach airway_

4. Dr. Lee performed the cardiogram. _heart activity record_

5. Dr. Raney is a hematologist. _blood Doctor_

6. Martin wants to be a gastroenterologist. *intestine & stomach specialist*

7. This patient will undergo a cystoscopy. *view a cyst*

8. Cardiomegaly can sometimes be identified by a chest x-ray. *heart picture record*

9. The blockage was found by an angiogram. *view/record of vessel*

10. Pathophysiology was one of the most interesting courses. *study of disease physical*

11. Thrombocytopenia causes excessive bleeding. *blood clot*

12. Dr. Pico treated Susan's erythroderma with a new salve. *red skin*

13. Fibrinolytic drugs can help dissolve blood clots. *fiber*

14. Bacteriostatic substances can help control infections. *capture of bacteria*

15. The exam was performed in cephalopelvic order. *head basin*

SUFFIXES

Many medical terms are formed by adding a suffix to a root or combining form. You already know that a root is the foundation of the medical term and is the source of a term's meaning. You may also recall that the suffix is an ending that adds information or modifies the meaning of the root or combining form. When you are studying or examining suffixes, pay particular attention to their spelling, since changing a single letter may change the meaning.

The following examples use the suffixes -logy and -logist to show how changing the suffix alters the meaning of the term.

Example: *nephr/o* (combining form meaning kidneys)
adding the suffix -logy (study of) creates nephrology (study of the kidneys)

Example: *cardi/o* (combining form meaning heart)
adding the suffix -logy (study of) creates cardiology (study of the heart)

Example: *nephr/o* (combining form meaning kidneys)
adding the suffix -logist (one who studies) creates nephrologist (one who studies the kidneys)

Example: *cardi* (combining form meaning heart)
adding the suffix -logist (one who studies) creates cardiologist (one who studies the heart)

Table 1.6 provides common combining forms and gives examples of how -logy and -logist can be used to form the names of body systems, medical specialties, and medical specialists. Study Table 1.6 to familiarize yourself with some of the combining forms used with -logy and -logist to name medical specialty areas and physician practitioners. Can you find the specialty and practitioner terms that use two combining forms in one term?

Table 1.6

Suffixes Used in the Names of Specialties and Practitioners

Combining form	Meaning	Term for specialty (using suffix -logy)	Term for practitioner (using suffix -logist)
arthr/o	joints	arthrology	arthrologist
cardi/o-	heart	cardiology	cardiologist
nephr/o-	kidney(s)	nephrology	nephrologist
pulmon/o-	lung(s)	pulmonology	pulmonologist
neur/o-	nerve	neurology	neurologist
gastr/o-	stomach	gastroenterology	gastroenterologist
enter/o-	intestines	gastroenterology	gastroenterologist
immune/o-	immune	immunology	immunologist
dermat/o-	skin	dermatology	dermatologist
oste/o-	bones	osteology	osteologist
path/o-	disease	pathology*	pathologist

*Note that, like so many English words, "pathology" has two definitions. One is the study of disease; the other refers to the manifestations of a disease or a deviation from what is normal. When we say that something is "pathological," we mean that it is not normal.

The term in this table that uses two combining forms plus a suffix is gastroenterologist.

Two or more suffixes can have the same meaning. In some cases, a group of suffixes may have related meanings. The language of medicine uses a large number of suffixes, and studying them in meaning groups can help you learn them. Each of the following tables presents groups of suffixes with the same or related meanings.

Table 1.7

Suffixes Meaning "Related to" or "Pertaining to"

Most of these suffixes form adjectives, but -e forms nouns.

Suffix	Example
-ac	cardiac
-al	caudal
-ar	vascular
-e (noun marker)	melanocyte
-eal	congeal
-ic	pelvic
-ose	cellulose
-ous	callous
-ry	secretory
-tic	arthritic

Many of the following suffixes can indicate a disease process or some type of pathology, but a few of the suffixes indicate only a condition. A condition can be something that is pathological or something that is an abnormality without any associated disease.

Table 1.8

Suffixes Indicating a Condition or Process

Suffix	Meaning	Example
-emia	condition of the blood	anemia
-ia	condition or process	insomnia
-ism	condition or process	aneurism *clot*
-itis	inflammation	phlebitis
-lysis	breakdown or dissolution process	hemolysis
-oma	tumor or neoplasm	sarcoma
-osis	condition	keratosis
-y	condition or process of	ambulatory

The next group of suffixes indicates shape, form, or size. These suffixes are important because medical language needs to communicate the size and shape of wounds, tumors, or abnormal formations. Note the similarities in the spelling of suffixes that mean "small."

Table 1.9

Suffixes Indicating Form, Size, and Formation

Suffix	Meaning	Example
-cle	small	auricle
-ole	small	arteriole
-ule	small	pustule
-ula	small	fistula
-megaly	enlargement *of liver*	hepatomegaly
-penia	abnormal reduction or lack of *cells*	cytopenia
-form	shape or resembling	vermiform
-asis	formation, presence of	lithiasis
-plasia	formation	achondroplasia
-trophy	development	dystrophy
-poiesis	formation	hematopoiesis

Identify the Suffixes

Exercise 3

Circle the medical term in each sentence, underline the suffix, and write the definition of the suffix.

1. The doctor said Joan's grandfather had carditis.   *inflamation of heart*

2. He was concerned about pulmonary complications.   *lungs / pneumonia*

3. Rheumatic heart disease is often coded incorrectly.   *pain inflamed joints, muscles ligaments*

4. The arthrosis has gotten worse.   *joint swelling*

5. Cardiomegaly can cause some distressing symptoms.   *enlarged heart*

6. The laboratory studies identified renal disease.   *kidney*

7. Anemia is often related to a poor diet.

8. Hypertrophy of the prostate sometimes required surgery.

9. The dysplasia was severe.

10. The pustule had to be opened and drained.

11. Once the arteriole was closed off, the bleeding stopped.

12. The macula was not damaged.

13. Lithiasis in the urine is not uncommon.

14. The vermiform portion of the structure was removed.

15. Hemolysis was the cause of death.

high white blood cell count
enlarged development
formation
skin eruption
small artery

condition of blood

Most medical procedures are either diagnostic (identifying what the problem is) or therapeutic (curing or treating the problem). The suffixes in the table immediately below describe diagnostic procedures.

Table 1.10

Suffixes Describing Diagnostic Procedures

Suffix	Meaning	Example
-gram	record	arteriogram
-graph	record or instrument used for making a record	electrocardiograph
-graphy	process of recording	amniography
-meter	measure or measurement	sphygmometer
-metry	process of measuring	spectrometry
-scope	instrument used for viewing	arthroscope
-scopy	process of viewing with an instrument	colonoscopy

The next table contains suffixes that describe some type of treatment or therapeutic procedure. Many of these suffixes indicate a procedure that is surgical in nature because surgery is frequently used to treat or restore damaged areas of the body.

Table 1.11

Suffixes Indicating Therapeutic Procedures

Suffix	Meaning	Example
-centesis	puncture to withdraw fluid or tissue	abdominocentesis
-desis	stabilization or binding	arthrodesis
-iatric	treatment	geriatric
-plasty	repair	angioplasty
-rrhaphy	suturing	hepatorrhaphy
-stomy or -ostomy	creation of an artificial opening	tracheostomy
-tomy	cut or incision	keratotomy
-tripsy	crushing	lithotripsy

Select the suffix that best fits the blank. Write it on the line to complete the word, then write the definition of the suffix.

centesis ✓	graphy	plasty	stomy
desis	iatric	rrhaphy	tomy
gram	meter ✓	scope	tripsy
graph	metry ✓	scopy	

1. During the first or second prenatal visit, the doctor performs pelvi *metry*. The doctor measures the pelvis.

   _____

2. A gluco *meter* measures glucose in the blood.

   _____

3. Russell underwent gastro *scopy* this morning. The technician looked into his stomach.

   _____

4. The test results of the electrical activity of Julie's heart, her electrocardio *gram*, was normal.

   _____

5. The procedure that uses x-rays to view the arteries of the heart, also called angio *graphy*, can help identify problems in the heart.

   _____

6. Jones-Swanson hospital is for treatment of mental disorders. This psych *iatric* hospital will soon expand.

   _____

7. The needle passed between Andrew's ribs to withdraw fluids. This procedure is called thora *centesis*

   _____

8. Louann's spine required arthro *desis* to fuse some vertebrae after the auto accident.

   _____

9. George's broken nose required rhino *plasty* to restore its original shape.

   _____

10. The surgeon sewed up Roger's ruptured stomach. She performed gastro *rrhaphy*

    _____

11. Creating an opening in the colon, or colo *stomy*, may be done as part of a cure for colon cancer.

    _____

12. Arthro _tomy_ opened the joint so the surgeon could drain it.

13. Stella's litho _tripsy_ treatments disintegrated her kidney stones.

14. An endo _scope_ is used to see into a body cavity.

15. The electroencephalo _graph_ is a sensitive instrument that measures brain wave activity.

The suffixes listed in Table 1.12 are widely used in describing procedures, actions, or structures.

Table 1.12

Commonly Used General Suffixes

Suffix	Meaning	Example
-blast	immature cell	osteoblast
-cyte	cell	leukocyte
-ium	tissue or structure	pericardium
-eum	tissue or structure	periosteum
-ize	make; use; subject to	anesthetize
-ate	make; use; subject to	intubate
-stasis	stop, stand	hemostasis
-algia	pain	neuralgia
-dynia	pain	arthrodynia
-cele	pouch _hernia_	cystocele
-emesis	vomiting	hematemesis
-oid	like, resembling	ovoid
-genic	origin	carcinogenic
-genesis	origin	lysogenesis
-oma	tumor	lymphoma
-phobia	fear	photophobia
-phile	affinity for _pedophile_	halophile
-malacia	softening	cardiomalacia
-pnea	breathing	apnea
-ptosis	drooping _falling_	blepharoptosis
-spasm	abrupt, forceful contraction _involuntary_	bronchiospasm
-rrhage	bursting forth or rapid flow	hemorrhage
-rrhagia	bursting forth or rapid flow	menorrhagia
-rrhea	bursting forth or rapid flow	diarrhea
-phage	eat, swallow	bacteriophage
-phagia	process of eating or related to eating	dysphagia

Select the word part from List A and the suffix from List B to form the word that best fits the blank in each sentence. Write the word in the blank. The meaning for the desired word is provided in brackets after each sentence.

List A	List B
an/esthet	blasts
arthro	cele
carcin/o	cyte
cephal	dynia
cyst/o	eum
erythr/o	genic
hem/o	gia
hem/o	ize
hemat/e	mesis
hepat	oid
ortho	oma
oste	phobia
oste/o	pnea
peri/ost	rrhagic
photo	stasis

1. Several _____ were found in the fluid. [immature cells associated with bone production]

2. The _____ ruptured when it was placed in the solution. [a red blood cell]

3. The _____ surrounds the bone. [fibrous sheath that covers bones]

4. The doctor will _____ the patient. [make unconscious]

5. _____ had to be achieved before the surgery could proceed. [procedure of stopping the flow of blood]

6. The patient required medication for severe _____. [headache].

7. _____ described the way the patient's knee felt. [pain in a joint]

8. A _____ often requires surgery. [herniation of the bladder]

9. _____ is an emergency condition. [vomiting of blood]

10. An _____ tumor was identified on x-ray. [bone matrix]

11. Some chemicals are _____. [capable of causing cancer]

12. A _____ involves the liver. [liver tumor]

13. Some drugs produce _____. [fear of light]

14. The patient's _____ required that he sit up all night. [difficulty breathing except when sitting straight or standing]

15. _____ diseases usually cause internal bleeding. [condition of blood escaping from blood vessels]

More About Suffixes

Some suffixes in medical terminology are technically compound suffixes; that is, one suffix with a second suffix added on. These suffixes are often found in terms relating to medical specialties, diagnoses, or procedures. The second suffix is usually only one letter and may simply function as a noun marker (a visual sign that the word is a noun), as in:

> **Example: erythrocyte (*erythr/o + -cyt + -e*)**
> *erythr/o* = red + *-cyt* = cell + *-e* = noun marker
> An erythrocyte is a red blood cell.

In the following example, part of the suffix is another single letter, a *y*:

> **Example: urology (*ur/o + -log + -y*)**
> *ur/o* = urine or the urinary tract + *-log* = to know (a derivative of the Greek word "logos") + *-y* = condition or process of
> Urology is the process of knowing urinary function and disease.

An analysis of the word *urology* points out a practice that occurs frequently in the formation of medical words: When two suffixes are combined, the resulting meaning is usually a shortened version of the two separate suffix meanings. Thus, *-logy* becomes "the study of" (shortened from "the process of knowing"). You will encounter many of these compound suffixes and usually learn the combined meaning. However, being aware of the individual suffix meanings may help you decipher new combinations of those suffixes in unfamiliar words.

PREFIXES

A prefix is a word part that comes before (*pre-* = before) the root or combining form and usually begins the term. Prefixes modify the root or combining form; they often give an indication of direction, time, or orientation.

> **Example: prenatal (*pre + natal*)**
> *pre-* = prefix for before
> *natal* = root meaning birth
> Prenatal means before birth.

> **Example: intra-abdominal (*intra + abdominal*)**
> *intra-* = prefix meaning within
> *abdomin* = root meaning abdomen
> *-al* = suffix meaning pertaining to
> Intra-abdominal means pertaining to the inside of the abdomen.

As with suffixes, there can be several prefixes associated with one meaning. A few prefixes have more than one related meaning. Watch the spelling as you study the tables on the next pages.

Table 1.13

Prefixes Related to Numbers or Amounts

Prefix	Meaning	Example
uni-	one, single	unilateral
mono-	one	mononucleosis
bi-	two, both	bilateral
di-	two	diplegia
ambi-	both	ambivalent
tri-	three	trivalent
quadra-	four	quadraplegic
tetra-	four	tetralogy
poly-	many	polycythemia
multi-	many, several	multiphasic
mega-	large, excessive	megaloblasts
olig-	few, scant	oliguria
micro-	very small	microtension
hemi-	half (usually right/left halves)	hemisphere
semi-	part of a whole	semifluent
a-	without	anemia
an-	without	anaerobic
tachy-	fast	tachicardial
brady-	slow	bradicardial
pan-	all	pandemic

Identify the Prefix

Study the sentences below. Write the appropriate prefix for the medical term related to the word or phrase in italics on the line.

1. The patient could only perceive *one*-color images. _mono_ chromatic

2. He had a hearing loss in *both* ears. _bi_ lateral

3. Some individuals are able to use *both* hands equally well. _ambi_ dextrous

4. The patient experienced several episodes of cardiac dysrhythmia in which heartbeats occur in *groups of three*. _tri_ geminy

5. Advances in technology have produced hope for paralysis of *all four limbs*. _quadra_ plegia

6. There is a new treatment for the condition marked by an *abnormally large number* of red blood cells in the circulatory system. _____cythemia

7. Teams with members from *several various* disciplines are common in health care. _____disciplinary

8. *Abnormally large* nucleated red blood cells are easily identified. _____blasts

9. *Abnormally slight or infrequent* urination is common in kidney failure. _olig_ uria

10. The baby was born with *abnormal smallness* of the heart. _micro_ cardia

11. A brain disorder sometimes produces paralysis *affecting only half* (one side) of the body. _hemi_ plegia

12. The patient's *cessation* of breathing during sleep was not easily diagnosed. _____pnea

13. A *rapid* heart rate is often associated with fear. _____cardia

14. Her *slow* heart rate was less than 50. _____cardia

15. The influenza epidemic was covering *a wide geographic area and affecting a large proportion of the population.* _____ demic

Table 1.14, below, lists prefixes that can either indicate amount or position/direction.

Table 1.14

Prefixes that Indicate Amount or Position/Direction

Prefix	Meaning amount	Example amount	Meaning position/direction	Example position/direction
hyper-	more, excessive, increased	hypertensive	above	hyperflexion
hypo-	less, deficient	hypoglycemic	below	hypodermic
infra-	less than	infrasonic	under, below	infrared
sub-	less than	subnormal	under, below	substernal
meta-	change	metastasize	behind	metacarpus
super-	excessive, more	supernumerary	above	superimpose
supra-	excessive, outside	supraliminal	beyond	suprarenal
ultra-	excessive	ultramodern	beyond	ultraviolet

Note how the definitions of the prefixes in Table 1.15 differ from those in table 1.14, above.

Table 1.15

Prefixes that Indicate Position/Direction

Prefix	Meaning	Example
ad-	toward, to, near	adhere
ab-	away from	absolve
anti-	against, opposed to	anticoagulant
contra-	against, opposed to	contraindicated
circum-	around, circular motion	circumcision
peri-	around	peritectomy
de-	not, from, down	descending
dia-	across or through	diagonal
trans-	across or through	transverse
dis-	separate, apart	distal
epi	upon, above	epiglottis
para-	along, beside	parathyroid

Some prefixes can indicate position or direction, or they can indicate time. Table 1.16 shows some of these versatile prefixes.

Table 1.16

Prefixes that Indicate Time or Position/Direction

Prefix	Meaning	Example time	Example position/direction
per-	through	permanent	percutaneous
post-	after	postsurgical	posterior
pre-	before	precursor	preaxial
re-	again, back	revive	recline
retro-	backward or behind	retrospective	retrobulbular

Identify the Prefix

Study the sentences below. From the list below, select the appropriate prefix to fill the blank in each sentence. The definition of the target word is given for each item. Write the prefix in the blank.

ab   epi   re
ad   hyper   sub
circum   hypo   super
supra   para   trans
de   post   ultra

1. The patient's _hyper_ kalemia was dangerous to his heart. (high levels of potassium)

2. The pain was located in the _sub_ gastric area. (lower part of the abdomen)

3. Some medications are intended for _hypo_ lingual use. (below the tongue)

4. The injuries were _super_ ficial. (on the surface; not deep)

5. The _supra_ clavicular tumors were easily felt. (situated above the clavicle)

6. _ultra_ sound helped identify the condition of the fetus. (a diagnostic technique that uses high-frequency sound waves)

7. _ad_ duction of the leg caused pain. (moving a limb toward the body midline)

8. The patient had only 10 degrees of _ab_ duction at the shoulder. (moving a limb away from the body)

9. The _circum_ oral burns made the doctor think the child had swallowed lye. (around the mouth)

10. The bone was severely _de_ mineralized. (removal of minerals)

11. Drugs are often delivered through the _trans_ dermal route. (through the skin)

12. The third degree burns destroyed the _epi_ dermis. (outer layer of skin)

13. The _para_ hepatic mass would be difficult to remove. (next to the liver)

14. Careful _post_ surgical monitoring was required. (after surgery)

15. The excess bone will be _re_ sorbed. (to absorb something again)

Prefixes in Table 1.17 are grouped by meaning. Study the groups and notice the differences and similarities in spelling. For example, the prefixes indicating "out" or "outside" all begin with *e*, and most have only one to three letters. The prefixes that mean "with" all contain either *n* or *m*. Noticing details can help you remember the prefixes and their spellings.

Table 1.17

Commonly Used Prefixes

Prefix	Meaning	Example
e-	out, outside, away	elevate
ec-	out, outside, away	eclabium
ex-	out, outside, away	external
ecto-	out, outside, away	ectoplasm
exo-	out, outside, away	exogenous
extra-	out, outside, away	extrapolate
en-	inside or in	endermic
endo-	inside or in	endodontic
in-	inside or in	interior
intra-	inside or in	intramuscular
ante-	before	anterior
pre-	before	preeclampsia
pro-	before	prophylactic
con-	with	connecting
syn-	with	synthetic
sym-	with	symbiosis
auto-	self	autoclave
bio-	life	biology
dys-	faulty, painful, difficult	dyspepsia
eu-	normal	eugenics
inter- *, intra,*	between *, within*	interstitial
mal-	bad, abnormal	malocclusion
neo-	new	neonatology
pachy- *tacky*	thick *fast*	pachycephalic

infra *beneath*

Match the Prefix with its Meaning

Exercise 8

Match the prefix with its meaning. Write the letter of the meaning on the line next to the prefix.

Prefix	Letter of Meaning		Meaning
1. ex-	*M*	a.	life
2. endo-	*O*	b.	thick
3. intra-	*I*	c.	normal

4. pre-   _J_   d. self

5. pro-   _____   e. with

6. sym-   _____   f. new

7. auto-   _D_   g. before

8. bio-   _A_   h. bad

9. dys-   _____   i. inside

10. eu-   _____   j. before

11. mal-   _H_   k. faulty

12. neo-   _____   l. away

13. pachy-   _B_   m. outside, away from

14. ecto-   _____   n. out, outside

15. extra-   _____   o. inside

FOUR WAYS TO COMBINE PARTS TO CREATE WORDS

A medical term can consist of a single word part, or a combination of several parts. Some terms are simply the roots (or combining forms) by themselves, while others consist of multiple roots, a prefix, and one or more suffixes. The following word constructions illustrate the standard four ways to combine word parts into terms. Study the examples and identify each part of the terms.

1. **root or its combining form**
   Example: phleb = vein

2. **root or its combining form + additional root or combining form**
   Example: thrombophleb = clot in a vein

3. **root or its combining form + additional root or combining form + suffix**
   Example: thrombophlebitis = inflammation of a vein with clotting

4. **prefix + root or its combining form + additional root or combining form + suffix**
   Example: postthrombophlebitis = after inflammation of a vein with clotting (recovery)

EXCEPTIONS TO THE RULES As with most languages, there are exceptions to the medical terminology rules that describe how terms are formed. You don't need to memorize each exception, but being aware of them will help you determine the meanings of words that seem to stray from the typical patterns. For example, terms consisting of a root and a suffix usually require a combining vowel to create a combining form of the root. However, this general rule has some exceptions, such as terms in which the suffix begins with a vowel, e.g., *ectomy* in *cardiectomy*. In addition, the combining vowel in a combining form and the final vowel in a root are both dropped before a suffix that begins with a vowel, e.g., *card* in carditis.

Word Play

Learning terminology doesn't have to be all pain and no play. In fact, playing with words can help you learn them. See how you do with the following "exercise."

Use your knowledge of word parts to answer these. You might need a dictionary for some of them.

1. Why do we call an elephant a pachyderm?
2. While we're on the subject, what's a pachycephalosaur?
3. What do these words have in common: clavicle, clavichord, conclave, and corn?
4. Can you use the words epidemic and epidermal and hypodermic in the same sentence? Try it.
5. What does bilateral have to do with being ambidextrous?
6. If erythroderma is reddening of the skin, why do we call St. Anthony's Fire "erysipelas"?
7. Go figure! What do you think a mal-leuko-melano-chromatic-scaled-clavichord player might be?
8. Why does "thrombosis" remind you of like a drumming sound? Or is it more like a bass fiddle? What image could you create to remind you that a thromb is a clot, not a sound?

(Possible) Answers

1. Because it has thick skin. Does that mean that because Uncle Joe is thick-skinned he's a pachyderm?
2. It's a medium-sized dinosaur that has a beaked mouth, rows of bumps on its head, and a *thick skull* (ten inches thick!) shaped like a dome. Met any lately?
3. The Latin word *clavus* means key. The clavicle bone is shaped like a key…well, somebody back then thought so. A clavichord is a keyboard instrument that makes sounds. (So's your computer. Hmm.) Conclave uses the prefix *con*, meaning with, and the root *clav-*, meaning key. So a conclave is a gathering together in a place or room that is locked *with a key*…although nowadays we don't lock people up when there's a conclave. And corn? We're talking about the medical term corn, the kind you get on your toes when your shoes don't fit. What's the connection? Yup. The other word for corn is, you guessed it, *clavus*.
4. Yes, of course the possibilities are limited only by your imagination. But here's one to get you started: The epidemic of epidermal spiderosis (Okay, name your own favorite skin thing.) could be treated only by hypodermic injections of antispiderosis serum.
5. Bilateral refers to something on two (both) sides, and ambidextrous refers to having dexterity with both hands. So bilateral ambidexterity is redundant, yes?
6. Erysipelas also means, literally, red skin … but erysipelas uses the prefix and root from the Latin, while erythroderma is from the Greek. The two words aren't synonyms, however. Erysipelas is the name of a specific disease, while erythroderma is a more general term for a condition. So you could say that patients with erysipelas (and some other diseases) suffer from erythroderma. Okay?
7. Let's translate. A bad white black toned scaled musical instrument player could be a sick pianist. Now you make up one. (It doesn't really have to make sense. It's to help you remember.)
8. Don't you think thromb sounds like thrum? And thrumming is a rhythmic strumming or drumming or humming. Can't you picture a guitar player with a big bowl of cottage (clotted) cheese? Or a drummer who cut himself shaving and the clot on his cheek shows? What would you invent for phlebitis? Can't you just see those fleas biting an affected leg? Now you invent one. Try making up one that will help you remember phlebitis!

Using the prefixes, roots, combining forms, and suffixes from the list below, create a term that matches the definition. You may use the same word parts in more than one term. Some terms use two parts; others use three parts. Write the term you create in the blanks at the end of the exercise.

Prefixes: neo-, pre-, dys-, peri-

Suffixes: -ectomy; -al; -ia; -rrhaphy; -osis; -ic; -oma; -ologist

Roots and Combining Forms: sarc/o; hepat/o; nat; phag; cephal/o; mast/o; cardi/o; necr

1. Removal of a breast   _____

2. Heart specialist   _____

3. Around the heart   _____

4. Connective tissue tumor   _____

5. Difficulty swallowing   _____

6. Pertaining to the head   _____

7. Suture of a liver wound   _____

8. Before birth   _____

9. Condition of dying cells or tissue   _____

10. Specialist in newborn babies   _____

LEARNING TO PRONOUNCE MEDICAL TERMS

When you work in a medical setting, you should be able to recognize and understand the most common medical terms by sound and by sight. Most of the terms you encounter will be ones you have seen or used before and are familiar with, but occasionally you will discover a new term. When you hear an unfamiliar word, repeat it aloud and listen for familiar word parts to help you determine the meaning of the entire term.

PRONUNCIATION IN THE WORKPLACE In the medical workplace, you will need to pronounce medical terms clearly and correctly so that others understand you precisely. Be particularly attentive to your pronunciation if you are speaking on the telephone, recording a voicemail message, or dictating for someone else to transcribe.

You will need to listen carefully to others; their pronunciation may be influenced by an accent or inflection. Listening to someone on the telephone or to voicemail or dictation may take practice and concentration. You will need to learn how others pronounce medical terms so that you do not misunderstand what they are saying.

PRONUNCIATION KEYS The tables in this text show the pronunciation of the term immediately below each word. The pronunciation is given in phonetic or "sounds like" syllables (see Table 1.18). When you encounter a new word, say the word out loud or to yourself several times; then if you are using the CD that accompanies this book, listen to the term and practice pronouncing it. Being able to speak the language you are learning is just as important as being able to spell the words correctly.

To help you with vocabulary words that might be difficult to pronounce, this textbook uses a phonetic pronunciation. The words are separated into syllables (indicated by hyphens), and **boldface** indicates which syllable should receive the emphasis when you say the word aloud. Note also that the word's plural spelling is shown only when it does not conform to the described plural rules. The following letters and letter combinations represent specific sounds in the phonetic pronunciations:

Table 1.18

Pronunciation Key

Letters and Combinations	Pronounced like
a	the short a as in can
ay	the long a as in cane
ah	a as in father
ai	ai as in fair
ar	ar as in far
aw	a as in fall
e	the short e as in pen
ee	the long e as in me
i	the short i as in pin
I	the long i as in pine
o	the short o as in not
O	the long o as in note
oo	oo as in food
or	or as in for
ow	ow as in cow
oy	oy as in boy
u	the short u as in run
yoo	the long u as in cube
zh	s as in casual

Example: artery is pronounced **ar**-ter-ee.

Learning How to Form Plurals and Adjectives

In medical terminology, plural word forms can be confusing. Some plural terms are formed based on Greek and Latin rules, while others are formed using English language rules. English usually forms plurals by adding *s* or *es* to the singular form (the plural of **vein** is **veins**). Latin- and Greek-based words form plurals by adding an ending based on the ending of the singular form. For example, many singular words ending in *a* add the letter *e* to create the plural form (**stria,** meaning a discolored stripe on the skin, becomes **striae** as a plural). Singular words ending in *um* replace the *um* with an *a* to create the plural form (**diverticulum,** a pouch or sac that has developed within the gut or bladder, becomes **diverticula** in the plural). Words ending in *nx* change the *nx* to *nges* in the plurals (**larynx,** part of the throat, becomes **larynges**).

Unfortunately, the rules do not apply consistently, and for that reason the best strategy is to memorize the plural spelling for each new word you learn. This text provides the plural spelling of terms in the tables only if the plural spelling differs from the guidelines described here. Whenever you are uncertain of the correct plural form of a term, consult your medical dictionary. Table 1.19 lists some of the common plural forms.

Table 1.19

Frequently Used Plural Forms

Singular	Ending	Plural
apex	-ex/-ices	apices
appendix	-ix/-ices	appendices
bacterium	-ium/-ia	bacteria
cardiopathy	-y/-ies	cardiopathies
condyloma	-a/-ata	condylomata
diagnosis	-is/-es	diagnoses
fungus	-us/-i	fungi
phenomenon	-on/a	phenomena
thorax	-ax/-aces	thoraces
vertebra	-a/-ae	vertebrae

ADJECTIVE ENDINGS Earlier sections of this chapter introduced a group of adjective suffixes (-ac, -al, -ar, -ary, -eal, -ic, -ous, and -tic) that, when added to the end of a noun, create the adjective form of a word. These suffixes generally mean "pertaining to," although they are not necessarily interchangeable. Other adjective suffixes include -genic (producing), -genous (produced by or from), -oid (resembling), and -ole or -ule (little). Creating adjectives from nouns often involves more than just adding an ending, however. Usually, the final letter in the noun is either dropped or changed to another letter. To help you learn the adjective forms of some common body system terms, the word tables in later chapters of this text sometimes include the adjective spelling.

SOUNDALIKES The correct spelling of a word can be critical in patient care. In some instances, two or more words may sound alike but be spelled differently and have different meanings. The difference of even one letter can make a dramatic difference in meaning. Consider the words **ilium** (a pelvic bone) and **ileum** (the terminal portion of the small intestine). These two words, very different in meaning, are pronounced the same and only differ by one letter in their spelling. Surgery to repair an ilium would be very different from that done to repair an ileum! Think about the words **osteal** (bony or bonelike) and **ostial** (relating to an ostium, an opening, as in the ostium of the eustachian tube). **Viscous** (sticky) and **viscus** (a hollow, multilayered, walled organ such as the heart) are two more terms that sound alike but are spelled differently and have different meanings.

Whenever you are uncertain about the spelling of a term, consult a reliable medical dictionary or other reference book. If you are not sure how to spell a drug name, look it up in the *Physicians' Desk Reference* or a similar drug reference book.

Read the sentences below, paying special attention to the medical terms. Some of the terms are spelled incorrectly. Identify the correctly spelled terms by writing "correct" in the blank next to the word. If the term is spelled incorrectly, write the correct spelling in the blank.

1. Larry will undergo a nephrectomy next week. _____

2. The physician performed a tracheaottomy. _____

3. Vanessa is studying to become a cardiolologist. _____

4. An abbonimoocentesis will remove the fluid. _____

5. Trachycardis is a condition of rapid heart rate. _____

6. A lipidoma is a fatty tumor. _____

7. The sarcoma was removed during surgery. _____

8. The cystoscopy found no abnormalities. _____

9. We viewed the leupkocites under the microscope. _____

10. The patient's cianocis, or bluish color, was remarkable. _____

Using a Medical Dictionary

Even with the best deciphering skills, your analysis of an unfamiliar term can sometimes produce a strange-sounding definition. If your word analysis result doesn't seem right, consult a reliable medical dictionary.

Looking up new terms in a medical dictionary is a smart strategy in general. Comparing definitions among different dictionaries takes your knowledge one step further. You may understand one definition better than another, or the combination of definitions may provide a more complete meaning. You may notice some minor differences among medical dictionaries. Sometimes the term you seek is not in one dictionary, but can be found in another.

If you have an idea of the correct spelling, of course, you can find the correct page easily. If you are uncertain of the spelling, concentrate on the sound of the first part of the word and look at the words that begin with that sound. Remember that c and s (and ps as in psychology) can sound alike, as can ph and f and a number of other letters and letter combinations. If you are working with a new or unfamiliar term and you don't know the spelling, try to visualize all the different possible spellings of the term and check your dictionary for each one.

A medical dictionary can be a great help even if you only need to *confirm* your understanding of a term's meaning. You may find some additional information that you were unaware of, or you may learn that your understanding of the meaning was inaccurate. Remember, if you don't find your term in the first medical dictionary you try, switch to a different one. Your time will be well spent because you will have looked up many different terms in the process of trying to find the one you need.

Don't overlook the resources on the Internet. Here are a few online medical dictionaries:

> http://medical-dictionary.com/
> http://www.nlm.nih.gov/medlineplus/dictionaries.html
> http://www.online-dictionary.net/medical/

The Internet changes frequently, so use a search engine, such as <u>Google.com</u> to find new or additional reference tools.

Word Analysis *Exercise 11*

Study the terms below. Use a diagonal line to break each word into its parts: prefix, suffix, and root or combining form. (Remember that not all medical terms have all word parts.) Write the meaning of each word part and try to combine those meanings into a definition of the term. Write your answer in the first blank, then look up the term in a medical dictionary and write the dictionary's definition in the second blank.

Term	Your definition	Dictionary definition
1. urologist	_____	_____
2. thrombocytosis	_____	_____
3. cephalic	_____	_____
4. extracellular	_____	_____
5. gastrorrhaphy	_____	_____
6. osteomyelitis	_____	_____
7. bradycardia	_____	_____
8. osteoma	_____	_____
9. necrotic	_____	_____
10. hypogastric	_____	_____

ABBREVIATIONS

In both written and oral communication, medical personnel use a large number of abbreviations to save time as well as to save space on forms. "HPI," for example, is much quicker and shorter to write than "history of present illness." Some abbreviations are immediately obvious or make sense; others are not. Personal medical history is often abbreviated "hx." Some common charting abbreviations are listed in Table 1.20, but many common medical abbreviations will be presented in Chapter 2. Moreover, each body system chapter includes a list of the abbreviations generally associated with that specialty. Remember that each hospital, clinic, or other healthcare setting has its own list of charting abbreviations. Be sure to request a list of accepted abbreviations for your particular workplace and use them accordingly. If you make decisions regarding charting in a setting that does not have an abbreviation list, prevent confusion and miscommunication by establishing a list for everyone to follow.

The abbreviations in Table 1.20 are widely used in the healthcare industry.

Table 1.20

Common Charting Abbreviations

Abbreviation	Meaning
BP	blood pressure
CC	chief complaint
CCU	coronary care unit
c/o	complains of (patient's report of a symptom)
CP	chest pain
D/C	discontinue
↓	decrease or decreasing
Dx	diagnosis
ETOH	ethyl alcohol (beverage alcohol)
♀	female
HEENT	head, eyes, ears, nose, throat
H&P	history and physical
HPI	history of present illness
hx	personal medical history
IMP	impression (related to diagnosis)
↑	increased or increasing
IP	inpatient
Ⓛ	left
Ⓡ	right
♂	male
NKA	no known allergies
NKDA	no known drug allergies
OP	outpatient
P	pulse
PAR	postanesthesia recovery
PERRLA	pupils equal, round, reactive to light and accommodation
PMH	past medical history
pt	patient
R	respirations
R/O	rule out
ROS	review of systems
RRR	regular rate and rhythm (refers to heart)
RTC	return to clinic
RTO	return to office
SOB	shortness of breath
T	temperature
Tx	treatment
VS	vital signs
WNL	within normal limits

Read the following list of abbreviations and definitions. Match the abbreviation with the correct definition by writing the letter for the definition in the blank beside the abbreviation.

Abbreviations	Definitions
1. SOB _____	a. within normal limits
2. RRR _____	b. temperature
3. CP _____	c. history
4. WNL _____	d. blood pressure
5. PAR _____	e. complains of
6. NKA _____	f. shortness of breath
7. c/o _____	g. patient
8. hx _____	h. respirations
9. BP _____	i. rule out
10. CC _____	j. treatment
11. T _____	k. regular rate and rhythm
12. Tx _____	l. chest pain
13. R/O _____	m. no known allergies
14. pt. _____	n. postanesthesia recovery
15. R _____	o. chief complaint

RTO
RTC

Performance Assessment 1

Proofreading

The progress note below contains ten spelling errors. There may be anywhere from no errors to five errors in a line. Find the errors, then write the progress note line number of the error and the correct spelling of the word on the lines provided.

Progress Note

1 Ms. Smith was seen today for complaints of stomach pain. There is a history of

2 gastraintestinel carcinomo in her family, and the patient herself has chronuc

3 hepatatis. Endoscepy indicated gustritis, with esophagal reflux. Biopsys of the

4 gastruc lining were obtained and sent to the patholugy lab. The patient was placed

5 on Prilosec and was scheduled to see a nutritionist in regard to an appropriate diet.

Line: _____ Word: _____

Line: _____ Word: _____

Line: _____ Word: _____

Line: _____ Word: _____

Line: _____ Word: _____

Line: _____ Word: _____

Line: _____ Word: _____

Line: _____ Word: _____

Line: _____ Word: _____

Line: _____ Word: _____

Proofreading

The progress note below contains ten spelling errors. There may be anywhere from one error to four errors in a line. Find the errors, then write the progress note line number of the error and the correct spelling of the word on the lines provided.

Progress Note

1 The patient is a 68-year-old male reporting musculoskleetal symtoms. He has

2 arthrodiynia with movement and AM stiffness in his left knee. X-ray reveals an

3 osteoam of the priximal tibia. History is significant for arhtroplasty of the right

4 knee, with complications of thrombsis and osteiitis. He will be referred to an

5 orthapedsit for arthrocsopy.

Line: _____ Word: _____

Line: _____ Word: _____

Line: _____ Word: _____

Line: _____ Word: _____

Line: _____ Word: _____

Line: _____ Word: _____

Line: _____ Word: _____

Line: _____ Word: _____

Line: _____ Word: _____

Line: _____ Word: _____

Word Maps

Organize each of the following word parts and abbreviations into one of the three categories by writing the part or abbreviation next to the category.

List of word parts:

ac

blast

centesis

cyte

eal

ETOH

hyper

infra

IP

meter

oma

plasty

SOB

super

tic

Category 1
Suffixes that indicate a treatment or test

_____

_____

_____

_____

Category 2
Common charting abbreviations

_____

_____

_____

_____

Category 3
Adjective endings

_____

_____

_____

_____

Category 4
Prefixes that can mean amount

_____

_____

_____

_____

Category 5
Commonly used medical suffixes

_____

_____

_____

_____

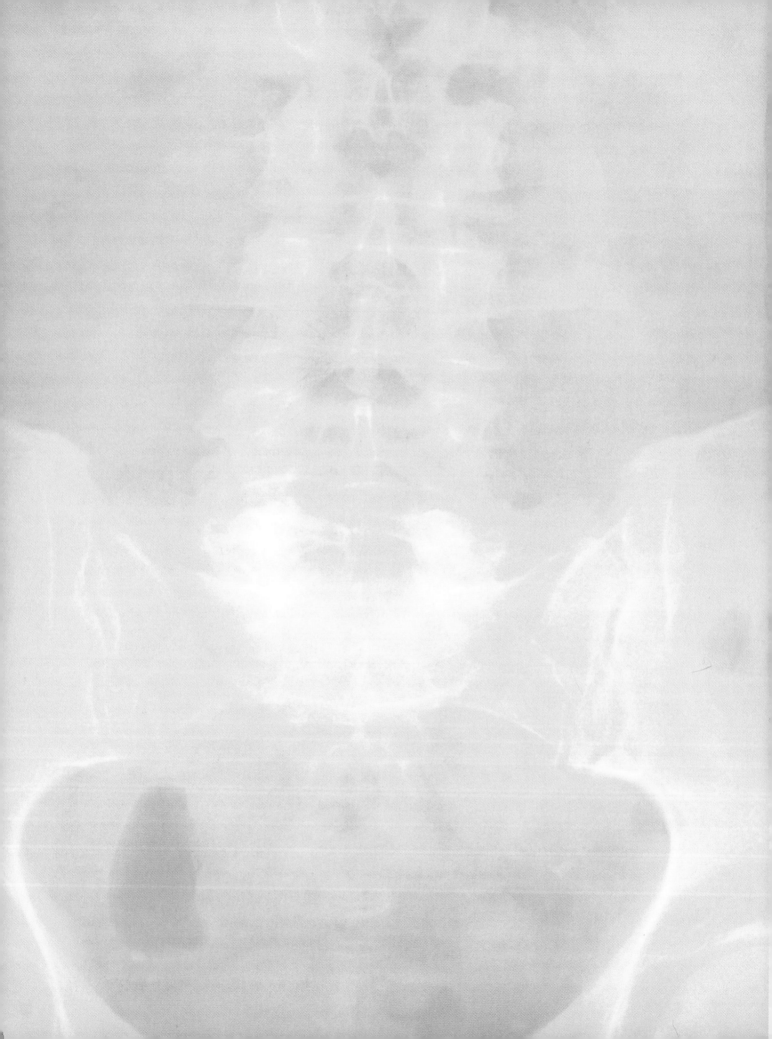

Chapter 2

Whole Body and Healthcare Systems Terminology

Learning Outcomes

Students will be able to:

- Explain the concept of levels of organization.
- Name the body systems and corresponding medical specialties.
- Label the areas, locations, and directions on the human body.
- Identify commonly used word parts used in medical imaging.
- Interpret medical records terminology and abbreviations for daily patient care, surgical and medical instruments, dates and times, and observations of color.
- Define some commonly used general lab, surgery, pathology, and pharmacology terms.
- Describe the apothecary system.
- Name the elements of a prescription.
- Distinguish among chemical, generic, and trade names of drugs.
- Interpret correctly the abbreviations commonly used in prescriptions.
- List and describe various routes of drug administration.
- Correctly spell and pronounce terminology related to body areas and directions, and general terms related to medical imaging, medical records, lab, and pharmacology.
- List and define the combining forms most commonly used to create terms related to the body areas, and directions and general terms related to medical imaging, medical records, lab, and pharmacology terms.

Much of your work learning medical terminology will happen in the separate contexts of the body systems. This chapter, however, brings together whole body areas, diagnosis of these areas using imaging technologies, and administration of drugs through various routes into the body. Begin with learning how the medical profession "organizes" its thinking about the body.

LEVELS OF ORGANIZATION

When Anton Van Leeuwenhoek invented the microscope in the late 1600s, the study of anatomy and physiology changed forever. The Dutchman's early search for a way to evaluate woven cloth had led him to experimentation that eventually produced a working, but crude, microscope. He refined his invention and, when he discovered "animacules" (little animals) in almost everything he viewed, the science of microbiology (the study of very small living things) was born.

Van Leeuwenhoek's discovery made it possible to study cells, the basic unit of life in the human body, which revolutionized the science of medicine. Researchers could now see how groups of cells make up a tissue, a group of tissues make up a body organ, and organs make up functional systems such as the nervous system, the gastrointestinal system, the urinary system, and others. This concept is known as "levels of organization" (see Figure 2.1). Note that each level becomes larger and

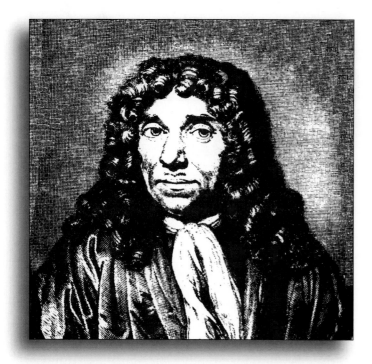

Van Leeuwenhoek

more complex than the one before it. The concept of levels of organization provides scientists with a useful tool for thinking about how all parts of the body function and how the functions are interrelated.

In this chapter you will develop a foundation for your study of body systems. You will learn the general, whole-body terminology that you need to build your vocabulary of individual body system words. As you read this chapter, notice the words such as bone, cartilage, nucleus, membrane, and tissue that do not combine as widely or as elegantly as the roots that make up so much of medical communication. We will refer to them as "non-combinable" words and—although not constructed of word parts—they will make up a significant portion of your medical vocabulary. Make a list of these terms, so that you can study them along with the combinable terms.

Figure 2.1 - Levels of Organization

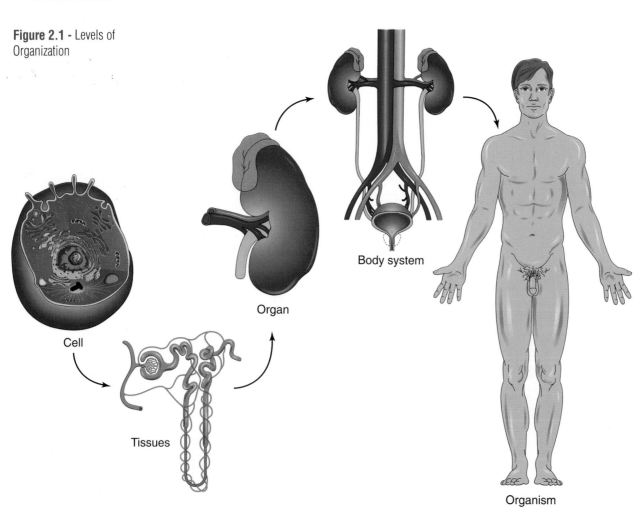

Cell

Tissues

Organ

Body system

Organism

Cells

Cytology is the study of cells, including their origin, structure, functions, and pathology. (Recall that the combining form *cyt/o* means "cell" and the suffix *-ology* means "study of.") The **cell** is the basic unit of all living things, the smallest unit capable of independent life and reproduction (see Figure 2.2). All cells have certain similarities: they have a nucleus, membrane, and protoplasm. The distinct outer membrane maintains the cell and controls passage of materials into and out of the cell. Inside the membrane is a substance called protoplasm, which contains cytoplasm and nucleoplasm. Cytoplasm is the area where structures called **organelles** do their work to help maintain the cell and assist with cell reproduction. There are several types of organelles, including the centrioles, endoplasmic reticulum, Golgi apparati, lysosomes, mitochondria, and ribosomes.

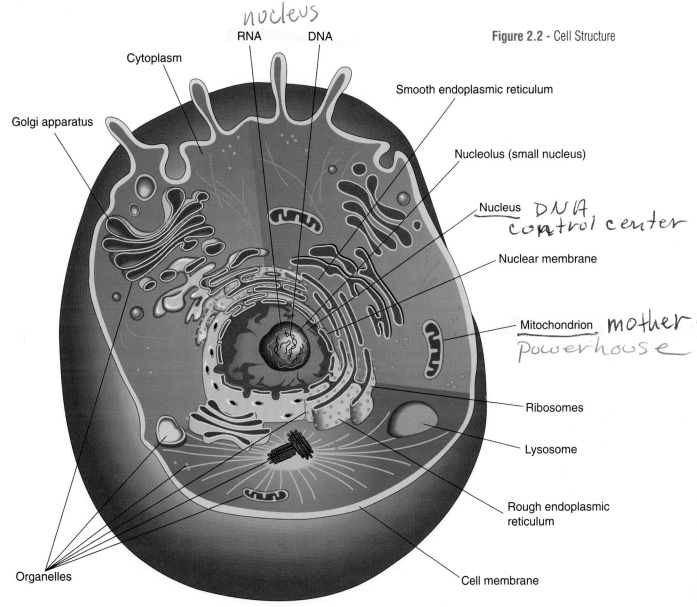

Figure 2.2 - Cell Structure

nucleus

RNA   DNA

Cytoplasm

Golgi apparatus

Smooth endoplasmic reticulum

Nucleolus (small nucleus)

Nucleus *DNA control center*

Nuclear membrane

Mitochondrion *mother powerhouse*

Ribosomes

Lysosome

Rough endoplasmic reticulum

Organelles

Cell membrane

Nucleoplasm (karyoplasm) makes up the cell's nucleus; it is surrounded by its own membrane. Nucleoplasm contains the genetic material needed for cell reproduction and for managing the cell's cytoplasmic activity. The genetic material in the nucleoplasm is deoxyribonucleic acid, or DNA. Compare the name of this material to the names of organelles and other cell parts. Do you see any sources for the abbreviation "DNA"?

Although cells share some structural similarities, they also have special characteristics that perform unique tasks depending on their location and purpose. A very general list of some cell types would include bone cells, blood cells, fat cells (these three are all associated with one general category), as well as skeletal and smooth muscle cells, nerve cells, and intestinal tract lining cells (of several types), sperm, ova, and many, many more. What follows is a description of how these form a higher level of organization.

Tissues

Human bodies consist of billions of cells that are grouped together and arranged to form tissues. A tissue is a collection of specialized cells with similar structures and functions. Some tissue is composed almost entirely of cells, whereas other types of tissue are largely composed of cells in an **intercellular matrix** that joins and supports the cells, fills the spaces between them, and helps hold them in position. This matrix contains special substances, such as electrolytes, salts, and fibers that give the tissue unique characteristics.

Histology is the branch of science specializing in the microscopic study of tissues. Tissues are grouped into four basic types—epithelial, connective, muscle, and nerve— and the entire body is made up of combinations of these tissues.

EPITHELIAL TISSUE found throughout the body covers internal and external surfaces. The skin and the linings of the digestive system, urinary system, and respiratory system are epithelial tissue. **Histologists** have identified several types of epithelial tissue, and they classify it according to the number of cell layers and the shape and characteristics of the surface layer.

CONNECTIVE TISSUE includes blood, bones, cartilage, tendons, ligaments, and fat. The human body has more connective tissue than any other tissue type. Connective tissue provides a framework for the body, holds organs in place, connects body parts, and allows for movement of joints. It also plays an important role in the body's immune system. Fat, or **adipose** tissue, is a type of connective tissue that cushions, stores energy, and insulates against heat loss.

MUSCLE TISSUE is categorized into three types: **smooth, skeletal** (or striated), and **cardiac**. All three types share the two primary muscle tissue activities: contraction and relaxation. Smooth muscle and cardiac muscle are considered **involuntary** (the individual has little or no control over the movement). Skeletal or striated muscle is considered **voluntary** (under the conscious control of the individual).

Smooth muscle is found in the walls of hollow internal structures, such as the bladder, intestines, blood vessels, and uterus. Skeletal muscles are attached to and move bones and joints. This muscle tissue is also called striated muscle because when viewed through a microscope it appears to have stripes, or *striae*. Chapter 4 presents more detail on muscle tissue.

Found only in the heart, cardiac muscle is specialized to conduct the electrical impulses that cause the heart to contract rhythmically. When seen close up, cardiac muscle tissue also has *striae*, but is distinguishable from skeletal muscle because of the impulse conduction system. We will discuss cardiac tissue in greater detail in Chapter 11.

NERVE TISSUE makes up the nervous system and is specialized to conduct nerve impulses, which are tiny electrical impulses. Nerve tissue comes in a variety of cell types, including those that support, maintain, and repair the nerves, and it comprises the brain and spinal cord, as well as nerves throughout the body. See Chapter 8 for more about nerve tissue.

Organs

The four tissue types—epithelial, muscle, connective, and nerve—combine in different ways to form organs, the essential body structures that work in harmony within body systems to perform specialized functions. Examples of organs are the small and large intestines, heart, liver, pancreas, lungs, stomach, and spleen. The body's internal organs are called visceral organs, or viscera. They are soft, and are generally located in one of the body cavities.

Not all organs are viscera. Some are not internal and not as localized as the heart or liver. For example, sweat glands, hair, and skin are all considered body organs, but they are not viscera.

Body Systems

A **body system** is comprised of several related organs that work together to perform a complex function. Figure 2.3 illustrates the body systems and lists the major structures and the corresponding medical specialties.

Where in the World Did That Term Originate?

Early Greek and Roman anatomists came up with the names for many body parts and diseases. For inspiration, they often turned to the natural world around them, as illustrated in the examples below.

Cochlea
Root: Cochlea (Latin for snail shell)
Named after the spiral structure of a snail's shell, this tube forms part of the inner ear. It is filled with fluid and houses the organ of Corti, a group of cells that convert sound vibrations into nerve impulses, which are then translated by the brain as sounds.

Ichthyosis
Root: Ichthys (Greek for fish)
Ichthyosis is the term for any one of a group of skin disorders characterized by a skin texture resembling fish scales. Most ichthyoses are hereditary.

Lupus
Root: Lupus (Latin for wolf)
A term dating to the thirteenth century, lupus originally denoted a type of localized skin lesion that resembled a wolf bite. Today, the term is paired with a range of modifiers to name a class of connective tissue disorders, each of which has a typical skin lesion.

Muscle
Root: Musculus (Latin for little mouse)
A muscle is a group of fibers that can contract and produce movement. Early anatomists thought the small mass moving under the skin when a person flexed an arm looked like a mouse scurrying back and forth; hence, they named this mass musculus.

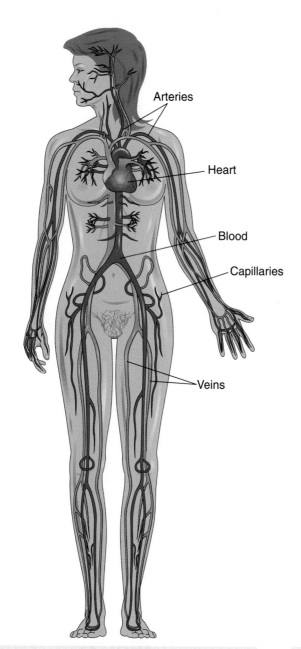

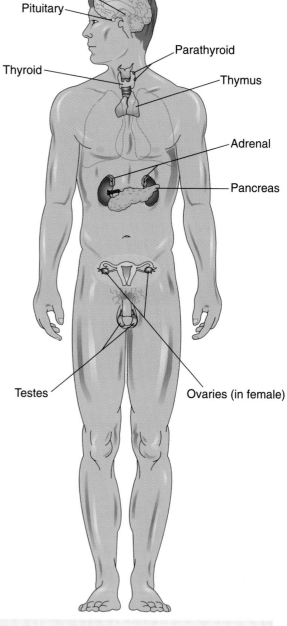

A. Cardiovascular or Circulatory System
Major structures:
    heart, blood vessels (arteries, veins, and
    capillaries), blood
Medical field/specialists:
    cardiology   cardiologist
    hematology   hematologist
    internal medicine internist
                                cardiovascular surgeon

B. Endocrine System
Major structures:
    thyroid gland, pituitary gland, testes and
    ovaries, adrenal glands, pancreas,
    parathyroid glands, pineal gland, thymus
    gland
Medical field/specialists:
    endocrinology   endocrinologist
    internal medicine internist

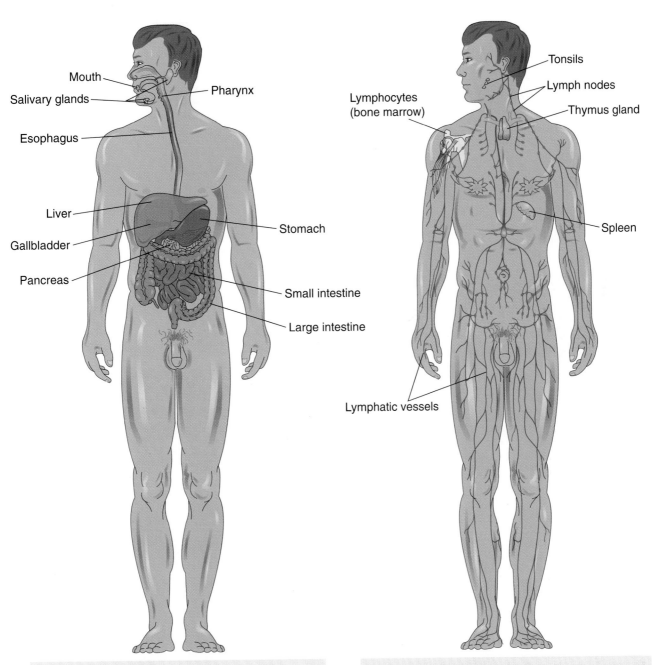

Mouth

Salivary glands

Pharynx

Esophagus

Liver

Stomach

Gallbladder

Pancreas

Small intestine

Large intestine

Tonsils

Lymph nodes

Lymphocytes (bone marrow)

Thymus gland

Spleen

Lymphatic vessels

C. Gastrointestinal or Digestive System
Major structures:
    mouth, pharynx, esophagus, stomach, small intestine, large intestine, liver, gallbladder, anus
Medical field/specialists:
    gastroenterology   gastroenterologist
    proctology   proctologist

D. Immune System
Major structures:
    lymphatic nodes, thymus gland, tonsils, spleen, lymphocytes (white blood cells), lymphatic fluid, lymph nodes, lymphatic vessels
Medical field/specialists:
    immunology   immunologist

Figure 2.3 - Body Systems, Including Major Structures and Medical Specialties

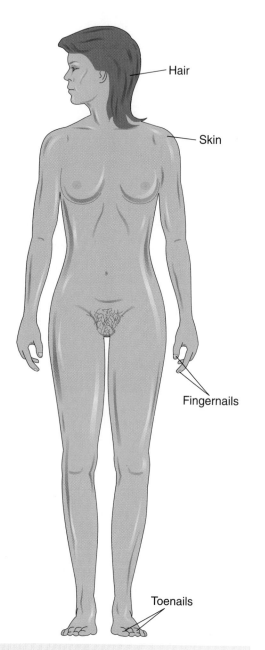

Hair

Skin

Fingernails

Toenails

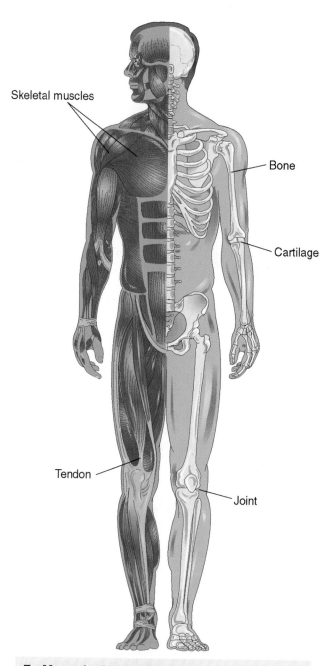

Skeletal muscles

Bone

Cartilage

Tendon

Joint

E. Integumentary System
   Major structures:
      skin, sweat glands, sebaceous (oil)
      glands, hair, fingernails, toenails
   Medical field/specialists:
      dermatology   dermatologist

F. Musculoskeletal System
   Major structures:
      muscles, tendons, bones, joints, cartilage
   Medical field/specialists:
      orthopedics   orthopedist
                        orthopedic surgeon

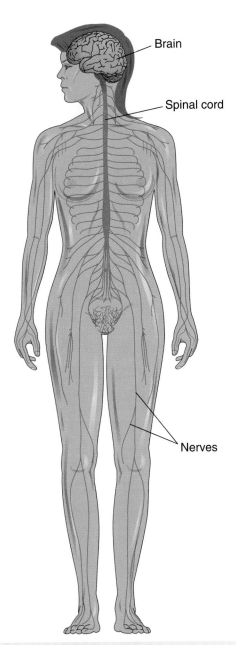

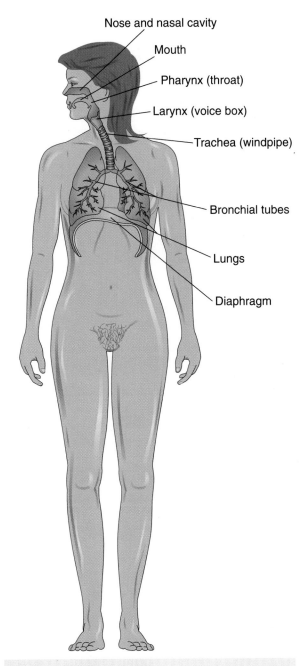

G. Nervous System
Major structures:
   brain, spinal cord, nerves
Medical field/specialists:
   neurology   neurologist
                      neurosurgeon

H. Respiratory System
Major structures:
   nose, pharynx, larynx, trachea, bronchial
   tubes, lungs, mouth, diaphragm
Medical field/specialists:
   pulmonology   pulmonologist
                      thoracic surgeon
                      allergist
                      internist

Figure 2.3 - Body Systems,
Including Major Structures and
Medical Specialties

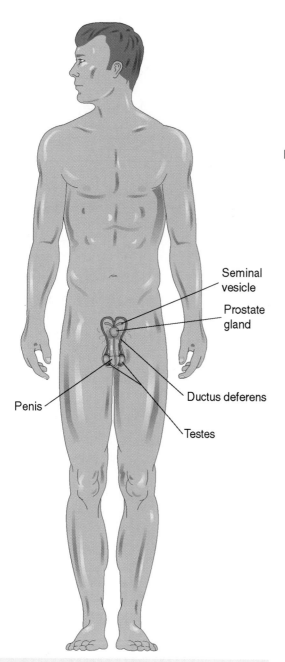

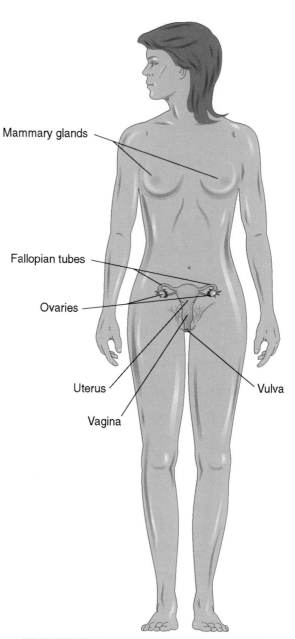

Mammary glands

Seminal
vesicle

Prostate
gland

Fallopian tubes

Ovaries

Ductus deferens

Penis

Uterus

Vulva

Testes

Vagina

I. Reproductive System (male)
Major structures:
testes, seminal vesicle, ductus deferens,
prostate gland, penis
Medical field/specialists:
urology   urologist

J. Reproductive System (female)
Major structures:
ovaries, fallopian tubes, uterus, vagina,
vulva, mammary glands (breasts)
Medical field/specialists:
obstetrics   obstetrician
gynecology   gynecologist

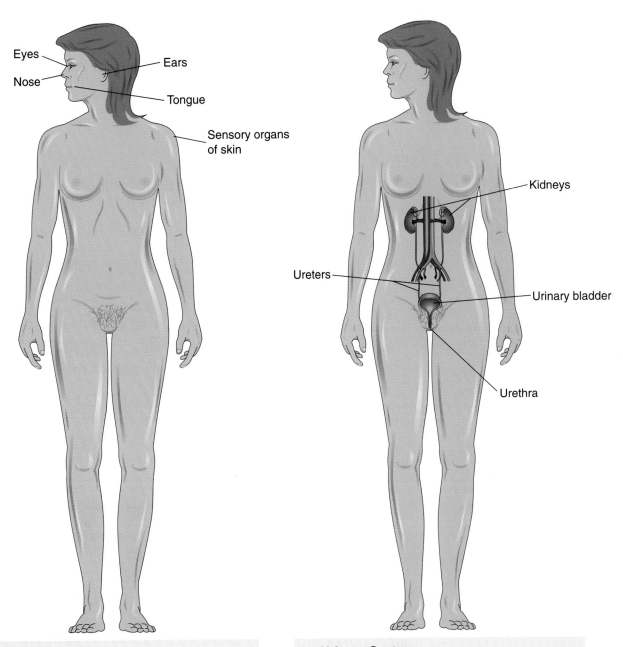

K. Special Senses

Major structures:

eyes, ears, nose, tongue, sensory organs of the skin

Medical field/specialists:

ophthalmology ophthalmologist

otolaryngology otolaryngologist

L. Urinary System

Major structures:

kidneys, ureters, urinary bladder, urethra

Medical field/specialists:

urology urologist

nephrology nephrologist

Match the terms in the first column with the meanings in the second column. Write the letter of the meaning in the blank beside the term. After you complete the matching, identify the three non-combinable terms in this exercise by circling them.

Term

1. cell   _____

2. tissue   _____

3. cytoplasm   _____

4. nucleus   _____

5. connective tissue   _____

6. epithelial   _____

7. voluntary   _____

8. viscera   _____

9. cytology   _____

10. body system   _____

11. muscle tissue   _____

12. intercellular matrix   _____

13. nervous tissue   _____

14. organs   _____

15. striated   _____

16. histology   _____

Meaning

a. under the conscious control of the individual

b. study of cells

c. study of tissues

d. internal organs

e. striped

f. comprised of several related organs that work together to perform a complex function

g. primary functions are contraction and relaxation

h. tissue that makes up covering of internal and external surfaces

i. structure that controls activities of cell; contains genetic material necessary for its reproduction

j. basic unit of living things; smallest unit capable of independent life and reproduction

k. essential body structures; work in harmony within body systems; carry on specialized functions essential to a human being

l. collection of specialized cells with similar structures and functions

m. conducts information relayed as tiny electrical impulses

n. nonliving material that joins/supports the cells, fills spaces between them, and helps hold them in position

o. provides framework for the body; holds organs in place; connects body parts; allows for movement of joints

p. cell substance; collection of organelles in fluid-like matrix

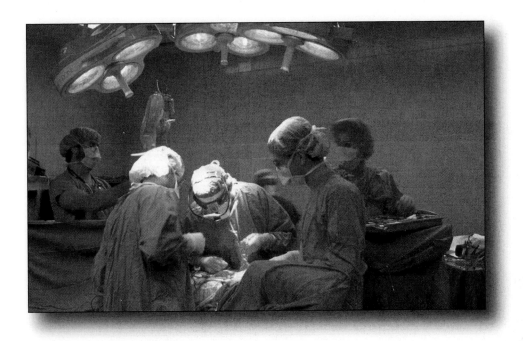

DIRECTIONAL AND POSITIONAL TERMS

Most people have used a map to establish directions, and know that when the map is held in the correct position, the top of the map represents north. However, the reference point of "north" can only be established if the map is held in the appropriate position. Like map readers and map makers who use commonly understood reference points and positions to make map reading easier, medical personnel use certain positions and reference points to insure accurate and quick communication about the human body. For example, read the following sentence, taken from a surgeon's report on a lung procedure. The surgeon uses three directional terms (italicized) that convey instantly and precisely to healthcare staff where the chest tubes were placed.

> "Two 32 French chest tubes were then placed *inferior* to the incision, directed both *anteriorly* and *posteriorly* toward the apex."

Using directional terms that are common knowledge among healthcare personnel gives the surgeon confidence that everyone who reads the report comes away with the same information. You will learn the meaning of these and other terms in the sections that follow.

Anatomical Position

A specific position, called "anatomical position," is used as a reference position in medical communication. Anatomical position assumes that the patient is standing, facing forward, with arms at the sides, palms facing forward, legs straight, and feet flat on the floor with toes pointing forward. Imagining a person in anatomical position provides uniform reference points for anyone describing areas of the body.

Figure 2.4 - Anatomical Position
(a) Frontal; (b) Side

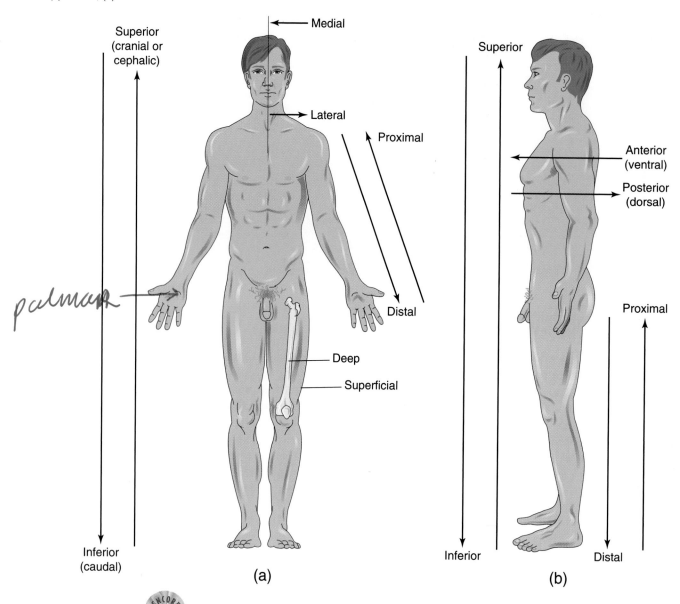

Superior
(cranial or
cephalic)

Medial

Lateral

Proximal

Distal

Deep

Superficial

palmar

Inferior
(caudal)

(a)

Superior

Anterior
(ventral)

Posterior
(dorsal)

Proximal

Distal

Inferior

(b)

Directional Terms

With the anatomical position as a base, a whole host of terms have been developed to describe the location of structures and **lesions** (injuries, defects, and pathological changes), as well as the direction of movements during a surgical procedure or physical exam. These terms are usually in pairs that have opposite meanings, such as terms that mean front and back, inside and outside, top and bottom. The following directional terms are part of the core medical vocabulary that is used to communicate about every body system. To learn the meaning of the directional terms, read each term and the sentence that accompanies it. Then look at Figures 2.4 (a) and 2.4 (b) to locate the anatomical parts mentioned and note how their locations relate to one another.

Superior or cranial or cephalic — toward the head or upper portion of the body. The heart is superior to the diaphragm.

Inferior or caudal — toward the feet or lower portion of the body. The kidneys are inferior to the adrenal glands.

Anterior or ventral — toward the front of the body ("Ventral" is frequently used in veterinary anatomy to indicate the underside of an animal.)
The sternum is anterior to the vertebral column.

Posterior or dorsal — toward the back ("Dorsal" is frequently used in veterinary anatomy to indicate the top of an animal.)
The shoulder blades are posterior in relation to the mammary glands.

Medial — toward the middle or center of the body or body part
The nose is medial in relation to the cheekbone.

Lateral — on or closer to the side
In anatomical position, the thumb is on the lateral aspect of the hand.

Proximal — nearer the point where a limb attaches to the body (toward the point of movement)
The proximal aspect of the femur is near the hip joint.

Distal — farther from the point where a limb attaches to the body (away from the point of movement)
The elbow is distal in relation to the shoulder.

Bilateral — pertaining to both sides of the body or structure
The patient had lesions on his nose, bilaterally.

Unilateral — pertaining to only one side of the body or structure
A stroke may cause unilateral paralysis—only the right side or the left.

Deep — toward the interior
The heart is deep to the ribcage.

Superficial — near the surface
The skin is superficial to the skeleton.

Parietal — the wall of a cavity
The parietal pleura lines the chest cavity and adheres to the chest wall.

Visceral — refers to the internal organs
The visceral pleura covers the lungs within the thoracic cavity.

Body Positions

Patients are placed on a bed, examining table or operating table in positions that make treatment, examination, or surgery easier. Ten commonly used positions are listed below and shown in Figures 2.5–2.14. Study each illustration along with the description and the examples of when the position is used.

Supine — patient lying on back with knees straight and arms at sides

The supine position may be used for examination of the anterior (front) body surfaces, breast examinations, x-rays, and some surgical procedures.

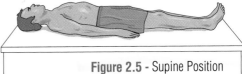

Figure 2.5 - Supine Position

Prone — patient lying on stomach, with knees straight; forearms may be under the head or at sides

The prone position may be used for examination of the posterior (back) body surfaces and for some operations.

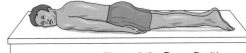

Figure 2.6 - Prone Position

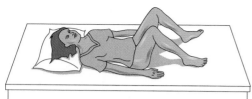

Figure 2.7 - Dorsal Recumbent Position

Dorsal recumbent — patient lying on back, with knees bent and feet flat on examination table, arms at sides

The dorsal recumbent position may be used for examination of the abdomen, occasionally for vaginal or rectal examinations, for childbirth, and for some surgical positions.

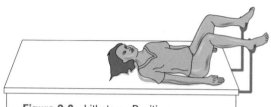

Figure 2.8 - Lithotomy Position

Lithotomy — patient lying on back, with knees bent, thighs abducted (apart) and feet resting in stirrups

The lithotomy position may be used for female pelvic examinations, rectal examinations, some operations, and sometimes in childbirth.

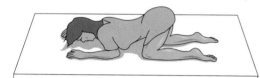

Figure 2.9 - Knee Chest Position

Knee-chest — patient's head, chest, and knees are flat against the examining table, knees are bent, and weight is resting primarily on the knees and chest

The knee-chest position may be used for rectal examinations, artificial insemination, and some surgical procedures. In some instances, the examination table may be contoured to facilitate positioning and to support the patient in this position.

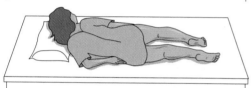

Figure 2.10 - Sims' Position

Sims' (or left lateral position) — patient lies on the left side, with left arm behind the back; left knee is slightly bent, and right knee is flexed rather sharply

Sims' position may be used for administering rectal suppositories and enemas, and for certain examinations and surgical procedures.

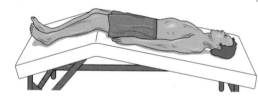

Figure 2.11 - Trendelenburg Position

Trendelenburg — the patient lies supine at an angle with the head lower than the trunk, knees bent, and feet below the level of the knees

The Trendelenburg position may be used to prevent and treat shock, for radiological examinations and procedures, and for some types of surgery.

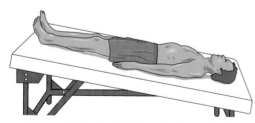

Figure 2.12 - Modified Trendelenburg Position

Modified Trendelenburg — the patient lies supine, with the head lower than the trunk, and the knees straight

The modified Trendelenburg position may be used to prevent and treat shock in trauma patients, for radiological examinations, or during some operations.

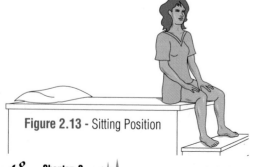

Figure 2.13 - Sitting Position

Sitting — the patient sits on the examining table, with knees bent; feet are often supported on a footrest

The sitting position may be used for auscultation of the heart and lungs, or for taking blood pressure readings; for head, eyes, ears, nose, and throat (HEENT) examinations, and for portions of a neurological exam.

Fowler's — the patient is sitting, with legs extended, and the trunk at a 90-degree angle; the back is supported, and sometimes the knees are elevated.

Fowler's position may be used for examination of the heart and lungs, to promote respiration in patients who have shortness of breath, and for examination of the feet and lower legs.

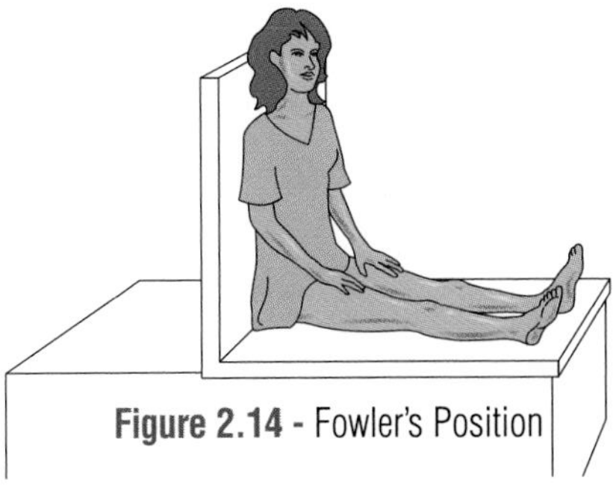

Figure 2.14 - Fowler's Position

Directional Planes

Another set of terms that describes the body and its parts is directional planes. The directional planes are imaginary slices through the body at specific points and in specific directions. Figure 2.15 illustrates the three planes.

1. The **sagittal plane** divides the body into two parts lengthwise, right and left, though not necessarily into halves. The term *midsagittal plane* refers to the sagittal plane dividing the body into equal parts, or halves.
2. The **frontal (or coronal) plane** divides the body into front and back sections from top to bottom. The front side is referred to as anterior, or ventral, and the back side is referred to as posterior, or dorsal.
3. The **transverse plane,** also called the horizontal plane divides the body into upper and lower portions. The upper portion is called superior or cephalic; the lower portion is referred to as inferior or caudal.

Figure 2.15 - Body Planes

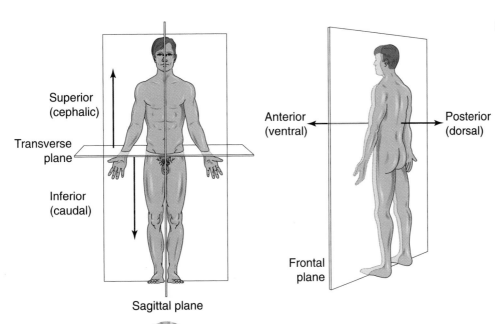

Superior (cephalic)

Transverse plane

Inferior (caudal)

Sagittal plane

Anterior (ventral)

Posterior (dorsal)

Frontal plane

Movement Terms

The following terms describe actions or movements of body parts. The terms are paired, that is, for almost every movement term, we have a term for the opposite movement. Read the terms, their descriptions, and the sentences using the terms in context. As you do so, examine the related illustration in Figure 2.16.

Flexion — bending of a joint
With the hand on the chest, the elbow joint is flexed.

Extension — straightening of a joint
When the hand is resting beside the thigh, the elbow is extended.

Figure 2.16 - Directional Terms

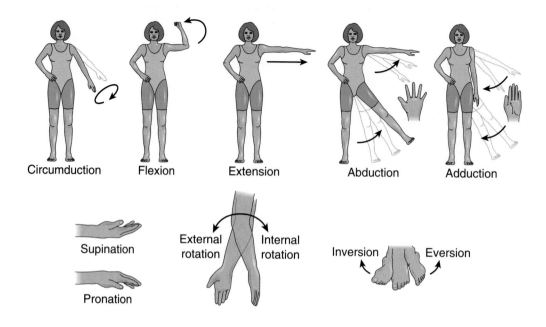

Abduction — joint movement that produces position of a limb away from the midline of the body
When the left leg moves away from the right leg, and to the side of the body, the thigh is abducted

Adduction — joint movement that produces position of a limb toward the midline of the body
When the legs are positioned together, side by side, the legs are adducted.

Circumduction — circular movement
Circumduction involves moving a body part (arm, leg, finger, etc.) to trace a circle.

Eversion — turned outward
When the feet are everted, they turn outward. This term is frequently used to describe turning the upper eyelid outward, to expose the inner side.

Inversion — turned inward
When a foot is turned inward, as to look at the thumbtack you stepped on, it is inverted.

Supination — turning the palm of the hand or the medial edge of the foot upward
If you wanted to hold soup in your hand, you would supinate your hand.

Pronation — turning the palm of the hand downward or raising the lateral edge of the foot
You may think of your hand in the prone position when you pronate your forearm.

Dorsiflexion — movement (rotation) of the foot upwards
To get a good look at your toenails, you would dorsiflex your foot.

Plantar flexion — movement (rotation) of the foot downward
Putting just your toes into the water may involve a plantar flexion of your foot.

Correct the spelling, if necessary, by writing the correct spelling of the underlined term above the term. Then write the term's meaning in the blank.

1. To test the range of motion of the hip joints, the patient's thighs were <u>abducted</u>.

_____

2. The <u>dorsal</u> aspect of the body was covered with second degree burns.

_____

3. The <u>mediam</u> aspect of the left thigh was swollen.

_____

4. The patient's injury was <u>superfecial</u>.

_____

5. The wrists were swollen <u>bilaterally</u>.

_____

6. The patient has a tattoo <u>distal</u> to his elbow.

_____

7. The <u>parietal</u> layer of the peritoneum was torn during surgery.

_____

8. Surgery was performed with the patient in the <u>pone</u> position.

_____

9. In a gynecologist's office, <u>lithetomy</u> position is frequently used.

_____

10. The patient was placed in <u>Trendelenburg</u> position to treat shock from blood loss.

_____

11. A <u>sagittal</u> section is a view of how the finger would look if it were cut in two lengthwise.

_____

12. The injured elbow had only ten degrees of <u>flexxion</u>.

_____

13. The orthopedic surgeon was unable to <u>extend</u> the patient's knee.

_____

14. The therapist wanted to improve the <u>adduction</u> of the shoulder.

_____

15. The eyelid was <u>everted</u> and the foreign particle was removed.

_____

BODY CAVITIES AND REGIONS

Medical language includes sets of terms to identify both general and specific areas of the body. Some general areas include body cavities, body regions, abdominopelvic regions and quadrants, and spinal column divisions. These terms are commonly used in both oral and written communication, and may accompany diagrams.

Body Cavities

Body cavities are areas that hold organs. The **cranial** cavity holds only the brain and the spinal cavity holds only the spinal cord. The other three cavities—the abdominal/abdominopelvic cavity, the pelvic cavity, and the thoracic cavity—hold various other organs. Study Table 2.1, which lists the major body cavities and the organs or structures they contain, and Figure 2.17.

Figure 2.17 - Body Cavities

Table 2.1

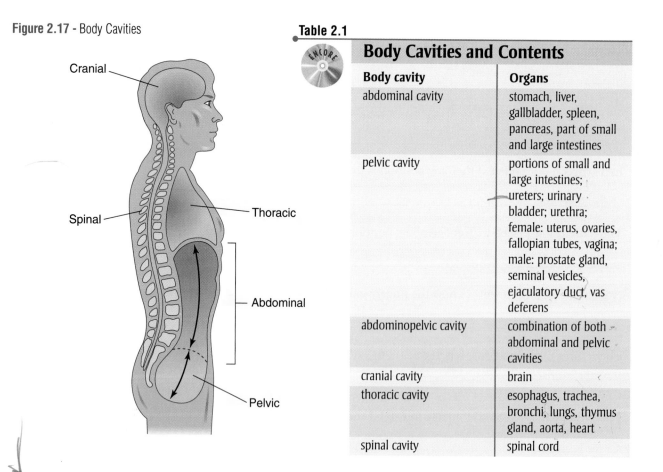

Body Cavities and Contents

Body cavity	Organs
abdominal cavity	stomach, liver, gallbladder, spleen, pancreas, part of small and large intestines
pelvic cavity	portions of small and large intestines; ureters; urinary bladder; urethra; female: uterus, ovaries, fallopian tubes, vagina; male: prostate gland, seminal vesicles, ejaculatory duct, vas deferens
abdominopelvic cavity	combination of both abdominal and pelvic cavities
cranial cavity	brain
thoracic cavity	esophagus, trachea, bronchi, lungs, thymus gland, aorta, heart
spinal cavity	spinal cord

Abdominopelvic Regions or Quadrants

The abdominopelvic region includes the abdominal cavity and the pelvic cavity. It is separated from the thoracic cavity by the diaphragm. Because the abdominopelvic area is quite large, we need to be able to indicate smaller areas so we can communicate more precisely. There are two separate division strategies for doing this: a division of nine regions and a division of four regions, or quadrants. Figures 2.18 and 2.19 show the abdominopelvic regions and the quadrants, respectively. Table 2.2 lists the regions and describes them. The abbreviations for the quadrants are also shown in Table 2.2.

Figure 2.18 - Abdominopelvic Regions

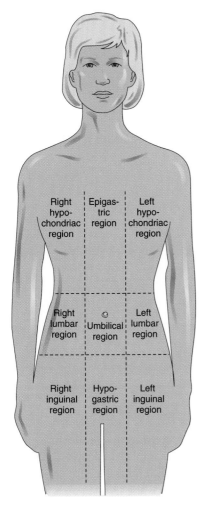

Table 2.2

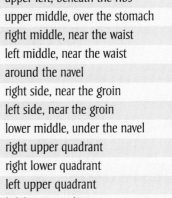

Abdominopelvic Regions and Quadrant Abbreviations

Right hypochondriac	upper right, beneath the ribs
Left hypochondriac	upper left, beneath the ribs
Epigastric	upper middle, over the stomach
Right lumbar	right middle, near the waist
Left lumbar	left middle, near the waist
Umbilical	around the navel
Right inguinal	right side, near the groin
Left inguinal	left side, near the groin
Hypogastric	lower middle, under the navel
RUQ	right upper quadrant
RLQ	right lower quadrant
LUQ	left upper quadrant
LLQ	left lower quadrant

Figure 2.19 - Body Quadrants

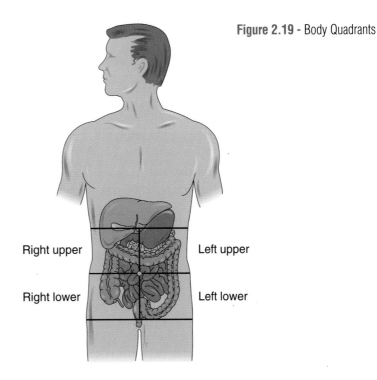

Divisions of the Spinal Columns

The back is divided into five regions, corresponding with the divisions of the spinal, or vertebral, column (see Figure 2.20): cervical, thoracic, lumbar, sacral, and coccygeal (or coccyx). The vertebral column consists of a series of twenty-four irregularly shaped bony structures, called vertebrae (singular form is vertebra) that encase and protect the spinal cord. Two sets of vertebrae are fused: five vertebrae are fused in the sacrum and four are fused in the coccyx. Physicians use the divisional terms to identify problems with the spine and resulting impairments in function. For example, a major spinal cord lesion in the cervical region (C1–C7) might tell a healthcare worker that the patient is a quadriplegic (paralysis in all four limbs), while a similar lesion in the lower thoracic area might produce paraplegia (paralysis in the lower part of the body). Table 2.3 lists the spinal divisions, their location, number of vertebrae, and abbreviations.

Figure 2.20 -
Spinal Column Regions

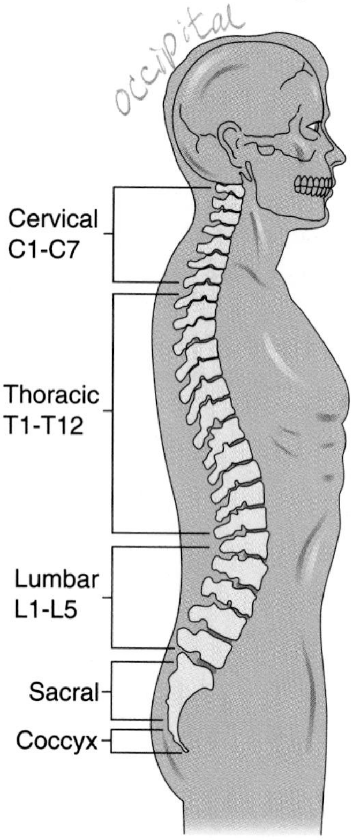

Cervical
C1-C7

Thoracic
T1-T12

Lumbar
L1-L5

Sacral

Coccyx

Table 2.3

The Vertebrae

Spinal division	Region of the back	Number of vertebrae	Abbreviation
cervical	neck	7	C (C1-C7)
thoracic	chest	12	T (T1-T12)
lumbar	loin	5	L (L1-L5)
sacral, sacrum	lower back	5 fused parts	S (S1-S5)
coccygeal, coccyx	tailbone	4 fused parts	

Table 2.4

Body Regions

Region name	Description
cranium	superior aspect of skull
cephalic	head
frontal	forehead
otic	ear
orbital	eye cavity
nasal	nose
buccal	cheek
cervical	neck
occipital	posterior of the head
mental	chin

Other Body Regions

Many regions of the body are named for the underlying bone. For example, the femur is the bone in the upper thigh, and the entire upper thigh area is referred to as the femoral area. This is not a rule, however. Some regions are named for a blood vessel that passes through the area; others are named for a prominent muscle or muscle group. For example, the brachial area refers to the upper arm. No bone has a corresponding name, but the brachial artery and brachial vein can be traced through the upper arm.

Study Table 2.4 to familiarize yourself with these additional terms for other areas of the body. Some of the terms and their regions are shown in Figure 2.21.

acromial	point of shoulder
thoracic	chest
pectoral	front of chest
sternal	anterior of rib cage
axillary	armpit
brachial	arm
cubital	elbow
antecubital	front of elbow
antebrachial	forearm
carpal	wrist
palmar	palm
digital	finger
coxal	hip
inguinal	groin
genital	external reproductive organs
perineal	between the thighs, the anus and the external reproductive organs
gluteal	buttocks
femoral	thigh
popliteal	back of knee
crural	shin
sural	calf of the leg
plantar	sole of the foot

Figure 2.21 - Body Regions

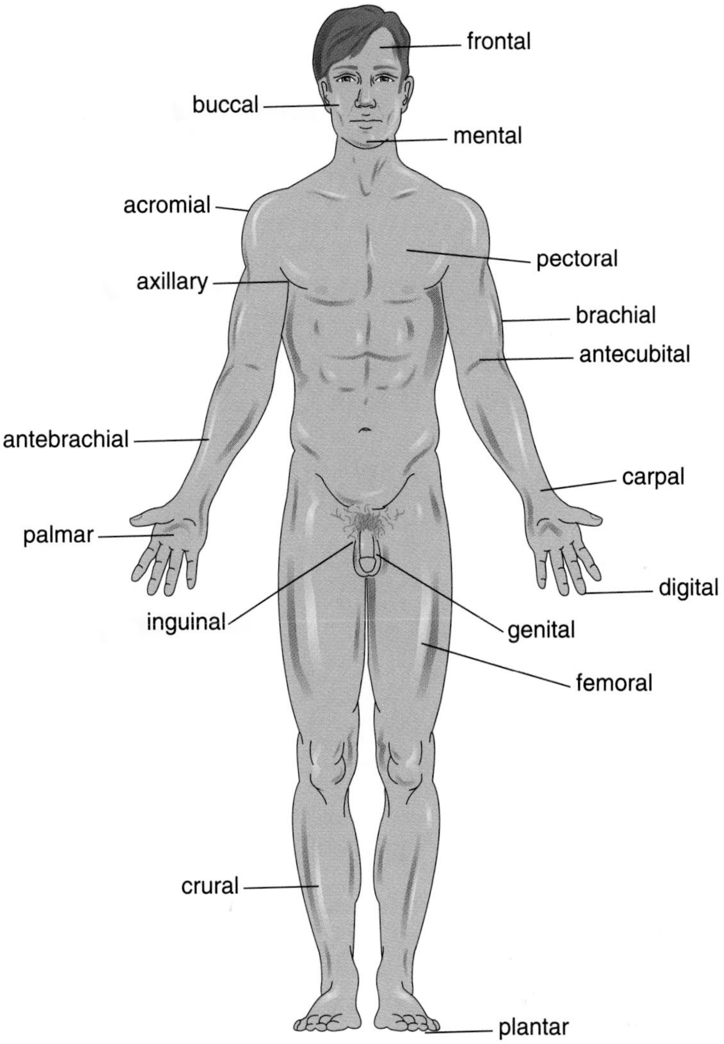

frontal
buccal
mental
acromial
axillary
pectoral
brachial
antecubital
antebrachial
palmar
carpal
inguinal
genital
digital
femoral
crural
plantar

Matching: Body Regions and Cavities

Exercise 3

Write the letter of the related definition in Column B on the line next to each item in Column A.

Column A

1. crural _____

2. coxal _____

3. popliteal _____

4. carpal _____

5. sternal _____

6. gluteal _____

7. cranial _____

8. spinal cavity _____

Column B

a. hip

b. wrist

c. shin

d. where the spinal cord is

e. upper middle, over the stomach

f. left side, beneath the ribs

g. back of knee

h. lower middle, under the navel

9. left hypochondriac   _____   i.   buttocks

10. epigastric   _____   j.   neck

11. hypogastric   _____   k.   front of ribs

12. cervical   _____   l.   top of skull

13. thoracic   _____   m. has five separate vertebrae

14. lumbar   _____   n. has five fused vertebrae

15. sacral   _____   o.   chest

Word Maps: Other Body Regions   *Exercise 4*

Write the appropriate term for each body area on the line provided.

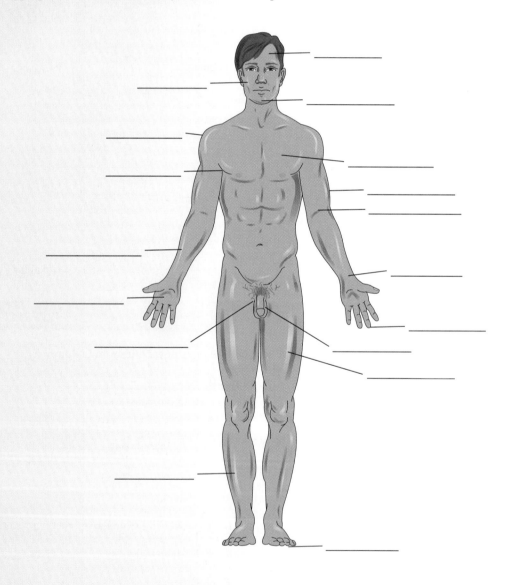

The squares below represent the abdominopelvic regions. Write the name of each region and its contents in the appropriate cell.

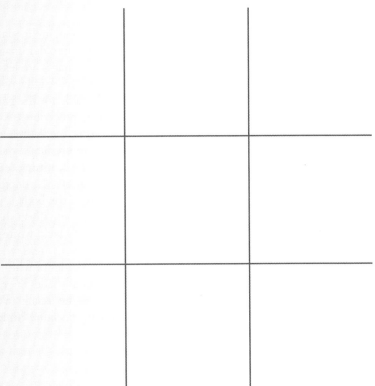

MEDICAL IMAGING TERMS

Medical imaging is a collective name for x-ray, computerized scans, and other techniques that permit visualization of the internal structures of the body. While they are often used for diagnostic purposes, these techniques may also be used to guide surgery or other procedures. Advances in medical imaging have made it possible for physicians to view refined, detailed pictures of the body's interior without touching a scalpel. The new equipment and techniques have revolutionized medicine and have made diagnosis safer, more accurate, and more comfortable for the patient.

The written results from medical imaging often appear in medical records as part of the diagnostic work, in the form of reports written by radiologists. While most paper-based chart formats have a separate section for radiology reports, with the actual images stored elsewhere, electronic medical records can accommodate both the reports and the images. These reports and images can be printed as often as necessary, eliminating the problem of original films being lost, damaged, or destroyed by exposure to chemicals or environmental conditions.

Radiological imaging includes conventional x-rays and fluoroscopy, sonography (or ultrasound), computed tomography (CT), magnetic resonance imaging (MRI), positron emission tomography (PET), and a variety of newer imaging techniques. New imaging technology is continually being developed, and older techniques are frequently updated to make them more effective. In some workplaces, the term nuclear medicine denotes the branch of medicine that uses radioactive emissions to produce images of the body for diagnosing and treating various illnesses. Also, some institutions group electrocardiograms, electroencephalograms, and similar image-producing techniques with x-rays and computerized scans under a single department referred to as medical imaging.

X-Rays

Radiology includes the study of x-rays and other imaging modalities used to screen for or diagnose abnormalities. Although x-rays are an older imaging technique, they are still useful for a number of applications. X-ray images are less detailed than many types of computerized scans, but they are inexpensive, readily available, and excellent as screening tools. X-rays are often more comfortable for the patient, and they carry less risk than some of the more advanced imaging procedures. X-ray techniques have been updated by the use of various types of contrast media injected intravenously or into a body cavity. These dye-enhanced x-rays can produce a quantity and quality of information that sometimes approaches that of the scanning techniques.

X-rays are produced by exposing sensitized film to the energy waves from an x-ray generator (a cathode ray tube). When part of the body is positioned between the generator and the film, the result is an image (actually, a shadow) of that body part. The resulting radiographs appear in shades of black, white, and gray. The areas where the x-rays strike the film directly appear black; areas where the x-rays are blocked by tissues of varying densities appear in shades of white or gray. As a result, soft tissue, which is less dense, appears on the film as shades of gray, and bone, which is more dense, appears as shades of white. The films are usually taken by a technologist and interpreted by a radiologist, a physician who specializes in radiology.

Fluoroscopy

Fluoroscopy is an imaging technique that uses a cathode ray tube to allow an observer to view a moving image. From the 1930s through the 1950s, shoe stores used a version of a fluoroscope to see feet inside shoes to assess fit. This popular use was discontinued because of the danger from the radiation exposure. Fluoroscopy is very similar to the traditional x-ray process, except that x-ray images are typically still, while fluoroscopy produces imaging of moving body parts. Fluoroscopy is particularly useful in diagnosing problems of the gastrointestinal system, joints, and mobile areas or organs. Fluoroscopy images can be recorded as either still pictures or moving images. Most fluoroscopy images today are digitized, and the recordings can be on videotape, motion picture film, compact discs, or other electronic media. See http://www.orau.org/ptp/collection/shoefittingfluor/shoe.htm for further discussion.

Ultrasound image of a fetus

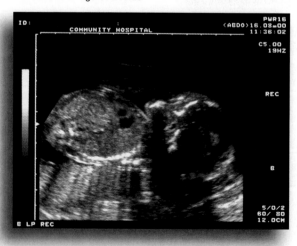

Sonography

Sonography, or ultrasound imaging, produces images of body structures by using sound waves above the frequency that can be heard by the human ear. A device that produces the ultrasound waves, called a *transducer,* is placed over the body part to be imaged, and the sound waves partially penetrate the structure to be examined. The sound waves are then reflected back to the transducer, which senses these echoes and converts them into an image. As with fluoroscopy, ultrasound can produce a moving image, and that image can be recorded as a still or a moving picture. Ultrasound is frequently used in obstetrics, and echocardiography is the form of ultrasound used to investigate cardiac problems.

Computed Tomography

Computed tomography (CT) is a medical imaging technique that uses computer interpretation of x-rays to produce images of structures inside the body. See Figure 2.22 for a simplified diagram of a CT scan. The body area is scanned in layers, using the x-rays to penetrate the various structures. Administering a variety of contrast media, sometimes called by the lay term "dye," may enhance the images. This media can include radioactive substances that are easy to detect on x-rays. The computer calculates densities and other information about the structures from the x-rays and displays the results as an image. Compiling individual scans of many very thin layers of a body area produces a highly accurate representation of that area. Positron emission tomography (PET) is one of several variations of computed tomography, and is frequently used for staging (describing the extent of spread within the body) of tumors or cancers.

Image from a CT scan

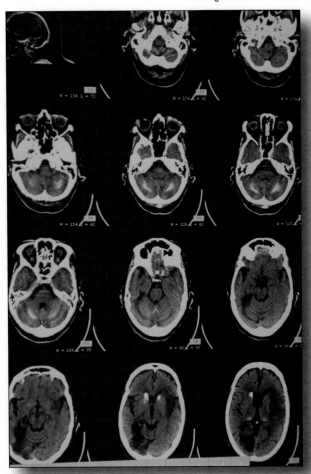

Image from a PET scan

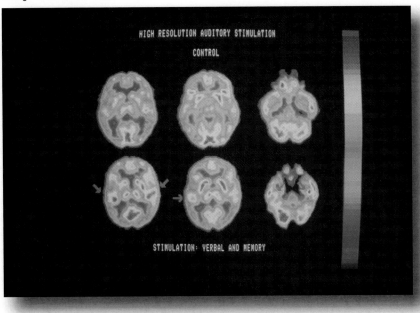

Figure 2.22 - CT Scan

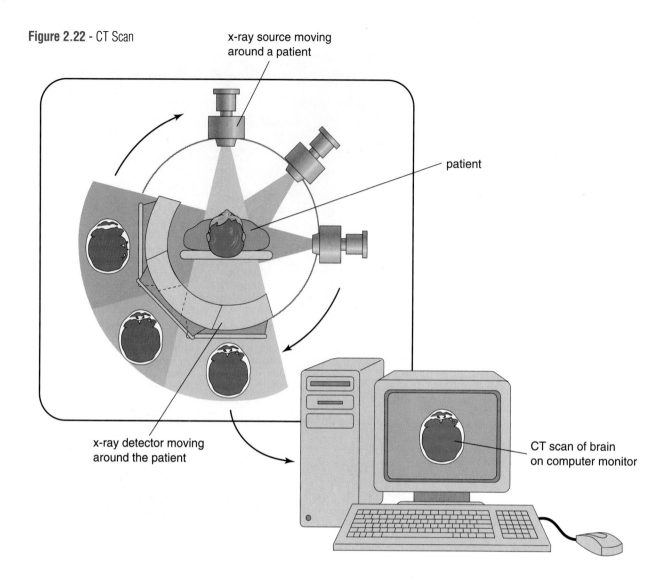

x-ray source moving around a patient

patient

x-ray detector moving around the patient

CT scan of brain on computer monitor

Magnetic Resonance Imaging

Magnetic resonance imaging (MRI), also called nuclear magnetic resonance (NMR), creates images from computer interpretations of the body's response to a strong magnetic field. The patient is placed within the magnetic field (see Figure 2.23), and the responses of the body's hydrogen atoms in the area being scanned are calculated by a computer to produce a highly accurate three-dimensional image. Since MRI is a relatively noninvasive procedure (introduction of the contrast media needed for some exams can be somewhat invasive, since it is usually accomplished through an intravenous injection, or IV), we can gather a great deal of information with low risk to the patient. MRI, like the other imaging techniques, is continually being refined and ongoing research is finding new applications for diagnosis and treatment.

Table 2.5 lists common terms associated with radiology, nuclear medicine, and diagnostic imaging. Notice that most of the procedural and diagnostic testing terms contain the suffixes *graphy* (process of recording), or *-gram* (record).

Figure 2.23 - MRI Imaging

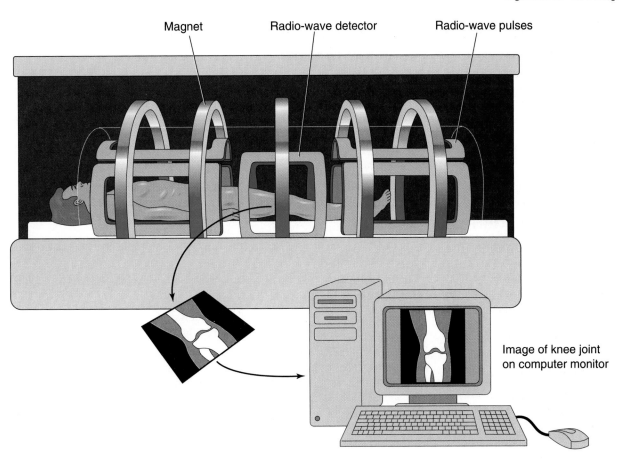

Magnet   Radio-wave detector   Radio-wave pulses

Image of knee joint on computer monitor

Terms Associated With Radiology and Nuclear Medicine

Materials and equipment terms	Meaning
barium	contrast medium or dye, frequently used to provide enhanced images of body structures of the digestive system
film	thin sheet of cellulose or plastic, coated with chemicals, used to take photos or x-rays
radioactive	emitting radiation energy
radiogram	image on x-ray film
roentgen	unit of exposure to radiation
shield	device used to protect against radiation
transducer	device for converting energy from one form to another
radiopaque	property of blocking the passage of x-rays

Diagnostic procedures terms

angiocardiography	process of viewing the heart and blood vessels by injecting radiopaque dye into circulating blood and exposing the chest to x-rays
angiography	process of recording a vessel through the use of radiopaque dye and x-rays
bronchography	process of viewing the bronchus by x-ray examination
cholangiogram	x-ray examination of the bile ducts
cholecystogram	x-ray examination of the gallbladder
echogram	examination of body structures using ultrasound imaging techniques
echocardiogram	ultrasound that records the function of the valves and flow of blood through the heart

fluoroscopy	examination of body tissues and deep structures by use of fluoroscope
lymphangiography	x-rays of lymphatic vessels
myelography	x-rays of the spinal cord
pyelography	x-rays of the kidneys and ureters
radiography	x-rays
radioimmunoassay	measurement of antigen-antibody interaction using radioactive substances
radiotherapy	treatment of disease using radioactive emissions; treatment for cancer
salpingography	x-rays of fallopian tubes
sonogram	image produced by sound waves reflected off body structures (examination of a part of the body using sound waves)
tomography	x-ray exam where the x-ray device is moved to view areas of the body
ultrasonography	imaging technique that uses sound waves to study a portion of the body

Directional terms in medical imaging

anteroposterior	front to back (direction of x-ray passing through the body when the patient is in a standard x-ray examination position)
posteroanterior	back to front (direction of x-ray passing through the body when the patient is in a standard x-ray examination position)
axial	around an axis
lateral	on or closer to the side (x-rays passing through the body from the side when the patient is in a standard x-ray position)
decubitus	lying down (describes patient position for an x-ray examination)

Medical imaging general terms

radiologist	physician who specializes in the use of x-rays and other imaging techniques; interprets x-rays
roentgenology	alternate term for x-ray technology
scan	repeated recording of emissions from radioactive substances onto a photographic film for one area of the body
scintiscan	image created by gamma radiation, indicating concentration within the body; an imaging technique that requires the injection of radioactive substances
sonolucent	permitting the passage of ultrasound waves
tagging	attachment of radioactive material to a substance that can be found as it moves through the body
technologist	one who is trained in the science and practice of using a technology
therapeutic	treatment of disease; curative
uptake	absorption of radioactive substance into tissue

Name That Term: Imaging Terms

Exercise 6

Read the definition provided and write the term it defines on the corresponding line. See if you can do it without looking it up in the table!

Definition   **Term**

1. process of recording a vessel (through the use of radiopaque dye and x-rays)   _____

2. process of viewing the bronchus (by x-ray examination)   _____

3. examination of body structures using ultrasound imaging techniques   _____

4. x-rays of the spinal cord _____

5. measurement of antigen-antibody interaction using radioactive substances _____

6. x-rays _____

7. x-rays of fallopian tubes _____

8. image produced by sound waves reflected off body structures _____

9. x-rays of the kidneys and ureters _____

10. examination of body tissues and deep structures by use of fluoroscope _____

GENERAL LABORATORY TERMS

Lab reports generally contain terms from the sciences of microbiology, microscopic analysis, and biochemistry, all of which use their own highly specialized language. For example, many of the terms microbiologists use are best learned in the context of the specific ways microbes survive, grow, flourish, and die. The other sciences have similar themes. Some of the frequently used general laboratory terms are defined in Table 2.6. Some of them have a common usage definition, but also have specialized meanings in the healthcare environment.

Table 2.6

General Laboratory Terms

Term	Meaning	Word Analysis	
asepsis	freedom from infection	*a*	not
		sepsis	putrefaction
CBC	complete blood count; calculation of numbers of red blood cells, white blood cells, and platelets (clotting cells)	N/A	
culture	a medium that encourages the growth of microorganisms, tissues, or cells	*cultura*	to till
differential	refers to white blood cell count; procedure that determines quantities of various types of white blood cells (WBCs)	*dif-fero*	to carry apart
hematology	the study of blood and its components	*hema*	blood
		logy	study
incubation	maintenance of near-ideal conditions for the growth of microorganisms	*incubo*	to lie upon
morphology	study of shape	*morph-*	form, shape
		logy	study
pathogens	disease-causing organisms	*path*	disease
		gen	to produce
resistant	refers to microbes that are completely or relatively unaffected by certain antibiotics	*re-sisto*	to stand back, withstand
sensitivity	state of being sensitive to a particular substance; refers to ability of certain drugs to inhibit the growth of a particular microorganism	*sensus*	to feel

serology	the study of serum (fluid portion of blood)	*ser*	serum
		logy	study
sterile	free from living organisms	*sterilis*	barren
urinalysis	laboratory study of the urine	*urin*	urine
		ana	up
		lysis	loosening

General Surgery Terms

Surgery has evolved from its earliest days of amputations without the benefit of painkillers or even the surgeon washing his hands. Tools for cutting, grasping, and connecting have been developed to meet very specific situations, but some widely used instruments are easily recognizable from their basic distinguishing characteristics. The art and science of surgery continues to change, as surgical procedures benefit from the use of computers, fiber optics, and the ingenuity of surgeons worldwide. Some of the common terms that describe surgery are shown in Table 2.7. One technology making a difference is **endoscopic** surgery, especially **laparoscopic** surgery, which has replaced many so-called "open" surgical procedures of the abdominal cavity. Laparoscopic surgery is safer, less time-consuming (and thereby less expensive), and results in a faster recovery time for the patient.

Table 2.7

Terms Related to Surgery

Term	Meaning	Word Analysis	
anesthesia	substance used to render a patient insensitive to pain	*an*	not
		(a)esthis	sensation
anesthetize	render a patient insensitive to pain	*an*	not
		(a)esthis	sensation
bandage	material used to cover dressing, to protect the dressing and hold it in place	*bande*	bandage
biopsy	procedure to remove tissue for diagnosis and/or treatment	*bios*	life
		opsis	appearance
cyberknife	combination of MRI and CT imaging technology that uses precisely aimed radiation to treat cancers	*kybernetica*	control or piloting
drain	device that establishes a channel for drainage of fluid or material from a cavity, wound, or infected area	*drehnian*	to draw off
drainage	material that exits a wound, cavity, or infected area	*drehnian*	to draw off
dressing	material used to cover a wound, protect it, and enhance healing	*drescer*	put right
excise	remove by cutting	*ex*	out
		cisio	cut
forceps	instrument with two blades, used for holding or grasping tissues, supplies, or other instruments	*formus*	warm
		capio	take or hold
hemostat	small surgical instrument used for clamping blood vessels	*hemo*	blood
		stat	stand
incision	surgical wound produced by cutting	*in*	into
		cisio	cut

intubation	insertion of a tube into the nose or mouth to provide for artificial breathing	*in* *tuba*	into tube
laparoscope	endoscope used to examine the abdomen that frequently includes capability of grasping and cutting; used for performing surgery of the gallbladder, appendix, uterus, and others	*lapara* *scope*	abdominal walls see
reduction	correction of a fracture; realignment of bone fragments	*re* *ductio*	back lead
resection	to surgically remove	*re* *seco*	back cut
retractor	instrument used to separate or hold tissues apart during surgery	*re* *traho*	back draw
scalpel	cutting instrument, usually consisting of a blade and a handle	*scalpellum*	knife
sponge	porous, absorbent material used to soak up fluids during surgery	*spongia*	aquatic organism that was the original source
suction	aspiration of gas or fluid by mechanical means	*suctum*	suck

General Pathology Terms

Although pathologists specialize in the study of disease processes, all healthcare practitioners need to know pathology to some degree. Much of pathology's language is specialized and best learned in the context of related diseases. However, many terms are important to know at every level of expertise. Some of them are included here in Table 2.8.

Table 2.8

Terms Related to General Pathology

Term	Meaning	Word Analysis	
epidemic	disease or illness afflicting many people in a geographical area at the same time	*epi* *demos*	upon people
etiology	the cause of an illness or disease	*etio-* *-logy*	cause study of
hyperplasia	uncontrolled overgrowth of tissue	*hyper* *plasia*	excessive formation
infection	invasion and growth of disease-causing microorganisms in body tissues	*in* *fect*	inside do or make
inflammation	response by the body to injury or disease	*in* *flammo*	inside flame or fire
lesion	area of pathological process or traumatic injury to a body part	*laesio*	hurt
pandemic	widespread epidemic	*pan* *demos*	widespread people
pathogenesis	origin of pathology; beginning of a disease process	*path* *genesis*	disease origin

General Pharmacology Terms

Every medical record contains pharmaceutical terms, either as part of the patient's history, the plan of treatment, or within a prescription. In addition to drug names, the vocabulary of pharmacology is replete with abbreviations and symbols for drug doses and regimens. Doctors, nurses, pharmacists, and pharmacy or medication technicians must know this language in detail so their communications to one another are accurately understood.

DRUG MEASUREMENT SYSTEMS Medical records use two drug measurement systems: the apothecary system (Table 2.9) and the metric system (Table 2.10). The apothecary system, developed by the earliest chemists and pharmacists (or apothecaries), bases liquid measurements on one drop and bases weight measurements on one grain of wheat. This system is rapidly giving way to the metric system, which has the advantages of being internationally recognized, easier to use, and more accurate. The metric system is a ten-based decimal system, which uses the following standard units:

Table 2.9

Units of Measure

To be measured	Metric unit	Abbreviation	Common US unit equivalent
length	meter	m	39.37 inches
volume	liter	L	1.0567 quarts
weight	gram	g	0.036 ounce

Table 2.10

Apothecary System

Unit	Abbreviation	Typical measurement
dram	dr	liquid medications
fluid ounce	fl oz	liquid medications
grain	gr	dry medications by weight
drop	gt (sing) or gtt (pl)	liquid medications for infants and medications applied to the eye and ear
pound (16 oz)	lb or #	weight of patient
ounce	oz	liquid medications
quart (32 oz)	qt	measurement of irrigation fluid

Table 2.11

The Metric System and Its Abbreviations

Unit	Abbreviation	Equivalent	Typical Measurement
cubic centimeter	cc	1 cc = 1 mL	liquid medications
centimeter	cm	2.54 cm = 1 inch	wound size
cubic millimeter	cu mm	1 cu mm = 0.001 cu m	laboratory measurement
gram	g or gm	1,000 gm = 2.2 lb	weight of a tumor
kilogram	kg	1 kg = 2.2 lb	weight of an infant
liter	L	1 L = 1.05 quarts	intravenous fluid measurement
milligram	mg	1 mg = 0.001 gm	dry medications
milliliter	mL	1 mL = 1 cc	liquid medications
millimeter	mm	1 mm = 0.001 m	size of skin lesion

PRESCRIPTIONS AND MEDICATION ORDERS Physicians, nurse practitioners, and physician's assistants write prescriptions and medication orders; healthcare team members dispense or administer the medication. No prescription is necessary if the physician administers the medication on a one-time basis, although an entry regarding the medication must be made in the patient's record. When delivered to the pharmacist, the prescription or medication order is an order to supply the patient with a certain drug of a given strength and quantity. The prescription also includes directions for administering the drug. If the drug goes directly to the patient, he or she follows the administration instructions; if the drug is supplied to the nursing staff of a hospital, it is indicated on a medication order, which includes administration instructions for nurses to follow in giving the drug to the patient.

ELEMENTS OF A PRESCRIPTION Federal regulations require that a prescription follow a specific format. The prescription must contain the following elements: doctor's or clinic's name, address, telephone number, and drug license or authorization number (DEA); name of the patient, date, drug name and strength, amount to be dispensed, instructions for administration, signature of the physician, permission for refills, and whether generic substitution is allowed, as shown in Figure 2.24.

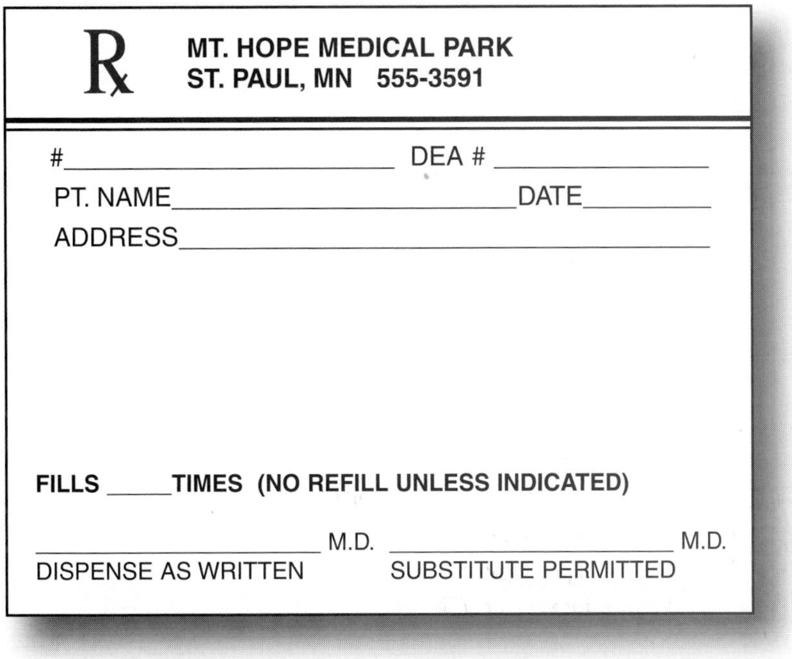

℞ MT. HOPE MEDICAL PARK
ST. PAUL, MN 555-3591

#________________ DEA # ____________

PT. NAME____________________ DATE________

ADDRESS______________________________

FILLS _____ TIMES (NO REFILL UNLESS INDICATED)

____________________ M.D. ____________________ M.D.

DISPENSE AS WRITTEN SUBSTITUTE PERMITTED

Figure 2.23 - Prescription Form

DRUG NAMES Drug names are written in one of three ways: the chemical name, the generic name, or the trade name.

Chemical name: the chemical formula for the drug written precisely according to its chemical structure. A chemical name can contain many syllables and numbers, which are often separated by commas or hyphens. A physician or pharmacist can use the chemical name to determine the composition of the drug.

Generic name: a name assigned by the manufacturer and generally accepted as a substitute for the chemical name. The generic name often indicates the drug classification, or general type. For example, phenobarbital is a generic name, and the compound phenobarbital is classified as a barbiturate drug. Drug classifications are important because most drugs in a given classification have similar actions, side effects, and precautions.

Trade name: the name under which the drug is marketed, usually a trademark. When a new drug is first developed, it has only a chemical name. The manufacturer gives the drug its generic name and a trade name. When the original manufacturer's patent on the drug expires, other drug companies can market the drug under brand names they provide. Consequently, one generic drug can have many trade or brand names.

ACCURACY IN DRUG NAMES   Although they may be difficult to spell, drug names must be recorded accurately. If you do not know how to spell or record the name accurately, find out! *The Physicians' Desk Reference* (PDR), published by the Medical Economics Company, contains detailed information on prescription drugs and is probably the most widely accepted drug reference book.

Medication Administration Terms

When a pharmacist fills a prescription, he or she translates the abbreviations into words that the patient can understand. Doctors use the same abbreviations and symbols when they write medication orders for hospitalized patients, although in a hospital setting, a nurse usually administers the medication. It is important to note that in many hospitals, medical and pharmacologic abbreviations are no longer allowed. Some abbreviations may be confusing to the practitioner and can cause inadvertent mistakes, or near errors to occur. Table 2.12 gives some common abbreviations and symbols related to medications. Note that the abbreviation letters often derive from the first letters of the Latin terms. Some of the abbreviations below are pronounced letter-by-letter. Those are marked with an asterisk.

Table 2.12

Common Abbreviations in Prescriptions

Abbreviation	Meaning	Latin term
ā	before	*ante*
a.c.	before meals	*ante cibum*
AD	right ear	*auricle dexter*
ad lib	as desired	*ad libitum*
a.m.	before noon	*ante meridiem*
amt.	amount	
aq	water	*aqua*
AS	left ear	*auricle sinister*
AU	both ears	*auris utraque*
Ⓑ	bilateral	
* b.i.d.	twice a day	*bis in die*
C	Celsius, centigrade	
c̄	with	
d.	day	*die*
F	Fahrenheit	
h.	hour	*hora*
h.s.	hour of sleep	*hora somni*
i	one	*uni*
ii	two	*bis*
iii	three	*ter*
OD	right eye	*oculus dexter*
ss	one-half	*semissem*
OS	left eye	*oculus sinister*
OU	both eyes	*oculi unitas*

p̄	after	*post*
p̄.c.	after meals	*post cibum*
per	by or through	*per*
p.m.	after noon	*post meridiem*
* p.o.	by mouth	*per os*
* p.r.	by rectum	*per rectum*
* p.r.n.	as needed	*pro re nata*
* q.	each or every	*quaque*
* q.d.	every day	*quaque die*
* q.h.	every hour	*quaque hora*
* q.2h.	every two hours	*quaque bis hora*
* q.i.d.	four times a day	*quater in die*
* q.o.d.	every other day	*quaque altera die*
q.s.	quantity sufficient	*quantum sufficiat*
Rx	prescription	recipe, take
sig.	label; instructions	*signa*
stat.	immediately	*statim*
* t.i.d.	three times a day	*ter in die*
s̄	without	*sine*
wk	week	
yr	year	
x̄	times or for	
>	greater than	
<	lesser than	

Routes of Medication Administration

Table 2.13 lists the routes by which medication is commonly administered. These terms and abbreviations often appear in physicians' prescriptions. See Figure 2.25 for an illustration of the different routes.

Table 2.13

Routes of Medication Administration

Route	Description	
inhalation	vapor or gas is inhaled through the nose or mouth and absorbed into the bloodstream through the lungs	
oral	drug is taken by mouth and is absorbed into the bloodstream through the stomach or small intestine (may also be called enteral administration)	
parenteral	drug is administered by injection using a needle and syringe or a needle and intravenous (IV) tubing	
	Types of parenteral injections	**Where injected**
	intradermal	within the layers of the skin
	intramuscular (IM)	into a muscle
	intravenous (IV)	into a vein
	subcutaneous (SQ)	beneath the skin
rectal	drug is in the form of a suppository or liquid and is inserted into the rectum	
sublingual	drug is placed under the tongue and is absorbed into the blood vessels there	
topical	drug is applied to a particular area for local action (generally lotions, ointments, and eye or ear drops)	
transdermal	drug is absorbed into the bloodstream through the skin by means of a controlled release patch	

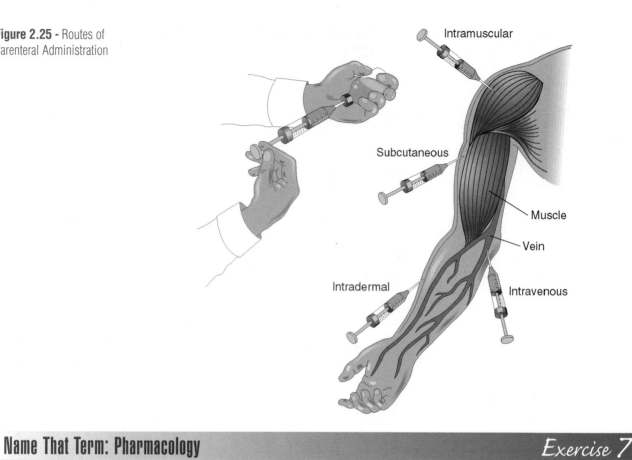

Figure 2.25 - Routes of Parenteral Administration

Intramuscular

Subcutaneous

Muscle

Vein

Intradermal

Intravenous

Name That Term: Pharmacology

Write the medical term for each definition.

1. analysis of urine to determine presence of abnormal substances _____

2. emitting radiation energy _____

3. cause of an illness or disease _____

4. response by the body to injury or disease _____

5. image on x-ray film _____

6. widespread epidemic _____

7. unit of exposure to radiation _____

8. encourage growth of bacteria _____

9. study of shape or form _____

10. material used to cover dressing, to protect the dressing and hold it in place _____

11. study of tissues _____

12. disease-causing organisms _____

13. study of serum (fluid portion of blood) _____

14. free from living organisms _____

15. absorbent material used to cover and protect a wound and enhance healing _____

WordPlay

1. If *intubation* means to put a tube in, why doesn't *incubation* mean put a cube in?
2. If *hypo* means under, and *chondros* means cartilage, and hypochondriac means under the ribs, why do we call a person who imagines illnesses a hypochondriac?
3. Long ago, persons who listened to gossip might have been in danger of having their left ear cut off. Can you guess why?
4. If a dram is a measure of liquid medication, then what's a "dram shop"?
5. Which term in this chapter might refer to the study of shape shifters?
6. Which imaging technique might we construe to be amusing, witty, sparkling, or clever?

Answers

1. The root for the word incubation isn't "cube." It is from a Latin word (*incubo*) that means "to hatch" or "to lie down."
2. The term first was used to describe persons with depression or melancholy without identifiable cause. Earlier beliefs held that the viscera of the hypochondriac were the location or source of melancholy.
3. The Latin for left ear will tell you—*auricle sinister*. Our derivative of *sinister* means evil or harmful.
4. Bet you're wrong. A dram shop is a legal term for the liability of one who serves liquor.
5. Yes, morphology. One use of the term morphing refers to changing the shape of something to make it something else.
6. A scintiscan. *Scinti* is from the Latin *scintilatum*, meaning sparkling. The technique is done using a scanning scintillation counter—a machine that counts "the sparks." The record it creates is a scintigram.

PUTTING IT TOGETHER

You will use the medical terms you have learned in this chapter again and again in your healthcare career, and they will be part of your vocabulary for the rest of your life. Healthcare workers rely on medical terminology to convey important information about patient care, health statistics, billing and reimbursement information, and research. In time, you will find yourself using this language, or parts of it, every day. Even if you are not working in healthcare, you will hear a word or a phrase that once was foreign, and you will understand its meaning.

The terminology you are learning is the English version of the medical language; other languages have different versions. Since many of the terms are derived from Greek and Latin (and the Greek/Latin influence is almost universal), many medical terms are recognizable in other languages. In addition, there are other vocabularies, or terminologies, in the language of medicine. The medical coding systems, ICD-9-CM (International Classification of Diseases — 9th version — Clinical Modification) and CPT (Current Procedural Terminology, revised every year) make up a type of language that is used primarily for gathering statistics and for health care reimbursement. The World Health Organization has completed work on creating ICD-10, but it is yet to be widely used.

One new terminology receiving a great deal of attention is SNOMED (Systematized Nomenclature of Medicine) and SNOMED CT (SNOMED Clinical Terms). SNOMED CT is a clinical reference terminology that bridges the communication gaps among healthcare workers, researchers, and patients through a common language. In some instances, SNOMED is almost like a translator, allowing the exchange of information between many different languages. The core vocabulary of SNOMED includes over 364,400 healthcare concepts and 984,000 descriptions. Combined with meanings and definitions, these are organized in ways that make SNOMED especially useful for electronic health records. It is anticipated that SNOWMED CT will also be used for such applications as ordering drugs and diagnostic tests, telemedicine, public health reporting, and clinical research.

Like the ICD coding systems, electronic health records, and the medical terminology you have been studying, SNOMED is an exciting part of healthcare. As your knowledge expands, watch for developments and changes in medical communication systems and be alert for the opportunities they provide. You can learn more about SNOMED at the SNOMED website, www.snomed.org

Performance Assessment 2

Crossword

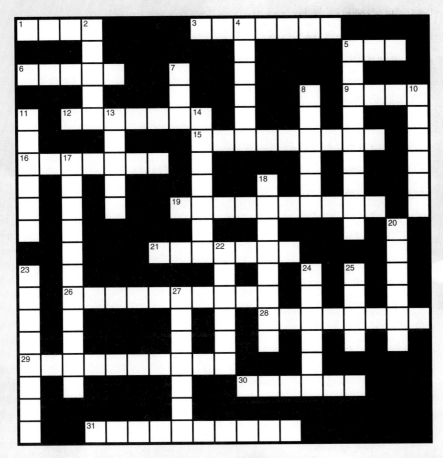

Across
1. toward the interior
3. cavity that holds the brain
5. coxal area
6. cubital area
9. position used for enemas
12. toward the front
15. straightening of a joint
16. side of the body
19. study of shape
21. internal organs
26. upper middle abdominopelvic region
28. groin area
29. tissue covering internal and external surfaces
30. toward the back
31. plane dividing the body into upper and lower

Down
2. lying on stomach
4. axillary area
5. microscopic study of tissues
7. deoxyribonucleic acid
8. far
10. lower back
11. cavity that holds the urinary bladder
13. a basic tissue type
14. injuries or defects
17. curative
18. cavity that holds the lungs
20. stripes
22. wrist
23. inside wall of a body cavity
24. essential body structures
25. mental
27. striae

Spelling Check

Read the following excerpts from a patient's chart and find the twelve medical terms that are spelled incorrectly. Each sentence contains one misspelled term. Circle the misspelled term and write the correct spelling, along with the definition, on the blanks following the record. One blank is provided for each sentence.

(1) The biopsy was performed and a sample of bicep miscle tissue was obtained.
(2) We will send the tissue sample to the hystology lab.

(3) The nurve conduction test revealed severe neurological disease. (4) The distel branch of the nerve was the most damaged.

(5) There is a bilataral vision loss.

(6) The viscara were examined and the abdominal wound was closed.

(7) The patient was found in the prone position and flection of the right knee appeared to be abnormal.

(8) The laceration began in the popleteal area, and spiraled around the leg, through the crural area. (9) It ended at the madial aspect of the ankle.

(10) The bullet entered through the umbilacal area. (11) It penetrated the abdominel cavity. (12) Finally, it exited through the lumbar region of the spinel cavity.

1. _____

2. _____

3. _____

4. _____

5. _____

6. _____

7. _____

8. _____

9. _____

10. _____

11. _____

12. _____

Name That Term

Write the medical term for each description or abbreviation.

1. pertaining to buttocks _____

2. wrist _____

3. below the stomach _____

4. MRI _____

5. PET _____

6. device used to protect against radiation _____

7. device for converting energy from one form to another _____

8. process of recording a vessel (through the use of radiopaque dye and x-rays) _____

9. treatment of disease using radioactive emissions _____

10. back to front direction of x-rays passing through the body _____

11. describing materials (such as lead) that are able to block x-rays _____

12. disease-causing organisms _____

13. freedom from infection _____

14. removal of a body part _____

15. process of introducing a tube into the patient's trachea _____

16. cause of an illness or disease _____

Analyzing Medical Records

Review the excerpts from physician's notes on Erica M, below, then answer the questions that follow.

Progress Notes

Date/Time	Patient Name: Erica M
7/13/XX	Office Visit #1
1500	This twelve-year-old female patient, diagnosed with Type I diabetes mellitus two years ago, is well known in this office. See previous records for prior histories. Today she is accompanied by her mother, who states that the child has not been checking her blood sugar correctly and has been self-administering her insulin incorrectly. Erica herself describes how she checks her blood sugar. She obtains a drop of blood from the superficial capillaries of the dorsal aspect of her lower arm. I observed evidence of pricks on her forearms, bilaterally. She states that she injects her morning and evening doses of insulin into the anterior femoral area of her legs, as she was instructed in the clinic. We discussed the fact that she should also use the abdominal areas, rotating injection sites between the RUQ, RLQ, LUQ, and LLQ, but avoiding the umbilical area.

Progress Notes

Date/Time	Patient Name: Erica M
9/13/XX	Office Visit #2
0900	I talked with the mother about the value of therapeutic exercise for Erica, since she is gaining weight rapidly. Erica describes pain and burning with urination, and we discussed the possibility that she might have a urinary tract infection, based on those symptoms. I will order a urinalysis, along with CBC and differential. If urinary pathogens are found, we will do a culture.

Progress Notes

Date/Time	Patient Name: Erica M
12/22/XX	Office Visit #3
1330	Today Erica had a small abscess on the left lateral
	aspect of her neck. It was incised, using a #22 scalpel,
	and drained under local anesthesia. A dressing of 2 x
	2s was applied.

Questions

1. What term describes the capillaries from which Erica obtains blood samples. Give the term's definition in plain language.

2. Where, on the lower arm, are the capillaries located? Write the medical term for the answer, then supply the definition.

3. Does Erica obtain blood samples from one arm or both arms? Write the term that answers this question and define it.

4. Where does Erica inject her insulin doses? Write the medical term(s), then provide a definition.

5. What other area does the doctor recommend for the insulin injections? Write the medical term the doctor used in the note and explain where the area is.

6. The doctor suggests "rotating injection sites" between what areas? Write the abbreviations used in the doctor's notes, then define the sites in your own words.

7. What area is Erica to avoid when administering her insulin injections? Write the medical term, then define it.

8. What kind of exercise did the doctor discuss in the notes for Office Visit #2? What does this term mean?

9. The doctor ordered a test because Erica described symptoms of pain and burning on urination. What was the test? Define the medical term for the test in your own words.

10. The doctor also ordered a CBC. What does this abbreviation mean?

11. The doctor ordered a differential. Define this term.

12. What is a culture?

13. On the office visit of 12/22/xx Erica had an abscess on her neck. Exactly where on her neck was the abscess, according to the doctor? Describe the location in your own words.

14. What did the doctor do about the abscess? In your own words, tell what "incised" means.

15. What was applied to the site of the abscess? Define the term.

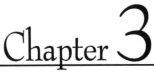

Chapter 3

The Integumentary System

Learning Outcomes

Students will be able to:

- Identify the structures of the integumentary system.
- Describe the functions of the skin.
- Identify and define the word forms most commonly used to describe the integumentary system.
- Name the terms that describe color, and identify the related color.
- Use the integumentary system vocabulary correctly in written and oral contexts.
- Correctly spell and pronounce integumentary system terminology.
- State the meaning of abbreviations related to the integumentary system.
- Name tests and treatments for major integumentary abnormalities.

Translation, Please? Translation, Please? Translation, Please?

Read this excerpt from a dermatology office note and try to answer the questions that follow.

Skin: Comedo formations on the nose. Several pustular lesions on the forehead. Smooth, erythematous rash over the neck and back. A small hyperpigmented nevus on the right breast.

1. Is a *comedo* a blackhead or a pimple?
2. What type of fluid is within a pustular lesion?
3. What color rash is on the neck and back?
4. What do you think a hyperpigmented nevus is?

Answers to "Translation, Please?"
1. A comedo is a blackhead.
2. A pustular lesion contains pus or serosanguinous fluid.
3. The rash is erythematous, which means red. Erythe is the Latin root for red.
4. A nevus is a beauty mark or a birth mark. Hyperpigmented means having excessive pigment. So the statement is referring to a dark, raised beauty or birthmark.

Identifying the Specialty

The System and Its Practitioners

The largest and most visible organ of the body is the skin. The skin and accessory organs (hair and nails) make up the **integumentary** system. The name comes from the Latin *integumentum* meaning, "cover." The average adult is covered by about two square yards of skin that weighs from eight to ten pounds. A person's skin reflects their general health and hygiene, and is usually the first thing the physician observes. The medical specialty concerned with the integumentary system is **dermatology**, and the physician who diagnoses and treats diseases and disorders of the skin, hair, and nails is a **dermatologist**. Dermatological treatments range from topical antibiotic and steroid creams, oral antibiotics and other pharmacological agents, to surgery for varicosities, cancer, and other problems.

Besides treating skin disorders and diseases, dermatologists also perform procedures to improve the skin, particularly on the face, and to remove the discomfort

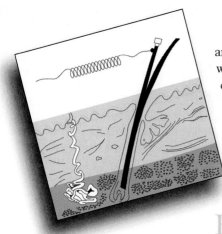

and disfigurement of varicose veins. Some of their procedures are now performed with laser surgery. Dermatology is a burgeoning field of medical practice that will continue to grow as society maintains its concern with outward appearances, and more people live longer.

When the skin is burned, or a restorative procedure needs to be performed, the patient is referred to a plastic surgeon. The plastic surgeon performs delicate and intricate surgery and is usually able to effect change with minimal scarring.

Examining the Patient ♂♀

Anatomy of the Skin, Hair, and Nails

Skin

The skin performs five main functions for the body:
- protection — against invasion by potentially harmful agents that could reach the deeper tissues
- regulation — by raising or lowering body temperature
- sensation —through millions of nerves that provide receptors for pain, touch, heat, cold, and pressure
- secretion — where specific types of glands secrete either perspiration or oil
- water retention — the skin acts as the barrier between the outside world and the internal organs

The external openings of the digestive, respiratory, and urogenital systems all interface with the skin. The skin is rich with nerve endings that relay the four **cutaneous** senses: touch pressure (sustained touch), cold, warmth, and pain.

Skin is made up of three layers: the outer layer or **epidermis**, the inner supportive layer called the **dermis,** and the lower **subcutaneous** layer (also called the hypodermis), which is made up in part of fatty tissue called **adipose** tissue. Figure 3.1 depicts the skin and its structures.

Figure 3.1 - Anatomy of Skin

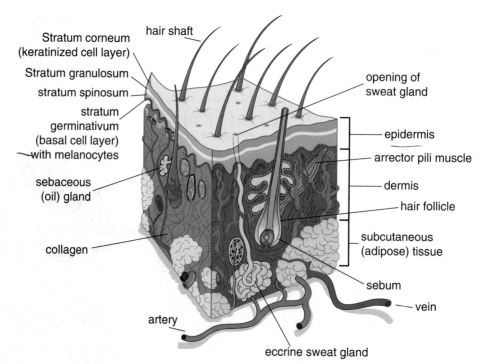

EPIDERMIS The epidermis, or outer layer of the skin, consists of five layers, from the innermost basal cell layer that forms new skin cells, called the **stratum germinativum**, to the outermost **stratum corneum**, sometimes referred to as the horny cell layer. New skin cells contain a protein called **keratin**, which provides tough, waterproof protection. Within the stratum germinativum are **melanocytes**, cells that produce the pigment **melanin**, which is what gives brown tones to the skin and hair. All people have the same number of melanocytes, so genetics, hormones, and the environment are responsible for the wide variation in human skin color,

New cells move from the basal layer to the stratum corneum as they die. Thus the stratum corneum is composed of dead keratinized cells that are continuously being shed and replaced by new cells. A person's skin is replaced about every four weeks, for a total amount of skin shed per year of about one pound. Millions of skin cells must reproduce daily to replace the millions that are shed.

DERMIS The upper region of the dermis is composed of peg-like projections called **dermal papillae**. Dermal papillae help keep the skin layers together and also form the ridges and grooves that make fingerprints.

The connective tissue, or **collagen** (from the Greek word for glue), in the dermis is a tough protein substance that prevents the skin from tearing. This elastic tissue within the skin allows it to stretch when the body moves, and it supports the blood vessels and nerves that pass through the dermis. Collagen is loose and delicate in the infant and hardens as the body ages. The dermis also contains the nerves, sensory receptors, blood vessels, lymphatics, and appendages of the skin: **hair follicles** and **sebaceous** and **sweat glands** (see subsequent paragraphs for more details).

SUBCUTANEOUS LAYER The subcutaneous layer stores fat for energy, provides temperature control, and cushions the body.

SKIN GLANDS The dermal layer also contains glands (Figure 3.1). The **sebaceous glands** secrete an oily substance, called **sebum**, into an area between each hair follicle and its hair shaft to make the hair soft and pliable. The sweat glands are classified into two categories: **eccrine** and **apocrine**. Eccrine sweat glands are all over the body and have ducts, or pores, that open directly onto the surface of the skin. The watery fluid they secrete is controlled by the sympathetic nervous system and is a method that helps eliminate waste products from the body and maintain body temperature. Approximately three thousand eccrine sweat glands occupy one square inch of the palm of the hand.

Apocrine sweat glands, found in the axilla and in the pigmented skin surrounding the genitals, become active during puberty. These glands secrete a milky sweat that causes an odor when it's broken down by bacteria.

Hair

Hair covers almost every part of the human body. It is formed within **follicles**, small tube-like structures within the dermis that develop early in fetal life. The lips, the palms of the hands, and the soles of the feet are the only areas of the body that do not have any hair. Examine Figure 3.2, which depicts the hair follicle and related structures.

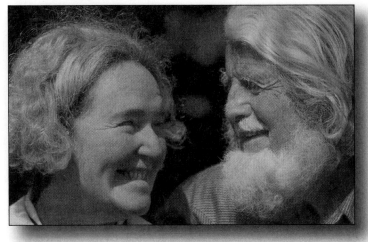

Hair growth begins in a cluster of cells called the **hair papilla**, found at the base of the follicle. The root is located within the follicle, and dermal blood vessels feed the papilla. The visible part of the hair is called the **shaft**. New hair will replace any hair that is removed as long as cells in the papilla are alive. Each hair is either in the growing phase, called **anagen**, or the resting phase, called **telogen**. About 80 percent of the hair on the scalp is in the anagen phase at any given time.

HAIR REMOVAL   Although it may seem to, hair does not grow faster when it is cut or shaved, because the actual area of growth is deeply embedded within the dermis and not at the epidermis. A **depilatory** is an agent (usually a cream) used to remove unwanted hair by dissolving the protein in the hair shafts. As with cutting, this process does not prevent hair from growing back because the follicle is not affected.

MUSCLES WITHIN THE DERMAL LAYER   There is a tiny smooth (involuntary) muscle attached to the base of the dermal papilla called the **arrector pili** muscle (Figure 3.2). Attached above and to the side of the hair follicle, it causes goose bumps by pulling straight up on the hair follicle and down on the skin when a person is frightened or cold.

Figure 3.2 - Hair Follicle and Related Structures

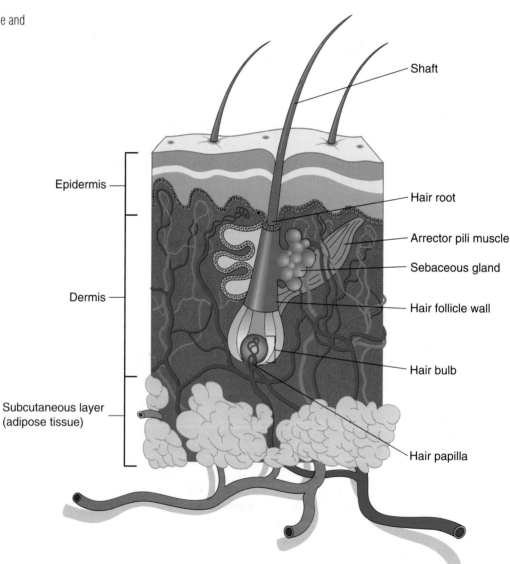

Epidermis

Dermis

Subcutaneous layer
(adipose tissue)

Shaft

Hair root

Arrector pili muscle

Sebaceous gland

Hair follicle wall

Hair bulb

Hair papilla

Nails

The nails, which are located on the dorsal side of the fingers and toes, are composed of hard keratin. Figure 3.3 depicts the nail, which is actually clear-colored but appears pink because the underlying **nail bed** of highly vascular epithelial cells shows through. The visible portion of the nail is called the **nail body**. Fine ridges run longitudinally the length of the nail body. The **lunula** is an opaque, white, crescent-shaped area at the proximal end of the nail. The lunula lies over the **root**, where new keratinized cells are formed. The **cuticle** is the fold of skin that covers the root. **Nail folds** overlap the nail borders.

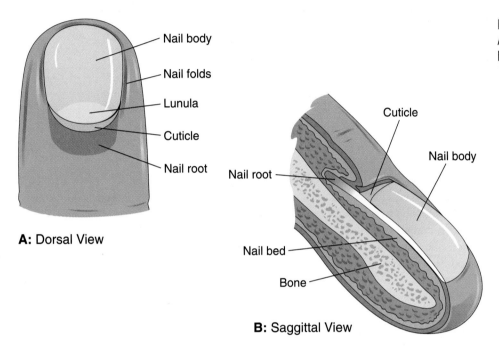

Figure 3.3 - The Fingernail.
A: Dorsal View.
B: Sagittal View.

A: Dorsal View

B: Saggittal View

PHYSIOLOGY OF THE SKIN

The skin has many functions, not the least of which is as an aid to identification. After all, each individual looks different because of facial characteristics, hair, skin color, and fingerprints. Communication is also an important function of the skin; it plays a role in expressing our emotions, such as when a person blushes from embarrassment or pales in fear. The sensory areas for touch, pain, temperature, and pressure lie within the skin. Another function of skin is production of vitamin D, produced using ultraviolet light. The most important function of skin is protection— the skin is the body's first line of defense against the outside world.

Protection

The skin is waterproof and tough, a nearly impervious barrier as long as there are no disruptions to its **integrity**. The **stratum corneum** protects against pathogenic and chemical entry and prevents tears. **Keratin** is the waterproofing agent that prevents excessive fluid loss from the body. **Melanin** prevents harmful ultraviolet rays from penetrating.

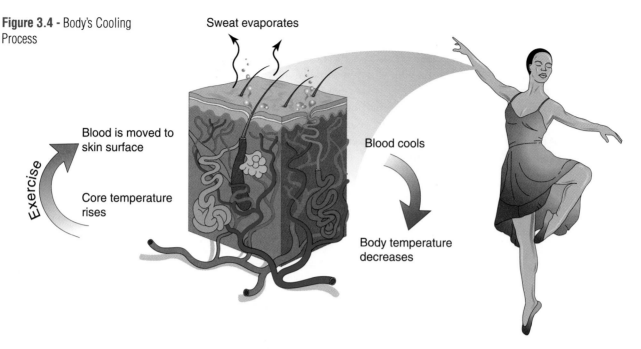

Figure 3.4 - Body's Cooling Process

Sweat evaporates

Blood is moved to skin surface

Exercise

Core temperature rises

Blood cools

Body temperature decreases

Temperature Control

Temperature regulation is a critical function of the skin. Subcutaneous insulation stores heat. The sweat glands of the skin function to release heat and, on a humid day, the skin can release enough calories of body heat to boil more than twenty liters of water. Such heat dissemination is achieved by regulation of sweat secretions and the blood flow close to the skin. As sweat evaporates on the skin, heat is lost. Figure 3.4 illustrates the body's cooling process.

Skeletal muscles produce heat during movement, which in turn increases the body's core temperature. The body can adjust blood flow to move the over-warmed core blood to the skin for cooling, which is why the skin becomes redder when people exercise. Sweat production increases during exercise as the three million sweat glands throughout the skin produce more sweat. The evaporation of sweat further cools the body. It is important to replace the fluids lost during exercise (up to about three liters per hour) to prevent dehydration.

INTEGUMENTARY SYSTEM COMBINING FORMS

As with the other body systems, a core of combining forms serves as the source for most of the medical words associated with the integumentary system. Table 3.1 lists common combining forms and their meanings, and Table 3.2 lists anatomy and physiology terms relating to the skin, hair, and nails.

Table 3.1

Combining Forms Relating to the Skin, Hair, and Nails

Combining form	Meaning	Example
adip/o	fat	adipose
cutane/o	skin	cutaneous
derm/o	skin	epidermis
dermat/o	skin	dermatology
hidr/o	sweat glands	hidrosis

ichthy/o	fish (scales)	ichthyosis
kerat/o	horny tissue (also refers to the cornea of the eye)	keratosis
lip/o	fat	liposuction
onych/o	nail	paronychia
pil/o	hair	pilonidal
seb/o	pertaining to secretion from the sebaceous glands (sebum)	seborrhea
squam/o	pertaining to scales	squamous cells

Table 3.2

Anatomy and Physiology Terms Relating to the Skin, Hair, and Nails

Term	Meaning	Word Analysis	
adipose **ad**-ih-pOs	fatty tissue	*adip/o* *-ose*	fat pertaining to
anagen **an**-ah-jen	the growth phase of hair cells	*ana-* *-gen(ous)*	up, back produced
apocrine **ap**-O-krin	relating to sweat glands; the cells separate and become part of the secretion	*ap/o* *-crine*	separate secrete
arrector pili ah-**rek**-tor pI-lI	muscles that cause the hair to raise when stimulated	*rectus* *pil/o (pil/i)*	to raise up hair
circumscribed **ser**-kum-skrIbd	having a boundary; confined	*circum* *-scribe*	surrounding write
collagen **kol**-ah-jen	a major protein within the body	*koila* *-gen*	glue producing
confluent kon-**floo**-ent	merging together	*con-* *-fluent*	with flowing
cutaneous kyoo-**tay**-nee-us	relating to the skin	*cutane/o*	skin
cuticle **kyoo**-tih-kl	the outer layer of skin that covers the root of the nail	*cutis*	skin
depilatory deh-**pil**-ah-tor-ee	an agent that removes hair	*de-* *pil/o*	away hair
dermatology der-mah-**tol**-ah-jee	the study of skin and its appendages	*dermat/o* *-logy*	pertaining to skin the study of
dermis **der**-mis	the skin	*derm/o*	pertaining to skin
eccrine **ek**-rin	denoting the flow of sweat	*ec-* *-crine*	out of; away from secrete
ephelis eh-**fee**-lis ephelides (pl) eh-**fel**-ih-deez	freckle; small, flat area of brown melanin-producing cells	*ephelis*	freckle
epidermis ep-ih-**der**-mis	the uppermost layer of skin	*epi-* *-dermis*	upon pertaining to skin
follicle **fol**-ih-kl	a spherical portion of cells that form a cavity	*follicle*	a small sac
integrity in-**teg**-rit-ee	soundness or firmness of a structure; as in skin integrity	*integritas*	wholeness, entirety
integument in-**teg**-yoo-ment	body's covering, which includes the skin, hair, and nails	*integument*	covering

keratin **ker**-ah-tin	the protein present in hair and nails	*kerat/o*	horny
lunula **loo**-nyoo-lah	the crescent-shaped white area at the proximal end of the nail	*lunar*	pertaining to the moon
melanin **mel**-ah-nin	the pigment within the skin	*melan/o*	black; dark hue
nevus **nee**-vus nevi (pl) **nee**-vI	a circumscribed, hyperpigmented area of the skin caused by a local overgrowth of melanin-forming cells	*nevus*	mole, birthmark
papilla pa-**pil**-ah	a small, nipplelike projection	*papilla*	nipple
root	the area where new cells are produced		
sebaceous gland sih-**bay**-shus gland	gland that produces oily secretion	*seb/o* *-aceous*	sebum pertaining to
sebum **see**-bum	the secretion of the sebaceous glands	*seb/o*	sebum
shaft (hair)	the portion of hair that protrudes above the skin		
stratum corneum **strat**-um **kor**-nee-um	the outer layer of skin	*stratum* *corne/o*	layer horny
stratum germinativum **strat**-um jer-min-ah-**tih**-vum	the layer of skin that produces new cells	*stratum* *germinativum*	layer bud
subcutaneous sub-kyoo-**tay**-nee-us	beneath the skin	*sub-* *cutane/o*	under; beneath pertaining to skin
telogen **tel**-O-jen	the resting phase of hair growth	*tel/o* *-gen*	distance; end producing

Word Analysis

This exercise lets you practice using roots. Identify the roots or combining forms in the following terms by drawing a box around them, then define the root word.

Example: dermatology   skin

Term	Definition
1. dermatology	_____
2. cutaneous	_____
3. dermatitis	_____
4. epidermis	_____
5. hidrosis	_____
6. keratin	_____
7. lipolysis	_____
8. melanocyte	_____

9. sebaceous _____

10. subcutaneous _____

Comprehension Check

This exercise provides practice in determining word meaning using its context. Circle the better word from the two choices in each sentence.

1. The adipose/exposed tissue underlying the dermis was damaged.

2. There were four confluent/congruent lesions on the left thigh.

3. The tuberculin skin test was given dermatitis/intradermally.

4. The young man's apocrine/eccrine glands became active at puberty.

5. Microbiology/Dermatology is the medical specialty concerned with skin disorders.

6. Intact intent/integument is one of the body's defenses against microorganisms.

7. Hair foliage/follicles are located within the dermis.

8. Turgor/Tremor refers to the natural motility, texture, and elasticity of the skin.

9. Stratum/Sebum is the oily secretion of the sebaceous glands.

10. Nevus/Nervous refers to a hyperpigmented area of skin.

Matching: Anatomical Terms

1. melanin   _____   a. loose connective tissue

2. keratin   _____   b. rigid shiny protein

3. subcutaneous   _____   c. cooling gland

4. dermis   _____   d. proximal end of nail

5. eccrine   _____   e. flow together

6. confluent   _____   f. moles

7. lunula   ____3____   g. inner skin

8. collagen   _____   h. freckles

9. nevi   ____1____   i. pigment

10. ephelides   ____8____   j. elastic protein fibers

Word Building

Build words to match the definitions provided. Use the roots (or combining forms) presented in this chapter plus prefixes and suffixes. Write the term in the space provided, with hyphens between the word parts.

1. pertaining to the skin _____

2. specialist in the skin and its appendages _____

3. the uppermost or outermost layer of skin _____

4. pertaining to innermost layer of skin _____

5. dissolution or breakdown of fat _____

6. pigment-producing cell within the skin _____

7. tissue layer beneath the skin _____

8. secretion of oil (from oil gland) _____

9. study of tissue _____

10. study of skin _____

Spelling Check

Practice editing for correct usage and meaning. Circle the correct plural or singular form for each word.

1. Several hyperpigmented nevus/nevi were noted on the right anterior chest.

2. The hair follicles/follicle on the entire right forearm were destroyed by burn injury.

3. Melanocytes/Melanocyte are dark-colored pigmentation cells.

4. Numerous papilla/papillae were noted along the right breast.

5. Ephelis/Ephelides are areas of brown melanin-producing cells.

6. The dermis contains many nerve/nerves.

7. Sensory receptor/receptors are important in the sense of touch.

8. Dermal blood vessels/vessel feed the hair papilla.

9. Hair growth is in two phase/phases: anagen and telogen.

10. The nail/nails are composed of hard keratin.

Learn the relationships among skin terms, structures, and functions. Label the illustration with the correct terms from the list, then write the letter of the corresponding physiological function beside each anatomical label.

Anatomical Structures

1. epidermis
2. dermis
3. subcutaneous tissue layer
4. hair follicle
5. basal layer of epidermis
6. sebaceous gland
7. sweat gland
8. dermal blood vessels
9. sensory receptors
10. melanocytes

Physiological Functions

a. stores fat for energy, provides temperature control, cushions
b. production of the pigment melanin
c. carry blood to nourish skin cells
d. site for formation of hair
e. reduction of body temperature through production of sweat
f. inner, supportive layer of skin
g. secretes oily substance
h. forms new skin cells
i. tough, outer skin layer
j. detect temperature, pressure, pain

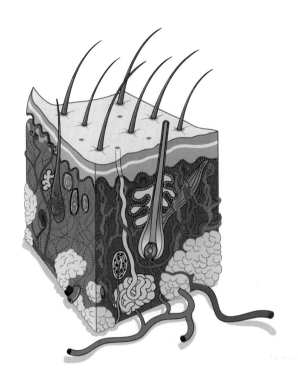

Assessing Patient Health

Wellness and Illness through the Life Span

Throughout one's life, skin appearance reflects the general health of the body. The physician's assessment of the skin involves the entire body and is usually accomplished during a complete physical examination. The examiner first inspects and palpates the patient's skin, mucous membranes, hair, and nails to determine appearance, color, temperature, and turgor. General hygiene is noted. The vascularity is noted, and a thorough inspection for abnormalities or lesions is performed. After the overall inspection, any area of special concern is viewed under high-intensity lighting.

Infants

The newborn is covered with a moist, white, cheese-like substance called the **vernix caseosa**, which protects its thin skin. The skin is covered with a fine, downy hair called **lanugo**. This hair, along with the hair on the head, may be lost in the first few weeks of life.

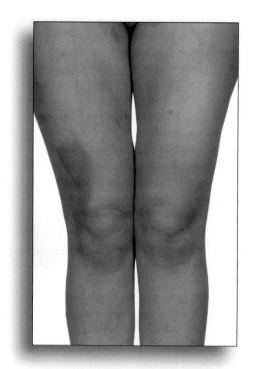

Café au lait spot

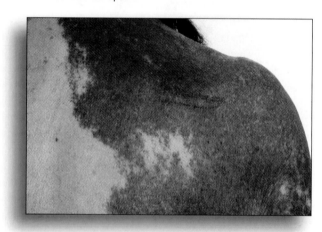

Port-wine stain

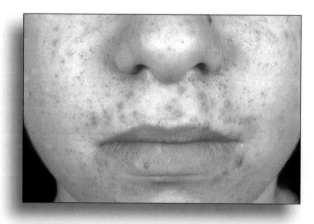

Acne

The skin color of African-American newborns is lighter than their parents' skin because the pigment function is not fully developed. The infant's full melanotic color is noted in the nail beds and, for males, in the scrotal folds. Native-American, Latin, Asian, and African-American infants commonly have a hyperpigmented blue-black to purple area on the sacrum or buttocks called a **Mongolian spot.** It is formed from the deep melanocytes and gradually fades during the first year of life.

Café au lait spots are round or oval areas of light brown pigmentation present at birth. A person with more than about five of these spots may have a condition called **neurofibromatosis.**

Port-wine stain, or **nevus flammeus,** is present at birth in some infants. It appears as a large, flat, red area sometimes covering the scalp or face. The area consists of capillaries and may darken with crying or exercise. This lesion will not fade with time, but may be diminished or removed with laser surgery.

Erythema toxicum is a common rash of infancy that appears within the first four days of life as a red, macular, papular rash of tiny bumps on the cheeks, trunk, back, and buttocks. There is no known cause and no treatment is necessary. **Acrocyanosis** is a bluish color around the lips, hands, fingernails, feet, and toenails. It may last for a few hours after birth but disappears when the newborn is warmed.

A common occurrence in newborns is **physiologic jaundice,** characterized by a yellowing of the skin, sclera, and mucous membranes because of the increased numbers of red blood cells that are broken down after the third or fourth day of life.

Adolescents

Acne (technically called **acne vulgaris**) is the most common skin problem of adolescence, occurring to some degree in nearly all teenagers. Sebaceous glands become more active during the early teenage years and produce excess oil. Acne usually appears on the face, but sometimes manifests on the chest, back, and shoulders. The two most common types blemish are: **open comedones** (blackheads) caused by a sebum plug partially blocking the pore, and **closed comedones** (whiteheads), when the pore becomes completely blocked. Severe acne includes **papules, pustules,** and **nodules,** more severe forms caused by bacteria that break down the sebum and produce inflammation in the surrounding tissue.

Pregnant Women

Pregnancy causes many changes. The skin stretches, and **striae**, or stretch marks, appear on the abdomen, the breasts, and sometimes the thighs. Striae result when the elastic collagen fibers break down. Striae usually fade after the delivery but do not disappear. A brownish-black line, the **linea nigra**, appears down the midline of the abdomen. A brownish hyper-pigmented patch called **chloasma** may appear on the face. These markings disappear after the mother gives birth. Many pregnant women develop **vascular spiders**, tiny red lines with radiating branches, on the face, neck, upper chest, and arms.

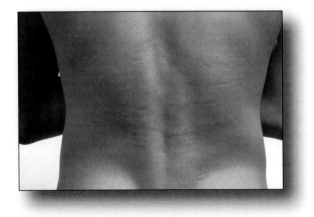

Striae

Middle-Aged Adults

Several skin changes appear as individuals age. **Cherry angiomas**, or **senile angiomas**, are small, punctate, slightly raised bright red dots that appear on the trunk. They are not malignant but may be profuse and cause the individual to feel self-conscious. Skin tags, or **acrochordons**, are overgrowths of normal skin that form on a stalk and have a small projection. They commonly appear on the eyelids, cheeks, neck, axillae, and trunk.

The growth rate of hair and nails slows down during middle age, and the amount of hair in axillary and pubic areas decreases. Menopausal women may develop hairs on the chin from a decrease in female hormones that allows the male hormones to produce these secondary male characteristics. Men may develop more hair in the ears, nose, and eyebrows but lose hair on the head. Male-pattern balding, or **alopecia**, is an inherited trait. In both men and women, the hair gradually turns gray from a decrease in melanocyte function.

Seniors

Age wreaks havoc on the skin. Daily exposure to the environment contributes to the skin's gradual breakdown. Aging skin loses elasticity and begins to sag. The stratum corneum and the dermis thin and flatten, causing wrinkling. The progressive loss of elastin, collagen, and subcutaneous fat coupled with decreased muscle tone increase wrinkling and decrease protection. Sebaceous and sweat glands secrete less (called **xerosis**), leaving the skin dry and diminishing its ability to maintain normal body temperature. This decreased temperature regulation can make the individual hypersensitive to heat; at the same time, loss of subcutaneous fat often makes the older person more sensitive to cold.

These changes cause the skin to become more fragile and break down more easily. Any trauma can produce **senile purpura,** purplish discolorations. **Senile lentigines**, or liver spots, appear as speckling in areas that were exposed to the sun, usually on the arms and hands. Some areas of the skin may appear yellowish and leathery. **Keratoses** are thick lesions with raised areas of pigmentation that usually appear on the trunk but may also be seen on the face. They rarely become cancerous. The risk of skin cancer increases with aging, particularly if there was significant sun exposure in childhood or young adulthood. One type of lesion that can become cancerous is **actinic keratosis**, which appears as a rough, raised, reddish-tan area, often with a silvery white scale attached to the plaque. These lesions can develop into **squamous cell carcinoma** (see the oncology information later in this chapter).

GENERAL SKIN CONDITIONS

Many illnesses are associated with the skin. One infectious disorder is **ringworm**, caused by a fungus. Ringworm can occur from the scalp to the feet, and the infection is named based on the site affected.

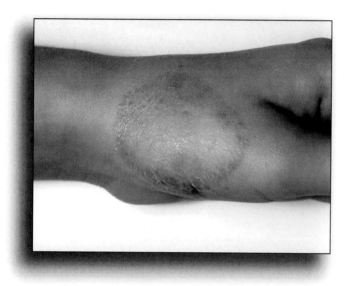

Ringworm

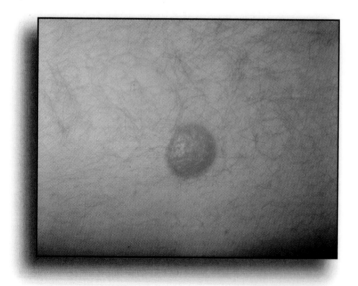

Hemangioma

One of the most common disorders is **dermatitis**, an inflammation of the skin that may be associated with an allergic reaction from contact with an allergen (**contact dermatitis**) or from ingestion of a particular food or drug. The area may be reddened and edematous, with lesions present. The rash may be **urticarial** (very itchy, hivelike) and weeping. Contact dermatitis often can be treated with corticosteroid cream applied topically, which relieves the pain and inflammation and may reduce the itching. An antihistamine may decrease the allergic response and provide relief from itching. A rash that becomes **excoriated** provides an opening for infection.

Atopic dermatitis is a chronic inflammation of the skin, usually caused by an allergy. **Psoriasis** is an example of atopia. **Seborrheic dermatitis**, or cradle cap, is a flattened, greasy patch on the scalp present in many infants, which can be removed by applying an oily substance to the scalp, leaving it on overnight, and then washing vigorously.

Several types of lesions appear as **nevi** (also known as birthmarks or beauty marks). Hairy nevi (singular, nevus) contain hair, and spider nevi have thin blood vessels near the skin's surface. A **hemangioma** is a collection of blood vessels near the epidermis that give a red appearance. These lesions may run very deep into the tissue, preventing removal.

Cancers of the Integumentary System

Skin cancers are the most prevalent of all cancers, and the majority of skin cancers are **basal cell carcinomas**. They usually begin as a skin-colored papule, often with telangiectasia, and can spread if not removed promptly. **Squamous cell carcinomas**, which have a scaly appearance and sharp margins, are less common. Areas that have been exposed to the sun, such as the hands, nose, and ears, are most vulnerable to this form of cancer. Most squamous and basal cell carcinomas are easily cured with surgery and radiation.

Malignant melanomas usually result from preexisting nevi, require more extensive surgery, and are often difficult to cure. These lesions are darkly pigmented, raised, and may have scaling. These cancerous cells can metastasize (spread) and must be treated promptly.

Primary Skin Lesions

Various skin lesions are described by specific terms. Early lesions that have not been changed by manipulation or natural development are called *primary* lesions. When primary lesions change or are manipulated, they become *secondary* lesions. Table 3.3 provides description of primary skin lesions and lists examples of infectious and noninfectious diseases and associated abnormalities.

Table 3.3

Primary Skin Lesions and Associated Abnormalities

Lesion	Description	Infectious type	Noninfectious type
bulla **bul**-lah	a fluid-filled lesion larger than 1 cm that is thin-walled and ruptures easily		blister contact dermatitis
cyst sist	an encapsulated, fluid-filled area in the dermis or subcutaneous layer		sebaceous cyst
macule **mak**-yool macular **mak**-yoo-ler	a round, flat, pigmented area	measles scarlet fever	freckles petechiae
nodule **nod**-yool nodular **nod**-yoo-ler	a solid, raised node-like lesion larger than 1 cm		xanthoma fibroma
papule **pap**-yool papular **pap**-yoo-ler	a palpable lesion (something that can be felt) that is rounded, solid, and raised (less than 1 cm)	molluscum rubella (German measles)	elevated nevus (mole)
plaque plak plaques (pl) plaks	an area of papules that are merged to form a lesion larger than 1 cm		psoriasis lichen planus
pustule **pust**-yool pustular **pust**-yoo-ler	a small, round, raised, pus-filled lesion	impetigo	acne
urticaria er-tih-**kayr**-ee-ah urticarial er-tih-**kayr**-ee-ahl	an intensely itchy (pruritic) area of wheals that have merged		severe allergic reaction
vesicle **ves**-ih-kl vesicular ve-**sik**-yoo-ler	a raised, clear fluid-filled lesion up to 1 cm in size	varicella (chickenpox) herpes zoster (shingles) herpes simplex	contact dermatitis poison ivy
wheal hweel	a raised, erythematous, irregularly shaped area that is transient		allergic reaction mosquito bite

Bulla

Cyst

Macule

Nodule

Papule

Plaque

Pustule

Urticaria

Vesicle

Wheal

Secondary Skin Lesions

Secondary skin lesions are primary lesions that have changed as a result of manipulation (scratching) or natural and/or pathologic progression. Table 3.4 describes these lesions and the diseases or conditions associated with them.

Table 3.4

Secondary Skin Lesions and Associated Abnormalities

	Lesion	Description	Infectious type	Noninfectious type
Crust	crust	a thickened, dried area from broken pustules or vesicles	impetigo varicella (at the end of the infection)	scab
Erosion	erosion ee-**rO**-zhun	a superficial, scooped-out area that does not extend into the dermal layer	herpesvirus	pemphigus
Excoriation	excoriation ek-skO-ree-**ay**-shun	reddened abrasions, usually from itching	scabies	insect bites
Fissure	fissure **fish**-er	a linear crack that extends into the dermis	athlete's foot	cheilosis (cracks in the corners of the mouth)
Keloid	keloid **kee**-loyd	excess scar tissue; most commonly seen in African-Americans		
Lichenification	lichenification lI-**ken**-ih-fI-**kay**-shun	thickened area of skin that forms after intense scratching		
Scale	scale	a flaky, dry, silvery or white form of shedding keratin cells	tinea corporis (ringworm of the body) tinea capitis (ringworm of the head) tinea pedis (ringworm of the foot)	eczema seborrheic dermatitis psoriasis ichthyosis
Scar	scar	connective tissue that remains after a skin lesion has healed	varicella (almost always leaves at least one pitted scar from a healed lesion)	acne
Ulcer	ulcer **ul**-ser	a deep depression that extends into the dermis	chancre (syphilitic lesion)	decubitus ulcers (pressure sores)

Bed sores

GENERAL CONDITIONS OF THE HAIR AND NAILS

Hirsutism is an abnormal growth of hair, particularly in areas where there is usually very little hair. Affected areas include the face (particularly in women), arms, back, and chest. **Alopecia** is the opposite of hirsutism: the absence of hair, or baldness. Alopecia can occur in men and women, and both hirsutism and alopecia may have psychological implications for the affected individual.

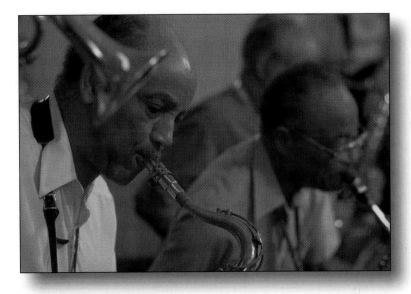

The nails and surrounding tissue are subject to inflammation and infection. A **paronychia** is a painful, red, swollen inflammation of the skin surrounding the nail. These inflammations can be caused by an infectious organism entering through the skin because of an improper removal of the cuticle. Herpetic paronychias also can develop when a person with a herpetic lesion of the lip bites his or her fingernails. Any opening in the skin can allow the herpes virus to enter the system in another location. **Onycholysis** is the loosening of the nail plate, beginning at the tip and progressing toward the root. Table 3.5 lists the major disease terms associated with the integumentary system.

Table 3.5

Wellness and Illness Terms Relating to the Integumentary System

Term	Meaning	Word Analysis	
acne **ak**-nee	an inflamed papular and/or pustular eruption	*akme*	blossoming
acrochordon ak-rO-**kor**-don	a papillomatous skin tag	*acr/o* *chord/o* *-on*	extremity; tip cordlike structure noun ending
acrocyanosis **ak**-rO-sI-ah-**nO**-sis acrocyanotic **ak**-rO-sI-ah-**not**-ik	a condition in which the hands and feet are cyanotic (blue-colored) because of the cold or decreased circulation; common in newborns	*acr/o* *cyan/o* *-osis*	extremity; tip pertaining to the color blue condition
actinic keratosis ak-**tin**-ik ker-ah-**tO**-sis	a pre-malignant lesion	*actin/o* *kerat/o* *-osis*	pertaining to rays or radiation or parts that radiate out horny condition
alopecia al-O-**pee**-shee-ah	baldness; hair loss	*alopecia*	fox mange
alopecia areata al-O-**pee**-shee-ah ahr ee-**ah**-tah	baldness in a circumscribed pattern, most commonly on the head	*areat/o*	pertaining to an area

Term	Definition	Word Parts	Meaning
angioma an-jee-**O**-mah	a tumor caused by increased filling of the blood vessels	angi/o -oma	pertaining to blood or lymph vessels pertaining to a tumor
atopic dermatitis a-**top**-ik der-mah-**tI**-tis atopia a-**tO**-pee-ah	an inflammation of the skin caused by an allergic response	atopy- dermat/o -itis	strange; without a place pertaining to skin inflammation
basal cell carcinoma **bay**-sl sel kahr-sih-**nO**- mah	a malignant tumor of the basal cell layer of skin	basal cella carcin/o -oma	relating to a base chamber cancer pertaining to a tumor
café au lait spot caf-fay-O-**lay** spot	a type of light brown lesion on the skin that resembles coffee with cream	café au lait	coffee with milk
carotenemia kar-ah-teh-**nee**-mee-ah	an orange pigment transported via the blood that results in change in skin color; produced by ingesting carrots or other foods high in carotene	carotene -emia	an orange pigment found in plants and animals pertaining to the blood
chloasma klO-**az**-mah	brownish, irregularly shaped patches, particularly on the faces of pregnant women	chloasma	to become green
comedo **kom**-eh-dO comedones (pl) **kom**-eh-dO-nes	blackheads (open); whiteheads (closed)	comedo	glutton
condyloma acuminatum kon-deh-**lO**-mah ah-kyoo-min-**ay**-tum condylomata (pl) kon-deh-**lO**-meh-tah	a contagious wart that appears on the external genitalia; genital warts	kondyloma accumino	knob pointed
dermatitis der-mah-**tI**-tis	inflammation of the skin	derm/o -itis	pertaining to skin a malignancy
ecchymosis ek-im-**O**-sis	black and blue mark caused by leakage of blood from the vessel	ec- chyme -osis	out of; away from juice condition
eczema **ek**-zeh-mah	a type of atopic dermatitis characterized by a rash that first is vesicular, then changes to an erythematous, papular, swollen rash; finally it becomes a scaling, crusted lichenification	eczema	to boil over
erythema toxicum er-ih-**thee**-mah **toks**-ih-kum	a red rash commonly seen on the newborn at about 3 or 4 days; there is no known cause and it disappears without treatment	erythema toxic/o	flush, redness of skin poison
eschar **es**-kar	a thick crust that forms on the skin after a burn	eschar	fireplace
exanthem eg-**zan**-them exanthema eg-zan-**thee**-mah	a rash, usually of viral origin	exanthem	eruption
folliculitis fol-lik-yoo-**II**-tis	an inflammation of the hair follicles	folliculus -itis	a small sac inflammation

hematoma hee-mah-**tO**-mah	an area of blood that has extravasated from the vessel and is confined in a space	hemat/o -oma	blood relating to a tumor
hidrosis hI-**drO**-sis	excessive sweating	hidr/o -osis	pertaining to the sweat glands condition
hirsutism **her**-soot-iz-em	excessive hair growth	hirsutism	shaggy
impetigo im-peh-**tI**-gO	contagious rash caused by *Staphylococcus aureus* (group A) streptococci that consists of vesicles that rupture and then form a crust	impetigo	an eruption that forms a scab
keratosis ker-eh-**tO**-sis	lesion formed from an overgrowth of the horny layer of skin	kerat/o -osis	horny cells condition
lanugo lan-**oo**-gO	the fine, downy hair covering the fetus from the end of the first trimester	lanugo	down; wool
lentigo len-**tI**-gO lentigines (pl) len-**tI**-jen-ees	a brownish spot on the skin; a freckle	lentigo	lentil
linea nigra **lin**-ee-ah **nI**-grah lineae nigrae (pl) **lin**-ee-ah **nI**-gree	the vertical line that appears on the abdomen of a pregnant woman	linea nigra	line black
melanoma mel-eh-**nO**-mah	a malignancy formed from the cells that produce melanin	melan/o -oma	black; extremely dark a malignancy
melanocyte mah-**lan**-O-sIt	the pigment-producing cells within the skin	melan/o -cyte	black; dark hue denoting a cell
milia (pl) **mil**-ee-ah	tiny white papules present on the face of the newborn; whiteheads	milium	millet
Mongolian spot mon-**gO**-lee-an spot	a variation of pigment often found on the sacrum and buttocks of African-Americans, Asians, Native Americans, and Latinos	Mongolian	relating to a person
nevus flammeus **nee**-vus **flam**-ee-us	a congenital nevus, bright red in color, found on the head	nevus flammeus	mole; birthmark flame
nodule **nod**-yool nodular **nod**-yoo-ler	a solid, raised nodelike lesion larger than 1 cm	nodule	node
onycholysis on-ih-**kol**-ih-sis	a loosening of the fingernail	onych/o -lysis	pertaining to the nail to kill
papule **pap**-yool papular **pap**-yoo-ler	a palpable lesion (something that can be felt) that is rounded, solid, and raised (less than 1 cm)	papule	pimple
paronychia par-O-**nik**-ee-ah paronychial par-O-**nik**-ee-ahl	a red, inflamed area around the nail, usually from an infection of the nail	para- onych/o -ia	around nail condition
petechia peh-**tek**-ee-ah petechiae (pl) peh-**tek**-ee-ee	small, round hemorrhagic spot	petechia	based on Italian *petecchie*

psoriasis sO-**rI**-eh-sis	condition characterized by round, reddish lesions with silvery scales	psoriasis	the itch
purpura **per**-pyoo-rah	areas of hemorrhage into the skin; they first appear red, then turn purplish	purpura	purple
pustule **pus**-tyool	a small, round, raised, pus-filled round lesion	pustule	pustule
seborrhea seb-O-**ree**-ah	overactivity of the sebaceous glands; lesions usually appear on the scalp	seb/o -rrhea	sebum flowing
squamous cell carcinoma **skway**-mus sel kar-sih-**nO**-mah	a scaly, cancerous lesion of the skin	squam/o carcin- -oma	scale tumor; cancer malignancy
stria **strI**-eh striae (pl) **strI**-ee	a stripe on the skin different in color from the area on which it appears	stria	channel
telangiectasia tel-**an**-jee-ek-**tay**-see-ah telangiectasis tel-**an**-jee-ek-**tay**-sis telangiectases (pl) tel-**an**-jee-ek-**tay**-sees	a condition characterized by the dilatation of small vessels, making them appear red	tel/o angi/o -asis	distance pertaining to blood condition
turgor **ter**-ger	the motility, elasticity, and texture of the skin	turgeo	to swell
vernix caseosa **ver**-niks kay-see-**O**-sah	the cheese-like substance covering the skin of the newborn	vernix caseose	varnish product resulting from digestion of casein in cheese
verruca ve-**roo**-kah	a wart; a small virus-induced lesion of the epidermal layer	verruca	wart
vitiligo vit-i-**lI**-gO	white patches (depigmented) on the skin; without melanocytes	vitiligo	blemish
xanthoma zan-**thO**-mah	a yellowish nodule of the skin	xanth/o -oma	yellowish tumor
xerosis **zee-rO**-sis	dry skin	xer/o -osis	dry condition

The Common Wart

There have been many treatments for *verruca vulgaris* (the common wart). Many physicians will use cryotherapy with liquid nitrogen. At home people will use salicylic acid and other over-the-counter remedies. One of the methods under investigation is the use of duct tape. The tape is cut to cover the wart and left on for six days. The tape is removed, the wart is filed down with an emory board, and the area is left uncovered overnight. Tape is re-applied and the same protocol is repeated as necessary for a maximum of two months. Since warts will abate on their own eventually (they are caused by the human papilloma viruses), unless they are unsightly or causing pain, it is probably not necessary to remove them at all.

This exercise provides practice in using roots. Break each word into parts, define the parts, and define the term.

Example:

angioma   *angi-* = blood vessel   tumor composed of blood vessels
               -oma = tumor

Term	Analysis	Definition
1. melanocyte	_____	_____
	_____	
2. ecchymosis	_____	_____
	_____	
3. cyanosis	_____	_____
	_____	
4. chronic	_____	_____
	_____	
5. pustule	_____	_____
	_____	
6. squamous	_____	_____
	_____	
7. xerosis	_____	_____
	_____	
8. onycholysis	_____	_____
	_____	
9. carcinoma	_____	_____
	_____	
10. dermatitis	_____	_____
	_____	

Circle the correct term in each sentence.

1. Physiologic jaundice/Lineae nigrae was observed in three of four infants in the neonatal intensive care nursery.

2. The capillary/erythema toxicum rash on the infant's cheeks will not require treatment.

3. We will recommend laser surgery to remove the nevus flammeus/Mongolian spot.

4. Ephelides/Striae, also called stretch marks, are common during pregnancy.

5. Increased activity in the sebaceous glands/stratum corneum frequently produces acne during the teenage years.

6. Whiteheads, or open comedones/closed comedones, may appear with teenage acne.

7. A brownish, hyperpigmented/hypopigmented patch known as chloasma may appear during pregnancy.

8. Xerosis is a condition of increased/decreased secretion from the sebaceous glands.

9. Loss of sebaceous/subcutaneous fat may make a person sensitive to cold.

10. Alopecia/Lanugo is an inherited trait.

Matching

Exercise 9

Match the terms in Column 1 with the definitions in Column 2. Write the letter of the definition in the space beside the term.

Column 1	Column 2
_____ 1. dermatoses	a. wart
_____ 2. angioma	b. skin inflammation
_____ 3. acrocyanosis	c. brownish, irregularly-shaped patches found on the face during pregnancy
_____ 4. nevus flammeus	d. tumor of blood
_____ 5. verruca	e. thick crust that forms on the skin after a burn
_____ 6. cholasma	f. premalignant skin lesions
_____ 7. actinic keratoses	g. vessel tumor
_____ 8. dermatitis	h. blue color of the extremities
_____ 9. eschar	i. bright red, congenital nevus found on the head
_____ 10. hematoma	j. conditions of the skin

In this exercise, you are to build words from combining forms, prefixes, and suffixes to fit the definitions given. Write the correct term in the space provided. Then, write the meaning of the root or combining form, the prefix, and/or the suffix for each term.

1. inflammation of the skin _____

   _____

2. pertaining to flow of oil _____

   _____

3. condition of blueness of the extremities _____

   _____

4. tumor of vessels _____

   _____

5. skin condition from orange pigment in the blood _____

   _____

6. inflammation of a small sac _____

   _____

7. collection of blood outside a vessel _____

   _____

8. condition of increased sweat _____

   _____

9. condition of horny skin cells _____

   _____

10. condition of dry skin _____

    _____

Spelling Check

On the line beside each term, write the correct spelling.

1. zerosis _____

2. senile purpera _____

3. exzema _____

4. linea nagra _____

5. impetago _____

6. nodlue _____

7. purtule _____

8. vewruca _____

9. xantoma _____

10. villigo _____

Word Maps

Learn the relationship between anatomical and diagnostic terms. Label the pictures with the term that corresponds to the description of the abnormality.

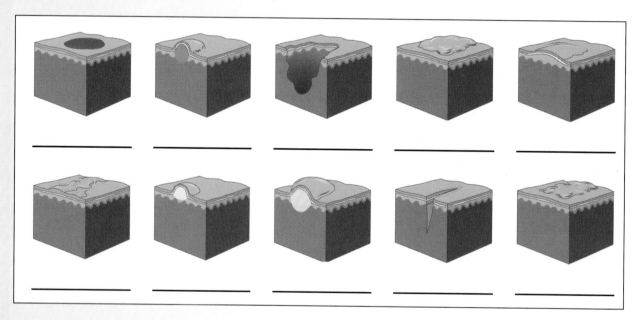

1. round, flat, pigmented area

2. palpable lesion that is rounded, solid, and raised <1 cm

3. deep depression that extends into the dermis

4. area of papules merged to form lesion >1 cm in diameter

5. transient, raised, erythematous area

6. pruritic area of merged wheals

7. raised lesion filled with clear fluid, up to 1 cm in diameter

8. round, raised, pus-filled lesion

9. linear crack that extends into the dermis

10. thickened area of skin that forms after intense scratching

Diagnosing and Treating Skin Problems

Tests, Surgical Procedures, and Pharmaceuticals

Various tests are used to diagnose skin problems. The most common ones are listed below.

- The most important tool for determining the diagnosis of a skin lesion is the **biopsy**. This procedure involves removing a sample of the affected tissue and examining it under the microscope. The physician administers a local anesthetic to numb the area and uses a surgical scalpel to remove the specimen. A hole-punch-type instrument is used to perform a **punch biopsy**. Often, special immunofluorescent tests are performed to assist with the diagnosis. A dye stains the specimen, and a diagnosis is made based on how the lesion absorbs the dye.
- A physician might perform a **Patch test** to identify a patient's particular allergies. Suspected allergens are placed on the surface of the skin and covered for several days to determine the reaction.
- A **scratch test** involves scratching the surface of the skin with an instrument coated with different serums that contain the essence of various allergens.
- **Intradermal** injections of allergens can be placed just below the epidermis using a very tiny needle. Any area that has a local inflammatory response is considered an allergen for that individual.
- A **Wood's lamp** is used to view skin or hair samples under an ultraviolet light to diagnose different species of tinea (ringworm).

Is Indoor Tanning Safe?

What is the truth about indoor tanning? Does tanning in the booth mimic the harmful effects of tanning on the beach? Questions about tanning salons abound. Americans have worshipped the sun and the beauty of a tanned body for decades. It is known today that sunlight contains dangerous ultraviolet rays—ultraviolet A (UVA) and ultraviolet B (UVB)—that can do long-term damage to the skin. Sun-blocking agents can decrease the damage caused by these rays if they are used properly.

Indoor tanning salons use UVA rays rather than UVB, claiming they are safer. However, UVA rays penetrate deeply and can break down the connective structures deep within the skin. It is believed that UVA exposure causes increased wrinkling in a person's later years because of the damage to the deeper layers. UVB rays actually burn the outer layers of the skin and may be even more dangerous.

Although required by the Food and Drug Administration (FDA) to offer protective glasses to customers, tanning salons often do not follow through. Without the special glasses, UVA rays can penetrate and harm the retinas of the eyes. It is important that the tanning salon program the lights to shut off automatically at a time appropriate for the client's skin type to minimize exposure.

Just as sun exposure increases the risk of skin cancer, liver spots, and other disorders later in life, certain medications and diseases can increase the risks for unforeseen complications and cancer many years after indoor tanning exposure.

Surgical Procedures

Some surgical procedures involving the skin attempt to improve or preserve the appearance of the individual. The Mohs technique, for example, surgically removes a cancer layer by layer and tests each layer before removing the next. When a layer's test finally shows no cancer, no more layers are removed. The technique minimizes the amount of skin removed while working to assure the cancer is completely removed. Several techniques are used to perform reconstructive surgery.

Burn victims undergo many **debriding** (from the French word *débride*, meaning unbridle) procedures to remove the burned skin, which is called **eschar**.

One of the most common procedures today is **laser treatment**, which uses a focused beam of light to remove skin lesions, unwanted hair, varicose veins, and other undesirable lesions. The procedure produces little pain or discomfort, and the area remains red for only a short period of time.

Dermabrasion is a procedure that rubs an abrasive device against the skin, similar to sanding a piece of wood to make it smooth. The rubbing can remove the upper layers of the skin and some scars, such as acne scars or tattoos. Another procedure is called a **chemical peel**. An acidic chemical is put on the skin of the face to burn the area. A new epidermis forms, and the burned skin is sloughed away. A chemical peel can remove small lines and scars on the face.

Table 3.6 describes procedures and surgeries related to the skin. Cosmetic surgery uses several methods to improve a person's physical appearance.

Cosmetic Treatments

Our society is vain when it comes to aging, body image, the clothing we wear, and what people think about us. Although wrinkles can reveal much of our life history—laughing, worrying, frowning, too much sun, cigarette smoking—we don't want others to use them when forming an opinion about us. There are many medical treatments for facial wrinkles in a burgeoning industry that's trying to keep up with our aging society. Table 3.7 describes some facial cosmetic treatments that may reduce the appearance of wrinkles.

Table 3.6

Procedures and Surgeries Relating to the Skin

Procedure	Meaning	Word Analysis	
debridement day-breed-**mon**	procedure to remove dead skin	*débride*	unbridle
dermabrasion der-mah-**bray**-shun	procedure using an abrasive device to remove scarring	*derm/o* abrasion	skin scraping off

Table 3.7

Cosmetic Treatments

Type of treatment	Treatment	What is it?	How does it work?
Fillers & injectables	*Botulinum* toxin type A (Botox)	Purified, low-dose form of toxin released by the bacteria that causes botulism	Immobilizes muscles that cause wrinkles
	Bovine collagen (Zyderm, Zyplast)	Protein that forms skin, bones & cartilage (purified from cow's tissue)	Replaces depleted collagen under wrinkles

	Fat transplantation (micro-lipoinjection)	Fat is removed from thigh, abdomen, or buttock, & re-injected into wrinkles	Fills in wrinkles
	Human-based collagen (Cosmoderm, Cosmoplast)	Identical to bovine collagen, but made from human sources	Replaces depleted collagen in wrinkles
	Hyaluronic acid (Restylane, Hylaform)	Natural sugar molecule that adds volume & shape to skin	Binds to water molecules in skin, plumping wrinkles
Topicals (available by prescription)	Tretinoin (Retin-A, Renova)	Vitamin A cream	Lightens skin & replaces old skin with new skin
Skin resurfacing	Chemical peels	Chemicals ranging from mild (glycolic acid) to harsh (phenol)	Dissolves old skin layers in order to reveal new smoother
	Dermabrasion	Sandpaper-like, high-speed rotary wheel	Sands down skin layers making wrinkles less visible
	Laser resurfacing	High-energy light beam lasers	Vaporizes outer skin layers; new skin grows back smoother & tighter
	Microdermabrasion	Device blows crystals onto skin	Gently abrades (polishes) skin surface, stimulating skin cell & collagen production
	Photorejuvenation	Low energy light beam from laser & non-laser sources	Stimulates new collagen formation
Surgery	Face lift (rhytidectomy)	Removal of excess fat; tightening of muscles & re-draping of skin across face	Lifts sagging skin, & areas of the face & neck

(Adapted from "Smooth moves" at http://www.mayoclinic.com)

Pharmaceutical Agents

Dermatological pharmaceutical preparations are mostly topical agents. Abradants contain substances that act as an abrasive to remove dry, calloused skin. Several acne preparations, primarily applied to the skin to dry lesions, are available over-the-counter or by prescription. Severe acne may be treated with a retinoid or antibiotics.

Topical antibacterial and antifungal creams and ointments are used to prevent infections and kill bacteria and fungi. The salves are usually rubbed into the wound and can be covered to provide a protective barrier in the case of small burns or cuts and scrapes. Atopic dermatitis is treated with anti-inflammatory agents, which decrease inflammation, control itch, and help to soothe the tissue.

Dandruff, seborrhea, and psoriasis can be treated with coal tar, zinc, and emollient (moistening) preparations. There are no topical agents for herpes lesions, but substances such as keratolytic and antimitotic agents used to treat external genital warts can interfere with the replication of the herpes virus.

BURNS

Burns are treated with agents that offer pain relief and encourage healing. These agents often provide antibacterial protection as well. Some agents, including iodine-based products or other antimicrobial solutions, are used for cleaning and sterilizing the skin. Antiseptic solutions are also used in the operating room to sterilize the skin before a surgical procedure.

Serious burns are described according to the amount of skin involved and the depth of skin damaged. The "rule of nines" is used to determine the extent of a burn injury. The body surface area is divided into eleven areas of 9 percent each, with the genitals representing the final 1 percent. Figure 3.5 depicts this rule, and Table 3.7 describes each burn and its symptomatology.

Figure 3.5 - Rule of Nines

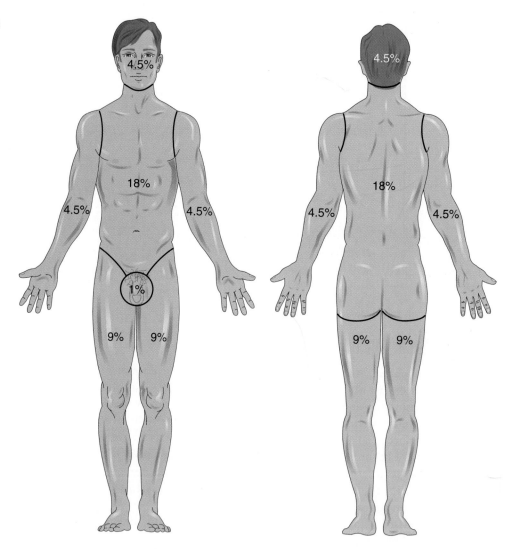

Table 3.8

Burn Types and Symptoms

Burn	Definition	Symptoms
first degree burn	surface layers of epidermis may peel, but there is minimal tissue destruction; can be a sunburn	Pain and redness of skin; soothing sprays or creams may decrease pain
second degree burn	extend to the deep epidermal layers; cause injury to upper layers of dermis; damage sweat glands, hair follicles, and sebaceous glands; do not cause complete destruction of the dermis	form blisters, severe pain, edema, fluid loss, and scarring; debridement necessary
third degree burn	complete destruction of the epidermis and dermis; tissue death extends into the subcutaneous tissue and may involve muscle and bone	may not cause immediate pain because of the damage to nerve fibers; serious fluid loss; excision of dead tissue and surgery with skin grafts is usually required

Table 3.9

Abbreviations

bx	biopsy
derm.	dermatology
FS	frozen section
I&D	incision and drainage
KOH	potassium hydroxide
subq; SQ	subcutaneous
ung.	ointment
UV	ultraviolet

Word Analysis   Exercise 13

Read each sentence carefully. Break each underlined word into its individual parts, using hyphens to divide the parts. Write a definition for the medical term.

1. The infant has insufficient <u>adipose</u> tissue. _____

    _____

2. A 15-year-old male presents with <u>dermatitis</u> on his face and hands. _____

    _____

3. The patient was shivering and <u>cyanotic</u> after exposure to the 18 degree temperature. _____

    _____

4. This 30 y/o male displays a <u>squamous</u> cell carcinoma. _____

    _____

5. A 5-year-old female child has a large <u>nevus</u>
    covering the right side of her face, neck, and shoulder. _____

    _____

6. The patient has contact dermatitis in the <u>antecubital</u> spaces bilaterally. _____

_____

7. The 93-year-old patient exhibited <u>actinic</u> <u>keratosis</u> on her legs and forearms. _____

_____

8. The young woman was diagnosed with a <u>melanoma</u> on the face. _____

_____

9. A patient has <u>vesicles</u>, redness, and crusting around the nose and mouth.
   He attends a day-care center that has experienced an outbreak of impetigo. _____

_____

10. The base of the nail appears red and swollen; the
    finger is warm to the touch. Impression is <u>paronychia</u>. _____

_____

Comprehension Check

Read each sentence. Answer the question after each statement, then write the meaning of the underlined words. You may need to use a medical dictionary for this exercise, but keep your answers brief.

1. The <u>debridement</u> procedure, although painful, was necessary for healing. Is debridement removal of hair or removal of dead tissue?

_____

2. The burn wounds were covered with a thick <u>eschar</u>. Is eschar a crust or an ointment?

_____

3. A chemical peel causes <u>sloughing</u> of damaged skin and formation of new epidermis. Does sloughing refer to dissolving or separating?

_____

4. The children received <u>first degree burns</u> when they played in the sun too long. Is sun exposure for the sake of tanning healthful?

_____

5. The <u>rule of nines</u> is a method of assessing burn injury. Does the rule of nines refer to depth of a burn or the area of the burn?

_____

6. <u>Third degree burns</u> require surgery and skin grafts. Are third degree burns the least burn or the worst burn?

_____

7. Antimicrobials are used on the skin before surgery. Are antimicrobials used to clean the skin or soften the skin?

_____

8. Abradants can often remove rough, thickened skin and some calluses. Are abradants chemicals or special lights?

_____

9. Dermatologists often prescribe topical agents for their patients. Are topicals applied on the skin or swallowed?

_____

10. The physician wrote a prescription for an antimitotic agent. Is an antimitotic agent for softening the skin or treatment of an infection?

_____

Matching

Exercise 15

Practice using the diagnostic terms below. Match the list of procedures and treatments in Column 1 with the diagnosis or reason for the treatment in Column 2. Write the letter of the diagnosis or problem in the space between columns.

Column 1		Column 2
1. biopsy	_____	a. remove eschar
2. débridement	_____	b. treatment of fungal infection
3. dermabrasion	_____	c. treatment of acne
4. laser treatment	_____	d. relieve itching
5. chemical peel	_____	e. treatment of bacterial infection
6. antibiotic ointment	_____	f. diagnose skin lesion
7. antifungal cream	_____	g. rub; remove some lines and scars
8. anti-inflammatory	_____	h. remove unwanted lesions and hair
9. retinoid and antibiotic	_____	i. acid burn; remove fine lines and scars
10. antipruritic	_____	j. relieve inflammation

Word Building

Exercise 16

Practice building words by combining roots, prefixes, and suffixes. Find word parts in your text and construct medical terms for the definitions that follow. Write the term on the blank beside the definition.

1. study of the skin _____

2. condition of numbness (without sensation) _____

3. flow of oil _____

4. within the skin _____

5. using an abrasive device to remove scars on the skin _____

6. pertaining to microbes _____

7. like or resembling retinol _____

8. against fungus _____

9. against bacteria _____

10. against sepsis _____

Spelling Check

Write the correct plural form for each term on the blank provided.

1. angioma _____

2. keratosis _____

3. carcinoma _____

4. comedo _____

5. condyloma _____

6. chemical peel _____

7. follicle _____

8. milium _____

9. linea _____

10. lentigo _____

Word Maps

Group the following conditions by the general age span during which they occur: newborns, pregnant women, and seniors. Then define each term and draw a box around its root(s).

alopecia   milia   vascular spiders   erythema toxicum

melanoma   chloasma   senile purpura   linea nigra

acrocyanosis

Newborns   **Pregnant Women**   **Seniors**

Performance Assessment 3

Crossword Puzzle

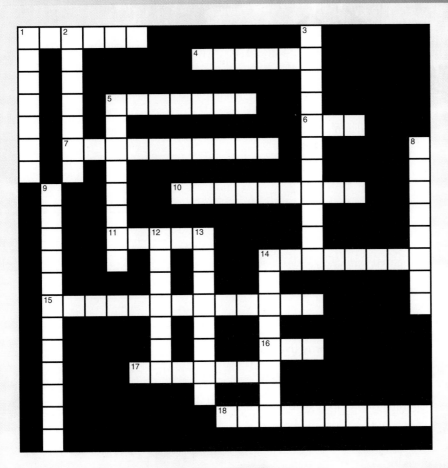

Across
1. small round elevation on the skin
4. a solid, raised area larger than 1 cm
5. dry skin
6. incision and drainage
7. the vertical line that appears on the abdomen of a pregnant woman
10. above the skin; outermost layer of skin
11. tiny white papules present on the face of the newborn; whiteheads
14. white patches (depigmented) on the skin; without melanocytes
15. surgical repair of the skin
16. abbreviation for ointment
17. on the surface of the body (skin)
18. a red, inflamed area around the nail, usually from an infection

Down
1. areas of hemorrhage into the skin
2. small round lesion containing pus
3. procedure to remove dead skin
5. a yellowish nodule of the skin
8. a malignancy formed from the cells that produce melanin
9. face lift
12. a brownish spot on the skin; a freckle
13. baldness; hair loss
14. pertaining to vessels

Build the Terms

Select word parts from the lists to build a complete medical term for each definition given. Note that some terms may not have all three word parts (combining form, prefix, and suffix).

Combining forms	Prefixes	Suffixes
dermat/o	hyper-	-itis
melan/o	epi-	-logy
cyan/o	sub-	-logist
physi/o	hypo-	-icle
adip/o	intra-	-ous
lip/o	dis-	-sis
seb/o	an-	-al
squam/o	pre-	-rrhea
cutane/o	de-	-ic
kerat/o	anti-	-in
onych/o	per-	-cyte
hidr/o	bi-	-lysis
ichthy/o		

1. study of the skin _____

2. breakdown of fat _____

3. pigmented skin cell _____

4. pertaining to scales _____

5. overaction of oil glands _____

6. skin condition of horny overgrowth _____

7. condition of excessive sweating _____

8. accumulation of excessive fat _____

9. bluish discoloration of skin _____

10. breaking down of the nail _____

Analyze the Terms

Read each sentence carefully. Then break each underlined word into its individual parts and write a definition for the whole term. Use hyphens to divide the words.

1. The <u>intradermal</u> injection is administered on the inner forearm.

2. Dr. Martin is the town's only <u>dermatologist</u>.

3. <u>Anti-inflammatory</u> agents are often used for atopic dermatitis.

4. A sample of tissue may be viewed under the <u>microscope</u>.

5. There is a small <u>hyperpigmented</u> area on the lower back.

6. The outer layer of the skin is the <u>epidermis</u>.

7. The patient has severe <u>facial</u> acne.

8. There were five to six <u>confluent</u> lesions on the upper abdomen.

9. The child's mother pointed out a collection of <u>pustules</u> around the external nares.

10. The parents were concerned about the disfiguring <u>hemangioma</u> that covered half of the face.

What Do These Abbreviations Mean?

Give the definition for each of the following abbreviations.

1. b.i.d. _____

2. hx _____

3. CXR _____

4. H&P _____

5. p.c. _____

6. dx _____

7. I&D _____

8. SQ _____

9. bx _____

10. ung. _____

What's Your Conclusion?

In this exercise, assume you work as a medical assistant. To prepare for equipment or materials that will be needed, you need to anticipate the physician's next step. Read each mini medical record and the two choices carefully, then select the best choice and write the letter of your answer in the space provided.

1. Mrs. Roberts has just given birth to a 4 lb. 8 oz. baby girl. When she is given the infant to hold for the first time, she begins to cry and calls for the nurse. "My baby has blue hands and feet. What's wrong?" You hear the nurse explain:

   A. Your baby has a serious condition called autosomal infant toxicum. She is scheduled for some tests.
   B. Your baby is slightly small and has a temporary condition called acrocyanosis. We will keep her warm and observe her carefully.

   Your choice:_____

2. Tommy has come to the clinic from the day-care center. He has fluid-filled vesicles, crusting, and excoriation in a 1 cm area around his left nostril and the left corner of his mouth. His mother reports that several children at the day-care center have pediculosis capitus. You understand that:

   A. These symptoms represent the illness mentioned.
   B. These symptoms may be common in day-care centers and require treatment.

   Your choice:_____

3. Mrs. Ellison is a 91 y/o female, brought to the hospital emergency room by her daughter, who became alarmed when she visited her mother in the nursing home. The daughter observed numerous large, purplish areas on Mrs. Ellison's forearms and is convinced that her mother has been physically abused. Mrs. Ellison is

alert and articulate. She states that "everyone at the home is good to me" and denies abuse by anyone. She reports that two days ago she lost her balance as she rose from her chair and an attendant caught her by her arms to keep her from falling. The physician will:

A. Reassure the daughter that it is unlikely Mrs. Ellison was abused. Explain to her that elderly people often have a condition called senile purpura that causes purplish discoloration of the skin—sometimes with just a touch. Tell her that an attendant catching Mrs. Ellison's arms to prevent a fall could easily have produced the discoloration.

B. File a report with the proper authorities, stating that Mrs. Ellison is the victim of abuse. Prescribe medication for Mrs. Ellison's confused mental state.

Your choice:_____

Records Analysis

Read the progress note on the next page; then answer the following:

1. Give the patient's age and gender.

2. What is the patient's CC?

3. Describe the patient's rash. Where is it located?

4. In addition to the rash, name one other objective finding.

5. In your own words, what is the diagnosis and what is the treatment?

6. Locate the four spelling errors in the document. Write the correct spelling of the term.

Hayes-Oakwood Clinic, Inc.
Department of Dermatology

407 S. Parkway, Accord City, KS 77709-4321
phone (333) 555-1122 fax (333) 555-1234

Physician's Progress Note

PATIENT: Kane, R. H.
DATE: February 11, xxxx

S: Patient is a 30 y/o professional accountant. He is unmarried and lives alone. He comes to the clinic today with an extensive rash over his forehead and ears. He reports that the lessions have been present in some degree for the past four to five months, but have become worse in the past few weeks. He has tried over-the-counter remedies, including various soaps, without relief. Mr. Kane is experiencing a great deal of stress from the breakup of a six-year relationship with a woman he had expected to marry and believes the stress contributes to his condition.

O: Eyrthema with greasy, yellow scales, across the entire forehead from hairline to eyebrows. External ears are similarly involved. There are patchy erythemateus lesions with scaling along the hairline at the back of the neck. Erythematous pupules are scattered across the face, and skin appears quite oily around the nostrils.

A: Seborrheic dermatitis.

P: Rx: hydrocortisone cream, 4%, 1 oz. tube.
Sig: apply to affected areas t.i.d.
Patient was counseled on avoiding stress and stress-relieving measures, since that aggravates his condition. He was instructed to avoid soap on the area and to use only an oatmeal cleansing bar on his face. He is to also avoid over-the-counter preparations. He is to RTC in four weeks if the condition is not greatly improved.

Using Medical References

In this exercise you will spell and define words not provided in the chapter. Use a medical dictionary to look up the correct spelling and definition of the words provided. Write the correct spelling beside the word, and write the definition on the line below each word.

1. dernoplasty _____

_____

2. trichorhexis _____

_____

3. scabbies _____

_____

4. cicattrix   _____

_____

5. desssication   _____

_____

6. pediculoisis   _____

_____

7. lipomta   _____

_____

8. excoriaiation   _____

_____

9. diaphoresisse   _____

_____

10. exfoliaiated   _____

_____

11. autograftt   _____

_____

12. homomograft   _____

_____

Short Answer

In your own words and using plain language, describe the components of the dermis and their function(s).

_____

_____

_____

_____

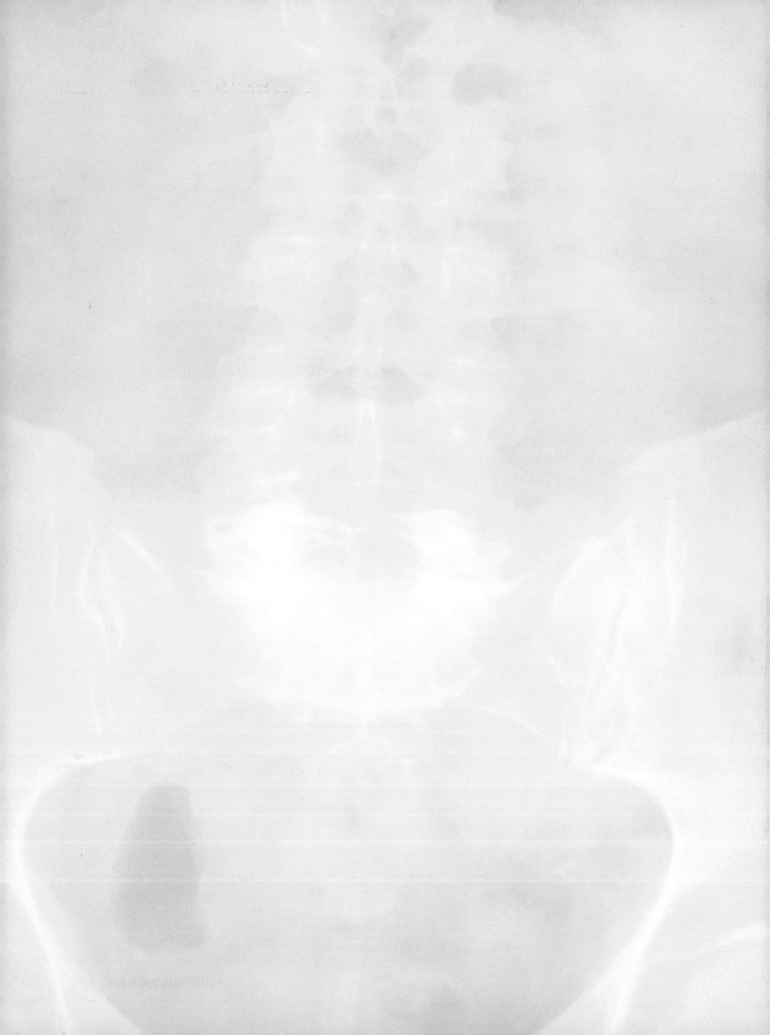

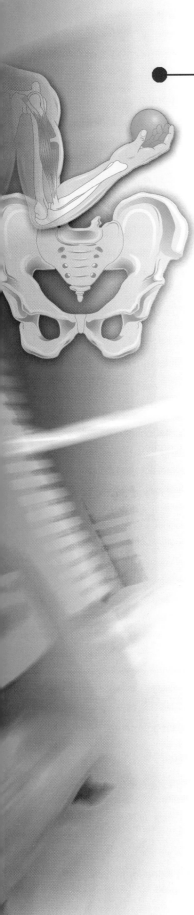

Chapter 4

The Musculoskeletal System

Learning Outcomes

Students will be able to:
- Identify the structures of the musculoskeletal system.
- Describe the functions of muscles and joints.
- Correctly use combining forms, prefixes, and suffixes in the analysis of musculoskeletal vocabulary.
- Correctly spell and pronounce terminology related to the musculoskeletal system.
- State the meaning of abbreviations related the musculoskeletal system.
- List and define the combining forms most commonly used to create terms related to the musculoskeletal system.
- Name tests and treatments for musculoskeletal system abnormalities or pathologies.
- Interpret medical records that document musculoskeletal conditions and treatments.

Translation, Please? Translation, Please? Translation, Please?

Read this excerpt from an orthopedist's records and answer the questions that follow.

She is status post THR and is able to ambulate well after physical therapy. In terms of her juvenile rheumatoid arthritis, she had arthroscopic surgery on the right knee, which is well healed, and she continues her Naprosyn 500 mg p.o. b.i.d. Previous surgery on third left metatarsal has healed completely.

1. Is THR a medication or a procedure?
2. Is arthroscopic surgery performed with a large or small incision?
3. How would metatarsals be related to tarsals?

Answers to "Translation, Please?"
1. THR is an abbreviation for *total hip replacement.*
2. Arthroscopic refers to a small incision. Remember the combining form *arthr/o* means joint and *scopic* means see. Arthroscopy is the process of looking into a joint with a tiny fiber optic tube.
3. *"Meta"* indicates beyond, so metatarsals are beyond—distal to—the tarsals. Similarly, a carpal is proximal to a metacarpal.

Identifying the Specialty

The System and Its Practitioners

The musculoskeletal system gives the body strength, structure, and the capability of movement. Think of the skeleton as similar to the framework of a house. The function of this framework is to support the internal components and to protect the contents from outside forces. The body's joints are the places where two pieces of the structure (bones) meet, and the ligaments connect them. Bone also is the site of blood cell formation and the storage place for minerals, such as calcium.

The field of medicine concerned with the musculoskeletal system is **orthopedics**, and the physician is an **orthopedist**. Another caregiver in this specialty is the **chiropractor**, who practices **chiropractic**, an area of medicine devoted to restoring health by optimizing the relationship between the musculoskeletal system and body

Figure 4.1 - Musculoskeletal System: Anterior View (A) and Posterior View (B)

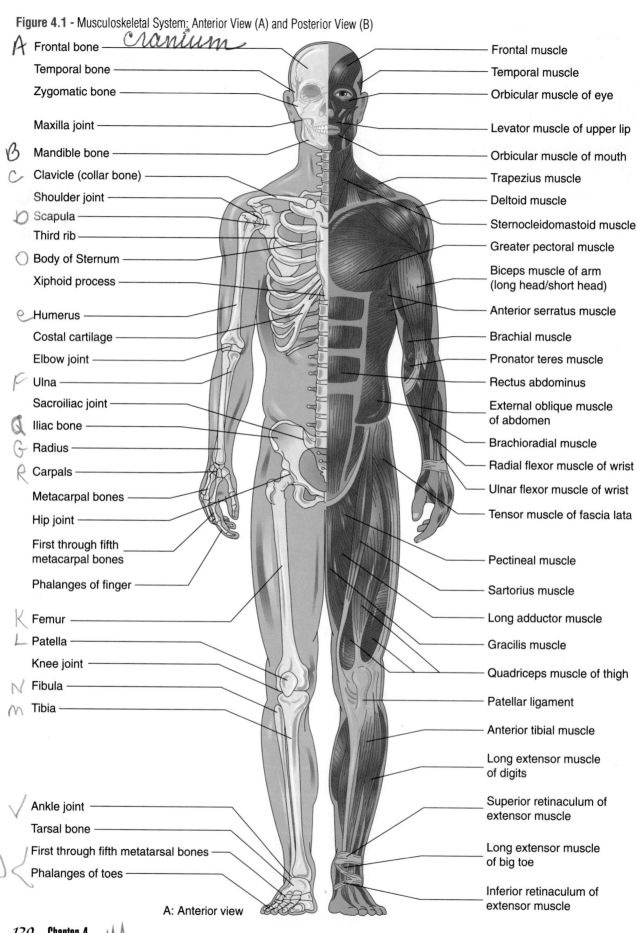

A Frontal bone *Cranium*
Temporal bone
Zygomatic bone
Maxilla joint
B Mandible bone
C Clavicle (collar bone)
Shoulder joint
D Scapula
Third rib
O Body of Sternum
Xiphoid process
e Humerus
Costal cartilage
Elbow joint
F Ulna
Sacroiliac joint
Q Iliac bone
G Radius
R Carpals
Metacarpal bones
Hip joint
First through fifth
metacarpal bones
Phalanges of finger
K Femur
L Patella
Knee joint
N Fibula
M Tibia
V Ankle joint
Tarsal bone
First through fifth metatarsal bones
W Phalanges of toes

Frontal muscle
Temporal muscle
Orbicular muscle of eye
Levator muscle of upper lip
Orbicular muscle of mouth
Trapezius muscle
Deltoid muscle
Sternocleidomastoid muscle
Greater pectoral muscle
Biceps muscle of arm
(long head/short head)
Anterior serratus muscle
Brachial muscle
Pronator teres muscle
Rectus abdominus
External oblique muscle
of abdomen
Brachioradial muscle
Radial flexor muscle of wrist
Ulnar flexor muscle of wrist
Tensor muscle of fascia lata
Pectineal muscle
Sartorius muscle
Long adductor muscle
Gracilis muscle
Quadriceps muscle of thigh
Patellar ligament
Anterior tibial muscle
Long extensor muscle
of digits
Superior retinaculum of
extensor muscle
Long extensor muscle
of big toe
Inferior retinaculum of
extensor muscle

A: Anterior view

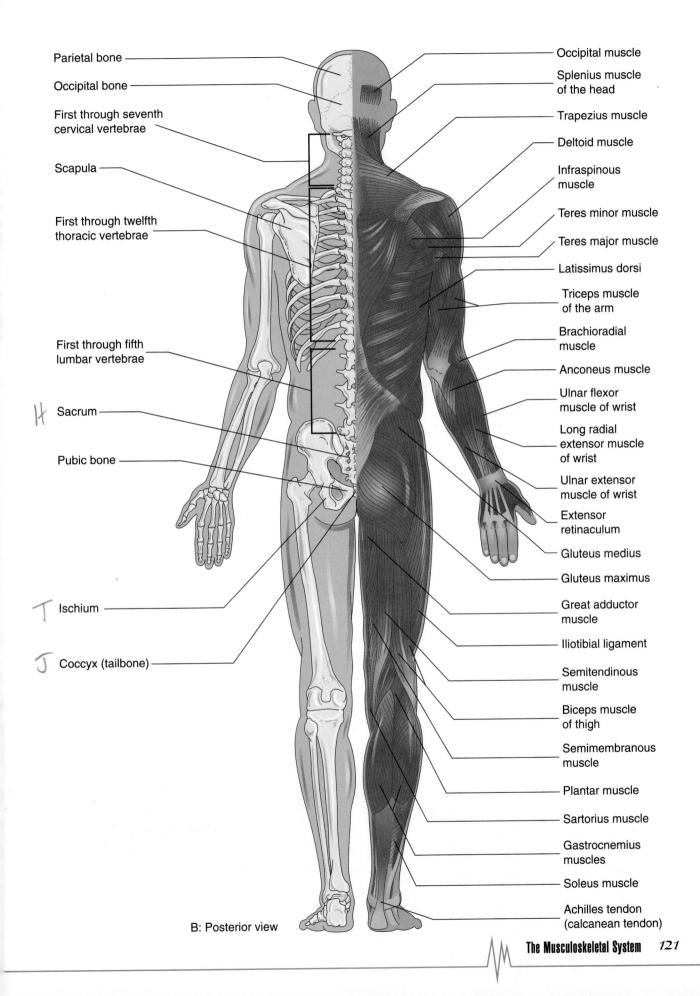

Parietal bone

Occipital bone

First through seventh
cervical vertebrae

Scapula

First through twelfth
thoracic vertebrae

First through fifth
lumbar vertebrae

Sacrum

Pubic bone

Ischium

Coccyx (tailbone)

Occipital muscle

Splenius muscle
of the head

Trapezius muscle

Deltoid muscle

Infraspinous
muscle

Teres minor muscle

Teres major muscle

Latissimus dorsi

Triceps muscle
of the arm

Brachioradial
muscle

Anconeus muscle

Ulnar flexor
muscle of wrist

Long radial
extensor muscle
of wrist

Ulnar extensor
muscle of wrist

Extensor
retinaculum

Gluteus medius

Gluteus maximus

Great adductor
muscle

Iliotibial ligament

Semitendinous
muscle

Biceps muscle
of thigh

Semimembranous
muscle

Plantar muscle

Sartorius muscle

Gastrocnemius
muscles

Soleus muscle

Achilles tendon
(calcanean tendon)

B: Posterior view

functions. An osteopathic physician is a Doctor of Osteopathy (DO). The DO is trained and educated much as an MD, but with the focus on treating health problems through the theory that the body is better able to heal itself when the bones are in proper alignment and the body is in a good nutritional state. **Rheumatologists** are physicians who treat patients suffering from diseases of the joints, connective tissues, and collagen, among other structures. A podiatrist (Doctor of Podiatry, DP) specializes in diagnosing and treating disorders of the foot.

This discussion of the musculoskeletal system is separated into sections, first describing the structure and function of the skeleton, then that of the muscles, and lastly their combined function.

Examining the Patient ♂♀

Anatomy and Physiology of the Skeletal System

The skeleton (Figure 4.1A-B) consists of 206 bones divided into four types based on their shape: (1) the long bones, such as the **humerus** in the arm or **femur** in the leg; (2) the short bones, such as the **carpals** in the hand; (3) the flat bones, such as the **sternum** in the chest; and (4) the irregular bones, such as the **vertebrae** in the spine. Because of their size and location, the long bones play a major role in supporting the body and facilitating movement. Studying the structure of the long bones (as shown in Figure 4.2) provides insight into the makeup of all bones.

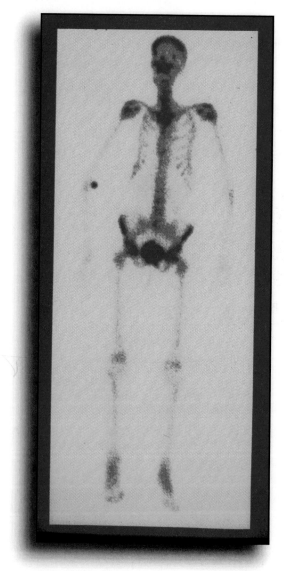

Total body bone scan

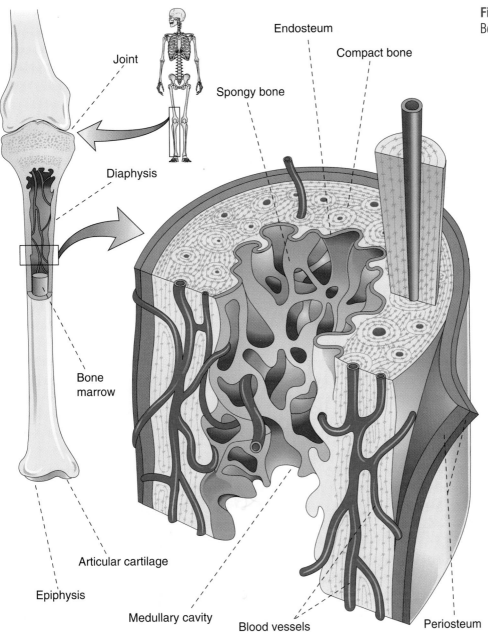

Joint

Endosteum

Compact bone

Spongy bone

Figure 4.2 - Structure of Long Bones

Diaphysis

Bone marrow

Articular cartilage

Epiphysis

Medullary cavity

Blood vessels

Periosteum

Structure of Long Bones

With the exception of any joint area, the outer surface of a long bone is covered by a dense, fibrous membrane called the **periosteum**, which contains nerves, blood, and lymph vessels. The **diaphysis** is the shaft of the bone, tube-shaped and made of hard, compact bone. It is strong but light, which allows for easy movement. Within the bone is the **medullary cavity**, which is lined with a fibrous membrane called the **endosteum**, and which contains **bone marrow**—a gritty, fatty substance that produces blood cells. (The function of bone marrow will be described further in Chapter 5.)

The **epiphysis**, found at either end of the bone, is the area where the bone **articulates**, or meets, with another bone or bones. The **epiphyses** are composed of spongy bone that is more porous than compact bone. Covering each epiphysis is a thin layer of cartilage called the **articular cartilage**, which functions as a cushion at the **joint** where two bones meet.

Bone Cells

A closer look at bone (Figure 4.3) reveals that it is not a lifeless structure. **Osteocytes** are the living cells of bone. They continually produce new bone, formed by **osteoblasts**, and **resorb** bone with cells called **osteoclasts**. These cells produce and resorb bone in response to exercise, activity, and hormonal stimulation to lay down the calcium salts needed to strengthen bone. Within spongy bone are the **trabeculae**, which provide the network of spaces that surround the open area filled with marrow. Blood vessels feed the bone and move blood cells in and out of the bone marrow.

Cartilage

Cartilage consists of collagen fibers embedded in a gelatinous substance that provides flexibility. Cartilage cells are called **chondrocytes**. Since cartilage does not contain blood vessels, nutrients pass through the **matrix** to the cells by a process called **diffusion**. This lack of blood supply causes cartilage to repair itself very slowly after injury.

Figure 4.3 - Microscopic View of Bone

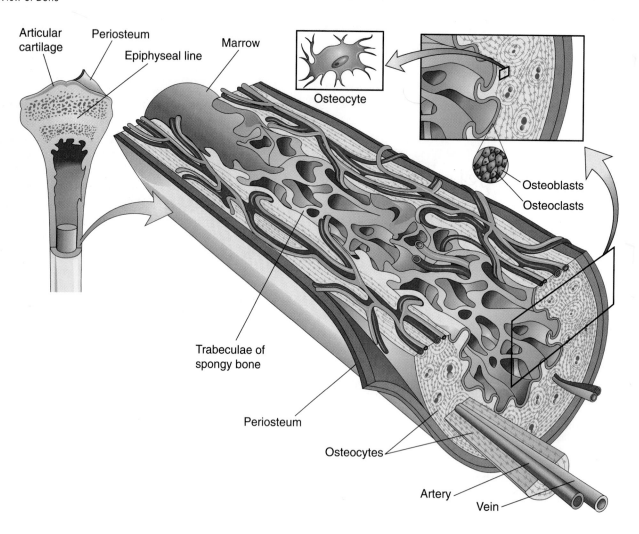

BONE GROWTH

Bone formation begins in the fetus, when the skeleton is composed of cartilage (1). The cartilage is bone-shaped and gradually becomes bone by a process called **endochondral ossification**. During ossification, the osteoblasts lay down calcium salts in the cartilage to form hardened bone (2-5). Osteoclasts resorb some of the hardened bone, which gives the bone its adult structure. As bone becomes **ossified**, the **epiphyseal plate** (6) gradually decreases and eventually leaves an **epiphyseal line**, indicating that bone growth is complete and the person has attained adult height (7).

A similar process, intramembranous ossification, takes place within connective tissue and also results in the formation of bone.

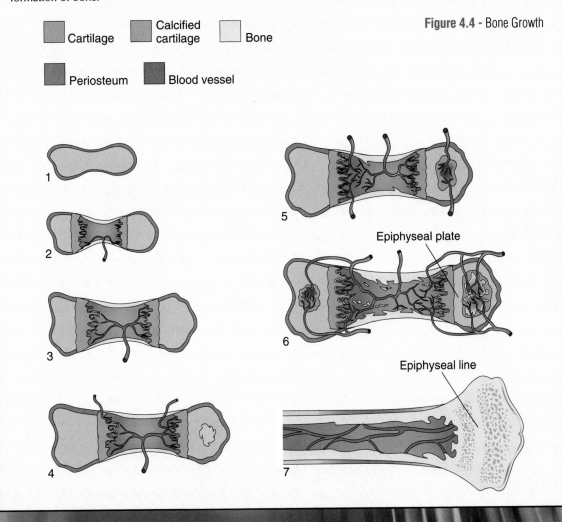

Cartilage
Calcified cartilage
Bone
Periosteum
Blood vessel

Figure 4.4 - Bone Growth

Epiphyseal plate

Epiphyseal line

1
2
3
4
5
6
7

Joints

Every bone in the human body, except the hyoid bone in the neck (to which the tongue is attached), meets with another bone and forms a **joint**. There are three types of joints, classified according to the movement they can achieve. **Synarthroses**, which join the skull bones, allow no movement. **Amphiarthroses** connect the vertebrae and provide slight movement. **Diarthroses** (synovial joints) allow free movement and connect most bones in the body.

Figure 4.5 - Diarthrotic Joint

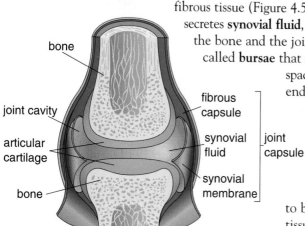

bone

joint cavity

articular cartilage

bone

fibrous capsule

synovial fluid

synovial membrane

joint capsule

To provide a smooth motion, diarthroses have a **joint capsule** made of a strong, fibrous tissue (Figure 4.5). The capsule is lined with a **synovial membrane**, which secretes **synovial fluid**, a smooth, slippery substance that prevents rubbing between the bone and the joint. Areas that support the most impact contain small sacs called **bursae** that are filled with synovial fluid. A joint cavity provides the space for the motion, and the articular cartilage covers the ends of the bones where it absorbs bumps and jolts.

There are several types of diarthroses: ball and socket, hinge, pivot, saddle, gliding, and condyloid. Figure 4.6 shows each type, its movement, and gives one or more examples of that type of joint in the body.

Tendons are like heavy cords that attach muscles to bones. They are composed of dense regular connective tissue that provides great strength at their attachment sites.

Ligaments are fibrous bands of dense regular connective tissue that run from one bone to another to support and strengthen joints and to prevent movement in the wrong direction.

COMBINING FORMS FOR THE SKELETAL SYSTEM

Table 4.1 lists the essential combining forms for the skeletal system, and Table 4.2 lists some anatomy and physiology terms related to the system. Refer to Figure 4.1 as you learn the skeletal combining forms.

Table 4.1

Combining Forms for the Skeletal System

Combining form	Meaning	Example
arthr/o	joint	arthritis
cervic/o	neck	cervical spine
crani/o	head	craniospinal
dactyl/o	fingers or toes	polydactyly
ili/o	ilium; hip	iliosacral
lumb/o	lower back	lumbosacral
mandibul/o	lower jaw	submandibular
orth/o	straight	orthopedic
osse/o	bony	osseous
oste/o	bone	osteoarthritis
pelv/o	pelvis	pelvimetry
pod/o	foot	podiatrist
sacr/o	sacrum	sacroiliac
scapul/o	scapula	scapulopexy
spondyl/o	vertebrae	spondylosis
stern/o	chest	sternocostal
tars/o	tarsal bones in the foot	tarsoclasis
tempor/o	temporal (a skull bone)	temporoauricular
vertebr/o	vertebra	vertebrocostal
zyg/o	a yoke; a type of joining; the cheek bone	zygomatic bone; zygomaticofacial

Figure 4.6 - Types of
Diarthroses and Their
Functions

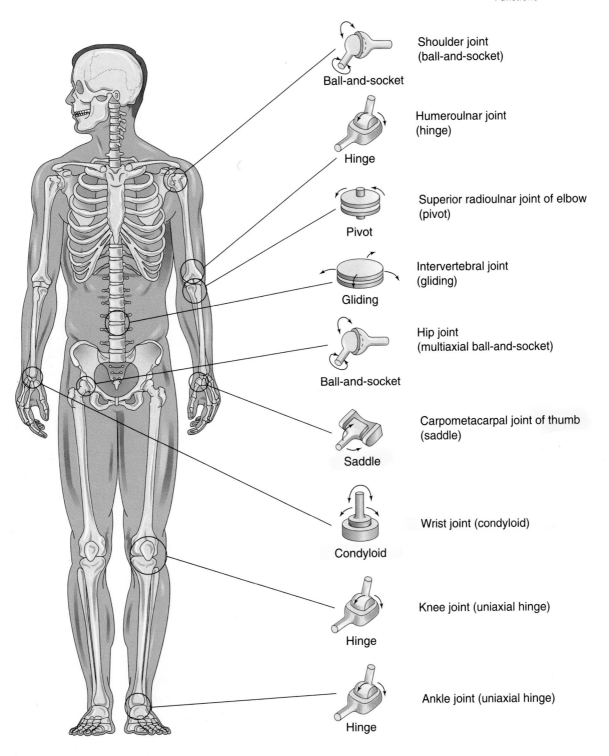

Ball-and-socket — Shoulder joint
(ball-and-socket)

Hinge — Humeroulnar joint
(hinge)

Pivot — Superior radioulnar joint of elbow
(pivot)

Gliding — Intervertebral joint
(gliding)

Ball-and-socket — Hip joint
(multiaxial ball-and-socket)

Saddle — Carpometacarpal joint of thumb
(saddle)

Condyloid — Wrist joint (condyloid)

Hinge — Knee joint (uniaxial hinge)

Hinge — Ankle joint (uniaxial hinge)

Table 4.2

Anatomy and Physiology Terms Relating to the Skeleton

Term	Meaning	Word Analysis	
amphiarthrosis **am**-fee-ar-thrO-sis	a fibrocartilaginous joining of two bones	amph/ arthr/o -osis	on both sides; around joint condition
articular cartilage ar-**tik**-yoo-lar **kar**-tih-lij	firm connective tissue covering the bone surface in a synovial joint	articular cartilage	a forming of vines gristle
articulate ar-**tik**-yoo-layt	to join or meet loosely in a way that allows motion	articulate	a forming of vines
bone marrow	gritty, fatty substance that produces red blood cells	mearh	for marrow
bursa **ber**-sah	a closed sac containing synovial fluid found in areas of the most friction	bursa	purse
carpal **kar**-pl	relating to the wrist bones	carpus	term
cartilage **kar**-tih-lij	a nonvascular, firm connective tissue	cartilage	gristle
chiropractic kI-rO-**prak**-tik	medical practice that teaches manipulation of the musculoskeletal system to restore health to bodily functions	chir/o practic/o	hand efficient
chiropractor kI-rO-**prak**-tor	the professional who practices chiropractic		
chondrocyte **kon**-drO-sIt	a cartilage cell within the matrix of cartilage	chondr/o -cyte	cartilage cell
diaphysis dI-**af**-ih-sis	shaft of a bone	diaphysis	growing between
diarthrosis dI-ar-**thrO**-sis	synovial joint	diarthrosis	articulation
diffusion dih-**fyoo**-zhun	movement of molecules from one area to another to produce a uniform population in both	diffusion	moving in different directions
endochondral en-dO-**kon**-dral	within the cartilage	end/ chondr/o	within cartilage
endosteum en-**dos**-tee-um	layer of cells lining the inner bone structure	end/o oste/o	within bone
epiphyseal line eh-ih-**fiz**-ee-al	an area of the long bone that remains after bone growth has ceased and epiphyseal plates are gone	epi- physis linea	upon growth string
epiphyseal plate eh-ih-**fiz**-ee-al	area of the long bone where growth takes place; it becomes the epiphyseal line after growth has ceased	epi- physis plate	upon growth flat, broad
epiphysis eh-**pif**-eh-sis	area of the long bone where growth takes place	epi- physis	upon growth
femur **fee**-mer	thigh bone	femur	thigh
humerus **hyoo**-mer-us	bone in the arm between the shoulder and elbow	humerus	shoulder
joint joynt	area where two bones meet	joindre	point of contact

joint capsule joynt **kap**-sl	area surrounding the joint that provides the fluid for movement and acts as a shock absorber	joindre capsule	point of contact box
ligament **lig**-ah-ment	band of strong, fibrous tissue that connects the bones and provides support	ligament	band
matrix **may**-triks	inner area of the bone where new cells are produced to form bone (including teeth or nails)	matrix	womb
medullary cavity **med**-yoo-lar-ee **kav**-ih-tee	area inside bone that contains bone marrow	medull/o cavity	marrow hollow

orthopedics
  or-thO-**pee**-diks
  (orthopaedics is the
  spelling some practitioners
  prefer)
orthopedist
  or-thO-**pee**-dist
	medical practice concerned with the form and function of the musculoskeletal system	orth/o-
		ped/o
			straight; normal
			child

ossification
  os-sih-fih-**kay**-shun
ossify
  os-sif-I
	process of forming bone from cartilage	osse/o	bony

osteoblast **os**-tee-O-blast	cell that produces bone	oste/o -blast	bone immature cell
osteoclast **os**-tee-O-klast	cell that resorbs bone to help shape new bone	oste/o -clast	bone broken
osteocyte **os**-tee-O-sIt	bone cell	oste/o -cyte	bone cell
periosteum per-ee-**os**-tee-um	outer covering of bone	peri/o oste/o	around bone
resorb ree-**sorb**	to absorb (as in an excretion)	re- sorb	again; back Latin for to suck back

rheumatology
  roo-mah-**tol**-ah-jee
rheumatologist
  roo-mah-**tol**-ah-jist
	study of conditions related to musculoskeletal movement	rheum/a
		
		-logy
			flux (a movement of fluid from a cavity)
			the study of

sternum **ster**-num	chest bone	stern/o	chest
synarthrosis sin-ar-**thrO**-sis	fibrous joint	syn- arthr/o	together joint
synovial fluid sih-**nO**-vee-al **floo**-id	fluid that bathes the joints to prevent friction	syn- ovum	together egg
synovial membrane sih-**nO**-vee-al **mem**-brayn	membrane that surrounds the synovial capsule	syn- ovum	together egg
trabecula trah-**bek**-yoo-la	spongy area inside bone	trabecula	beam
vertebra **ver**-teh-brah	bone of the spine	vertebr/o	to turn

Identify the anatomical structures on the skeleton opposite. Write the letter of the correct term beside the bone; on the line next to the bone name, write the root from which the term is formed.

A. cranium _____

B. mandible _____

C. sternum _____

D. ribs _____

E. scapula _____

F. humerus _____

G. radius _____

H. ulna _____

I. ilium _____

J. femur _____

K. patella _____

L. tibia _____

M. fibula _____

N. tarsal bones _____

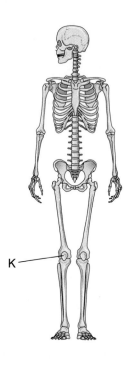

K

Define the Problem *Exercise 2*

Match the list of terms in Column 1 with the definition in Column 2. Write the letter of the definition in the space beside the term.

Column 1

1. humerus _____

2. scapula _____

3. sternum _____

4. periosteum _____

5. osteocytes _____

6. chondrocytes _____

7. diaphysis _____

8. ossification _____

9. endochondral _____

10. bursa _____

Column 2

a. outer covering of bone

b. bone cells

c. shaft of a long bone

d. cartilage changes to bone

e. bone of the upper arm

f. within cartilage

g. breastbone

h. sac of synovial fluid

i. shoulder blade

j. cartilage cells

Word Building

Use roots, combining forms, prefixes, and suffixes to construct a medical term to match each definition. Separate the parts of the term with a plus (+) sign.

1. study of rheumatic conditions _____

2. field of medicine concerned with the musculoskeletal system _____

3. examination of a joint using an instrument _____

4. process of becoming ossified _____

5. pertaining to the epiphysis _____

6. pertaining to a joint _____

7. inflammation of a bursa _____

8. condition of straight (also: brace or splint) _____

9. study of bone _____

10. pertaining to fiber _____

Spelling Check

Using contextual clues to determine meaning, circle the correct plural or singular form in each word pair.

1. Ligamenti/Ligaments are fibrous bands between bones.

2. The vertebra/vertebrae are poorly aligned.

3. Osteoblastum/Osteoblasts are immature bone cells.

4. Both scapula/scapulae are fractured.

5. Several phalanges/phalange on the right hand are missing.

6. Trabecula/Trabeculae are a network of spaces within spongy bone.

7. Synarthroses/Synarthrosis are joints that connect the bones in the skull.

8. Carpal/Carpals are bones in the wrist.

9. Several rheumatologists/rheumatologi attended the conference.

10. Fasciculus/Fasciculi is a term for a bundle of muscle fibers.

Examining the Patient ♂♀

Anatomy and Physiology of the Muscular System

The three types of muscle tissue are skeletal, smooth, and cardiac. **Skeletal muscle** is also called **voluntary muscle**, and is under the person's direct control.

Figure 4.7 - Major Skeletal Muscles and the Movements They Control

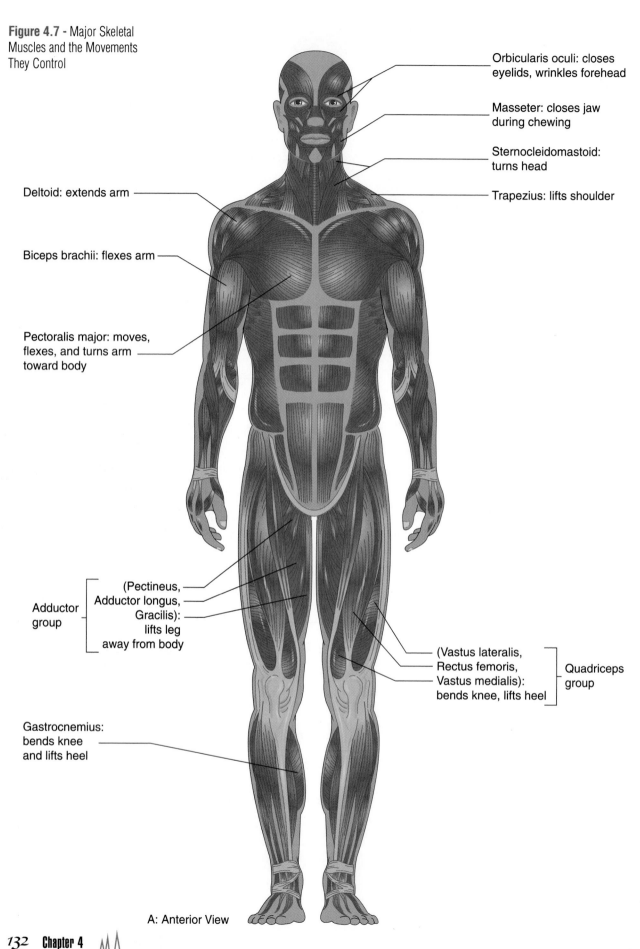

Orbicularis oculi: closes eyelids, wrinkles forehead

Masseter: closes jaw during chewing

Sternocleidomastoid: turns head

Trapezius: lifts shoulder

Deltoid: extends arm

Biceps brachii: flexes arm

Pectoralis major: moves, flexes, and turns arm toward body

Adductor group

(Pectineus, Adductor longus, Gracilis): lifts leg away from body

(Vastus lateralis, Rectus femoris, Vastus medialis): bends knee, lifts heel

Quadriceps group

Gastrocnemius: bends knee and lifts heel

A: Anterior View

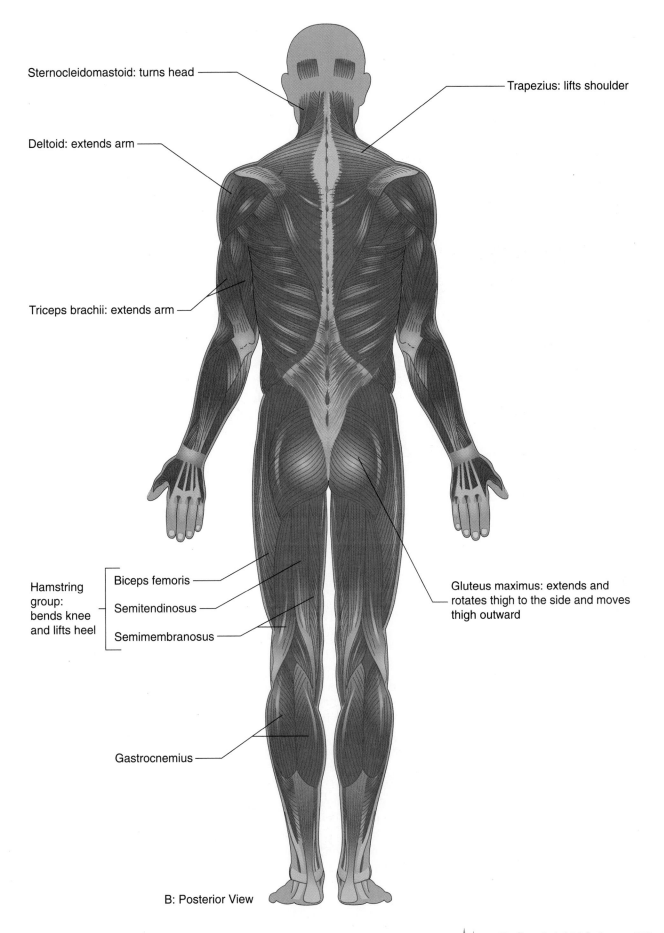

Sternocleidomastoid: turns head

Trapezius: lifts shoulder

Deltoid: extends arm

Triceps brachii: extends arm

Hamstring group: bends knee and lifts heel

Biceps femoris

Semitendinosus

Semimembranosus

Gluteus maximus: extends and rotates thigh to the side and moves thigh outward

Gastrocnemius

B: Posterior View

Figure 4.8 - Structure of Skeletal Muscle

Bundles of muscle fibers (fasciculi)

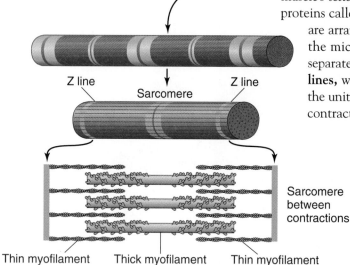

Bone

Tendon

Muscle fiber

One myofibril

Z line

Sarcomere

Z line

Thin myofilament (actin)

Thick myofilament (myosin)

Thin myofilament (actin)

Sarcomere between contractions

Sarcomere contracted

Smooth muscle, or involuntary muscle, is found in organs such as the stomach, and functions through involuntary stimulation. Specific involuntary muscles are described in subsequent related chapters. **Cardiac muscle,** found only in the heart, is described more fully in Chapter 11.

More than 40 percent of the body's weight comes from skeletal muscle. Skeletal muscle provides movement, helps maintain the body's posture, and produces the heat necessary to maintain the body's temperature. Figure 4.7A-B shows the major skeletal muscles and the movements they control.

Skeletal muscle is composed of **striated muscle** (muscle with stripes called **striations**) and connective tissue. The striated muscle tissue is composed of contractile cells called muscle fibers, as shown in Figure 4.8. These fibers are arranged in bundles called **fasciculi,** which lie parallel to one another between the muscle's tendinous ends. Muscle fibers are composed of proteins called thick and thin **myofilaments,** which are arranged into units called **sarcomeres.** Under the microscope, sarcomeres appear as stripes separated from each other by dark bands called **Z lines,** which form the striations. Sarcomeres are the units of muscle fiber that help an entire muscle contract, or shorten, when stimulated.

Muscle Functions

Skeletal muscle connects two or more bones and is divided into three parts: (1) the **origin,** which is attached to the more stationary bone; (2) the **insertion,** or the area where the muscle attaches to the more movable bone, and (3) the **body** of the muscle (see Figure 4.9). Muscles move bones by pulling them. Usually, the insertion bone moves toward the origin bone, producing a coordinated, smooth motion. Posture is a kind of movement maintained by the musculoskeletal system pulling just enough to overcome the force of gravity. In proper posture, the head is

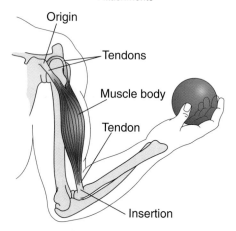

Figure 4.9 - Skeletal Muscle Attachments

Origin

Tendons

Muscle body

Tendon

Insertion

held high, with the chin parallel to the ground in a tucked inward position. The shoulders are pulled back, the stomach and buttocks are pulled in, and the knees are slightly bent. Correct posture decreases the risk of deformities and provides adequate working space for the heart, lungs, and other internal organs.

Heat production is another function of muscle. Muscle contraction releases energy stored in the muscles and generates the heat required to maintain the normal body temperature of approximately 98.6°F (37°C).

About Exercise

Muscles contract during exercise using stored energy and oxygen. The increase in activity increases the heart rate, which increases the blood flow. The increased blood flow brings additional oxygen to the muscle tissues. The rate and depth of respiration increases to maintain the amount of oxygen dissolved in the blood, and to blow off carbon dioxide. The entire process is an example of how the body always tries to maintain **homeostasis.** Insufficient oxygenation during exercise results in a buildup of **lactic acid,** which causes muscle pain. Lactic acid is carried off to the liver where it is converted to glucose, which can be used by exercising muscles.

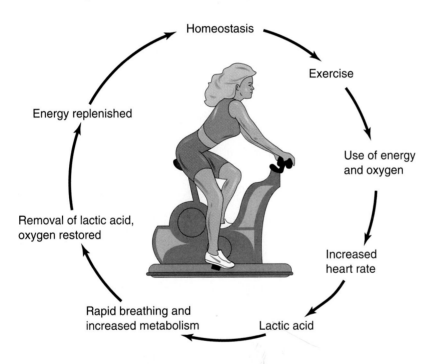

Figure 4.10 - How the Body Uses Energy During Exercise

COMBINING FORMS FOR THE MUSCULAR SYSTEM

Table 4.3 displays the essential combining forms for the vocabulary of the muscular system, and Table 4.4 lists important anatomy and physiology terms related to muscles.

Table 4.3

Combining Forms for the Muscular System

Combining form	Meaning	Example
-algia	pain	neuralgia
ankyl/o	crooked, fusion, stiffness	ankylosis
arthr/o	joint	arthritis
articul/o	joint	articulation

asthen/o	loss of strength	myasthenia gravis
chondr/o	cartilage	chondritis
fibr/o	fiber	fibrosis
kinesi/o	pertaining to movement	kinesthesia
muscul/o	muscle	musculature
my/o	muscle	myofilament
tend/o; tendin/o	tendon	tendinitis

Table 4.4

Anatomy and Physiology Terms Relating to the Muscles

Term	Meaning	Word Analysis	
fasciculus fah-**sik**-yoo-lus	a bundle of muscle fibers	*fasciculus*	bundle
homeostasis **hO**-mee-**os**-tas-is	state of having all body functions in balance	*home/o* *-stasis*	alike stop
insertion in-**ser**-shun	attachment of a muscle to a more movable part	*insertion*	a planting
involuntary muscle in-**vol**-un-tar-ee **mus**-sl	muscle that cannot be controlled by the person; smooth muscle	*in-* *voluntas* *-ary*	not will relating to
lactic acid **lak**-tik **as**-id	a chemical substance released by muscle cells during increased activity	*lact/o* *acid*	milk sour
ligament **lig**-ah-ment	band of strong, fibrous tissue that connects the bones and provides support	*ligament*	band
myofilaments mI-O-**fil**-ah-ments	microscopic threads that make up striated muscle	*my/o* *filament*	muscle thread
origin **or**-ih-jin	the less movable area of the points of attachment of bones	*origin*	source, beginning
sarcomeres **sar**-kO-meers	area of striated muscle found between Z lines	*sarc/o* *-mere*	muscular substance part
skeletal muscle **skel**-eh-tl **mus**-sl	striated muscle fibers connected to the bones of the body, voluntary muscle	*skeletos* *musculus*	dried up little mouse
smooth muscle	muscle fibers of the internal organs; involuntary muscle	*musculus*	little mouse
striated muscle **strI**-ay-ted **mus**-sl	voluntary skeletal muscle with striations	*stria* *musculus*	channel little mouse
voluntary muscle **vol**-un-tar-ee **mus**-sl	muscle that can be controlled (moved) by the person	*voluntas* *-ary* *musculus*	will relating to little mouse
Z lines	bands of tissue that separate sarcomeres		named for their resemblance to the letter Z under the microscope

Comprehension Check

This exercise provides practice in determining word meaning according to context. Circle the better word from the two choices in each sentence.

1. The periosteum/ pericardium was dissected away from the bone.

2. The metatarsal/medullary cavity was found to contain minimal marrow.

3. It is apparent that much of the articular cartilage/atrial cartilage is worn away.

4. The humerus and the ulna articulate/fibrilate.

5. The symbiotic membrane/synovial membrane was torn, and synovial fluid/syntactical fluid was absent.

6. The lumbosacral area/limbic system was tender to palpation.

7. Jana's parents were told that the fracture in her tibia occurred in the epidermal plate/epiphyseal plate.

8. Mrs. Hamby had previously seen a local chiropractor/contractor, who treated her back pain successfully.

9. The joint was examined with the limb in both full extension/examination and full fusion/flexion.

10. Muscle was dissected away from the bone at the insertion/disertion point.

Name That Term

Write the medical term for the underlined word, phrase, or abbreviation in each sentence.

1. Nearly all persons over the age of 60 have signs of a non-inflammatory, progressive disorder that eventually causes deterioration of the articular cartilage in the hands, feet, hips, spine, and other places.

_____

2. The physician indicated that the bundle of muscle fibers was inflamed.

_____

3. Establishing and maintaining a state of equilibrium among body systems is always a goal of treatment.

_____

4. This connective tissue is like heavy cords and attaches muscles to bones.

_____

5. The uterus is composed of smooth muscle.

_____

6. The fibrous bands that prevent joints from moving in the wrong direction were badly torn in the accident.

_____

7. The living bone cells in the tissue sample were disrupted.

_____

8. After running, her legs were sore from the chemical substance released by muscle cells during increased activity.

_____

9. The <u>specialist</u> treats conditions related to disorders of the foot.

_____

10. Striated muscle has <u>stripes</u>.

_____

Word Maps

The chart below is designed to group muscles by type, location, and type of nerve control. Fill in the blank spaces with the appropriate terms.

Muscle Type	skeletal		smooth
Location		heart	
Type of Nerve Control		involuntary	

Word Puzzle

Use these misspelled clues to write the correctly spelled terms in the puzzle.

Across

Ostoclast
Stermun
Epifisi
Stirations
Femor
Carnium
Sinoviul
Dharthrosis
Chartalige
Sarchomires
Facsiculous

Down

Perinostiume
Scalpula
Tribecola
Reumotology
Bon
Miofilaments
Bhurssa
Illium
Ostify
Karpl

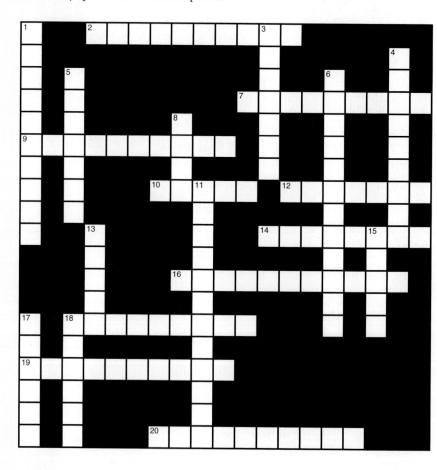

Wellness and Illness through the Life Span

A person with a problem or complaint such as a fracture, pain, swelling in a joint or muscle, or a skeletal malformation is referred to a specialist in the field. The physical examination of the musculoskeletal system includes an assessment of the patient's posture, standing and walking movements, and mobility of the joints and extremities. The examiner elicits full range of motion (ROM) activities from each muscle group. Asymmetry of an area's range of motion indicates a problem; obvious malformations such as scoliosis and kyphosis are noted. All joints are inspected for pain, swelling, or redness, any of which would indicate a problem.

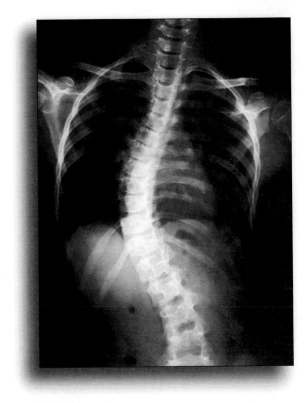

X-ray of Scoliosis

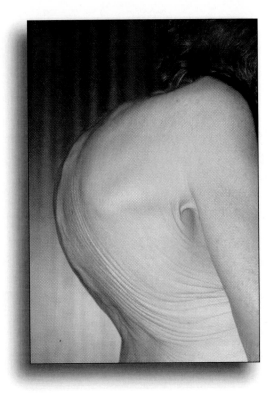

Kyphosis

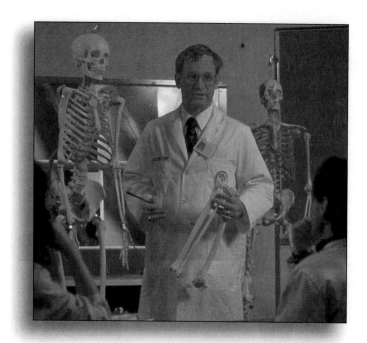

During the physical examination, the health professional palpates for certain landmarks that can be touched and identified through the skin. These landmarks, called bone markings, are specific locations on different bones and each provides reference points for the examiner and may be noted in the patient's chart. Table 4.5 describes these landmarks and their associated structures. Review Figure 4.11 and locate each landmark.

Table 4.5

Palpable Bony Landmarks

Landmark	Location
various bones of the skull	example: zygomatic bone
acromion process of scapula	the highest corner of the shoulder
spinous processes	vertebrae
medial and lateral epicondyles of the humerus	area where the upper arm and forearm connect
styloid process of the radius	projection on the bone on the thumb side of the lower arm
styloid process of the ulna	projection on the bone on the medial side of the lower arm
anterior superior iliac crest	upper portion of hip bone on anterior aspect of body
posterior iliac crest	upper portion of hip bone on posterior aspect of body
patella	kneecap
anterior crest of the tibia	shinbone
lateral malleolus of fibula	outside bone of fibula; lateral projection at ankle bone
medial malleolus of tibia	inside bone of the tibia; medial projection at ankle bone
calcaneus	heel bone

Infants

By about two months' gestation, the fetal skeleton is a miniature of the actual skeletal form, but is composed of cartilage. As the fetus develops, the cartilage begins to **ossify** (to become hardened bone) and grow into the shape of the true bone. After birth, the infant grows rapidly. The bones are soft, and the newborn seems almost foldable. When an infant breaks a bone, the fracture does not extend completely through the bone but has the appearance of the bend or break of a young—sometimes referred to as green—piece of wood, and is therefore called a greenstick fracture. These fractures most often occur as a result of trauma to the newborn.

The bones of the skull also change from fetal to infant life. At birth the newborn's head measures between 32 and 38 cm and is about 2 cm larger than the chest circumference. The newborn head has palpable **suture lines**, the areas where the

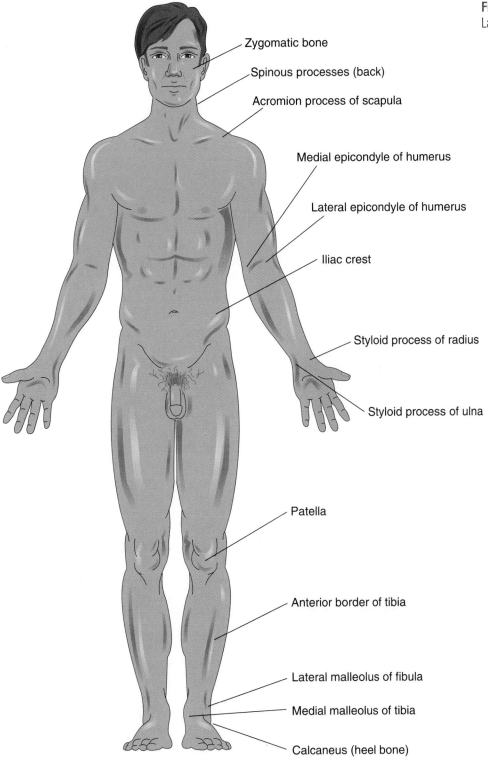

Figure 4.11 - Palpable Bony Landmarks

Zygomatic bone

Spinous processes (back)

Acromion process of scapula

Medial epicondyle of humerus

Lateral epicondyle of humerus

Iliac crest

Styloid process of radius

Styloid process of ulna

Patella

Anterior border of tibia

Lateral malleolus of fibula

Medial malleolus of tibia

Calcaneus (heel bone)

bones meet. Spaces, called **fontanels**, between the posterior sutures and the anterior sutures are called the posterior and anterior fontanels, respectively. The posterior fontanel may be palpable at birth but completely closes within one to two months. The anterior fontanel is larger and usually does not close until almost one year later, and possibly as long as two years. The fontanels provide space for the growing brain.

Infants cannot control their heads at birth. In about two weeks, they can turn their heads from side to side, but they are unable to hold them erect until after about four months. Muscle movement is involuntary and uncoordinated at birth. Newborn movements are a result of reflexes, described more fully in Chapter 8.

The infant's cranial bones may become molded during the passage through the birth canal. This molding, which may cause an initial asymmetry of the infant's head, is caused by the cranial bones overlapping each other, and can be palpated as irregularly shaped ridges.

Congenital Disorders

At birth the newborn is assessed for musculoskeletal development, beginning at the feet and working upward. Some deformities may originate from the fetus' position in the womb, and it is important to determine whether these deformities are positional (i.e., correctable) or permanent. The first assessment also reveals whether the infant has **metatarsus varus** (an adduction and inversion of the forefoot), **metatarsus valgus** (where the feet are turned outward), or neither.

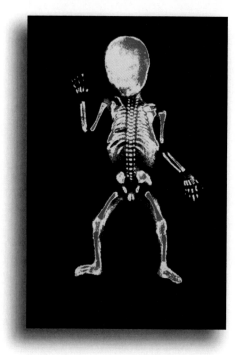

X-ray of newborn

The hips are checked for congenital dislocation by performing the Ortolani maneuver. This procedure involves appropriate positioning of the examiner's hands and abduction of the infant's knees apart and downward until the lateral aspects of the knees touch the examining table. The motion should feel smooth and be noiseless. The Allis test checks for hip dislocation by comparing leg lengths. The examiner checks the appearance of the folds of the legs: the anterior and posterior folds of the knees, and the symmetry of the gluteal folds.

Congenital malformations, such as **syndactyly** (webbed or fused fingers or toes) and **polydactyly** (extra digits on the hands or feet), are also noted. These deformities may be corrected by reconstructive surgery. **Talipes equinovarus**, or clubfoot, is a congenital, rigid malposition of the foot and a common birth defect (one to three out of every thousand live births), with twice as many incidents in males as in females. This deformity may be corrected with casting in infancy or surgical intervention.

The newborn should have full ROM of the arms. A frequent birth injury is a fractured clavicle from passage through the birth canal. The examiner traces the length of the spine with two or three fingers to detect spinal deformities. There is a normal "C" curve of the newborn's spine that remains until the head can be lifted at about two months. Thereafter, the concave anterior cervical spinal formation normal in childhood is present.

Toddlers and School-Aged Children

The child develops length from the skeletal system, and muscles grow as the child gains motor skills. Spinal curvature development continues from twelve to about eighteen months, when the child begins to walk, and develops an anterior curve in the lumbar region.

Commonly, the child may have **genu varum** (bowleg), or **genu valgum** (knock-knee). These abnormalities should disappear by the age of about three years. Often children this age have **pes planus** (flatfoot), because of the wide-based stance they must use to maintain balance. Young children may also appear to have pigeon toes, or toeing in, which usually corrects itself by the time they are about three years old.

Tibial torsion is the twisting of the tibia. This condition can be present at birth from intrauterine position, but it becomes problematic when the child sits in a way such that the buttocks are flat on the floor and the lower legs are positioned behind and outward.

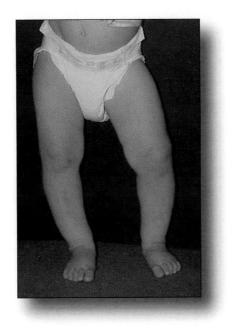
Genu Varum

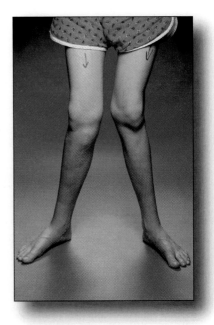
Genu Valgum

Legg-Calvé-Perthes disease occurs most commonly in males between three and twelve years of age (with most cases occurring at six years). An inflammatory stage causes decreased blood supply to the femoral head, a condition called **avascular necrosis**. The area eventually re-vascularizes, but often with residual deformity and loss of function.

Adolescents

The period of adolescence is characterized by a growth spurt, resulting from rising hormone levels (to be discussed further in Chapter 7), which cause significant linear (height) and muscular growth. Bone continues to expand until the epiphyseal plates close at about twenty years.

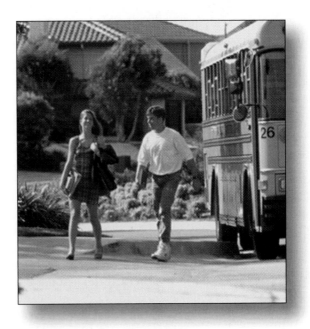

Adolescents frequently have poor posture, in part because they are self-conscious about their changing bodies. Girls may be uncomfortable about developing breasts or, if they mature later than their peers, non-developing breasts. Boys may feel that their thin, lanky shape is not attractive. Also, carrying heavy books in front of the body can lead to poor posture. Therefore, it is not uncommon to see **kyphosis**, a spinal deformity sometimes called humpback, in teenagers. Adolescence is the period when **scoliosis** is most commonly diagnosed. A familial trait, scoliosis is most commonly seen in girls and may cause spinal deformity if not surgically corrected.

Osgood-Schlatter disease occurs during the growth spurt, particularly in males, as a result of stress on the patellar tendon. It is characterized by painful swelling of the tibial tubercle, just below the knee, and may be brought on by biking, bending, kneeling, or climbing stairs. It is self-limiting and resolves with rest.

Sports injuries are common in the adolescent. Approximately 30 million children and adolescents participate in organized sports in the United States. Nearly 3 million injuries occur annually. In fact, musculoskeletal complaints account for 20 percent of the visits to primary care physicians and 80 percent of the visits to sports medicine clinics.

Fractures, **sprains**, **ligament tears**, and other injuries, most commonly to the knees and ankles, are part of the active teenager's life. Low back pain in adolescent athletes is a commonly seen problem in both sports medicine and general pediatrics and should be taken seriously as a significant problem.

Pregnant Women

Pregnancy brings about increased levels of the hormones estrogen, relaxin, and corticosteroids (discussed more fully in Chapter 16). These hormones cause an increase in the mobility of the joints of the pelvic bones, allowing the pelvic outlet to expand during labor and delivery. A woman's posture changes during pregnancy, with a gradual **lordosis** or swayback, to compensate for the growing fetus. Consequently, the pregnant woman must shift her center of gravity.

Male and female pelvic bones have some significant differences, as depicted in Figure 4.12. The female pelvis is structured to carry a fetus; it is broader and shallower, and the inlet and outlet are wider than the male's. A wider pubic angle in women allows for childbirth.

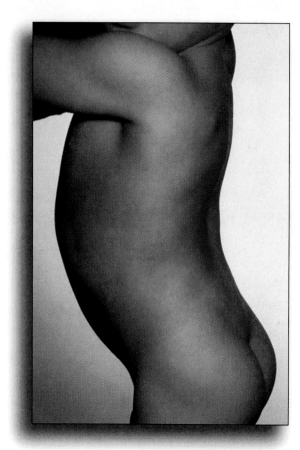

Lordosis

Adults

Inflammatory conditions of the joints, bones, and surrounding connective tissues usually begin in young adults, although children and adolescents can have these conditions (e.g., **juvenile rheumatoid arthritis**, or JRA). **Arthritis** and **rheumatoid arthritis** are **chronic** (i.e., constant and continuous), although there may be periods of regression of symptoms. A thickening of the synovial membranes leads to **fibrosis**, resulting in limited and painful motion. **Ankylosis** is often the result.

Ankylosing spondylitis is a chronic, progressive, inflammatory disease of the spine, sacroiliac, and larger joints of the extremities. The process leads to ankylosis and eventually deformity. Males are affected by ankylosing spondylitis more often than females by a ratio of ten to one.

Osteoarthritis is a noninflammatory, progressive disorder that eventually causes deterioration of the articular cartilage, with formation of new bone, at these joints. Nearly all persons over the age of sixty have signs of osteoarthritis in the hands, feet, hips, spine, and other places. The symptoms include pain, redness, swelling, stiffness, and often, decreased range of motion.

Gout, or **gouty arthritis**, is actually a metabolic disorder caused by hyperuricemia, an increase in uric acid, one of the body's necessary chemicals. Uric acid accumulates in the joints and surrounding tissues, causing damage and even destruction of the articular cartilage or synovial membrane. Gout is characterized by severe pain and

Figure 4.12 - Comparison of Male and Female Pelvises

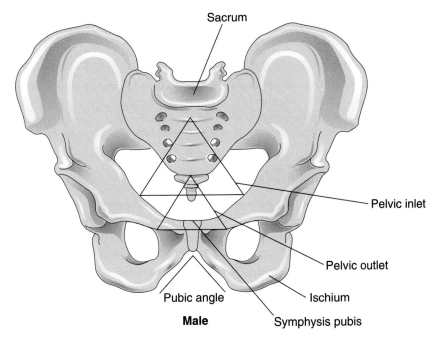

Male

Sacrum

Pelvic inlet

Pelvic outlet

Ischium

Pubic angle

Symphysis pubis

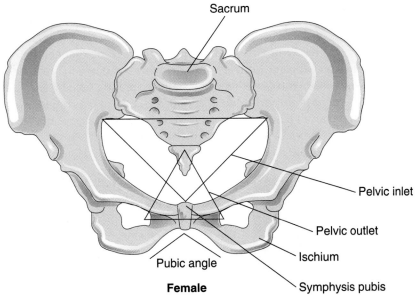

Female

Sacrum

Pelvic inlet

Pelvic outlet

Ischium

Pubic angle

Symphysis pubis

inflammation and most often affects the great toe, causing a condition called **podagra,** pain in the foot. Gout is most common in men over the age of forty.

Seniors

The aging adult shows changes in **physique,** that is, the physical, structural body, including a decrease in height, with a lengthening of the arm-trunk axis; the shortening of the trunk makes the arms appear longer in comparison. It is common to see **kyphosis,** with the head jutting forward and the hips and knees flexing for balance.

   Osteoporosis occurs when bone mass decreases because the rate of bone resorption is greater than that of bone formation. The bone becomes weak, and fractures in the hip and vertebrae are common. Postmenopausal women are most commonly affected by osteoporosis, because of the decrease in the female hormones estrogen and progesterone.

The most common orthopedic operation performed in the older adult population is the **total hip replacement** (THR), with more than 200,000 performed annually in the United States. The procedure has advanced continually since 1953, when it was introduced. Osteoporosis and use weaken the juncture at the hip joint where the femoral head joins the acetabulum of the hip. The THR involves replacing the femoral head with a metal **prosthesis** and inserting a polyethylene cup into the acetabular socket. Bone growth eventually occurs over the porous coating that covers these prostheses.

General Musculoskeletal System Illnesses

Thanks to the current emphasis on physical fitness, many people are very active and exercise regularly. Injuries due to exercise are treated by orthopedists; the field of sports medicine has also developed to treat such patients. Table 4.6 lists terms used to describe some common conditions of the musculoskeletal system.

One of the most typical musculoskeletal problems is **epicondylitis**. The common name "tennis elbow" is a misnomer, since it is possible to develop epicondylitis from any activity that involves excessive and repeated pronation and supination of the forearm with the wrist extended. The actual injury includes chronic pain at the lateral epicondyle of the humerus, which may radiate down the arm.

Carpal tunnel syndrome is a repetitive motion injury seen in people who do the same activities daily. It is common in typists, carpenters, and other such workers who use their hands in the same manner all day. Characterized by an inflammation of the tendon sheath, **tenosynovitis** produces pain and swelling that can limit the movement of the affected part. Although tenosynovitis can occur in any tendon, carpal tunnel syndrome involves the tendon sheath around the tendons in the wrist, limiting the movement of the wrist, hand, and fingers. Edema puts pressure on the median nerve, and pain radiates to the thumb and up the arm. Anti-inflammatory agents, such as corticosteroids, are injected into the area, but it is often necessary to surgically remove the swollen tissue pressing on the nerve.

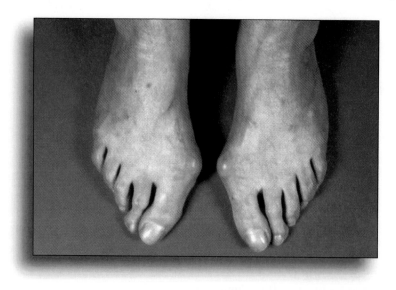

Bunions

The tendon sheath near the ankle can become inflamed and produce a tenosynovitis called **Achilles tenosynovitis,** named for its presence in the Achilles tendon. Swelling and tenderness along the route of the tendon make movement very painful and limited.

Bunions are a common deformity appearing on the medial prominence of the head of the first metatarsal (the side of the great toe). The bunion is actually an inflamed bursa that forms at the point of most pressure. The stress of walking (often in improperly fitted shoes) puts pressure on the great toe, which pushes off to produce each step and precipitates bunion formation. Bunions are characterized by swelling and pain. Callus formation, hammer toes, and joint **subluxation** are chronic sequels to bunions.

Hammer toes are deformities usually found in any or all of the second, third, fourth, and fifth toes. They include hyperextension of the metatarsophalangeal joint, the joint between the foot bones and the toes, and flexion of the proximal interphalangeal joint, the joint nearest to the body that moves the toes.

Fibromyalgia is a constellation of symptoms that includes chronic musculoskeletal pain as well as abdominal pain, headaches, muscle soreness, and stiffness lasting for more than six months. The American College of Rheumatology has strict criteria for diagnosis. There must be eleven of eighteen tender or trigger points on the body that are painful under pressure. Often the diagnosis is made after exclusion of several other conditions, such as depression, hypothyroidism, growing pains, chronic fatigue syndrome, and other systemic illnesses. Treatment includes medication, physical and occupational therapy, behavior modification, using techniques such as hypnosis, exercise, relaxation training, and/or biofeedback. Other typical musculoskeletal ailments include:

- **Dislocations**, which are injuries that involve the displacement of a bone from the joint. A **subluxation** is an incomplete dislocation, where some articulation between the bone and the joint is present.
- **Bursitis**, which is an inflammation (either acute or chronic) of a bursa, caused by trauma, chronic overuse, or infection. It can occur in any joint that has a bursa, and involves swelling, pain, tenderness, and inflammation of the area.
- A **ganglion** is a fluid-filled cyst (a rounded nodule) that appears over a tendon, most commonly in the wrist. It typically occurs and remits spontaneously.

Cancers of the Musculoskeletal System

Osteosarcoma is a malignancy arising from bone. It occurs most commonly during puberty, but can also be found in young adults. **Ewing's sarcoma** develops in the soft tissue and/or the bones. These tumors are usually treated with surgery and chemotherapy. **Rhabdomyosarcoma** is a malignant tumor, most commonly found in young children, which can occur in soft tissues and originates from embryonic muscle cells. Often surgery is not possible, so radiation and chemotherapy are used to shrink and/or eradicate the tumor. Synovial cell **sarcoma** occurs in the synovia that lines the joints.

Table 4.6

Wellness and Illness Terms Relating to the Musculoskeletal System

Term	Meaning	Word Analysis	
Achilles tenosynovitis a-**kil**-eez ten-O-sl-nO-**vI**-tis	inflammation of the heel and the surrounding tissue and tendons	Achilles	the mythical Greek warrior who was defeated only when wounded in the heel—his only weak spot
		ten/o	tendon
		synovia	fluid surrounding the joint
		-itis	inflammation
ankylosing spondylitis an-kih-**IO**-sing spon-dih-**II**-tis	stiffening and later fixation of the bones of the spine	ankyl/o	crooked; fusion
		-os	bone
		spondyl/o	vertebra
		-itis	inflammation
ankylosis an-kih-**IO**-sis	stiffening and later fixation of a joint caused by fibrosis	ankyl/o	crooked; fusion
		-os	bone
		-osis	condition
arthritis ar-**thrI**-tis	inflammation of a joint; usually a chronic condition	arthr/o	joint
		-itis	inflammation
avascular necrosis ah-**vas**-kyoo-lar neh-**krO**-sis	condition resulting from lack of blood supply, which leads to erosion and destruction of a joint	a-	without
		vascul/o	blood vessel
		necr/o	death
		-osis	condition

bunion **bun**-yun	inflammatory condition of the bursa of the first metatarsophalangeal joint	*bunion*	bump on the head
bursitis ber-**sI**-tis	inflammation of a bursa	*bursa* *-itis*	purse inflammation
carpal tunnel syndrome **kar**-pl **tun**-nl **sin**-drOm carpus carpi (pl)	condition of weakness, pain, or numbness resulting from pressure on the median nerve in the carpal tunnel (wrist)	*carpal*	relating to the wrist
dislocation dis-lO-**kay**-shun	displacement of a body part	*dis-* *location*	separation place
epicondylitis ep-ih-kon-dih-**lI**-tis	inflammation of the projection on a long bone near the articulation	*epi-* *condyle* *-itis*	upon knob inflammation
fibromyalgia **fI**-bro-my-al-gee-ah	condition characterized by chronic musculoskeletal pain, abdominal pain, headaches, muscle soreness, and stiffness lasting more than 6 months	*fibr/o-* *my/o-* *-algia*	fiber muscle pain
fibrosis fI-**brO**-sis	reparative or reactive tissue	*fibr/o* *-osis*	fiber condition
fontanel fon-tan-**el**	membranous area between the cranial bones of the infant	*fontanel*	fountain
fracture **frak**-cher	a break	*fracture*	break
ganglion cyst **gang**-lee-on ganglia **gang**-lee-ah ganglions (pl)	cyst usually found in the dorsal aspect of the wrist	*ganglion*	swelling; knot
genu valgum **jee**-nyoo **val**-gum genus (sing) genua (pl)	knock-knee	*genu* *valgum*	knee joint turned outward
genu varum **jee**-nyoo **vay**-rum	bowleg	*varum (varus)*	bent inward
gout	disorder characterized by an increase in uric acid, resulting in crystal formation in the articular cartilage; causes pain and inflammation; may be inherited (usually found in men)	*gout*	drop
greenstick fracture	incomplete fracture of a bone; bending of the bone	*green stick*	like the bending of young, green wood
kyphosis kih-**fO**-sis	spinal deformity characterized by an extreme flexion; humpback	*kyphosis*	bent
Legg-Calvé-Perthes disease leg-cal-**vay**-**per**-tez	aseptic necrosis of the epiphysis of the femur; named for the surgeons who identified the problem concurrently	*Legg* *Calvé* *Perthes*	U.S. surgeon French surgeon German surgeon
lordosis lor-**dO**-sis	anteroposterior curvature of the lumbar spine	*lordosis*	bending backward

Term	Definition	Word Parts	Meaning
metatarsus valgus met-ah-**tar**-sus **val**-gus metatarsus (sing) met-ah-**tar**-sus metatarsi (pl) met-ah-**tars**I metatarsal met-ah-**tar**-sal	deformity of the foot that causes the toes to face outward	meta tars/o valgus -	behind bones of the instep turned outward
metatarsus varus met-ah-**tar**-sus **vay**-rus	deformity of the foot that causes the toes to face inward	meta- tars/o varus	behind bones of the instep bent inward
Osgood-Schlatter disease **oz**-good-**shlah**-ter	aseptic necrosis of the tibial tubercle	Osgood Schlatter	U.S. orthopedic surgeon Swiss surgeon
osteoarthritis os-tee-O-ar-**thrI**-tis	arthritis characterized by destruction of the articular cartilage	oste/o arthr/o -itis	bone joint inflammation
osteoporosis os-tee-O-pah-**rO**-sis	reduction in the thickness of bone	oste/o por/o -osis	bone pore condition
pes planus pes **play**-nus pedes (sing) **pee**-deez pedi (pl) **pee**-dI	flatfoot	pes plan/o	foot flat; level
physique fih-**zeek**	the physical body type; the build	physi/o	physical
podagra pO-**dag**-rah	severe pain in the foot	pod/o -agra	foot sudden pain
polydactyly pol-ee-**dak**-tih-lee	extra fingers or toes	poly- dactyl/o	many fingers (digits)
rhabdomyosarcoma **rab**-dough-my-**oh**-sar-coma	malignant tumor of striated muscle	rhabd/o myo/o	rod-shaped pertaining to muscle
rheumatoid arthritis **roo**-mah-toyd ar-**thrI**-tis	painful condition affecting articulations; immunologic disorder causing pain and inflammation of the joints	rheuma arthr/o -itis	flux joint inflammation
sarcoma sar-coma	type of cancer derived from connective & supportive tissue	sarc/o -oma	denoting muscular substance denoting flesh tumor
scoliosis skO-lee-**O**-sis	abnormal lateral curvature of the spine	scoliosis	crookedness
sprain	injury to a ligament		
subluxation sub-luks-**ay**-shun	dislocation	sub- luxation	below dislocation
suture lines **soo**-cher	a fibrous joint between two bones that was formed in a membrane	suture	seam
syndactyly sin-**dak**-tih-lee	webbed or fused fingers or toes	syn- dactyl/o	together fingers or toes (digits)

talipes equinovarus **tal**-ih-peez ee-**kwI**-nO- **vay**-rus	clubfoot; the foot is plantar flexed, inverted, and adducted	*talipes* *equine* *varus*	ankle horse bent inward
tenosynovitis ten-O-sI-nO-**vI**-tis	inflammation of the tendon and its covering	*ten/o* *synovia* *-itis*	tendon fluid surrounding the joint inflammation
tibial torsion **tib**-ee-al **tor**-shun tibia **tib**-ee-ah tibiae (pl) **tib**-ee-ee tibial **tib**-ee-al	a twisting of the tibia (shinbone)	*tibi/o* *torsion*	tibia twist

Word Analysis

Read each sentence carefully, then break each underlined word into its parts and write a definition for the medical term. Divide the term into its parts by using plus (+) signs.

Example: arthroscopy arthro + scopy examination of interior of a joint using an instrument

1. The fibrosis of the muscle tissue in the shoulder girdle was widespread.

   _____   _____

2. The patient's arthritis limits her ability to use the telephone.

   _____   _____

3. Mr. Kelly has severe bursitis in his left hip.

   _____   _____

4. Necrosis in the head of the femur required a prosthetic replacement.

   _____   _____

5. The disarticulation of the knee required surgery.

   _____   _____

6. Janice has severe osteoporosis and could break a bone in a fall.

   _____   _____

7. The infant was born with polydactyly of the right hand.

   _____   _____

8. Terri Cramer has difficulty dressing due to ankylosis of her elbow.

   _____   _____

9. The child fractured his right <u>tibia</u> when he fell from the swing in the park.

_____   _____

10. We will request a consult for the patient's suspected <u>epicondylitis</u>.

_____   _____

Comprehension Check

Circle the correct word or phrase from the two choices in each sentence.

1. Carpal tunnel syndrome/Genu varum is an example of a repetitive motion injury.

2. The fontanels/suture lines are palpable in an infant's head and are areas where the bones of the skull meet.

3. We will recommend surgery to correct the calcaneus/syndactyly.

4. Tibial torsion/Tendinitis is a twisting of the tibia.

5. In bursitis/osteoporosis there is a decrease in bone mass.

6. Fluxion/Flexion of the joint results in sharp pain.

7. An inflammation of the tendon sheath is known as tendinitis/tenosynovitis.

8. Arthrography/Arthrodynia is pain in a joint.

9. A ganglion/gang is a rounded nodule over a tendon.

10. Achilles/Avascular refers to a condition involving lack of blood supply.

Name That Term

Write the medical term for the underlined word, phrase, or abbreviation in each sentence.

1. <u>Stiffening and later fixation of a joint</u> may be associated with aging.

_____

2. An <u>inflamed bursa on the side of the great toe</u> may be aggravated by poorly fitting shoes.

_____

3. The child displayed severe <u>humpback</u>.

_____

4. A 70-year-old woman is referred for treatment of a <u>decrease in bone mass</u>.

_____

5. The patient is a 30-year-old carpenter with a fracture of the <u>heel bone,</u> the result of a fall.

_____

6. Joan's baby has <u>feet turned outward</u> and she was referred for evaluation and treatment.

_____

7. Dr. Murrow will perform an <u>examination of the interior of a joint</u> tomorrow.

_____

8. Impression: <u>JRA</u>

_____

9. The surgery was performed to correct the <u>abnormal lateral curvature of the spine</u>. _____

10. The baby's <u>bone fracture</u> had the appearance of a broken piece of wood. _____

Word Building

Use prefixes, root words, combining vowels, and suffixes to create medical terms for the definitions given. Write the term in the space beside the definition.

1. inflammation of a bone and bone marrow _____

2. pertaining to the femur _____

3. pertaining to the skeleton _____

4. bone tumor _____

5. bone pain _____

6. inflammation of a fluid-filled sac over a joint _____

7. lack of blood supply _____

8. inflammation of a joint _____

9. surgical repair of a bone _____

10. against inflammation _____

Spelling Check

Write the correct spelling of the underlined terms on the line that follows each entry. Note: some underlined terms are already spelled correctly.

1. Several <u>biopsy</u> will be necessary to accurately diagnose the problem. _____

2. An <u>antigens</u> is a protein. _____

3. Mr. Archer has multiple <u>diagnosis</u>. _____

4. The <u>metatarsus</u> of the left ankle were crushed in the accident. _____

5. The two <u>fontanel</u> in the child's head were closed. _____

6. The <u>ganglions</u> was present on the left wrist. _____

7. There was inflammation of the <u>bursae</u> in the right shoulder. _____

8. <u>Dislocations</u> is an injury to a joint. _____

9. Margit fell on the ski slope and fractured both <u>tibia</u>. _____

10. He suffers from <u>genua vulgum</u> in both legs. _____

For each condition listed below, write a one- or two-sentence explanation of the cause. Then circle the area of the body where the condition occurs. Write the number of the condition in the circle, and also indicate if the condition occurs most frequently in infants, adolescents, adults, or seniors. (Some body areas may have more than one circle and number.)

1. kyphosis

2. costochondritis

3. scoliosis

4. Osgood-Schlatter disease, right

5. ankylosing spondylitis

6. left podagra

7. gout

8. osteoporosis

9. polydactyly

10. carpal tunnel syndrome

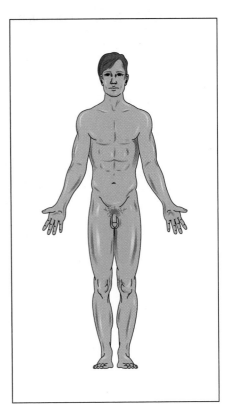

Tests, Surgical Procedures, and Pharmaceuticals

Treating injuries of the musculoskeletal system often requires visualizing the inside of the body using one of the radiographic techniques described in Chapter 2. One of the most frequently used diagnostic imaging tools is **arthrography**, which involves injecting a radiopaque contrast medium into a joint and taking an x-ray picture.

Certain blood tests assess how well the body is functioning and can help the practitioner make a diagnosis. An **erythrocyte sedimentation rate (ESR)**, also known as a *sed rate*, is a nonspecific blood test used to assess an inflammatory process. Although the sed rate is elevated in a variety of illnesses, it is used to diagnose rheumatoid arthritis if other signs and symptoms are present.

The **rheumatoid factor** is an antibody found in the serum of persons with rheumatoid arthritis. The **serum calcium** indicates if the mineral calcium is being released into the blood, and is a measure of bony destruction. An elevated calcium level is called **hypercalcemia**.

Human leukocyte antigen (HLA) B-27 is a protein present on the white blood cells of persons with arthritic conditions such as ankylosing spondylitis. A blood test called **serum alkaline phosphatase** can determine the levels of HLA B-27 in the body. Although the chemical is necessary to build new bone, conditions such as osteomalacia and rheumatoid disease may cause an elevation in its levels. Serum **creatine phosphokinase (CPK)** is an enzyme found in skeletal and cardiac muscle. An elevation of CPK in the serum may indicate muscular dystrophy, certain malignancies, and other illnesses.

Arthrocentesis is a procedure in which synovial fluid is removed and examined to diagnose a musculoskeletal disorder such as arthritis or gout.

Bone marrow aspiration and **biopsy** are procedures in which a long, thick needle is inserted through the skin and into the posterior iliac crest; a small amount of bone marrow is aspirated through the needle. A biopsy involves examining a small piece of the core of the bone marrow to diagnose certain diseases, such as malignancies and infections.

An **electromyograph** is a test of muscle strength that measures muscular contractibility by electrical stimulation. Bone density is measured by **photon absorptiometry**, which determines whether a person has osteoporosis.

Surgical Procedures

Fusing or connecting joint structures to make them immobile is called **fixation**. **Arthrodesis**, the surgical procedure for fixating joints, is performed in patients with severe arthritis or joint injuries in order to promote new bone formation.

Arthroplasty is the name for the procedure that involves placing a prosthesis consisting of the movable parts of the joint in the joint capsule, and it is used in many areas of the body to replace damaged joints, such as a **resection** of bone to remove a malignant lesion, for instance. Then, a **bone graft** taken from another site or a cadaver bone may be inserted at the site to maintain the graft and provide stability.

A **fracture**, or break in a bone, must be returned to normal alignment and then **immobilized** in a cast to promote correct new bone growth and healing. The method to realign the bone structures is called **reduction**. Several methods are used:

- Bones can be realigned by using **traction** to pull the fragments (each piece of a broken bone) into proper position. A pulley and weight are used to pull the distal end of the bone into realignment with the proximal end.

- A **closed reduction** is performed using either local or general anesthesia, since the procedure can be painful. The ends of the fractured bone are manually manipulated, externally, to position them into proper physiological alignment.
- An **open reduction** is a surgical procedure performed in the operating room. An incision is made, and the injury is repaired directly. After the repair is made, the patient's wound is sutured.
- When there has been considerable damage to the bone, such as being crushed in an accident, it may be necessary to perform an **internal fixation**. Screws, pins, and rods may be used to hold the pieces together and promote healing.

Table 4.7

Tests and Procedures Relating to the Musculoskeletal System

Term	Meaning	Word Analysis	
arthrocentesis ar-thrO-sen-**tee**-sis	aspiration of fluid from a joint	arthr/o centesis	joint puncture for removal of fluid
arthrodesis ar-**throd**-eh-sis	surgical procedure whereby a joint is fused	arthr/o -desis	joint binding
arthrography ar-**throg**-raf-ee	x-ray during which radiopaque dye is injected to visualize a joint	arthr/o -graph/o	joint radiograph, x-ray
arthroplasty **ar**-thrO-plas-tee	surgical procedure to create an artificial joint or to restore an injured joint	arthr/o -plasty	joint surgical repair or reconstruction
arthroscopy ar-**thros**-kah-pee	examination of the interior of a joint using an endoscope	arthr/o -scopy	joint examination
calcium (serum) **kal**-see-um	test that measures the amount of calcium in the blood	calc/i -um	lime noun ending
electromyography ee-lek-trO-**mI**-O-graf	method to measure muscle strength by testing muscular contractibility using electrical stimulation	electr/o my/o -graph	electric muscle recording
erythrocyte sedimentation rate er-**ith**-rO-sIt sed-ih-men-**tay**-shun rayt	laboratory test by which the number of erythrocytes (red blood cells) that fall from the plasma are measured over time	erythr/o -cyte sediment rate	red cell cell settle measurement
human leukocyte antigen B-27 **hyoo**-man **loo**-kO-sIt **an**-tih-jen	designation of genetic makeup on chromosomes helpful in determining transplant matching and associated with certain diseases, in particular arthritis	leuk/o -cyte antigen	white cell substance that produces an immunogenic response
photon absorptiometry **fO**-ton ab-sorp-shee-**om**-ah-tree	a test to measure bone density	phot/o absorption -metry	a particle of light incorporation; taking in the process of measuring
resection ree-**sek**-shun	to surgically remove	re- -sect	again to cut
rheumatoid factor **roo**-mah-toyd **fak**-tor	antibody found in the serum of a person with rheumatoid arthritis	rheuma -toid	movement relating to
serum alkaline phosphatase **seer**-um **al**-kah-lIn **fos**-fah-tays	laboratory test on the serum of the blood that measures whether there is an excess of new bone formation		chemical name

| serum creatine phosphokinase
seer-um **kree**-ah-tin fos-fO-**kI**-nays | laboratory test on the serum of the blood that may indicate certain illnesses and diseases; an enzyme found in skeletal and cardiac muscle | chemical name |
| uric acid test
yoo-rik **as**-id test | test of the blood or urine to determine the amount of this chemical salt present | |

Pharmacologic Agents

The agents used in orthopedics often are aimed at relieving pain and decreasing inflammation (see Table 4.8). The most common analgesic agents are **nonsteroidal anti-inflammatory drugs (NSAIDs)**, such as **ibuprofen**, and **salicylates**, such as **aspirin**. These drugs are prescribed for arthritis, bursitis, and muscle aches and pains. **Steroids** are sometimes injected directly into the affected joint. Many analgesics are currently being developed, and new ones are becoming available quickly.

Severe rheumatoid arthritic conditions may require treatment with **gold compounds** and **immunosuppressants**, since these conditions may have an immunologic component. **Muscle relaxants** are used for muscle spasms and the associated muscle pain. Specific agents promote skeletal muscle relaxation.

Gout is treated with **uricosuric agents**, which lower the uric acid level in the blood, and NSAIDs; some are manufactured with an analgesic already combined.

Table 4.8

Pharmacologic Agents

Drug classes	Use	Generic names	Brand names
antigout preparations	used to decrease the uric acid in the blood	allopurinol probenecid colchicine	Zyloprim Col-Probenecid
immunosuppressants	rheumatoid arthritis	gold sodium thiomalate	Aurolate
antineoplastic agent	rheumatoid arthritis	methotrexate	Rheumatrex
muscle relaxants	relaxes skeletal muscle and relieves pain	baclofen chlorzoxazone cyclobenzaprine hydrochloride	Lioresal Parafon Forte DSC Flexeril
nonsteroidal anti-inflammatory agents	used to decrease pain and inflammation from diseases such as rheumatoid arthritis, sprains, strains, and sports injuries	ibuprofen indomethacin ketorolac tromethamine	Motrin, Advil Indocin Toradol
salicylates	used to decrease pain and inflammation from diseases such as rheumatoid arthritis, sprains, strains, and sports injuries	aspirin	Anacin, Bufferin
steroids	used to decrease pain and inflammation from diseases such as rheumatoid arthritis, sprains, strains, and sports injuries	hydrocortisone injection	A-HydroCort

Table 4.8

Abbreviations

AE	above the elbow amputation
AK	above the knee amputation
AP	anteroposterior
AROM	active range of motion
BE	below the elbow amputation
BK	below the knee amputation
C1, C2, etc.	cervical vertebrae (numbered according to area of the spine)
CDH	congenital dislocation of the hip
DIP joint	distal interphalangeal joint
DJD	degenerative joint disease
EMG	electromyography
fx	fracture
HD	hip disarticulation
HNP	herniated nucleus pulposus (disk)
HP	hemipelvectomy
IP	interphalangeal joint
IS	intracostal space
KD	knee disarticulation
L1, L2, etc.	lumbar vertebrae
MCP joint	metacarpophalangeal joint
OA	osteoarthritis
ortho	orthopedics
PIP joint	proximal interphalangeal joint
PROM	passive range of motion
RA	rheumatoid arthritis
ROJM	range of joint motion
S1, S2, etc.	sacral vertebrae
SD	shoulder disarticulation
T1, T2, etc.	thoracic vertebrae
TENS	transcutaneous electric nerve stimulation
THA	total hip arthroplasty
THR	total hip replacement

Word Building

Exercise 15

Read each sentence, noting the partially completed medical term. Supply the missing part to complete the term.

1. A physio_____ is someone who studies the functions
   of the body.   _____

2. Arthro_____ allows the physician to view the inside
   of the joint through a flexible, lighted instrument.   _____

3. Myo_____means "pathology or disease of a muscle." _____

4. _____itis means inflammation of cartilage.   _____

5. Vascul_____ means "pertaining to vessels." _____

6. Kine_____ means "pertaining to movement." _____

7. Osteo_____ means inflammation of bone. _____

8. Tars_____ means pertaining to the tarsal bones _____
   (bones of the ankle).

9. Fibr_____means like or resembling fiber. _____

10. Burs_____means inflammation of a bursa. _____

Comprehension Check

Exercise 16

Read each sentence and write the meaning of each underlined word on the line below the sentence, keeping your answers brief. You may need to use a medical dictionary for this exercise.

1. Mr. Osborne is scheduled for an <u>electromyogram</u> this afternoon.

_____

2. This patient is being referred to an <u>orthopedist</u>.

_____

3. The <u>periosteum</u> was dissected away to reveal the diaphysis.

_____

4. Microscopic examination of the material revealed several <u>osteocytes</u>.

_____

5. <u>Endochondral ossification</u> has begun in the long bones.

_____

6. The <u>bursa</u> has ruptured.

_____

7. An <u>osseous</u> projection is apparent in the wound bed.

_____

8. This patient's <u>lordosis</u> is severe, making ambulation difficult.

_____

9. There is an apparent <u>fracture</u> of the right femur.

_____

10. Dr. Hardesty has prescribed <u>salicylates</u> for pain and inflammation.

_____

Match the list of procedures and treatments in Column 2 with the diagnosis or reason for the procedure in Column 1. Write the number of the diagnosis or problem in the space beside the name of the treatment or procedure. Note that some entries in Column 2 are diagnostic procedures.

Column 1		Column 2
1. fx	_____	a. photon absorptiometry
2. scoliosis	_____	b. HLA B-27
3. ankylosing spondylitis	_____	c. uricosuric agents
4. osteoma	_____	d. fracture reduction and casting
5. crushing fracture	_____	e. sed rate or ESR
6. muscle strain	_____	f. resection of bone and grafting
7. Osgood-Schlatter disease	_____	g. open reduction/internal fixation
8. gout	_____	h. brace for torso
9. RA	_____	i. rest
10. osteoporosis	_____	j. NSAIDs

Find word parts in this chapter to construct medical terms for the definitions that follow. Write the term in the blank beside the definition. Separate the parts with a hyphen or plus sign.

1. study of bone   _____

2. without blood supply   _____

3. condition of death   _____

4. within cartilage   _____

5. inflammation of tendon   _____

6. pertaining to cartilage   _____

7. like or resembling bone   _____

8. like or resembling a knot or swelling   _____

9. pertaining to against inflammation   _____

10. to cut again   _____

Spelling Check

Indicate whether the underlined term is plural or singular (write P or S). For each plural term, provide the singular form; for each singular term, give the plural.

1. The <u>erythrocyte</u> count was abnormal. _____ _____

2. Three surgeons participated in the <u>resection</u> of the diseased bone. _____ _____

3. The structure of the <u>myofilaments</u> was examined. _____ _____

4. There were a number of <u>grafts</u> performed from a single donor. _____ _____

5. The patient had three separate <u>sprains</u>. _____ _____

6. The child's <u>tibia</u> was malformed at birth. _____ _____

7. Some bone <u>diseases</u> can be difficult to detect. _____ _____

8. The <u>osteocytes</u> were vertically oriented. _____ _____

9. The <u>ligaments</u> in the joint had been damaged by stretching. _____ _____

10. The patient's <u>bunion</u> made walking difficult. _____ _____

Word Maps

Rearrange the following terms to create three flowcharts. For each chart, begin with a body part, then add a related disease or condition, a test or procedure for that condition, and finally a drug treatment for the disease.

feet	JRA	gout	immunosuppressants
arthrocentesis	allopurinol	ESR	osteoporosis
joints	calcium supplements	spine	photon absorptiometry

Performance Assessment 4

Crossword Puzzle

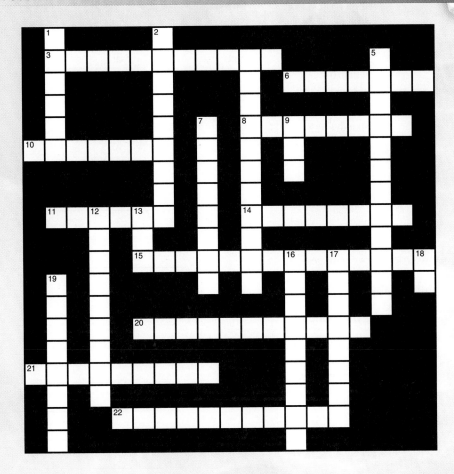

Across

3. extra fingers or toes
6. bone of the lower arm
8. inflammation of a bursa
10. bending at a joint
11. fingers and/or toes
14. pertaining to cartilage
15. physician specializing in the diagnosis and treatment of joint disorders
20. areas where bones of a newborn's skull meet
21. setting a broken bone
22. bones of the hand

Down

1. pertaining to the spine
2. heelbone
4. pertaining to both the lumbar and sacral areas of the spine
5. joint
7. physical, structural body
9. range of motion
12. bowleg
13. total hip replacement
16. bone at the back of the skull
17. inflammation of bone
18. first thoracic vertebra
19. pertaining to the skeleton

In this exercise you will construct words from roots, prefixes and suffixes. Select word parts from the lists to build a complete medical term for each definition given. Note that not all terms will have a root or combining form, prefix, and suffix. Some word parts may be used more than once.

Combining forms	Prefixes	Suffixes
arthr/o	hyper-	-itis
tendon/o	epi-	-logy
articul/o	sub-	-logist
physi/o	hypo-	-icle
oste/o	intra-	-ous
orth/o	dis-	-sis
burs/o	an-	-al
femur/o	pre-	-ar
chondr/o	de-	-ic
osse/o	anti-	-in
spondyl/o	per-	-cyte
mandibul/o	bi-	-lysis

1. study of the body's function _____

2. bony _____

3. breakdown of cartilage _____

4. inflammation of vertebrae _____

5. pertaining to the mandible _____

6. condition of straight _____

7. inflammation of cartilage _____

8. pertaining to inside a joint _____

9. bone cell _____

10. under cartilage _____

Word Maps

Identify the anatomical structures by number on the accompanying diagram and write the combining form on the line under each structure name.

1. cranium

   _____

2. mandible

   _____

3. humerus

   _____

4. metacarpal bones

   _____

5. vertebral column

   _____

6. femur

   _____

7. patella

   _____

8. tibia

   _____

9. tarsal bones

   _____

10. metatarsal bones

    _____

11. phalanges of lower extremity

    _____

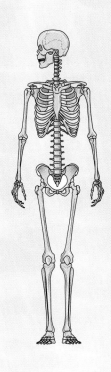

What Do These Abbreviations Mean?

Give the correct terms for the following abbreviations.

1. AK _____

2. AROM _____

3. DJD _____

4. EMG _____

5. fx _____

6. CDH _____

7. HD _____

8. OA _____

9. PROM _____

10. SD _____

What's Your Conclusion?

Read each mini medical record carefully. Then select the response that describes the physician's logical next step. Write the letter of your answer in the space provided.

1. Mary T. was brought to the hospital emergency room by ambulance after she slipped on a wet floor at a nearby supermarket. She has pain, erythema, and a great deal of edema in her right metatarsal and calcaneus. The physician will:

   A. Stabilize the foot and ankle and elevate it on a pillow. Prepare to send Mary to the x-ray department for films of the right foot and ankle.
   B. Call the surgery department and request that Mary be scheduled for a BKA.

   Correct response: _____

2. Sylvia U. has been referred to the clinic for evaluation and treatment because her family physician suspects that she may have osteoporosis, although no tests have been performed. Sylvia is 73 years old and appears thin and frail. She has had two hip fractures during the past eighteen months. She is accompanied by her daughter. The physician will:

   A. Prescribe a calcium dietary supplement, schedule hip x-rays, and order a walker to help Sylvia with ambulation.
   B. Examine Sylvia carefully, then schedule her for photon absorptiometry.

   Correct response: _____

3. Keith M. is a 12 y/o male who was brought to the office by his mother. He has pain and swelling in the area of the tibial tubercle, just below his right knee. Keith says that his favorite activities are bike riding and wrestling. About a week ago Keith saw Dr. Whiteside, who diagnosed Osgood-Schlatter Disease. Keith's mother says, "Dr. Whiteside said that Keith has a disease; then he refused to do anything about it. He said that Keith should just take ibuprofen and rest the knee. Keith needs surgery for this disease, and pain-killers." You realize that:

A. Osgood-Schlatter is self-limiting and resolves with time. The accepted treatment is rest and nonsteroidal anti-inflammatory agents, such as ibuprofen.

B. Keith will require arthroscopic surgery and will need to be away from school for approximately two weeks.

Correct response: _____

Analyzing Medical Records

In this exercise you will practice interpreting and extracting information from realistic medical documents. Read the progress note on the following page. Then answer the following questions:

1. What is the age and the gender of the patient?

2. Where was the patient seen?

3. Describe the findings from the physical examination.

4. What is the assessment? Is this an infectious disease?

5. List three tests that are to be performed.

Hayes-Oakwood Clinic, Inc.
Department of Orthopedics

407 S. Parkway, Accord City, KS 77709-4321
phone (333) 555-1122 fax (333) 555-1234

Physician's Progress Note

PATIENT: Juan L.
DATE: June 29, xxxx

S: Patient is a 5 y/o. He comes to the clinic today accompanied by his mother, who is quite concerned about her son's symptoms. Mother states that her son has always been a healthy child, and has had no problems until recently. He has been seen in the clinic here for check-ups and immunizations. She reports that over the past few months he has become quite clumsy, falling down, dropping things, etc. Pt. admits to some muscle weakness and feeling "trembly" in his legs. He says, "I'm tired."

O: Examination of the HEENT is WNL. T 98.6, P 68, R 15, BP 90/64. Auscultation of the precordial area reveals RRR, without murmurs. Lungs clear. Neurological exam is generally WNL. Skeletal muscles in the extremities appear hypertrophic and firm. Grip strength is somewhat ^, and biceps strength appears less than expected. No contractures noted at this point.

A: Possible muscular dystrophic disorder.

P: Admit to Accord City General Hospital for:
   1) Muscle biopsy.
   2) EMG.
   3) 24-hour blood samples for CPK.
   4) 24-hour urine collection for creatinine.

_____

C. L. Parton, MD

Using Medical References

The following sentences contain medical terms that were not addressed on the charts in this chapter. Use medical reference books, your medical term analysis skills, and/or a medical dictionary to find the correct definition of each underlined word. Write the definition on the line below each sentence.

1. Although the <u>leiomyoma</u> may produce symptoms, it is not ultimately fatal.

   _____

2. The patient is an 18 y/o male with a diagnosis of <u>osteogenic sarcoma</u>.

   _____

3. Mrs. Clarke's <u>hypotonia</u> has become progressively worse over the past two weeks.

   _____

4. X-ray films reveal a large transverse <u>medial malleolar</u> fracture.

_____

5. Imp: <u>Lumbar spondylosis</u> with narrowing of the disc spaces.

_____

6. The patient has elected not to terminate the pregnancy, even though she has been diagnosed with <u>rhabdomyosarcoma</u>.

_____

7. After the suggestions from the physical therapist during case conference, Dr. Maloney prescribed <u>ROM</u> exercises for all his elderly patients.

_____

8. The pathologist reported finding several <u>myelocytes</u> on the slide.

_____

9. Mr. Horton will be fitted with a <u>prosthesis</u>.

_____

10. The right arm was <u>flaccid</u>, and the patient was unable to grasp my fingers.

_____

11. The patient's <u>orthosis</u> had to be replaced after it was damaged in an accident.

_____

12. Many children in Third World countries suffer from <u>rickets</u> because of inadequate nutrition.

_____

Short Answer

In plain language, describe Legg-Calve-Perthes disease.

_____

_____

_____

_____

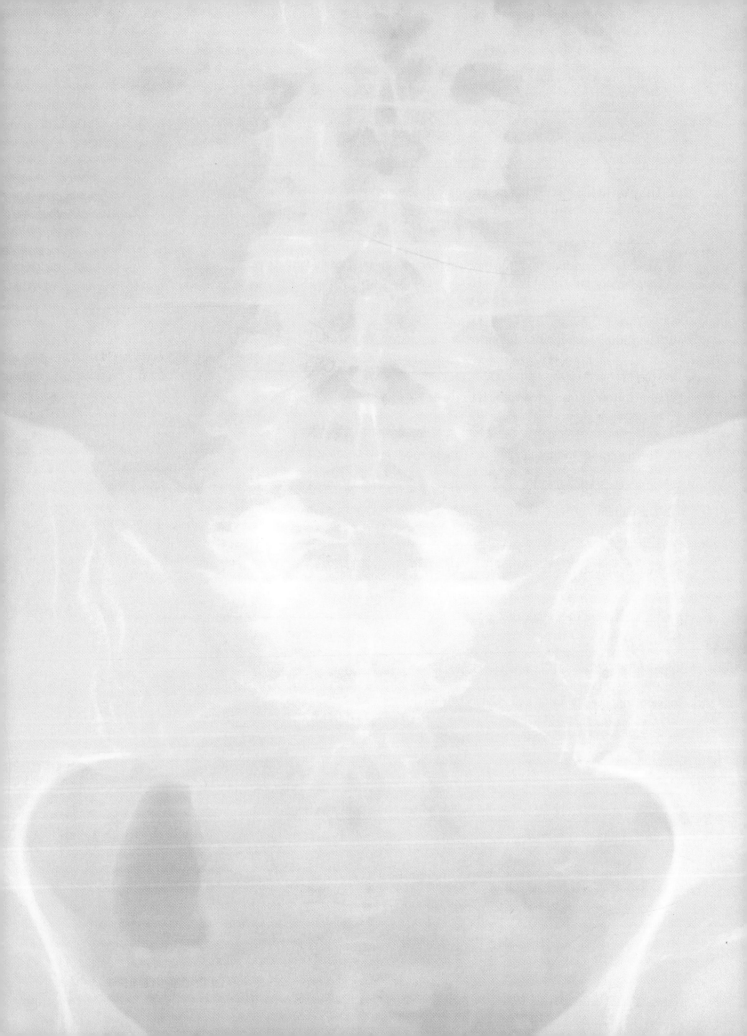

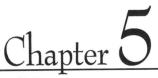

Chapter 5

Hematology and Oncology

Learning Outcomes

Students will be able to:
- Describe the structure and function of the blood cells.
- Recognize the word forms that are commonly used to characterize blood and its components.
- Explain the process of hematopoiesis and the growth and maturation of blood cells.
- Differentiate the characteristics of normal and malignant cells.
- Indicate the importance of blood and its components in maintaining hemostasis.
- Use the language of hematology correctly in written and oral communication.
- Correctly spell and pronounce hematology and oncology terminology.
- State the meaning of abbreviations related to hematology and oncology.
- List and define the combining forms most commonly used to create terms related to hematology and oncology.
- Name and describe tests and treatments related to hematology and oncology.

Translation, Please? Translation, Please? Translation, Please?

Read this excerpt from a physician's report and try to answer the questions that follow it.

It was discovered that the fetus had erythroblastosis fetalis. Treatment was started in utero, and the infant was delivered prematurely. An exchange transfusion was administered immediately after birth. The platelet count was 12,000 mm³. There were petechiae and ecchymoses over the body. The rest of the examination was normal. Treatment was started to attempt to correct the thrombocytopenia.

1. To what blood cell line does erythroblastosis fetalis refer: red blood cells or blast cells?
2. What is an exchange transfusion?
3. Do you think a platelet count of 12,000 mm³ is lower or higher than normal?
4. Using the word analysis skills and the word parts you have learned in previous chapters, which parts of *thrombocytopenia* can you decipher?

Answers to "Translation, Please?"
1. Erythroblastosis fetalis refers to red blood cells.
2. Most of the patient's blood is replaced with donor blood.
3. A normal platelet count is 150,000 to 300,000 mm³, so a count of 12,000 is lower than normal.
4. *Thromb/o* = clot; *cyt/o* = cell; and *-penia* = lack of or abnormal reduction. Thrombocytopenia means decreased platelets.

Identifying the Specialty

The System and Its Practitioners

Hematology is the study of blood and its components. Blood is the fluid that transports nutrients, gases, hormones, and cells throughout the body. Because blood plays a critical role in the function of all body systems, references to blood-related words, tests, and procedures appear throughout all types of medical communication. The physician who specializes in the field of hematology is a **hematologist**. A physician who is trained in hematology is usually trained in oncology as well (*onc/o*, pertaining to cancer), so the practice is often called hematology-oncology. This chapter is divided into two sections: the first section describes hematology, and the second section addresses oncology.

Examining the Patient ♂♀

Anatomy and Physiology of the Blood

Blood is a fluid that contains so many millions of floating cells that it is almost impossible to imagine the total number of blood cells in the human body. When a **complete blood count** (a standard blood analysis, usually referred to by its initials, CBC) is performed, one drop of blood is placed on a glass slide and viewed under the microscope. The normal CBC has approximately 5,000,000 red blood cells, 300,000 platelets, and nearly 10,000 white blood cells in 1 mm^3 of blood—remember, that is one drop of blood!

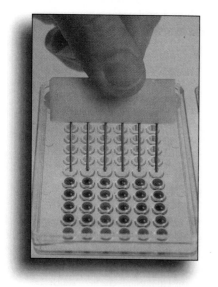

Blood is composed of a fluid portion called **plasma** and a cellular portion called **formed elements**. Plasma holds the cellular portion and also carries nutrients, electrolytes (salts), hormones, and waste products. Important plasma proteins include blood clotting factors; **albumin** that thickens the blood; and **globulins**, which provide protective **antibodies** against foreign invaders.

The human body contains between four and six liters of blood, accounting for about 8 percent of a person's weight. The plasma portion of the blood is approximately half the volume of the whole blood and about 4 to 5 percent of body weight. **Serum** is plasma without the **fibrinogen**, a globulin that helps to produce clotting. Serum is used to provide antibodies to patients whose own bodies are not producing enough of a specific type of antibody. To obtain serum, whole blood is allowed to stand in a tube or container until it clots and drops to the bottom of the container. The fluid that remains on top is the serum.

The volume of blood and its cellular components changes over an individual's life span. As a person grows and more tissue mass develops, the proportion of blood decreases. Table 5.1 depicts these changes and translates the amounts into household measurements.

Table 5.1

Blood Volume by Age

Age	Weight (kg)	Total blood volume (mL/kg)	Measurement (cup(s))
Premature infant	2.4	90-105	0.95
Newborns	3.3	78-86	1.1
1-year-old	9.6	73-78	3
5-year-old	18.0	80-86	6.15
Adult (male)	70.0	68-88	22

Hematopoiesis

Blood and bone marrow contain three main types of blood cells: (1) **erythrocytes**, also called red blood cells; (2) **leukocytes**, or white blood cells; and (3) **thrombocytes**, or platelets. Leukocytes have two subgroups: (1) **granulocytes**, which include **neutrophils**, **eosinophils**, and **basophils**; and (2) **agranulocytes**, which include **lymphocytes** and **monocytes**. Table 5.2 lists the cell groups along with their normal values (number or percentage in a given amount of blood fluid), functions, life spans, and associated illnesses.

Hematopoiesis (sometimes spelled *hemopoiesis*), or blood cell formation, begins in the bone marrow with the stem cell, which is called "uncommitted" because it can become any type of cell as it matures and differentiates. Special **hormones** called **colony-stimulating factors** are released in response to the body's needs for blood cells. The process is not well understood, but the factors influence the number and rate at which specific blood cells are produced. The factors are probably released in response to a feedback mechanism to ensure that the body has an appropriate supply of the various blood cells.

Table 5.2

The Blood Cells

Blood cell	Normal value	Function	Life span	Associated illnesses
erythrocytes (red blood cells, or RBCs)	4.0-5.5/mm^3	carry oxygen and carbon dioxide	120 days	hemorrhage; chronic anoxia
leukocytes (white blood cells, or WBCs)	5,000-10,000/mm^3	defend the body against outside invaders		infection, bone marrow failure
Subgroup granulocytes				
neutrophils	50-70%	seek, ingest, and kill bacteria	6 hours	acute infection
eosinophils	1-4%	defend against parasites and allergens	unknown	allergic reactions; parasites
basophils	0.4%	contain histamine and heparin, but role is uncertain	7 days	
Subgroup agranulocytes				
lymphocytes (lymphs)	20-40%	play key role in immunity by producing antibodies		
monocytes	2-8%	phagocytic cells that engulf and kill bacteria and play a role in killing tumor cells		
thrombocytes (platelets, or Plts)	140,000-450,000/mm^3	promote hemostasis by forming a plug (clot) at the site of an injury to a blood vessel	7 days	

Erythrocytes (Red Blood Cells)

The production of red blood cells (RBC) is called **erythropoiesis**, and it is controlled by the hormone **erythropoietin**. When the body requires more RBCs—for example, in conditions such as hypoxia (decreased oxygen level) and anemia (decreased number of RBCs)—cells in the kidney secrete erythropoietin. During the process of differentiation, a stem cell becomes a particular type of blood cell. In one of the steps in forming an erythrocyte the nucleus of the cell is lost and hemoglobin (HGB), the oxygen-carrying pigment, is formed and becomes the primary component. The new RBC then enters the body's circulation.

The RBC is biconcave in shape, meaning it resembles a caved-in disk. It is thick around the rim, thin in the middle, soft, and pliable. RBCs carry oxygen to the cells in the form of **oxyhemoglobin**, the molecule formed when oxygen and hemoglobin meet. RBCs also transport the waste product carbon dioxide away from the cells and to the lungs, where it is exhaled.

Blood Types

Each person has a particular blood type (A, B, AB, or O), depending on the kind of antigens (proteins) located on the surface of their RBCs. The body recognizes antigens that belong in the host body, as well as antigens invading from the outside. To protect itself from foreign antigens, the body produces substances called **antibodies**, which reside in blood plasma. When antibodies react with RBC antigens, they may **agglutinate**, or clump together (see Figure 5.1). These RBC antibodies are called **isohemagglutinins**.

Figure 5.1 - Agglutination

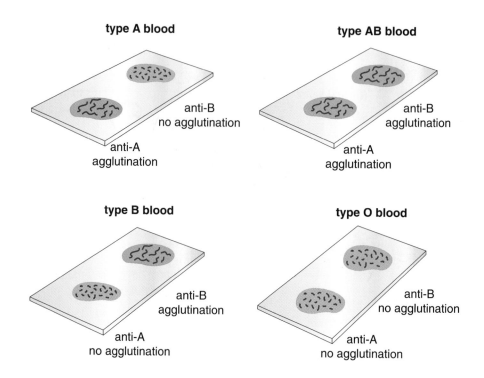

Blood type letters represent the antigens on the surface of the RBCs. Persons with blood type A do not have antibodies, or agglutinins, against A, but do have them against B (anti-B); persons with type O blood have anti-A and anti-B agglutinins; persons with type AB blood have no circulating agglutinins. Agglutinins are inherited, but may be produced by exposure to the RBCs of another person, either through a transfusion or during pregnancy. Table 5.3 lists blood types and compatibilities.

Blood is also classified by the Rh system, so named for the *Rhesus* monkey in which it was first studied. The Rh system is composed of many antigens, with D being the most antigenic (having the most antigens). Therefore, an Rh-positive individual has the agglutinogen D. An Rh-negative person does not have the agglutinogen D but reacts by forming antigens against D if exposed to Rh-positive blood cells. In addition to the ABO and Rh systems, there are many other antigenic systems based on the characteristics of RBCs.

Before blood is **transfused** to a person, the donor's blood is typed and cross-matched with that of the recipient. A sample of each is mixed together to determine whether the blood types are compatible. If they are not, the mixture will clump, or agglutinate.

Table 5.3

Blood Types and Transfusions

If a person's blood type is	Agglutinins in plasma	Frequency of occurrence	Can be safely transfused with (receive)
type A	anti-B	40%	types A, O
type B	anti-A	10%	types B, O
type AB	none	4%	types A, B, AB, O (universal recipient)
type O	anti-A, anti-B	45%	type O (universal donor)
Rh positive	none	85%	should receive Rh-positive blood but may receive Rh-negative blood if necessary
Rh negative	anti-D	15%	may receive only Rh-negative blood

Blood typing determines compatibilities.

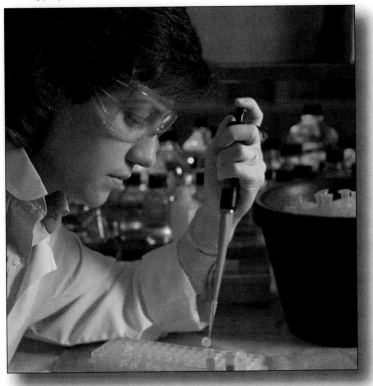

Leukocytes (White Blood Cells)

The leukocytes (white blood cells or WBCs) are the body's soldiers, ready and able to attack and destroy bacteria and other foreign invaders. Named for their nearly white appearance under the microscope, WBCs cannot be viewed unless a stain is first applied to the slide. Normally there are 5,000-10,000 WBCs per microliter of blood.

The WBCs are divided into two primary groups: **granulocytes** (so-named because of a grainy appearance when properly stained and seen under a microscope); and **agranulocytes** (without a grainy appearance). Each of these groups has subgroups, as shown in Figure 5.2. The granulocytes are sometimes called **polymorphonuclear leukocytes**, PMNs, polys, or segs. The three types of granulocytes are neutrophils, eosinophils, and basophils, and each has a particular defensive function (see Table 5.2). The agranulocytes include lymphocytes and monocytes, each with their own unique defensive mission.

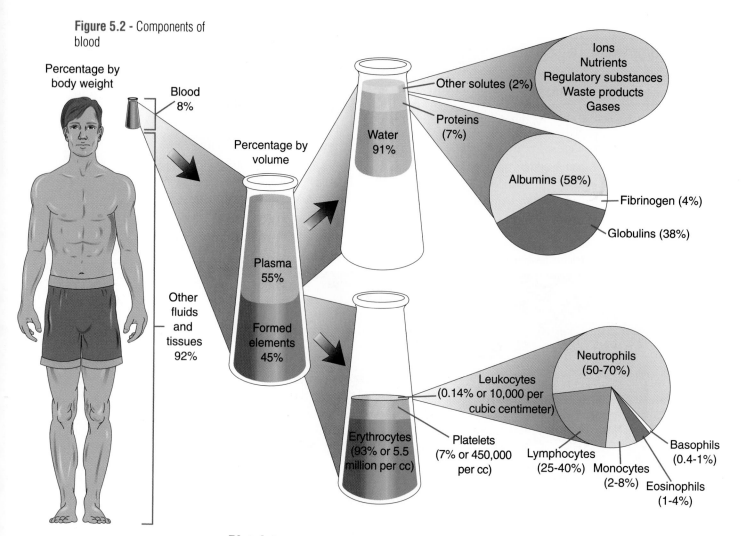

Figure 5.2 - Components of blood

Percentage by body weight

Blood 8%

Other fluids and tissues 92%

Percentage by volume

Plasma 55%

Formed elements 45%

Water 91%

Other solutes (2%)

Ions
Nutrients
Regulatory substances
Waste products
Gases

Proteins (7%)

Albumins (58%)

Fibrinogen (4%)

Globulins (38%)

Leukocytes (0.14% or 10,000 per cubic centimeter)

Erythrocytes (93% or 5.5 million per cc)

Platelets (7% or 450,000 per cc)

Neutrophils (50-70%)

Lymphocytes (25-40%)

Monocytes (2-8%)

Basophils (0.4-1%)

Eosinophils (1-4%)

Platelets

Platelets are small cells that form in the bone marrow from **megakaryocytes,** or giant cells. Each microliter of circulating blood contains about 300,000 platelets, which live about seven days. Platelets rush to the site of an injury and adhere to the blood vessel wall, helping the body form a clot. The hormone that regulates platelet production is **thrombopoietin.** (Immunoglobulins and lymphocytes are discussed further in Chapter 6, "The Immune System.")

Clotting

As part of the body's work to maintain normal functioning of the blood (hemostasis), it immediately reacts to stop the bleeding when a blood vessel is damaged. It does so by launching three processes: (1) vascular constriction (of small blood vessels) to decrease blood flow; (2) platelet plug formation; and (3) local blood coagulation, leading to a fibrin thrombus formation (blood clot).

The clotting process begins when the damaged tissue exposes collagen to the circulating blood. This collagen exposure causes certain clotting factors and platelets to come to the site of the injury. As the platelets arrive, they become sticky and form a temporary hemostatic plug. These platelets also release chemicals that stimulate the **prothrombin** activator, which, when combined with calcium in the blood, triggers a series of events known as the clotting cascade (Figure 5.3). This process forms a stable clot in less than fifteen minutes.

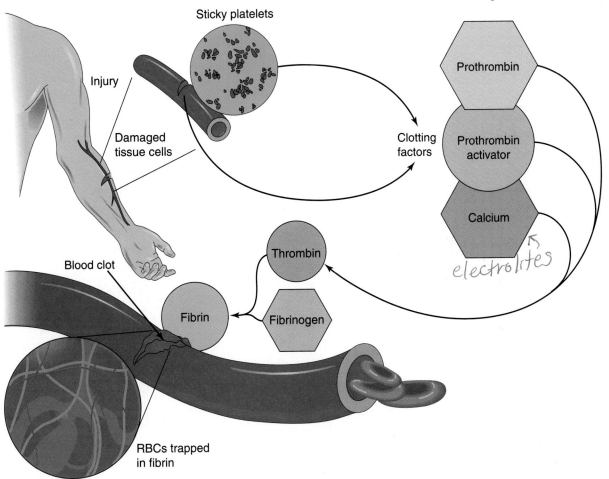

Figure 5.3 - Clotting Cascade

Table 5.4 lists common combining forms for hematology, and Table 5.5 presents anatomy and physiology terms related to the field.

Table 5.4

Combining Forms Relating to Hematology-Oncology

Combining form	Meaning	Example
anis/o	unequal	anisocytosis
bas/o	Greek for base, basis	basophil
blast/o	immature cell	blastogenesis
-blast	immature cell	myeloblast
chrom/o	Greek for color	chromatography
cyt/o	Greek for cell	cytospin
-cyte	Greek for cell	lymphocyte
echin/o	prickly	echinocyte
erythr/o	red	erythrocyte
granul/o	granular, granules	granulocyte
hemat/o	blood	hematologist
hem/o	blood	hemolysis
kary/o	nucleus	megakaryocyte
leuk/o	white	leukocyte
lymph/o	lymph	lymphadenopathy

continued on next page

morph/o	shape	morphology
myel/o	bone marrow	myelofibrosis
neutr/o	neutral	neutrophil
nucle/o	nucleus	nucleoli
onc/o	tumor	oncologic
organ/o	organ	organomegaly
phag/o	eating	phagocytosis
plasm/o	formed; plasma	plasmapheresis
-poiesis	production	hematopoiesis
poikil/o	irregular	poikilocytosis
reticul/o	reticulum (a fine network of cells)	reticulocyte
schist/o	split	schistocyte
ser/o	serum (fluid part of blood)	serous
sider/o	iron	siderosis
spher/o	sphere-shaped	spherocyte
splen/o	pertaining to the spleen	splenectomy
stomat/o	mouth	stomatocytosis
thromb/o	blood clot	thrombosis

Table 5.5

Anatomy and Physiology Terms Relating to the Blood

Term	Meaning	Word Analysis	
agglutinate ah-**gloo**-tih-nayt	to adhere and form clumps	a- gluten	to glue
agranulocyte **A-gran**-yoo-lO-sIt	WBC that does not have a granulated appearance when a stain is applied	a granul/o -cyte	without granular cell
albumin al-**byoo**-min	protein in the blood	albumin	white of the egg
anemia ah-**nee**-mee-ah	condition of decreased hemoglobin level	an- hem/o -ia	without blood condition of
antibody **an**-tih-bod-ee	immunoglobulin in the blood that is produced in response to an antigen; a protective protein produced by the body	anti- body	against body
antigen **an**-tih-jen	substance that produces an immune response	anti- -gen	against to produce
basophil **bay**-sO-fil	WBC that contains histamine and heparin; its role is uncertain	bas/o -phil	base affinity for; fondness
catalyst **kat**-ah-list	substance that accelerates a chemical reaction	cata- -lyze	down to break up
coagulation kO-ag-yoo-**lay**-shun	to cause clotting	coagulate	to curdle
corpuscle **kor**-pus-sl	blood cell	corpuscle	body
differentiate dif-er-**en**-shee-ayt	to produce more than one characteristic; having more than one characteristic	differentiate	to carry apart

Term	Definition	Word Parts	Meaning
eosinophil e-oh-sin-oh-fill	WBC that defends against parasites and allergens	eosin phil	a dye fond
erythrocyte er-ih-thrO-sites	blood cells that carry oxygen and carbon dioxide	erythr/o cyte	red cell
erythropoiesis er-ih-thrO-poy-**ee**-sis	process of producing RBCs (erythrocytes)	erythr/o -poiesis	red making; producing
erythropoietin er-ih-thrO-**poy**-et-in	hormone that simulates RBC production	erythr/o -poiesis	red making; producing
fibrin **fI**-brin	elastic protein that is part of the clotting mechanism	fibr/o	fiber
fibrinogen fI-**brin**-O-jen	globulin within the blood that helps to produce a clot	fibr/o -gen	fiber to make
globulin **glob**-yoo-lin	protein in the serum	globulin	globule
glycoprotein **glI**-kO-**prO**-tee-in	substance of combined carbohydrate and protein	glyc/o prōtos	pertaining to sugar first
granulocyte **gran**-yoo-lO-sIt	WBC that has a granulated appearance when a stain is applied	granul/o -cyte	granular cell
hematopoiesis **hem**-ah-tO-poy-**ee**-sis	formation and maturation of blood cells	hemat/o -poiesis	blood making; producing
hemoglobin **hee**-mO-**glO**-bin	protein in the RBC that carries oxygen	hem/o -globin	blood globule
hormone **hor**-mOn	chemical substance secreted by specific organs and/or glands and carried into the bloodstream to stimulate another organ	hormone	to set in motion
hypochromic hI-pO-**krO**-mik	RBC that has decreased hemoglobin	hyp/o -chrom -ic	under, less color pertaining to
hypoxia hI-**poks**-ee-ah	having too little oxygen	hyp/o -oxy -ia	under, less oxygen condition of
index **in**-deks indices **in**-dih-seez	standard; refers to the measurements of the size and amount of oxygen of the RBC in relationship to the total volume of the blood specimen	index	to point out
isohemagglutinin I-sO-hem-ah-**gloo**-tih-nin	antibody against a specific RBC antigen	is/o hem/o ad- gluten	equal blood to glue
leukocyte **loo**-kO-sIt	WBC that defends the body against outside invaders	leuk/o -cyte	white cell
lymphocyte **lim**-fO-sIt	WBC involved in immunity	lymph/o -cyte	pertaining to lymph cell
macrocyte **mak**-rO-sIt	large RBC	macro- -cyte	large cell
megakaryocyte meg-ah-**kar**-ee-O-sIt	young cell that produces the thrombocyte (platelet)	mega- kary/o -cyte	large nucleus cell
microcyte **mI**-krO-sIt	small RBC	micro- -cyte	small cell

continued on next page

monocyte **mon**-O-sIt	one of the WBCs found in lymph nodes, the spleen, and bone marrow; a phagocytic cell that engulfs and kills bacteria and plays a role in tumor cell kill	mono- -cyte	one cell
neutrophil **noo**-trO-fil	WBC that seeks, ingests, and kills bacteria	neutron phil	neutral (dye) fond
oxyhemoglobin oks-ee-hee-mO-**glO**-bin	combination of oxygen and hemoglobin; oxygenated blood of the arteries	oxy- hem/o globin	oxygen blood globule
plasma **plaz**-mah	non-cellular portion of the blood	plasma	formed
platelet **playt**-let	blood cell that helps form the plug that stops bleeding at the site of an injury	platelet	flat
polymorphonuclear leukocyte (PMN) **pol**-ee-mor-fO-**noo**-klee-ar **loo**-kO-sIt	variety of leukocytes that have various forms of nuclei	poly- morph/o nucle/o -ar leuk/o -cyte	many shape nucleus pertaining to white cell
prothrombin prO-**throm**-bin	protein necessary for clot formation	pro- thromb/o	before blood clot
serum **seer**-um	fluid portion of the blood	ser/o -um	serum structure
thrombin **throm**-bin	enzyme that is the final step in the formation of a clot	thromb/o	blood clot
thrombocyte **throm**-bo-site (platelet)	blood cell that helps form the plug that stops bleeding at the site of an injury	thrombo cyte	clot cell
thrombopoietin throm-bO-**poy**-eh-tin	hormone that stimulates platelet cell formation	thromb/o -poiesis	blood clot making; producing
thrombopoiesis throm-bO-poy-**ee**-sis	process of platelet formation		
transfusion trans-**fyoo**-zhun	process of moving a blood product from one person's body to another	trans- fusion	across; transfer to connect

Word Analysis

Exercise 1

Separate the terms into their word parts and give a definition for each whole term. Use hyphens to separate the word parts and label each part (P = prefix, R = root, S = suffix, CV = combining vowel).

	Word analysis	Definition
1. anemia	_____	_____
2. microcytic	_____	_____
3. hypochromic	_____	_____
4. nuclear	_____	_____
5. splenectomy	_____	_____
6. hepatomegaly	_____	_____

7. granulocyte _____ _____

8. blastogenesis _____ _____

9. hematologist _____ _____

10. erythrocyte _____ _____

Comprehension Check

Read each sentence and circle the term that is most appropriate.

1. Erythropoiesis/Hematopoiesis means formation of red blood cells.

2. Hypoxia/Hyperoxia means decreased oxygen.

3. Microcytic/Macrocytic means "pertaining to large cells."

4. Leukocytes/Melanocytes/erythrocytes are white blood cells.

5. Phrenology/Hematology/Oncology is the study of the blood.

6. Hypermegaly/Organomegaly means an enlarged organ.

7. Oncocytosis/Phagocytosis means "cell-eating."

8. The term reticulocytes/remocytes refer to a network of cells.

9. Hemostasis/Homeostasis is a condition of appropriate blood clotting.

10. Dermatophylic/Hematophylic means "attraction to blood."

Matching

Match the term or abbreviation in Column 1 with the correct definition in Column 2. Write the letter of the definition on the line beside the term.

Column 1		Column 2
1. antibodies	__8__	a. protein substance against which antibodies are produced
2. antigen	__10__	b. abbreviation for red blood cell
3. oxyhemoglobin	__2__	c. provide antibodies against foreign invaders
4. hemoglobin	__1__	d. protect the body from foreign antigens
5. catalyze	__9__	e. abbreviation for complete blood count
6. serum	__3__	f. combination of oxygen and hemoglobin
7. plasma	__4__	g. oxygen-carrying pigment in red blood cells
8. globulins	__6__	h. plasma without fibrinogen
9. CBC	__5__	i. to speed up
10. RBC	__7__	j. fluid that contains cellular components of blood

Word Building

Supply roots, combining forms, or word parts to create a term that completes each sentence.

1. Blasto_genesis_ means immature cell origin.

2. A _Leuko_cyte is a white cell.

3. Phago_cyto_sis means cell eating.

4. _____ous means pertaining to serum.

5. Baso_phil_ is an affinity for alkaline (base) dye.

6. Hepato_megaly_ refers to enlargement of the liver.

7. A hemato_logist_ is one who studies the blood.

8. Chromato_gram_ is the process of recording color.

9. A _megalocyto_phage is a large eating (cell).

10. Schisto_cyte_ means split cell.

Spelling Check

Choose the correctly spelled word from each pair in the following sentences.

1. To obtain serum/serium, the cellular components of blood are allowed to clot, leaving only the fluid.

2. Plasma/Pilazma is the fluid portion of the blood.

3. Albumin/Albuminum and globulins/gobulines are plasma proteins.

4. Oxyhemoglobin/Oxihemaglobin is the molecule formed when oxygen and hemoglobin join.

5. Large RBCs are called macrocytes/macrocysts; small RBCs are called microcytes/microcysts.

6. Hypoxia/Hyproxia is a condition of decreased oxygen.

7. Plataletes/Platelets have a life span of about seven days.

8. Thrombocytes promote homostansis/hemostasis by forming a plug at the site of injury to a blood vessel.

9. Leukocytes/Luekocytes defend the body against outside invaders.

10. Vascular constriction/vescular construction is among the first of the body's responses to a blood vessel injury.

Draw a simple diagram of lines and boxes that shows the relationships among the following terms. *Hint:* Think in terms of groups and subgroups.

WBCs   RBCs   thrombocytes
cellular components   serum   plasma
fibrinogen   whole blood

glob for clot

Assessing Patient Health

Wellness and Illness through the Life Span

The status of a patient's blood system is best evaluated by laboratory tests. However, certain aspects of patient history and physical examination can provide insight into the hematological system. For example, the examiner queries the patient about activities: "Do you get out of breath when walking up stairs?" If the answer is "yes," it might mean that the patient is out of shape, or the patient may be anemic. The examiner also observes the coloring of the patient, including the lips, the inside of the mouth, the mucous membranes of the lower inner eyelid, and the nailbeds. These areas should be pink. If any are pale, the condition is noted as **pallor**, which may indicate **anemia**.

The physician pays particular attention to the liver and spleen. An enlarged liver, **hepatomegaly**, may suggest **hemolysis** (destruction of RBCs), congestive heart failure, or **extramedullary hematopoiesis** (blood cell production in sites other than the bone marrow). **Splenomegaly**, or enlarged spleen, may indicate that blood cells are being **sequestered**, or trapped, in that organ, or it may point to extramedullary hematopoiesis or hemolysis.

Fetuses, Infants, and Children

Specific kinds of blood cells can be recognized in the fetus by the third week of gestation. As blood vessels develop, stem cells migrate to the future sites of blood production. The liver is the main site of blood cell production from the second to sixth month of gestation, at which time blood formation starts in the bone marrow. During fetal life, the spleen, lymph nodes, and thymus are also sites of hematopoiesis (see Figure 5.4).

Figure 5.4 - Hematopoiesis Tree

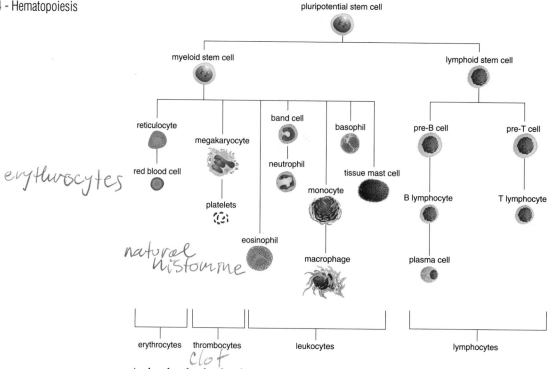

erythrocytes

natural histamine

clot

At birth, the body's bone marrow is the chief factory for blood production. The liver ceases to produce blood cells two weeks after birth. In infants, blood cells are actively produced in the medullary cavities of all of the bones (red marrow). During childhood, active marrow in the long bones is replaced by fatty tissue (yellow marrow), so that by the time a person reaches their 20th birthday, active blood production takes place only in the skull, vertebrae, sternum, ribs, clavicles, scapulae, and pelvis. However, in disease states such as **sickle cell anemia** (abnormally low levels of hemoglobin produced by sickle-shaped RBCs) or **myelofibrosis** (the forming of fibrous tissue in the bone marrow), the yellow marrow and fetal hematopoietic organs can resume active hematopoiesis. When fetal hematopoietic organs resume making blood cells, it is called **extramedullary hematopoiesis**.

As mentioned earlier, a person's blood group and Rh type are inherited from the parents. This inheritance becomes significant when an Rh-negative mother is carrying an Rh-positive fetus. The Rh factor on the fetal red cells may stimulate the mother's body to form anti-D antibodies. The production of anti-D antibodies may not be a problem for the first pregnancy, but if the Rh-negative mother carries another Rh-positive fetus, her antibodies may cause **erythroblastosis fetalis**, a severe, life-threatening anemia, in the baby. Treatment consists of **intrauterine** (inside the womb) **transfusions** or **exchange transfusions** with Rh-negative blood immediately after birth. Today, Rh-negative mothers who carry Rh-positive fetuses are given a protein marketed as RhoGAM. This drug prevents the mother's body from forming anti-D antibodies, thus preventing harm to any subsequent Rh-positive baby.

The most common hematologic disorder in infancy and childhood is dietary **iron deficiency**, since the human diet during the first year contains very few foods rich in iron. The infant's rapid growth during the first year of life depletes iron stores, leaving the baby dependent on iron from foods. Dietary iron deficiency is common from about nine to twenty-four months of age.

The possibility of **occult blood loss** must be considered in every child with iron deficiency anemia. Gastrointestinal bleeding can be caused by a peptic ulcer, Meckel's diverticulum (a pouch or sac in the intestine remaining from a stage of embryonic development), or polyps (see Chapter 12). In infants, gastrointestinal bleeding may result from intolerance to cow's milk.

Many childhood diseases associated with the blood system are of genetic origin, meaning that they are passed from the parent to the child through the genes. Table 5.6 lists the major hereditary blood diseases.

Table 5.6

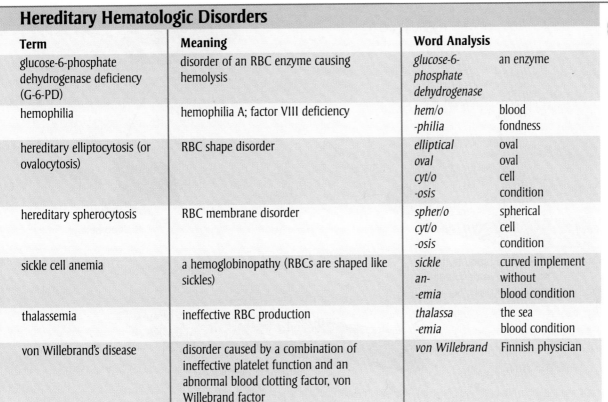

Hereditary Hematologic Disorders

Term	Meaning	Word Analysis	
glucose-6-phosphate dehydrogenase deficiency (G-6-PD)	disorder of an RBC enzyme causing hemolysis	glucose-6-phosphate dehydrogenase	an enzyme
hemophilia	hemophilia A; factor VIII deficiency	hem/o	blood
		-philia	fondness
hereditary elliptocytosis (or ovalocytosis)	RBC shape disorder	elliptical	oval
		oval	oval
		cyt/o	cell
		-osis	condition
hereditary spherocytosis	RBC membrane disorder	spher/o	spherical
		cyt/o	cell
		-osis	condition
sickle cell anemia	a hemoglobinopathy (RBCs are shaped like sickles)	sickle	curved implement
		an-	without
		-emia	blood condition
thalassemia	ineffective RBC production	thalassa	the sea
		-emia	blood condition
von Willebrand's disease	disorder caused by a combination of ineffective platelet function and an abnormal blood clotting factor, von Willebrand factor	von Willebrand	Finnish physician

Sickle cell anemia is a hereditary disorder that has been well publicized through medical articles in newspapers and magazines. It is the most common **hemoglobinopathy** (hemoglobin-related disease) in the United States, but it also occurs widely throughout Africa, the Mediterranean, and the Middle East. Sickle cell anemia is caused by an abnormal hemoglobin that makes the RBCs assume a sickle shape. These sickle-shaped cells are less pliable and get caught in the blood vessels, causing painful crises (episodes) that may lead to inadequate blood circulation and tissue death in the affected body part. Typical sites of vessel-blocking crises include: (1) the bones of the hand and foot, resulting in the **hand-foot syndrome**, which commonly occurs in infants during the first year of life; (2) other bones throughout the body; (3) the central nervous system, producing **cerebral thrombosis** (stroke) and **hemorrhage**; (4) the abdomen; (5) the chest, sometimes resulting in **acute chest syndrome**, a severe, life-threatening **infarction** of the lung; and (6) the penis, where **priapism** (prolonged penile erection) can occur. Figure 5.5 illustrates the path of a sickle cell crisis. Trace the pathway of events leading to the blocking of the blood vessel.

Figure 5.5 - Vaso-Occlusive
Crisis

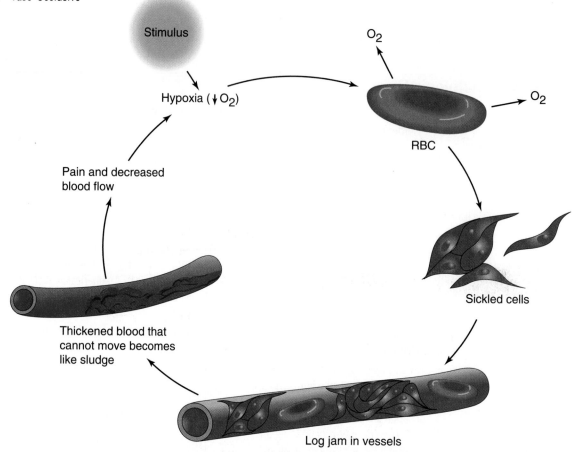

Stimulus

Hypoxia ($\downarrow O_2$)

O_2

O_2

RBC

Pain and decreased
blood flow

Sickled cells

Thickened blood that
cannot move becomes
like sludge

Log jam in vessels

The enzyme **glucose-6-phosphate dehydrogenase (G-6-PD)** is found in all cells. A deficiency of this enzyme in the red blood cell results in **hemolytic anemia**, or G-6-PD deficiency, in which the red blood cells are rapidly destroyed, or **hemolyzed**. Glucose-6-phosphate dehydrogenase deficiency is a hereditary disorder that can be triggered by exposure to certain foods, infections, and medications.

Hereditary spherocytosis occurs in 1 of every 5,000 individuals. It is a disorder of the RBC membrane that causes the cell to assume a sphere-shape (hence their name, *spherocytes*). Spherocytes become sequestered in the spleen, resulting in hemolysis, anemia, and splenomegaly.

Thalassemia becomes evident clinically in the second half of the first year of life when the infant loses his or her fetal hemoglobin. Pallor, splenomegaly, and decreased appetite are the typical presenting signs. Thalassemia is caused by an inequal production of alpha and other globin chains, which results in ineffective production of RBCs. Extramedullary hematopoiesis produces progressive enlargement of the spleen and liver. Treatment involves administering RBC transfusions to maintain a fairly normal hemoglobin level, but iron overload, or **hemosiderosis**, from repeated blood transfusions is a side effect that involves every organ in the body. Death from cardiac hemosiderosis usually occurs during the second or third decade of life.

Another hereditary disorder, **von Willebrand's disease**, is caused by abnormal platelet function and a decreased level of von Willebrand factor. The disorder is characterized by easy bruising, **epistaxis** (nosebleeds), bleeding from gums, oozing from cuts, **menorrhagia**, and severe bleeding after trauma or surgery.

Hemophilia is a genetic disorder that often first becomes apparent when an infant boy bleeds excessively after circumcision. It is caused by a decreased or dysfunctional factor VIII that is carried by the female and transmitted to the male. Hemophilia is linked to the X chromosome. A female carrier has a 50:50 chance that each son will have hemophilia and a 50:50 chance that each daughter will be a carrier. A hemophilic male cannot transmit the disease to his sons, but all of his daughters will be carriers.

Fanconi's anemia is a hereditary condition associated with congenital anomalies, including **microcephaly**, **microphthalmia**, absence of radii and thumbs, abnormalities of heart and kidney, short stature, and hyperpigmentation of the skin. The average age at onset is 6 to 8 years; bruising due to **thrombocytopenia** may be the first symptom. In about 5 to 10 percent of cases, acute myelogenous leukemia will develop.

Adults

Iron deficiency as a result of gastrointestinal bleeding occurs in the adult. There may be an underlying problem such as an ulcer, gastrointestinal cancer, polyps, or other GI disorders (discussed in Chapter 12, "The Gastrointestinal System").

Myelodysplasia, or **myelodysplastic syndrome**, occurs most frequently in adults. Patients with ineffective hematopoiesis produce fewer circulating blood cells. The cells the body can produce may be abnormal in shape and appearance. Myelodysplastic syndrome is usually associated with a preleukemic state.

Vitamin B_{12} deficiency, also known as **pernicious anemia**, causes **megaloblastic anemia**. A healthy diet should contain enough B_{12} to maintain normal metabolic functions, but if a deficiency or a problem with absorption in the gastrointestinal tract exists, the body cannot form enough blood cells. Erythrocytes, which become larger than normal but fewer in number, are most frequently involved, and the imbalance causes the anemia.

Seniors

Polycythemia vera is a disorder associated with a high hemoglobin level that arises from an increase in total RBC volume. Often a sign of a preleukemic state, this disorder is potentially dangerous because it causes an increase in blood **viscosity**, or thickness, and the heightened risk of **thrombosis** (see below).

General Illnesses

When blood leaks outside a blood vessel, either from a traumatic injury or from spontaneous causes, an **ecchymosis** is formed. Usually an ecchymosis (plural: ecchymoses) will change color from the immediate reddish-purple spot, fade to brown, and then disappear, as the collected blood under the skin is cleared away by the body's own mechanisms. A severe injury may result in a **hematoma** (a large, firm collection of blood) that may require surgical intervention if it does not resolve on its own. The disorder **immune thrombocytopenic purpura (ITP)** can occur at any age; the acute form is seen most often in children, while the chronic form, defined as lasting at least one year, is more common in adults. ITP occurs when the spleen destroys platelet-antibody complexes, resulting in a low platelet count. The body's decreased clotting ability places the patient at risk for life-threatening bleeding. Treatment consists of drugs that fool the immune system into slowing the destruction of platelets, but if treatment does not maintain a safe platelet count the patient may need to undergo a **splenectomy**.

Aplastic anemia is often **idiopathic** (of an unknown cause), but may be the result of ionizing radiation, chemotherapeutic agents, benzene, or other agents. Many factors can decrease bone marrow function and the production of blood cells.

An autoimmune disorder is one that occurs when the body forms antibodies against itself. **Autoimmune hemolytic anemia** is caused by antibodies that destroy RBCs, which leads to anemia.

Thrombosis is a condition of increased clotting that occurs within the blood vessels. The clot is called a **thrombus**, and when a thrombus forms in a vital organ, such as the brain or heart, its effects can be life threatening. A stroke may be caused by a thrombus. If the thrombus dislodges and travels through the bloodstream, it is called an **embolus**.

Many abnormalities of the blood are defined by the number, size, and shape, or morphology, of the blood cells. Tables 5.7 through 5.10 list the terms for these abnormalities. Table 5.11 lists common wellness and illness terms associated with the hematologic system.

Table 5.7

Abnormalities in the Number of Blood Cells

Type and subtype	Too few	Too many
leukocytes (white blood cells)	leukocytopenia	leukocytosis
granulocytes	granulocytopenia	granulocytosis
neutrophils	neutropenia	neutrophilia
eosinophils		eosinophilia
basophils		basophilia
agranulocytes		
lymphocytes	lymphocytopenia	lymphocytosis
monocytes		monocytosis
erythrocytes (red blood cells)	erythrocytopenia	erythrocytosis polycythemia
reticulocytes		reticulocytosis
thrombocytes (platelets)	thrombocytopenia	thrombocytosis

Table 5.8

Abnormalities in the Color of Blood Cells*

Term	Meaning	Word Analysis	
hypochromia hI-pO-**krO**-mee-ah	too little hemoglobin	hypo- chrom/o -ia	less than color condition of
polychromasia **pol**-ee-krO-**may**-zee-ah	purple-tinged when stained; young red blood cell that is seen with increased red blood cell production as in pernicious anemia or any hemolytic anemia or in response to any blood loss	poly- chrom/o -ia	many color condition of

*Refers to the amount of hemoglobin in the red blood cells

Table 5.9

Abnormalities in the Size of Blood Cells

Term	Meaning	Word Analysis	
microcyte **mI**-krO-sIt microcytic mI-krO-**sit**-ik	small RBC	*micro-* *-cyte*	small cell
macrocyte **mak**-rO-sIt macrocytic mak-rO-**sit**-ik	large RBC	*macro-* *-cyte*	large cell

Table 5.10

Abnormalities in the Morphology of Red Blood Cells

Term	Meaning	Word Analysis	
anisocytosis **an**-is-O-sI-**tO**-sis	variation in the size of cells	*anis/o* *cyt/o* *-osis*	unequal cell condition
echinocyte ee-**kI**-nO-sIt	loss of fluid of the RBC causes the cell to have a spiny appearance	*echin/o* *-cyte*	spiny cell
elliptocyte eh-**lip**-tO-sIt	elliptical-shaped cell	*ellipt/o* *-cyte*	ellipse cell
helmet cell	helmet-shaped cell	*helmet*	shape
ovalocyte **O**-vah-lO-sIt	oval-shaped cell	*oval* *-cyte*	oval cell
poikilocyte poy-**kil**-O-sIt	irregularly shaped cell	*poikil/o* *-cyte*	irregular cell
rouleaux roo-**lO**	a stack of RBCs	*rouleaux*	to roll
schistocyte **skis**-tO-sIt	oddly shaped cell	*schist/o* *-cyte*	cleft cell
sickle cell	sickle-shaped cell	*sickle*	shape
spherocyte **sfee**-rO-sIt	sphere-shaped cell	*spher/o* *-cyte*	globe cell
stippled cell	speckled cell	*stippled*	appearance
stomatocyte **stO**-mah-tO-sIt	mouth-shaped pallor in the center of RBC	*stomat/o* *-cyte*	mouth cell
target cell	target-like; bulls-eye in the center of RBC	*target*	shape

Table 5.11

Wellness and Illness Terms Relating to the Blood

Term	Meaning	Word Analysis	
anemia ah-**nee**-mee-ah	condition of decreased hemoglobin level	*an-* *-emia*	without blood
anomaly ah-**nom**-ah-lee	condition or appearance that is different from normal	*anomaly*	irregular
aplasia ah-**play**-zha	defective development of a blood cell line	*a-* *-plasia*	without formation

continued on next page

Term	Definition	Word Parts	
autoimmune aw-tO-ih-**myoon**	process in which the person's immune system turns against itself (relating to antibodies that attack the cells of the body producing them)	auto immun/o	one; oneself free from catching a specific infectious disease
ecchymosis ek-im-**O**-sis	black and blue mark caused by leakage of blood from the vessel	ec- chyme -osis	out of; away from juice condition
embolus **em**-bO-lus	clot that has broken loose within the body	embolus	a plug
epistaxis ep-ih-**staks**-is	nosebleed	epi- -stazo	upon to fall in drops
erythroblastosis fetalis **er**-ih-thrO-blas-tO-sis fee-**tay**-lis	life-threatening disorder caused by an incompatibility between mother and fetal blood *RH*	erythr/o blast/o -osis fetalis	red young cell condition of the fetus
extramedullary eks-trah-**med**-yoo-lar-ee	outside the bone marrow cavity	extra- medulla -ary	beyond the marrow space pertaining to
hematoma **hee**-ma-tO-mah	an area of blood that has extravasated from the vessel and is confined in a space	hem/o -oma	blood tumor
hemoglobinopathy hee-mO-glO-bin-**op**-ah-thee	disease caused by a problem with the hemoglobin	hem/o globin -pathy	blood globule disease
hemolysis hee-**mol**-ih-sis hemolyze **hee**-mO-lIz	destruction of the RBC	hem/o -lysis	blood destruction
hemorrhage **hem**-ah-rej	uncontrolled bleeding	hem/o -rrhage	blood to burst forth
hemosiderosis hee-mO-sid-er-**O**-sis hemosiderin **hee**-mO-**sid**-er-in	accumulation of a greenish- yellow substance caused by iron in the blood	hem/o sider/o -osis	blood iron condition
hepatomegaly **hep**-ah-tO-**meg**-ah-lee	enlarged liver	hepat/o -megaly	pertaining to the liver large
immune thrombocytopenic purpura im-**myoon** throm-bO-sI-tO-**pee**-nik **per**-pyoo-rah	autoimmune disorder that produces platelet antibodies and results in the destruction of the body's own platelets	immune thromb/o cyt/o -penic purpura	free from catching a specific infectious disease blood clot cell pertaining to deficiency purple
lymphoma limf-**Oh**-mah	malignancy of lymph tissue that can be localized or systemic	lymph/o -oma	pertaining to lymph tumor
megaloblastic anemia **meg**-ah-lO-**blas**-tik ah-**nee**-mee-ah	condition of enlarged erythrocytes	megal/o blast/o -ic an- -emia	large young cell pertaining to without blood

menorrhagia men-or-**raj**-ee-ah	increased or excessive menstrual flow	*men/o* *-rrhagia*	menstruation to burst forth
morphology morf-**ol**-ah-jee	study of shape	*morph/o* *-ology*	shape the study of
myelodysplasia **mI**-el-O-dis-**play**-see-ah	abnormality of the bone marrow	*myel/o* *dys-* *-plasia*	bone marrow separation formation
myelofibrosis mI-lO-fI-**brO**-sis	fibrosis of the bone marrow	*myel/o* *fibr/o* *-osis*	bone marrow fibrous condition
occult ok-**kult**	hidden	*-cultus*	to cover
pallor **pal**-or	pale appearance	*pallor*	pale
pancytopenia pan-sI-tO-**pee**-nee-ah	severe reduction of all blood cell lines	*pan-* *cyt/o* *-penia*	all, entire cell deficiency
polycythemia vera pol-ee-sI-**thee**-mee-ah **vee**-rah	condition of increased RBCs	*poly-* *cyt/o* *hem/o* *vera*	many cell blood true
splenomegaly **splee**-nO-**meg**-ah-lee	increased size of the spleen	*splen/o* *-megaly*	spleen large
thrombocytopenia throm-bO-sI-tO-**pee**-nee-ah	decreased platelets	*thromb/o* *cyt/o* *-penia*	platelet cell deficiency
thrombosis throm-**bO**-sis	clot formation in the blood vessels	*thrombosis*	clot

Cancers of the Hematopoietic System

The physician who treats cancers of the hematopoietic system is a **hematologist-oncologist**. These types of cancer usually arise in the bone marrow, the body's blood-making organ. **Leukemia** is the most common malignancy of the hematopoietic system. There are different types of leukemia, depending on the blood cell line that develops the malignant abnormality. Leukemia is manifested by the proliferation (multiplication) of abnormal blood cells within the bone marrow. For instance, acute lymphoblastic leukemia is manifested by an abnormal population of lymphoblasts in the bone marrow. Eventually, the bone marrow space becomes overpopulated by malignant cells, and the cells are pushed out of the bone marrow where they can be seen in the peripheral blood on a CBC with a differential.

The patient with leukemia may present with pallor, ecchymoses, petechiae, fatigue, history of recurrent illness, pain, and fever. All of the signs and symptoms occur because the normal blood cells are being crowded out of production by the very fast growing leukemia cells. Table 5.12 describes the types of leukemia, the cell line from which it arises, and the typical age of diagnosis.

Many of the leukemias, especially those diagnosed in childhood, are treatable and potentially curable with **chemotherapy** (*chemo*, meaning chemical; *therapy*, meaning treatment) and/or biotherapy.

Table 5.12

Types of Leukemia

Type of leukemia	Cell line	Most common age at presentation
Acute lymphoblastic leukemia	Lymphoid	Childhood
Acute myelogenous leukemia	Myeloid	Late teens-adulthood
Acute monocytic leukemia	Monocyte	Adulthood
Acute promyelocytic leukemia	Promyelocyte	Young adults
Chronic myelogenous leukemia	Myeloid	Late teens-adulthood
Chronic lymphocytic leukemia	Lymphoid	Older age

Lymphomas are a type of malignancy that affects the tissues of the lymphatic system, and they are often classified as hematologic malignancies. There are two major categories of lymphoma: **Hodgkin's**, named for the British physician who first identified it; and **non-Hodgkin** lymphoma, often classified by the specific cell type of origin. **Multiple myeloma** is a malignancy affecting plasma cells.

Word Analysis

Exercise 7

Identify the root or combining form in each of the following terms by drawing a box around it, and then supply the definition of the root and the definition of the entire term.

1. Splenomegaly can indicate that blood cells are trapped in the spleen.

    Definition: _____

2. Hemoglobinopathy is detected by laboratory tests.

    Definition: _____

3. The red blood cells are destroyed in the process of hemolysis.

    Definition: _____

4. Erythroblastopenia, a childhood disorder of red blood cell production, is transient.

    Definition: _____

5. Bruising due to thrombocytopenia may be an early manifestation of a hereditary anemia.

    Definition: _____

6. Hypopigmentation of the skin may be indicative of certain disorders.

    Definition: _____

7. The patient has severe menorrhagia.

    Definition: _____

8. Certain blood disorders can place a patient at increased risk for <u>thrombosis</u>.

Definition: _____

9. <u>Intravascular</u> coagulation refers to clotting in a specific part of the body.

Definition: _____

10. <u>Hemorrhage</u> is a life-threatening condition.

Definition: _____

Comprehension Check

Select the correct medical term from the list to substitute for the underlined definition in each sentence.

epistaxis	polycythemia vera
erythroblastosis fetalis	splenomegaly
embolus	hemolysis
occult	anomaly
anemia	autoimmune disease
myelofibrosis	menorrhagia
hematologist	hemosiderosis

1. The patient is a 60-year-old male who was diagnosed with <u>a condition of decreased hemoglobin</u>. _____

2. The child was brought to the office with severe, recurrent <u>nosebleeds</u>. _____

3. Katherine has come to the clinic today because of pronounced <u>increased menstrual flow</u>. _____

4. Plan: stool specimen for <u>hidden</u> blood. _____

5. There is no evidence of <u>increased size of the spleen</u>. _____

6. Impression is <u>a condition of increased blood cells</u>. _____

7. Postmortem laboratory studies revealed widespread <u>destruction of red blood cells</u>. _____

8. Impression is life-threatening disorder caused by <u>an incompatibility between maternal and fetal blood</u>. _____

9. Disorders of the blood are diagnosed and treated by <u>a blood specialist</u>. _____

10. The patient has <u>a process in which the person's immune system turns against itself</u>. _____

Matching

Match the term or abbreviation in Column 1 with the correct definition in Column 2. Write the number of the term on the line beside the definition.

Column 1   **Column 2**

1. hemoglobinopathy   _____   a. increased menstrual flow

2. hemosiderin   _____   b. hidden

3. morphology   _____   c. pale appearance (color of skin)

4. occult   _____   d. iron in the blood

5. epistaxis   _____   e. defective development of a blood cell line

6. extramedullary   _____   f. disease caused by problem with hemoglobin

7. menorrhagia   _____   g. study of shape

8. aplasia   _____   h. condition of increased RBCs

9. polycythemia   _____   i. outside the bone marrow

10. pallor   _____   j. nosebleed

Word Building

Supply roots, combining forms, or word parts to create a term that completes each sentence.

1. _____venous means within a vein.

2. Hemo_____ means pertaining to flow of blood.

3. Thrombo_____ is a condition of blood clot.

4. An_____ means without blood (deficiency of iron in the blood).

5. Morpho_____ is the study of shape or form.

6. _____chromic refers to less-than-sufficient color (deficiency of hemoglobin).

7. _____cyte is a large cell.

8. _____cytopenia means too few white blood cells.

9. Granulocyto_____ is a condition of granulocytes (too few granulocytes).

10. _____immune means immune to self.

Find the misspelled medical terms in each sentence, then rewrite the terms correctly and define them on the blanks provided.

1. Mr. Knowles was admitted with a diagnosis of hemesiderosus. _____

_____

2. Microscopic studies revealed widespread hemmolysis. _____

_____

3. Acute chest syndrome is an acute life-threatening infearction of the lung. _____

_____

4. Sickle cell anemia is the most common hemogloboniopathy in the United States. _____

_____

5. The infant has been diagnosed with a hereditary hemotalogic disorder. _____

_____

6. Extrmedulary hematopoiesis results in progressive enlargement of the spleen and liver. _____

_____

7. Spleenomegaly and hepatamegaly may indicate a hematologic disorder. _____

_____

8. In sickle cell anemea, the RCBs are shaped like a sickle. _____

_____

Place the appropriate term or group of terms in each of the boxes that follow. Fill in the symptom boxes first, then add the diagnostic terms and diseases or effects terms that relate to each symptom.

> anemia
> splenomegaly
> enlarged liver
> hemolysis, congestive heart failure, extramedullary hematopoiesis
> hepatomegaly
> pale lips, nailbeds, and inside of mouth
> enlarged spleen
> pallor
> sequestered blood cells, extramedullary hematopoiesis, hemolysis

Symptom

Diagnostic term

Disease or effects

Diagnosing and Treating Problems

Tests, Procedures, and Pharmaceuticals

The hematopoietic system is evaluated by three major laboratory tests: (1) **complete blood count (CBC)**, (2) **white blood cell count with differential**, and (3) **peripheral blood smear**. Several additional procedures evaluating blood cell production and clotting properties are used to diagnose a variety of abnormalities.

Complete Blood Count (CBC)

The CBC includes various tests. In addition to the count of the RBCs and the WBCs, there are also measurements of a patient's RBC size and hemoglobin content, (called the RBC **indices**) which serve as indicators of health or illness. Cell size is represented as mean corpuscular volume (MCV). The amount of hemoglobin carried in the RBC is called the mean corpuscular hemoglobin (MCH). The MCH concentration (MCHC) represents the concentration of hemoglobin within the average RBC. There may also be a platelet count included. Production of RBCs is assessed by the **reticulocyte** (young RBC) count. If the hemoglobin value is decreased, a high reticulocyte count would suggest that young RBCs are being produced.

White Cell Count with Differential

The count of the WBC line is called the differential. The number of these cells changes normally from newborn through adolescence, when the values reach the adult range.

Peripheral Blood Smear

The smear is a specimen of blood placed on the slide and viewed under the microscope. This is a test of the size and appearance of blood cells, as well as the presence of abnormally shaped cells. Any abnormal value in the CBC or abnormal morphology seen on the peripheral smear is an indication that something is wrong. Change can also be the result of abnormal production or increased destruction of normal blood cells.

Additional Blood Tests and Procedures

Table 5.13 lists common tests and procedures related to the blood. A patient's production of neutrophils, platelets, and RBCs may be assessed using a **bone marrow aspiration,** a test performed by pushing a special needle through the skin into the bone marrow cavity and drawing some fluid (bone marrow) into the syringe. A **bone marrow biopsy** consists of taking a small specimen, or core, of the bone marrow. Each of these tests is usually performed on the posterior superior iliac crest. The specimen is viewed under the microscope to determine numbers of blood cells.

A **pheresis** is a procedure that involves removing some blood into a special centrifuge that separates the cells. Blood components that can be separated by pheresis are the WBCs (leukapheresis), the plasma (plasmapheresis), and the platelets (plateletpheresis).

Blood clotting can also be evaluated with specific tests. A **bleeding time** is used to measure the time it takes for clotting to occur after a small wound is made on the skin. The **prothrombin time (PT)** and the **activated partial thromboplastin time (PTT)** are additional tests used to assess clotting.

Coombs' test can determine whether the patient has an autoimmune hemolytic anemia. The test detects antibodies in the serum that react with antigens on the patient's RBCs.

Table 5.13

Tests and Procedures Relating to the Blood

Term	Description
activated partial thromboplastin time	A test of clotting
blood smear	A drop of blood is spread thinly on a glass slide. The slide is bathed in a stain and when dry is viewed under the microscope. Each cell absorbs the stain.
bone marrow aspiration and biopsy	A special needle (Jamshidi or Illinois) is inserted through the skin into the bone marrow space of the bone (posterior superior iliac crest in most cases, anterior iliac crest and sternum less commonly). A sample of the fluid portion of the bone marrow is drawn into a syringe. The biopsy is a small core of bone marrow.
complete blood count and differential	The complete blood count is a test performed on blood to determine the value of each of the blood cells. Usually, computerized equipment (e.g., a Coulter counter) analyzes the blood sample. The differential is the measure of the WBCs.
Coombs' test	A test to detect antibodies in the serum that react with antigen on the patient's RBCs; used to determine whether the patient has an autoimmune hemolytic anemia. (Note: Coombs was an English immunologist.)

continued on next page

pheresis	Blood is removed through a special intravenous catheter, a machine (centrifuge) separates the components of the blood, the needed component is removed, and the remainder of the blood is returned to the donor.
prothrombin time	A test of clotting; prothrombin is a glycoprotein necessary for clotting.
reticulocyte count	Test to determine the number of young cells that will become RBCs.

Pharmaceutical Agents

Only a few classes of pharmacologic agents are used in hematology (see Table 5.14). **Thrombolytic** agents such as streptokinase and urokinase break down clots that have formed. **Antithrombotic** agents, also called **anticoagulants**, prevent clots from forming; these medications include warfarin, heparin, and aspirin. Agents that promote clotting are called **coagulants**. Several products known as antihemophilic factors are used to replace the factors that cause hemophilia. Antifibrinolytic agents prevent clots from breaking down.

Growth factors are agents used to stimulate the growth of specific cells in the bone marrow and include granulocyte colony-stimulating factor (G-CSF), granulocyte-macrophage colony-stimulating factor (GM-CSF), and erythropoietin (EPO). Much research is under way to find other growth factors to stimulate hematopoietic cells within the bone marrow.

Table 5.14

Pharmacologic Agents Relating to the Blood

Drug classes	Use	Generic name	Brand names
anticoagulant (antithrombotic)	prevents blood from clotting	heparin warfarin sodium	Hep-Lock Coumadin
antihemophilic factors	promote clotting	factor VIII human antihemophilic factor human factor IX complex	Humate-P, Koate-DVI, Monoclate-P Konyne
biological response modifier: interferon	stimulate the body's own immune system	interferon alfa-2b interferon gamma-1b	Intron Actimmune
colony-stimulating factor	stimulates RBC production	epoetin alfa, erythropoietin	Epogen, Procrit
granulocyte colony-stimulating factor	stimulates the formation of neutrophils	filgrastim	Neupogen
granulocyte-macrophage colony-stimulating factor	stimulates the formation of myeloid cells in the bone marrow	sargramostim	Leukine
hemostatic/synthetic ADH	promotes clotting	desmopressin	DDAVP
hemostatic/antifibrinolytic	prevents the breakdown of a clot	aminocaproic acid	Amicar
thrombolytic	breaks down clots	streptokinase urokinase	Streptase Abbokinase

Table 5.15

Hematology Abbreviations

AHF	antihemophilic factor VIII
AHG	antihemophilic globulin factor VIII
ALL	acute lymphoblastic leukemia
AML	acute myeloblastic leukemia (also known as acute myelogenous leukemia)
ANC	absolute neutrophil count
APML	acute promyelocytic leukemia
baso	basophil
CBC	complete blood count
CLL	chronic lymphocytic leukemia
CML	chronic myelogenous leukemia
diff	differential
eosin/eos	eosinophil
ESR	erythrocyte sedimentation rate
HCT/Hct	hematocrit
HGB/Hgb	hemoglobin
ITP	immune thrombocytopenic purpura
lymphs	lymphocytes
MCH	mean corpuscular hemoglobin
MCHC	mean corpuscular hemoglobin concentration
MCV	mean corpuscular volume
mono	monocyte
plts/PLT	platelets
PMN	polymorphonuclear neutrophil
polys	polymorphonuclear neutrophils
PT	prothrombin time
PTT	partial thromboplastin time
RBC	red blood cell
sed rate	sedimentation rate
segs	segmented neutrophils
WBC	white blood cell

Give the definition of the following combining forms, then build a term with each and use the term in a sentence.

	Definition	Term

1. erythr/o _____ _____

_____

2. splen/o _____ _____

_____

3. hem/o _____ _____

_____

4. thromb/o _____ _____

_____

5. cyt/o _____ _____

_____

6. blast/o _____ _____

_____

7. ser/o _____ _____

_____

8. leuk/o _____ _____

_____

9. hepat/o _____ _____

_____

10. morph/o _____ _____

_____

Circle the term that best completes each sentence.

1. Lydia is a plasmapheresis/electrophresis donor.

2. Janice is being referred to a hematologist/hematosiologist.

3. Hattie's prothrombin/thrombopoietin time was evaluated yesterday.

4. Dan's Coombs test detected the antibodies/hormones.

5. A bone marrow aspiration and biopsy will be done to assess Timmy's bone marrow/white blood cells.

6. The patient's reticulocyte/marrowcyte count was quite high.

7. Dr. Petenski has ordered a CBC/RBC and a chest x-ray for the patient.

8. Coumadin is an example of a coagulant/an anticoagulant.

9. After the line was flushed with normal saline, hemosiderin/heparin was injected.

10. The patient was given streptokinase/streptococcus in the emergency room.

Matching

Match the abbreviations in Column 1 with the definitions in Column 2. Write the number of the abbreviation in the space beside the definition.

Column 1		Column 2
1. PTT	_____	a. platelets
2. CBC	_____	b. white blood cell
3. sed rate	_____	c. partial thromboplastin time
4. AHF	_____	d. lymphocytes
5. plts	_____	e. differential
6. ITP	_____	f. sedimentation rate
7. baso	_____	g. antihemophilic factor VII
8. WBC	_____	h. basophil
9. diff	_____	i. complete blood count
10. lymphs	_____	j. immune thrombocytic purpura

Word Building

Supply roots, combining forms, or word parts to create a term that completes each sentence.

1. Pro_____in time is a test of blood clotting.

2. Mono_____ means one cell (type of white blood cell).

3. _____lytic is a breakdown of blood clots.

4. Hemato_____ is the formation of blood.

5. A granulo_____ is a granular cell (type of white blood cell).

6. _____coagulant means against clotting.

7. _____thrombotic prevents clots from forming (same as anticoagulant).

8. An _____cyte is a red blood cell.

What Does This Abbreviation Mean?

Write the correct definition for each abbreviation on the blank provided.

1. Hct   _____

2. Hgb   _____

3. MCH   _____

4. mono   _____

5. polys   _____

6. PT   _____

7. ANC   _____

8. MCV   _____

9. RBC   _____

10. segs   _____

Complete the following table of medications using terms from the list that follows.

thrombolytic
streptokinase, urokinase
hemostatic
prevents blood from clotting

Humate-P, Koate, Konyne
DDAVP
hemostatic
aminocaproic acid

prevents the breakdown of a clot
antihemophilic factors
Hep-Lock, Coumadin
desmopressin

Drug class	Use	Generic name	Brand name
anticoagulant	_____	heparin	_____
antithrombotics	_____	warfarin sodium	_____
_____	breaks down clots	_____	Streptase, Abbokinase
antifibrinolytic	_____	_____	Amicar
_____	_____	factor replacements named for the factor they replace	_____
_____	promotes clotting	_____	_____

ONCOLOGY

As described at the beginning of this chapter, a physician who is trained in hematology is usually trained in oncology (pertaining to cancer) as well. Cancer refers to a large group of diseases that have malignant properties—that is, a tendency to grow and spread. Some 900,000 new cancer cases are diagnosed in adults each year in the United States. Each type of cancer is identified by the site and/or cell type from which it begins. For example, colon cancer starts in the colon; breast cancer starts in the breast. The physician who specializes in the treatment of cancer is called an oncologist.

The cause of cancer remains something of a mystery. Carcinogenesis may result from exposure to **carcinogens**, a damaged immune system, or a genetic predisposition. For some cancers in adults, alterations in personal lifestyle or environmental factors can increase or decrease the incidence, prevalence, morbidity, and mortality of cancer.

Anatomy of Cancer Cells

Cancer cells differ in appearance from normal cells and from one another as well. Normal cells are well organized, having the same size, shape, and color when stained and viewed under the microscope. Cancer cells also behave differently from normal cells, and their ability to recognize other cells is altered. Contact inhibition of movement and cell division are affected which leads to invasion of organs and **metastasis** or spreading to other parts of the body (Figure 5.6).

Figure 5.6 - The Metastatic Sequence

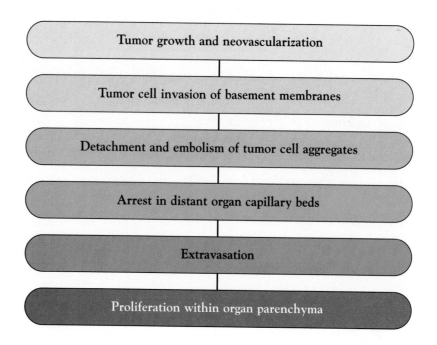

Cell Development

In normal cell development, all cells that come from one fertilized egg carry identical DNA (deoxyribonucleic acid) molecules. As the organism develops, the cells differentiate, developing for specific purposes. Cancer cells are less differentiated than normal cells. Interruption of the differentiation process can occur at any time in cell development. The result is cells that range from well-differentiated to anaplastic, or undifferentiated. During this change from normal to malignant cells, alterations in surrounding tissue also occur (Figure 5.7).

Figure 5.7 - Change from Normal Cell to Malignant Cell

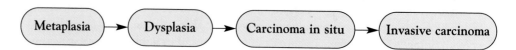

Cell Metabolism

Biochemically, the metabolism of a cancer cell differs from a normal cell. Surface enzymes produced by cancer cells aid in invasion (of surrounding tissue) and metastasis. Decreased production of glycoproteins contributes to the loss of contact inhibition, which is the signal to the cell to stop dividing. Cancer cells lose the surface antigens that normally identify a cell and replace them with new tumor-associated antigens.

Risk Assessment

The successful management of cancer focuses on assessing patient risk factors and on prevention and early detection. Assessing a patient's cancer risk is typically part of a thorough physical examination. After taking a complete health history, including information on cancer occurrences in the family tree, the healthcare professional inspects the patient from head to toe. The thorax, liver, spleen, abdomen, and rectum are palpated in all patients. Further palpation of the female anatomy includes manual examination of the breasts, vagina, cervix, uterus, and ovaries. In male patients, the prostate and testes are palpated for abnormalities. The lungs and abdomen are auscultated and percussed in all patients. After the physical examination is completed, specific attention is paid to any area in which an abnormality is suspected.

Diagnostic Tests and Procedures

Once an abnormality is detected, it must be further evaluated using a series of diagnostic tools. Radiographic techniques, nuclear medicine techniques, ultrasonography, and magnetic resonance imaging produce images that are used to locate, diagnose, and stage disease. Invasive procedures such as endoscopy and biopsy allow the physician to visualize a tumor and to take tissue samples for histologic or cytologic examination and diagnosis.

Tumor Staging

Confirmed solid tumor malignancies are graded and staged to provide prognostic information and to assist in planning and evaluating treatment. **Grade** (typically ranging from 1 to 4) refers to the tumor cells' degree of maturity; **stage** refers to the extent of spread within the body. Several tumor classification systems are used, depending on the body area affected. For example, Dukes' staging is used for colon cancer, and Jewett's staging is used for bladder cancer. The most widely used classification is based on three factors and is called the TNM (primary **T**umor, lymph **N**ode, and **M**etastasis) system:

T (T1–T4)	Extent of the primary tumor
N (N0–N3)	Extent of regional lymph node involvement
M (M0–M1)	Presence or absence of distant metastasis

Table 5.16

General Cancer Terms

Word	Meaning	Word analysis	
aggregates **a**-greg-gates	groupings of particles or components to form a mass	ag- gregare	to to herd
anaplastic **ann**-ah-plas-tic	reversion of a cell to a more primitive form; loss of differentiation	ana- plas- -ic; -tic	backward formation having the characteristic of
benign bee-**nine**	not cancerous	ben	well
carcinogen kar-**sin**-oh-gen	cancer-causing substance	carcin/o genesis	cancer origin
carcinogenesis kar-**sin**-oh-**gen**-ih-sis	process of starting and promoting cancer	carcin/o genesis	cancer origin
carcinoma **kar**-sin-oh-ma	type of solid tumor cancer derived from epithelial tissue; constitutes about 90 percent of all cancers	carcin/o oma	cancer tumor
carcinoma in situ **kar**-sin-oh-ma in **sigh**-too	premalignant process that has not invaded the basement membrane but shows characteristics of cancer	carcin oma in situ	cancer tumor "in the original place"
contact inhibition **con**-tact **in**-hib-ish-shun	signal of the cell to stop cell division	con- tact in hib tion	with or together touch in hold indicator of a noun

continued on next page

differentiation dif-fur-**rent**-she-ay-shun	developmental process in which unspecialized cells achieve specialized form, function, and properties	*differentiation*	distinction
dysplasia dis-**play**-she-ah	abnormal development of tissue	*dys* *plasia*	difficult or painful development or formation
embryonal **em**-brie-on-al	relating to an organism in the earliest stages of life	*embryo* *nal; al*	embryo adjective
extravasation ex-tra-**vay**-shun	passage or escape into tissue	*extra* *vas* *tion*	out vessel noun
host	an organism in which another organism lives	*hospes*	host
hyperchromatic **hi**-per-**crow**-mat-ick	having a greater density of color or pigment	*hyper-* *chrom/a* *tic*	more, greater color adjective
immunotherapy **im**-u-no-**there**-a-pea	administration of antibodies produced by another individual to stimulate a response	*immun/o* *therapia*	safe to treat
induction in-**duct**-shun	administration of chemotherapy, causing severe bone marrow hypoplasia	*in* *duc* *tion*	in, into lead noun
invasive carcinoma in-**vase**-of kar-sin-**oh**-ma	malignant neoplasm that invades and destroys surrounding tissue	*in* *vas* *ive* *carcin/o* *oma*	in, into vessel adjective cancer tumor
local **lo**-cal	treatment to a specified area	*local*	place or position
malignant ma-**lig**-nant	tending to grow and spread (metastasize)	*mal*	bad, evil
metaplasia met-ah-**play**-zee-ah	conversion of normal tissue to abnormal tissue	*meta-* *plasia*	change development, formation
metastasis met-**tas**-ta-sis	process by which malignant cells spread to other parts of the body	*meta-* *stasis*	change; beyond control
mitosis my-**toe**-sis	cell division process resulting in 2 cells with the same number of chromosomes as the parent cell	*mit-* *-osis*	thread condition
neoplasm **knee**-oh-plaz-em	abnormal growth of new tissue	*neo-* *plasm*	new a thing formed
neovascularization **knee**-oh-vas-que-lar-eh-zay-shun	development of a new blood supply	*neo-* *vascul* *ization*	new small vessel making of
neuroblastoma **nur**-oh-blast-**oh**-ma	malignant tumor of the sympathetic nervous system arising from primitive cells	*neuro* *blast* *oma*	nerve cell tumor
pleomorphic plea-oh-**more**-fic	describing cells of variable sizes and shapes	*pleo-* *morph* *-ic*	many shape adjective indicator
prognosis **prog**-no-sis	indication of possible outcome	*pro-* *gnosis*	ahead, before knowledge

proliferation pro-lif-er-**a**-shun	reproduction of similar forms	*prole* *fer* *ation*	offspring bear, carry making of
retinoblastoma **ret**-in-oh-blast-**oh**-ma	cancer of the retina	*retin/o* *blast-* *oma*	retina cell tumor
rhabdomyosarcoma **rab**-dough-my-**oh**-sar-**coma**	malignant tumor of striated muscle	*rhabdo* *myo* *sarc* *oma*	rod muscle tissue tumor
sarcoma sar-**coma**	type of cancer derived from connective and supportive tissue	*sarc* *oma*	tissue tumor
survivorship	living or remaining disease-free five years after completion of cancer therapy	*sur-* *vivi* *ship*	beyond life noun indicator
systemic sis-**tem**-ick	pertaining to the whole body	*system* *-ic*	system adjective indicator

Cancer Treatment Goals And Options

The three possible goals in the treatment of cancer are to cure the disease, control the malignancy, or palliate the symptoms. Treatment options include surgery, radiation (see terms in Chapter 2), chemotherapy (including hormonal therapy), and biological therapy. Combining treatment strategies is called **multimodal** (multimethod) therapy.

SURGICAL PROCEDURES Surgery may provide a successful outcome for several early-stage cancers; it also plays a role in diagnosing and preventing disease.

STEM CELL TRANSPLANTATION Hematopoietic stem cell transplantation is performed by giving very high dose chemotherapy to a patient and then giving the patient either their own or a donor's stem cells to rescue the patient from the toxic side effects of the chemotherapy. The stem cells are harvested (gathered) through the use of a machine called a pharesis machine that will remove the young stem cells from the donor. The stem cells are stored until the patient has received the chemotherapy, and then the cells are infused into the patient. Donor stem cells can take weeks to months to become active in the host.

CHEMOTHERAPY Chemotherapy is the use of antineoplastic and hormonal agents to treat cancer. The goal of chemotherapy is to kill as many cancer cells as possible without causing unmanageable toxicity. Combining several chemotherapy drugs with different mechanisms of action and side effects is the hallmark of treatment. Antineoplastic agents are classified according to their chemical structure, cell cycle activity, and mechanism of action.

Table 5.17

Common Chemotherapy Regimens

Acronym	Agents
ABV	Adriamycin, bleomycin, vinblastine
CAF	cyclophosphamide, Adriamycin, 5-fluorouracil
CAV	cyclophosphamide, Adriamycin, vincristine
CHOP	cyclophosphamide, hydroxydaunorubicin, Oncovin, prednisone

continued on next page

COD	cyclophosphamide, Oncovin, DTIC
CytaBOM	cytarabine, bleomycin, Oncovin, methotrexate
DCTER ("doctor")	dexamethasone, cytosine arabinoside, thioguanine, etoposide, rubidomycin
DECAL	daunomycin, etoposide, cyclophosphamide, Ara-C, L-asparaginase
FAM	5-fluorouracil, Adriamycin, mitomycin C
HiDAC ("high dak")	high dose Ara-C
MACOPB ("May-cop-B")	methotrexate, Adriamycin, cyclophosphamide, Oncovin, prednisone, bleomycin
MOPP	mechlorethamine, Oncovin, prednisone, procarbazine
ProMACE	prednisone, methotrexate, Adriamycin, cytarabine, etoposide
VAD	vincristine, Adriamycin, dexamethasone

Biologic Therapy

Biologic therapy (also called biotherapy) uses agents derived from the body's own sources to modify the response to a tumor. Immune system defenses in particular can be used to locate and kill cancerous cells, such as interferon, which is made by the lymphocytes in the blood. The knowledge that has been gained in the field of cancer therapy has improved the cure rate for most cancers.

Biologic therapies have not only been used singly, but with other medications and modalities to further improve treatment. Some new therapies include treatments that attach directly to cancer cells and cause them to be destroyed. Other agents decrease the blood supply to cancer cells, thus preventing them from growing and multiplying. New agents continue to be developed to prevent and treat cancers.

Table 5.18

Oncology Abbreviations

AFP	alpha fetoprotein
BMT	bone marrow transplant
BRM	biologic response modifier
CEA	carcinoembryonic antigen
CSF	colony stimulating factor
DIC	disseminated intravascular coagulation
DRE	digital rectal examination
GVHD	graft-versus-host disease
HLA	human-leukocyte antigen
NSCLC	non-small cell lung cancer
PSCT	peripheral stem cell transplant
SCC	spinal cord compression
SCLC	small cell lung cancer
SIADH	syndrome of inappropriate antidiuretic hormone
SVCS	superior vena cava syndrome

Select from the list of suffixes to build a word that fits each definition.

Suffixes	-cyte	-rrhage
-ic	-ia	-ology
-osis	-philia	-megaly
-oma	-poiesis	

1. Hemat_____ is the study of blood.

2. Hemo_____ means literally "an affinity for blood."

3. Thromb_____ means literally "condition of a clot."

4. Hemat_____ means "tumor of blood."

5. Mono_____ means one (or a single) cell.

6. Hemato_____ means formation of blood.

7. Microcyt_____ means pertaining to a small cell.

8. Spleno_____ means enlargement of the spleen.

9. Hypochrom_____ means pertaining to decreased hemoglobin.

10. Hemo_____ means literally "bursting forth of blood".

Use these misspelled clues to write the correctly spelled terms in the puzzle.

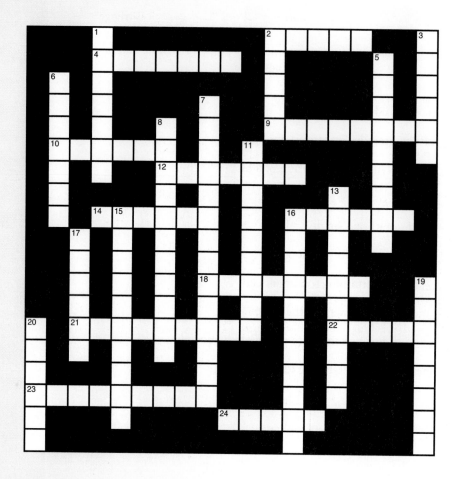

Across
2. fulid
4. emobulus
9. sinddroam
10. paller
12. antomy
14. plazma
16. amenia
18. oncylogy
21. mkcorcyte
22. orgin
23. palatlets
24. ackute

Down
1. vessiles
2. fetis
3. kindey
5. hemalisis
6. perpera
7. megokaryacytes
8. transifuzion
11. corpussel
13. hemagoguin
15. luekoncites
16. aglutanite
17. enzime
19. sindrom
20. biopcy

Performance Assessment 5

Crossword Puzzle

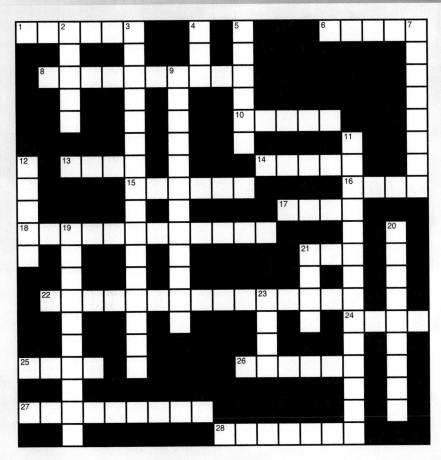

Across
1. hidden
6. stomat/o
8. uncontrolled bleeding
10. white
13. combining form for blood
14. echin/o
15. test to detect autoimmune hemolytic anemia
16. blood condition
17. elliptical
18. chemical treatment
21. erythr/o
22. "defenders of the body"
24. many
25. embolus
26. fluid portion of the blood that contains the cellular components
27. nosebleed
28. defective development of a blood cell line

Down
2. schist/o
3. decreased platelets
4. thalassa
5. Jamshidi
7. "tumor of blood"
9. enlargement of the liver
11. abnormality of the bone marrow
12. chyme
19. black-and-blue mark caused by leakage of blood from a vessel (bruising)
20. destruction of red blood cells
21. rouleaux
23. cyte

Build the Terms

Construct words from roots, prefixes, and suffixes.

Select word parts from the lists to build a complete medical term for each definition given. Note that not all terms will have a root or combining form, prefix, and suffix, and some word parts may be used more than once.

Combining Forms	Prefixes	Suffixes
hem/o	hyper-	-ia
medull/o	epi-	-logy
splen/o	sub-	-logic
ox/o	hypo-	-oma
poikil/o	extra-	-ous
hemat/o	dis-	-sis
spher/o	an-	-al
blast/o	pre-	-ary
chrom/o	de-	-ic
leuk/o	anti-	-in
erythr/o	per-	-cyte
nucle/o	bi-	-lysis

1. study of the blood   _____

2. deficient color (lack of sufficient hemoglobin)   _____

3. breakdown of red blood cells   _____

4. insufficient oxygen   _____

5. pertaining to study of the blood   _____

6. irregularly shaped cell   _____

7. tumor of immature bone cells   _____

8. pertaining to outside bone marrow   _____

9. white (blood) cell   _____

10. red (blood) cell   _____

Using Medical References

The following sentences contain medical terms that may not have been included on the tables in this chapter. Use medical reference books, your medical term analysis skills, and/or a medical dictionary to find the correct definition of each underlined word. Write the definition on the line below the sentence.

1. Mr. Breyer's laboratory tests revealed an unexplained <u>erythrocytosis</u>.

  _____

2. Microscopic examination shows <u>polymorphonuclear leukocytes</u>.

  _____

3. Please call the lab and ask if they can give us Lisa's most recent <u>erythrocyte count</u>.

_____

4. This patient has been treated successfully with an <u>antihyperlipidemic agent</u>.

_____

5. Dr. Terryien has ordered a <u>Schilling test</u> for Mr. Braun.

_____

6. Mrs. Thompson will be injected with <u>RhoGAM</u> to protect future pregnancies.

_____

7. The lab technician is here to draw blood for Theresa's <u>lipid profile</u>.

_____

8. We have begun teaching Amanda's parents about her diagnosis of <u>leukemia</u>.

_____

9. Call Dr. Levin at home as soon as Jennifer's <u>cytology</u> report arrives from the lab.

_____

10. Mr. Dennison receives <u>heparin</u> to prevent <u>thrombus</u> formation.

_____

11. The plasma globulins will be separated by <u>electrophoresis</u>.

_____

12. <u>Agglutination</u> was observed when the two blood samples were mixed in the laboratory.

_____

What Do These Abbreviations Mean?

Write the definition of the abbreviation on the line provided.

1. Hgb _____

2. ALL _____

3. CBC _____

4. RBC _____

5. ESR _____

6. lymphs _____

7. PMN _____

8. plts _____

9. PT _____

10. sed rate _____

Build the Terms

Select from the roots and combining forms given to make a term for each definition. Write the term on the line beside the definition.

Roots/Combining Forms

hemo	mono
hemat	micro
erythro	blasto
onco	cyto
lympho	organo

Definitions

1. Immature cell _____

2. Enlargement of an organ or organs _____

3. Specialist in the study of cancer _____

4. Study of the blood _____

5. Tumor of blood _____

6. Red blood cell _____

7. Pertaining to a very small cell _____

8. Cancer of the lymphatic system _____

9. One cell (a single cell) _____

10. Study of cells _____

What's Your Conclusion?

In this exercise you will practice selecting the correct explanation. Read each mini medical record or scenario carefully, and select the correct response. Write the letter of your answer in the space provided.

1. This 18-year-old male has a history of sickle cell anemia with many past vaso-occlusive crises requiring hospitalizations two or three times per year. Yesterday was a hot day, and the patient admitted to not drinking enough fluids. Today, he has severe pain in many bones and in his abdomen. The nature of the pain is similar to past crises. He denies any fever. You understand that:

   A. The patient will be admitted and given IV hydration and parenteral analgesics.
   B. The patient will be sent home and told to take ibuprofen. If his pain does not resolve within three days, he is instructed to come to the ER.

   Your response: _____

2. On the third postnatal day, Baby Thomas has a yellowish tinge to his skin and sclerae. His mother expresses concern and requests information on her child's condition. The physician will:

   A. Tell her that babies who have problems involving their eyes always look yellow.
   B. Explain to her that the baby may have hyperbilirubinemia and that phototherapy, or exposing the baby to bright light, is often an effective treatment.

   Your response: _____

3. Your grandfather was recently diagnosed with a pulmonary embolism and admitted to the hospital. The family has been given little information, and everyone is puzzled by the words the doctor used. He explained that grandfather was experiencing hypoxia as evidenced by cyanosis, and would require treatment with thrombolytic agents. Your family is wondering what is wrong with grandfather and they request an explanation from you.

   A. Explain that "pulmonary" refers to the lungs, and "embolism" is a word for a blood clot that has dislodged from its original site and traveled through the bloodstream. Tell them that it is a serious problem that has produced a lack of oxygen, and because of this your grandfather has a bluish tinge to his lips and fingernails. Explain that grandfather will be treated with drugs to dissolve the clot.
   B. Tell them they should ask the doctor to let them read grandfather's chart so that they have a better understanding of the situation.

   Your response: _____

Analyzing Medical Records

Read the chart below. Then answer the following questions:

1. Describe in your own words the patient's initial presenting symptoms.

2. What were the results of the physical examination?

3. How did Michelle's WBC and platelet counts compare to normal values?

4. What was the diagnosis following the bone marrow examination?

5. Summarize the treatment regimen and the results.

Chart Summary

Patient Michelle W.
Date 2/2/xx

Michele is an 11-year-old who presented at 8 years of age with fever, bruising, and generalized pain. The physical examination was pertinent for pallor, petechiae, shotty lymphadenopathy, and a palpable spleen tip. The CBC revealed a WBC 5000, H/H 7.0/21.0, and platelet count 85,000. There were 70 % lymphocytes and 30% lymphoblasts on the peripheral smear. A bone marrow examination was diagnostic of ALL, FAB L1 morphology, cALLa positive, and a hyperdiploid karyotype. A chest x-ray was normal. The lumbar puncture was negative for leukemic cells.

She was placed on induction therapy with vincristine, prednisone, L-asparaginase and intrathecal methotrexate. Following the third dose of L-asparaginase, Michelle developed an anaphylactic reaction which was successfully treated. Induction therapy was continued with a single dose of PEG-L-asparaginase being substituted for the remaining six doses of native L-asparaginase, without further untoward events. By day 28, she was in bone marrow remission.

She continued on chemotherapy with consolidation and interim therapy. Delayed intensification was given with the BFM regimen. A single dose of PEG-L-asparaginase was substituted for native L-asparginase, again without further hypersensitivity reactions. Subsequently, she received maintenance therapy for two years. Michelle has now been off all treatment for one year, is doing well, and remains in complete continuous remission.

S. Burkowitz, MD

Short Answer

Describe the clotting cascade in your own words.

_____

_____

_____

_____

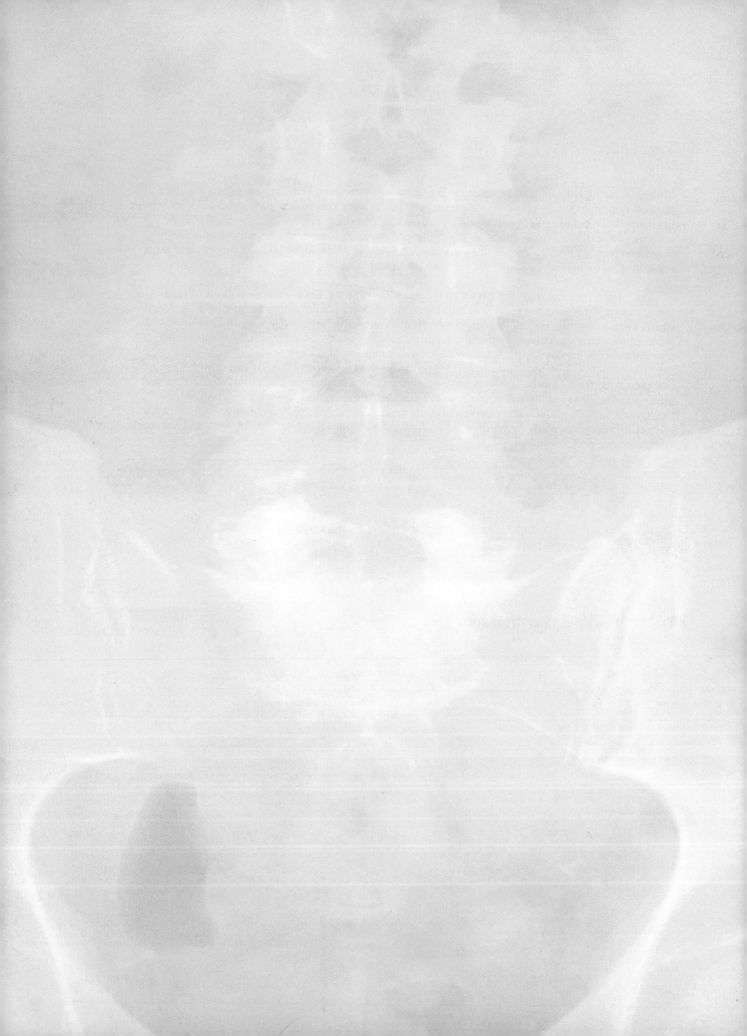

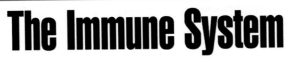

Chapter 6

The Immune System

Learning Outcomes

Students will be able to:
- Identify the organs of the immune system.
- Explain the elements of immunity.
- Describe the role of lymphocytes in the body's defense mechanism.
- Delineate the function of immunization in protecting the body.
- Use the terminology of the immune system into written and oral communication.
- Correctly spell and pronounce immune system terminology.
- State the meaning of abbreviations related to the immune system.
- List and define the combining forms most commonly used to create terms related to the immune system.
- Name tests and treatments for major immune system abnormalities.

Translation, Please?Translation, Please?Translation, Please?

Read the following excerpt from a medical record and try to answer the questions that follow.

Since his previous examination, the patient has continued to have active medical problems. With regard to his HIV infection, he continues to have a decreasing CD4 count. He continues his AZT therapy. His physical examination revealed palpable lymph nodes in the cervical, axillary, and inguinal areas.

1. HIV is the abbreviation for human immunodeficiency virus. True or false?
2. Is AZT a type of exercise or a type of medication?
3. What is the location of the lymph nodes mentioned?

Answers to "Translation Please?"
1. True. HIV is the abbreviation for human immunodeficiency virus.
2. AZT is a type of medication.
3. The lymph nodes mentioned are in the neck (cervical), under the arm (axillary), and in the groin (inguinal).

Identifying the Specialty

The System and Its Practitioners

Tiny, microscopic enemies lurk everywhere in your environment. Harmful toxins, bacteria, viruses, and even cells within the body can attack a person and cause a host of problems ranging from mild reactions such as sneezing and rashes to life-threatening illnesses. Fortunately, the body has a protective mechanism that fights these dangers and often wins the battle. This defense is called the **immune system.**

The emergence of acquired immunodeficiency syndrome (AIDS) in the 1980s prompted extensive research that generated an expanded understanding

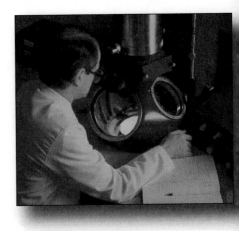

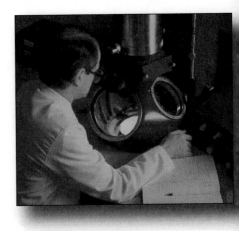

of the immune system. The area of practice concerned with the functioning of the immune system and the interrelationships between this system and the rest of the body is called **immunology.** The specialist in the field is the **immunologist.**

Examining the Patient ♂♀

Anatomy and Physiology of the Immune System

The immune system is composed of specialized organs, ducts, and cells located throughout the body. The organs of this system include the **thymus, tonsils, lymph nodes,** and **spleen,** as shown in Figure 6.1. The immune system is responsible for protecting and defending the body from the outside world and from internal mechanisms that cause the body to turn against itself.

Figure 6.1 - Components of the Lymphatic System

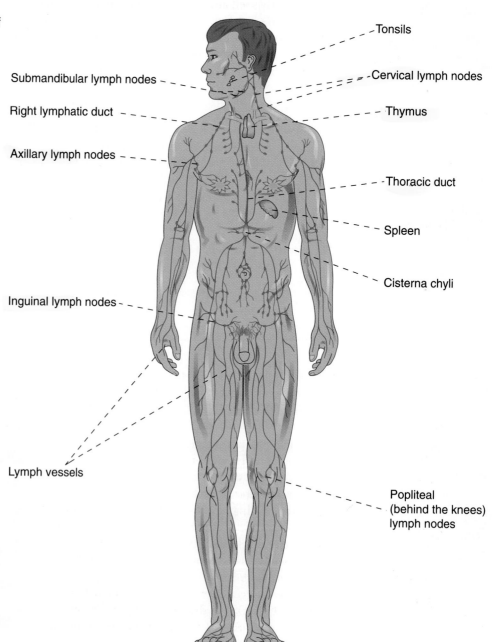

Tonsils

Cervical lymph nodes

Submandibular lymph nodes

Thymus

Right lymphatic duct

Axillary lymph nodes

Thoracic duct

Spleen

Cisterna chyli

Inguinal lymph nodes

Lymph vessels

Popliteal
(behind the knees)
lymph nodes

Organs of the Immune System

The **thymus** is an organ located in the anterior portion of the chest known as the **mediastinum**. The thymus is composed of epithelial tissue that is present in the fetus. Its major function is to produce lymphocytes, the cells responsible for protecting the body from pathogens. The thymus develops throughout childhood, reaching maximum size during the adolescent years, when it weighs between 35 and 40 g (just over an ounce). After puberty, the thymus begins to shrink and eventually becomes fatty tissue by a process called **involution.**

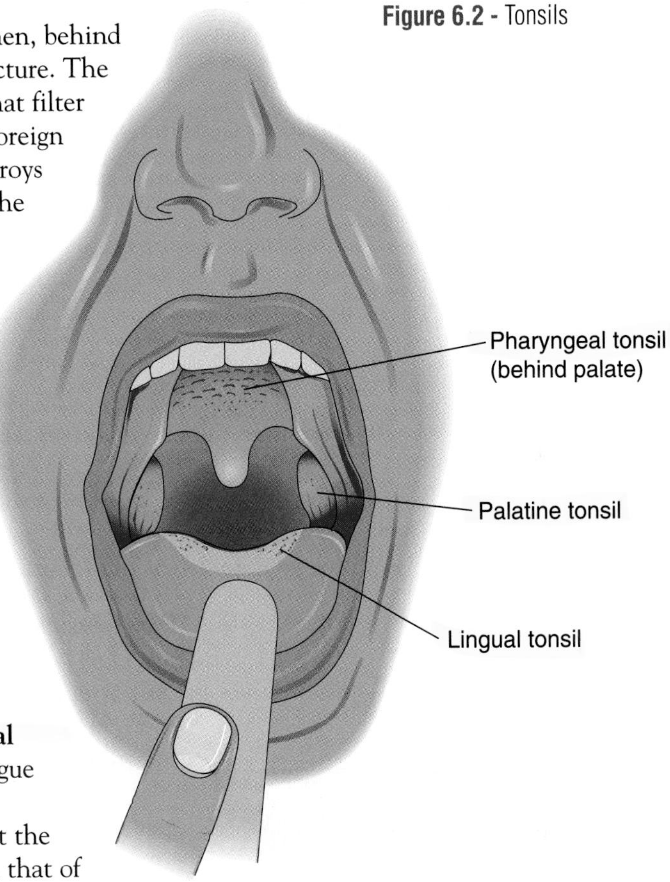

Located in the upper left quadrant of the abdomen, behind the stomach, the **spleen** is the largest lymphoid structure. The spleen contains dense populations of lymphocytes that filter and **phagocytose** (ingest and destroy) bacteria and foreign substances. It filters red blood cells (RBCs) and destroys the old ones. The remaining RBCs are returned to the system. The spleen, rich with blood, can contain more than 1 pint of blood at any time. Therefore, any injury to the spleen can cause serious blood loss, and removal of the spleen may be necessary to stop the bleeding.

The **tonsils** are structures made up of lymphoid tissue. They form a protective ring in the mouth and back of the throat, where they filter invasive particles from the nose and mouth. Because they are the first line of defense against the outside environment, the tonsils often become infected. The three sets of tonsils are: (1) the **palatine tonsils,** located on each side of the throat; (2) the **pharyngeal tonsils,** or **adenoids,** located in the posterior opening of the nasopharynx (the area connecting the nose and throat); and (3) the **lingual tonsils,** located on both sides of the base of the tongue (see Figures 6.1 and 6.2).

Lymph nodes are located in clusters throughout the body, as shown in Figure 6.1. Their sizes range from that of a pinhead to that of a lima bean. Lymph nodes in the head, arms, and legs are close to the surface. The nodes in the neck are equally divided between surface nodes and deeper nodes. In the trunk and internal organs, the nodes are very deep within the body. The lymph nodes serve as the filtration system of **lymph**, a specialized fluid containing lymphocytes, which flows from specific areas of the body.

Figure 6.2 - Tonsils

Pharyngeal tonsil (behind palate)

Palatine tonsil

Lingual tonsil

Lymph Vessels

The lymph nodes are drained by a system of lymph vessels separate from the vessels of the circulatory system (the system that carries blood throughout the body). The lymph fluid flows into two vessels, the **right lymphatic duct** and the **thoracic duct,** which eventually empty their lymph into the veins of the neck. The largest lymphatic vessel is the thoracic duct, which drains about three-fourths of the body. The right lymphatic duct drains lymph from the right upper extremity and the right side of the head, neck, and upper torso (Figure 6.1).

The vessels of the lymphatic system have one-way valves to maintain the flow of lymph in one direction. Lymph in the abdomen is often referred to as **chyle**. The thoracic duct in the abdomen contains the **cisterna chyli**, a pouchlike structure that stores lymph as it moves toward the venous system.

Lymph Node Filtering System

The filtering process begins when lymph enters the node through the **afferent** (toward) lymph vessels and is filtered of bacteria and other dangerous particles. After these organisms are removed, the lymph then exits through the **efferent** (away) lymph vessel. The one-way flow mechanism prevents bacteria from flowing through the entire body. The entry and exit of lymph through the nodes are important to the clinical care of a patient. For instance, if a patient had an ear infection in the left ear, the drainage of the bacteria would cause the lymph nodes of the left side of the neck to swell, because they are filled with the dead bacterial cells.

Immune System Cells

The cells of the immune system include the phagocytic cells of the white blood cell line: neutrophils, monocytes, and macrophages. Also included are the B and T lymphocytes. **Neutrophils** and **monocytes** circulate in the blood and move into the tissues when needed to fight infection. Once inside the tissues, the monocytes mature into phagocytic cells called **macrophages**.

B CELLS Lymphocytes, or B cells, are found in large numbers throughout the body. **B lymphocytes** secrete antibodies into the blood in response to the presence of foreign substances. When an antigen, or substance that the body sees as foreign, is sensed, the B cells change into plasma cells, which produce proteins called **immunoglobulins**. These immunoglobulins help to destroy the antigens. Because the immunoglobulins are released into the body's blood and lymph fluids (referred to as humors), the process is known as **humoral immunity**.

T CELLS The **T lymphocytes**, also called T cells, directly attack virus-infected and cancerous cells, providing **cell-mediated immunity**. As they mature, they migrate to the lymph nodes and lymphoid organs. When a virus invades the body, the T cells

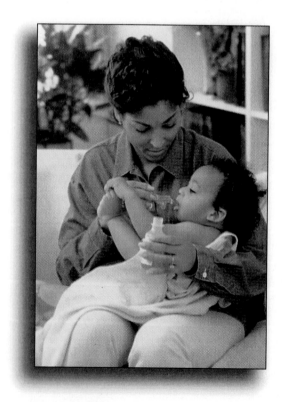

respond by multiplying rapidly. Then the antigen binds to the protein on the surface of the T cell, making it a sensitized T cell (Figure 6.3). These sensitized cells kill invading cells by releasing substances that are deadly to the invaders. As a final step, macrophages move to the area and phagocytose the invading cells.

The T lymphocytes (the *T* stands for *thymus*) are produced in the thymus under the stimulation of **thymosin**, the hormone secreted by the thymus. These lymphocytes eventually leave and circulate to the other lymphatic organs and tissues. T lymphocytes are responsible for antibody production, discussed later in this chapter. T4 helper cells, also known as CD4 cells, help by activating B cells and other T cells and macrophages. T8, or CD8, cells are cytotoxic, or killer, cells that suppress T4 function. They directly attack cells in the body that are infected or malignant. T8 cells also are responsible for graft and tissue rejection in patients undergoing organ transplants. T4 and T8 cells work together as a balance for one another.

T cells produce small proteins called **interferons**. These proteins interfere with the replication of viruses and other cells that invade the body. Pharmaceutical companies manufacture interferon in large quantities as a treatment for certain cancers, some types of hepatitis, and other conditions that appear to respond to its effects.

Figure 6.3 - T-Cell Function

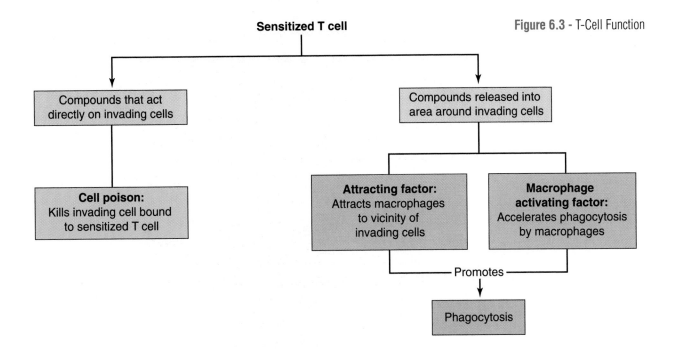

Figure 6.3 - T-Cell Function

Kinds of Immunity

The immune system has two types of defenses: nonspecific immunity and specific immunity. Specific immunity is developed by the body after exposure to an individual virus or another substance. **Nonspecific immunity** is provided by the skin and mucous membranes, which prevent outside organisms from entering the body. Additional mechanical barriers include tears and mucus. Tears wash foreign invaders out of the eyes, and mucus traps antigens before they enter the respiratory system.

NONSPECIFIC IMMUNITY Another part of nonspecific immunity is the **inflammatory response** that occurs when the body is damaged or when foreign organisms enter it. Tissue damage triggers the release of **mediators**, substances that activate immune cells. First to arrive at the scene are the white blood cells (WBCs). Their accumulation causes the external signs of inflammation: heat and redness from the increased blood flow, and swelling and pain from the damaged tissue. The WBCs enter the tissue and begin the process of **phagocytosis**. Bacteria and damaged cells are destroyed, and the increased blood flow promotes tissue repair.

COMPLEMENT PROTEINS Within the nonspecific immunity system is a group of proteins carried by the blood that assist with protection and immune function. These proteins are called **complement proteins,** and they are activated during the formation of antigen-antibody complexes. Specific antigen-antibody complexes cause **complement fixation,** the process that kills the foreign substances.

SPECIFIC IMMUNITY The second form of protection is **specific immunity,** which includes the specialized T- and B lymphocytes that "remember" and recognize substances to which they have previously been exposed. A virus entering the body for the first time may make the person sick, but the second time it appears, the organisms are destroyed and the individual does not have any symptoms. The person is then said to be **immune** to the organism. Table 6.1 summarizes the subgroups of specific immunity.

Acquired immunity is a natural immunity that occurs when a person has had the illness and will no longer become ill from the same organism. **Artificial active immunity** occurs when the exposure is deliberate, as in an **immunization.** A

Figure 6.4 - Inflammatory Response

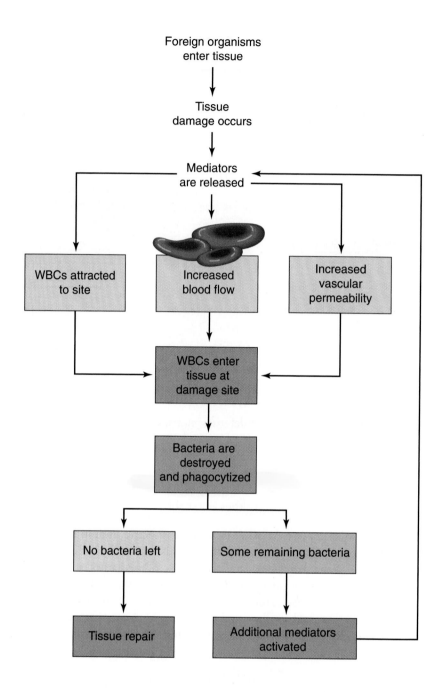

Foreign organisms
enter tissue

Tissue
damage occurs

Mediators
are released

WBCs attracted
to site

Increased
blood flow

Increased
vascular
permeability

WBCs enter
tissue at
damage site

Bacteria are
destroyed
and phagocytized

No bacteria left

Some remaining bacteria

Tissue repair

Additional mediators
activated

nonaggressive, or **attenuated**, form of the organism or toxin is injected into the person, allowing the individual to produce protective antibodies. **Maternal immunity** occurs passively with the transfer of antibodies through the placenta or the mother's milk. This immunity provides protection until the infant's immune system is mature enough to produce its own antibodies.

Passive artificial immunity occurs when antibodies produced in other persons are injected into an individual. The antibodies are usually given in the form of an immune globulin (see Chapter 7). Additionally, humans inherit immunity to certain diseases that affect animals. This protection is known as **species immunity**.

Table 6.2 lists common combining forms for the immune system, and Table 6.3 presents wellness and illness terms related to the field.

Table 6.1

Types of Specific Immunity

Type	Description
active immunity	immunity developed through exposure to a disease; antibodies are produced that protect the body upon second exposure
artificial active immunity	immunity provided by an immunization made from the causative agent in a mild form; the person's body makes antibodies against the causative agent
maternal immunity	immunity received when a mother passes her antibodies to the fetus through the placenta and to the newborn through her breast milk; the baby is immune to these diseases for a few months until able to develop his or her own antibodies
artificial passive immunity	immunity provided by an injection or infusion of antibodies developed from another person's exposure to the disease
species immunity	genetic immunity to animal diseases

Table 6.2

Combining Forms Relating to Immunity

Combining form	Meaning	Example
aden/o	gland	adenoids
auto-	self	autologous
bacteri/o	bacteria	bacteriology
immun/o	immune	immunity
lymph/o	lymph	lymphedema
macro-	large	macrophage
path/o	disease	pathology
splen/o	spleen	splenectomy
thym/o	thymus	thymocyte
tox/o	poison	toxic

Table 6.3

Anatomy and Physiology Terms Relating to Immunity

Term	Meaning	Word analysis	
adenoid **ad**-ah-noyd	lymph organs (glands) located in the back of the throat	aden/o -oid	gland resembling
afferent **af**-er-ent	toward; flowing in	afferent	to bring to
antibody **an**-tih-bod-ee	immunoglobulin in the blood that is produced in response to an antigen; a protective protein produced by the body	anti- body	against body
antigen **an**-tih-jen	substance that produces an immune response	anti- -gen	against producing
cisterna chyli sis-**ter**-nah **kI**-lI cisternae chyli (pl) sis-**ter**-neeh **kI**-lee	drainage sac for the lymph of the abdominal and lumbar lymphatics	cisterna chyli	reservoir body fluid
complement **kom**-pleh-ment	substance present in the body; can destroy dangerous cells	complement	complete
efferent **ef**-er-ent	outward; flowing away from	efferent	to bring out

humor **hyoo**-mer	watery fluid in the body	*humor*	liquid
immune im-**myoon** immunity im-**myoon**-ih-tee	not susceptible	*immun/o*	immune; free
immunoglobulin im-myoo-nO-**glob**-yoo-lin	protein in the body that helps to destroy antigens	*immun/o* *globulin*	immune globule
immunology im-myoo-**nol**-ah-jee	practice and study of the immune system	*immun/o* *-logy*	immune study of
inflammatory response in-**flam**-ah-tor-ee	bodily response produced when an injury occurs; the area becomes inflamed with the characteristic signs: swelling, redness, warmth, and pain	*in-* *flamma* *-ory*	in, into flame condition
interferon **in**-ter-**fer**-on	glycoprotein that helps the body fight viruses; also involved in regulation of other cells in the body	*interferon*	to interfere
involution in-vO-**loo**-shun	return of an organ or tissue from enlarged to normal size	*in-* *volution*	within to roll up
lymph node limf	collection and filtration capsule of the lymphatic system located in the lymph vessels	*lymph/o* *node*	lymph knot
macrophage **mak**-rO-fayj	phagocytic cell in the tissues	*macro-* *-phage*	large to eat
mediastinum **mee**-dee-as-**tI**-num	central area of the chest that separates the two sides and includes all internal structures except for the lungs	*mediastinum*	middle
monocyte **mon**-O-sIt	one of the WBCs found in lymph nodes, the spleen, and bone marrow; a phagocytic cell that engulfs and kills bacteria and plays a role in tumor cell kill	*mono-* *-cyte*	one cell
neutrophil **noo**-trO-fil	WBC that seeks, ingests, and kills bacteria	*neutro-* *-phil*	neutral abnormal attraction or fondness toward
palatine tonsil **pal**-ah-tIn **ton**-sil	lymphoid tissue located on either side of the pharynx	*palat/o* *-al* *tonsil*	pharynx pertaining to stake
phagocytosis fag-O-sI-**tO**-sis phagocyte **fag**-O-sIt	process of ingesting cells or foreign substances	*phag/o* *cyt/o* *-osis*	eat cell condition
pharyngeal tonsil far-**in**-jee-al	lymphoid organ located at the back of the throat; one of the body's defenses that prevents foreign substances from entering the system	*pharyng/o* *-al* *tonsil*	pharynx pertaining to stake
spleen	organ located in the left upper quadrant of the abdominal cavity; consists of lymphatic tissue with a large quantity of macrophages; a blood-forming organ in childhood and then a repository for RBCs and platelets; filters blood to eliminate old and destroyed cells	*splen/o* *-e*	spleen noun marker

thoracic duct thO-**ras**-ik dukt	largest lymph vessel in the body; drains most of the body	*thorac/o* *-ic* *duct(us)*	chest pertaining to duct (vessel)
thymosin **thI**-mO-sin	hormone of the thymus gland that stimulates the thymus to release its hormones	*thym/o*	thymus
thymus **thI**-mus	lymphoid organ located behind the mediastinum; functions in the development of the immune system until puberty	*thym/o*	thymus
tonsil	lymphoid tissue located throughout the oropharyngeal cavity	*tonsil*	stake

Word Building

Write the number of the five anatomical structures on the appropriate location on the accompanying diagram. Then write the combining form on the first line under each structure name. On the second line, write another word created from the combining form.

1. thymus

   _____

   _____

2. tonsils

   _____

   _____

3. inguinal lymph nodes

   _____

   _____

4. spleen

   _____

   _____

5. lymphatic vessels

   _____

   _____

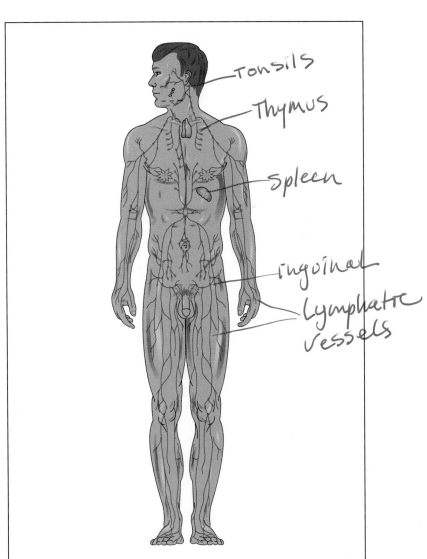

Tonsils
Thymus
spleen
inguinal
Lymphatic
Vessels

Read each sentence and correct the spelling of the underlined word or words; then supply a definition.

1. The <u>mediastunim</u> was opened and the thymus gland located. _____

_____

2. The <u>pharyngel tonsins</u> were found to be enlarged. _____

_____

3. The <u>palatin tonsuls</u> were covered with thick exudate. _____

_____

4. The <u>splen</u> is the largest <u>limpoid</u> structure. _____

_____

5. The <u>spleenectomy</u> was performed by Dr. Bright last week. _____

_____

6. The bacteriology report showed that *Staphylococcus aureus* was found in the <u>lynph node</u>. _____

_____

7. There were many <u>macrofages</u> in the tissue surrounding the wound. _____

_____

8. This patient is being referred to an <u>imunlogist</u> at Children's Hospital. _____

_____

9. The patient was told that a repeat exposure to this <u>antegen</u> could prove fatal. _____

_____

10. There was a great deal of tissue destruction, and the <u>inflamatory response</u> was widespread. _____

_____

Word Building

Provide the missing word parts to create the correct term for the definition provided.

1. _____osis means condition of cell eating.

2. _____itis refers to inflammation of cells.

3. _____ectomy is surgical removal of the spleen.

4. _____pathy refers to disease of the lymph gland.

5. _____ology is the study of bacteria.

6. _____logous means referring to the self.

7. _____atic means pertaining to lymph.

8. _____cyte means thymus cell.

9. Patho_____ is the study of disease.

10. _____toxic means poisonous to tissue.

Matching

Select a term from Column 1 to match each definition in Column 2. Write your choice on the line beside the definition.

Column 1	Column 2
1. Thymus gland _____	a. located on either side of the throat
2. Immunology _____	b. type of large white blood cell that devours invading cells and debris
3. Immunodeficiency _____	c. area connecting the nose and throat
4. Palatine tonsils _____	d. small proteins produced by T cells
5. Macrophage _____	e. gland of the immune system located in the mediastinum above the heart
6. Nasopharynx _____	f. study of bacteria
7. Artificial immunity _____	g. study of the immune system
8. Phagocytosis _____	h. type of immunity acquired through deliberate exposure (immunization)
9. Interferons _____	i. lacking in one or more components of the immune system
10. Bacteriology _____	j. "cell eating"

Word Building

Use roots, combining forms, prefixes, and suffixes to construct a medical term to match each definition provided.

Definition	Term
1. study of tissues	_____
2. study of shape and form	_____
3. large eating (cell)	_____
4. protein that helps destroy antigens	_____
5. pertaining to lymph	_____
6. pertaining to the spleen	_____
7. attraction for neutral (type of cell)	_____
8. one cell (type of WBC)	_____
9. lymphatic cell	_____
10. pertaining to watery fluid in the body (humor)	_____

Spelling Check

Correct the misspelled words in the following sentences.

1. Interfreons interfere with the replication of viruses. _____

2. Thymorsin is secreted by the thymus gland. _____

3. Macrophanges are a type of white blood cell. _____

4. Surgery on the cisterni chyli is the subject of the study. _____

5. Cayle flows from the abdominal lymph system. _____

6. The thyamus gland is located above the heart. _____

7. The palantine tonsils are on either side of the throat. _____

8. Imunogoblins help to destroy antigens. _____

9. The imunnologist is examining the patient. _____

10. Active artificial immuenity is given to an individual to prevent disease. _____

The diagram that follows shows various types of immunity and how each originates. Complete the diagram by providing the missing information.

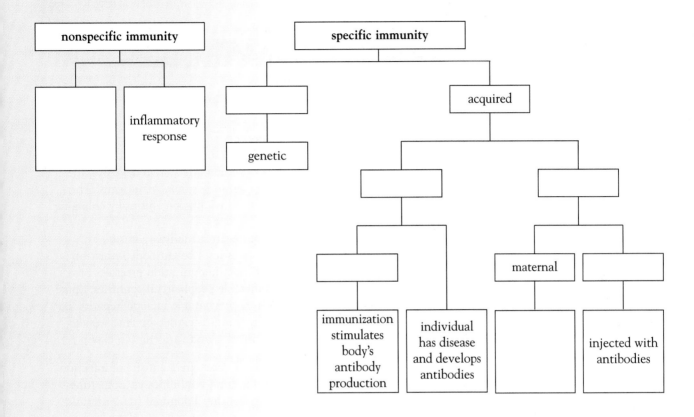

Assessing Patient Health

Wellness and Illness through the Life Span

The immune system undergoes many changes throughout the lifetime of the individual. Lymphoid tissue is the only tissue in the body that reaches adult growth during childhood, usually by age 6. It then continues to develop rapidly, surpassing adult size by puberty, when it slowly begins to decrease. This phenomenon is believed to occur because the child must produce antibodies and fight numerous antigenic stimuli.

The physician assesses the immune system by obtaining a complete history, performing a physical examination, and ordering laboratory tests. Frequent illness may suggest that the person has an incompetent immune system. The examiner palpates all areas containing superficial lymph nodes (refer to Figure 6.1). Enlarged lymph nodes, or swollen glands, can sometimes indicate an infection. Nodes that have responded to infection or cleared other substances feel spongy or like hard pellets (**shotty**). These **reactive nodes** are freely movable under the examiner's touch. Firm, fixed lymph nodes may signal an infection, a serious disorder, or a cancerous node. An enlarged liver or spleen may suggest an abnormality.

Controversy rages about immunizations. Side effects and toxicities of certain immunizations may cause serious, life-threatening and/or long-term effects. Some parents believe that the immunizations are unwarranted given that many of the diseases for which an infant is being immunized are uncommon today. On the other side of the argument are those who believe that the illnesses can cause a real threat to the particular child, as well as to society at large if the general population were not immunized.

Infants and Children

The infant is born with his or her mother's immunity, which provides protection for several months. The newborn acquires further immunity from the rich stores of bacterial and viral antibodies in breast milk. As the immune system develops, the child begins to produce antibodies of his or her own in response to antigens. The lymph nodes are large in childhood and respond to invading organisms by enlarging further.

In the early months, the child is immunized against many organisms. Immunizations are usually given in several doses to stimulate antibody formation and memory within the T cells. Stringent worldwide immunization practices have eliminated many diseases that once killed innumerable people in all countries. Some of the deadly diseases that are now almost entirely preventable include hepatitis B, diphtheria, tetanus, pertussis, pneumonia and meningitis caused by *Haemophilus influenzae* type b (Hib), polio, measles, mumps, rubella, and varicella (chickenpox).

COMMON CHILDHOOD INFECTIONS The tonsils are a frequent site of infection in youngsters who have upper respiratory infections and viral illnesses. Sometimes abdominal pain is associated with lymph drainage of the abdominal (mesenteric) lymph nodes.

Although young children may experience many upper respiratory illnesses, they usually do not develop serious bacterial infections unless they have an underlying condition, such as **immunodeficiency**. Children who are small for their age (a syndrome called failure to thrive) also should be tested for immunodeficiency. Primary immunodeficiency is inherited and may affect any part of the immune system. (Secondary immunodeficiency occurs as a result of an infection or virus, such as HIV, which is discussed later in this chapter.)

HEREDITARY IMMUNE SYSTEM DISEASES **Severe combined immunodeficiency (SCID)** is a life-threatening, hereditary condition that incorporates the failure of several aspects of immune function. Children with SCID cannot make antibodies and have incompetent lymphoid tissues. A bone marrow transplant from a matched donor is the only available cure.

Ataxia telangiectasia is another hereditary disease affecting the nervous system. Children with this disease experience decreased T-cell function and immunoglobulin deficiencies. **Wiskott-Aldrich syndrome** is a hereditary immunodeficiency disorder characterized by ineffective antigen response.

Adults and Seniors

With age, the immune system seems to function less efficiently. As an individual approaches his or her 60s and 70s, various illnesses tend to appear. One group of illnesses is the autoimmune disorders, characterized by a clinical syndrome in which there may be autoantibodies (antibodies against one's self) or specifically sensitized cells. Table 6.5 lists the most common autoimmune disorders and their antigens (the cells that the body turns against and attempts to destroy).

Table 6.4

Autoimmune Disorders and Their Antigens

Disorder	Age at onset	Antigen
diabetes (type 1)	any age	insulin, islet cell (pancreas)
glomerulonephritis (Goodpasture's syndrome)	any age	basement membrane (kidney)
Graves' disease (thyrotoxicosis)		follicle membrane (thyroid)
Hashimoto's thyroiditis	any age	thyroglobulin (thyroid)
hemolytic anemia	any age	RBCs
immune thrombocytopenic purpura	any age	platelets
multiple sclerosis	young adults	nerve myelin
myasthenia gravis	older	myoneural junction (nerve cells)
pernicious anemia	older	intrinsic factor
rheumatoid arthritis (excluding juvenile rheumatoid arthritis, a systemic autoimmune disorder in children)	older	immunoglobulin G (IgG)
scleroderma	older	unknown
systemic lupus erythematosus (SLE)	young adults, most commonly females	DN

ALLERGIES   Allergies are among the most common problems requiring people to visit the doctor or pharmacy. Hay fever, certain types of asthma, and hives are the major types of allergic reactions. As a group, allergies produce a range of responses from the minor annoyances of a runny nose and itchy eyes to potentially fatal, life-threatening reactions. In the Unites States between 1991 and 2001, there were 2,281 cases of allergic reactions reported out of the 1.9 billion doses of vaccinations administered. By way of comparison, the estimated incidence in the pediatric population of allergic reactions to food of any kind is approximately 6 to 8 percent; the incidence of allergy to an antibiotic in the same population is reported to be about 7.3%. The most common allergy is **hay fever,** which was first named by Blakley in England in 1865 after an illness known as farmer's lung, which was prevalent in the farmlands at that time. It was caused by an allergic reaction to the fungi and spores in the hay. Thus, the name *hay fever* was coined for the symptoms produced by the illness.

Allergic reactions occur because of the antibody immunoglobulin E (IgE) and are believed to be genetic. The first time an allergy-prone person encounters a substance to which he or she is allergic (an allergen), the body produces large amounts of IgE. Also involved in the allergic response are mast cells and basophils, a type of white blood cell in the circulating blood that migrates to the tissues. The IgE molecules attach to the surfaces of the mast cells and basophils. Mast cells are found in large quantities in the lungs, skin, tongue, and linings of the nose and intestinal tract.

The second encounter with an allergen produces a type I allergic reaction. Immunoglobulin E signals the mast cells or basophils to release their chemicals, including histamine, heparin, and other substances. These substances cause the telltale allergy signs: runny nose and eyes, itching, sneezing, and so forth. If the reaction is severe, it may result in **anaphylactic shock,** swelling of the tissues, including the throat, and a rapid drop in blood pressure. **Asthma** is actually a local anaphylactic reaction resulting from swelling within the respiratory tract. Type I reactions can be induced by certain foods, air contaminants, cosmetics, cleaning products, animals, flowers, trees, grasses, insects, drugs, and other substances.

Figure 6.5 depicts the chain reaction resulting from a bee sting in a susceptible person. This type I response can cause a local or severe allergic reaction, including anaphylaxis.

Figure 6.5 - Reaction From a Bee Sting

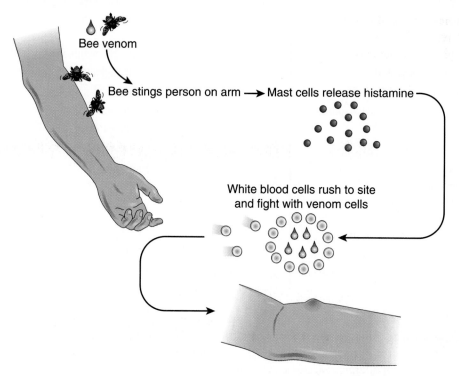

Bee venom

Bee stings person on arm → Mast cells release histamine

White blood cells rush to site and fight with venom cells

Causes inflamation, redness, swelling, warmth, and pain to ward off antigens (bee venom)

HUMAN IMMUNODEFICIENCY VIRUS **Human immunodeficiency virus (HIV)** is (globally) most commonly transmitted from mother to child during prenatal development, delivery, and breast feeding. It can also be transmitted by other body fluids including blood, semen, vaginal fluids, saliva, and wound drainage. It is a **retrovirus,** HIV-1, that can cause **acquired immunodeficiency syndrome (AIDS).** The virus enters the cells and, by a process called reverse transcription, becomes part of the cell's deoxyribonucleic acid (DNA), the compound within a cell that controls cellular reproduction. The viral DNA begins to produce (synthesize) its own ribonucleic acid (RNA), the chemical responsible for passing the genetic code to the cell, thereby taking over the cell. The T cells in the host, the person who has the virus, are affected and destroyed. As the cells are destroyed, the retrovirus spreads throughout the body. T-cell destruction leads to immunodeficiency, making the person susceptible to many infectious pathogens, classified as opportunistic infections. The body is also at risk for certain cancers: when the number of T cells is reduced, the immune system does not destroy and clear away cancer cells. Table 6.5 lists some of the illnesses associated with AIDS.

Table 6.5

Malignancies and Opportunistic Diseases Associated with AIDS

Disease	Description	Organism
Malignancies		
Kaposi's sarcoma	malignancy, particularly of skin and lymph nodes, most commonly found in older men but now seen in persons with AIDS	human herpesvirus 8
lymphoma	malignancy of lymph tissue that can be localized or systemic	N/A
Infections		
candidiasis	fungus normally found in the gastrointestinal tract that can cause systemic infection in an immunocompromised host	*Candida albicans*
Pneumocystis carinii pneumonia (PCP)	parasite found endemically that causes a particularly virulent type of pneumonia in the immunocompromised host	*Pneumocystis carinii*
tuberculosis (TB)	*Mycobacterium* that causes infection, usually in the lungs but sometimes disseminated, particularly in the immunocompromised host	*Mycobacterium tuberculosis*
Mycobacterium avium–intracellulare (MAI) complex	*Mycobacterium* that usually affects birds and fowl but has recently been found to be an opportunistic infection in AIDS patients	*Mycobacterium avium–intracellulare* complex
cytomegalovirus (CMV)	herpesvirus that infects humans and animals, causing swelling in the cell or organ in which it is found; particularly dangerous to the unborn child of an infected mother	Herpesviridae

PREVENTING THE SPREAD OF HIV The spread of HIV can be curtailed by avoiding contact with other people's bodily fluids. Using a condom when having sexual relations and avoiding contaminated needles are the major preventive measures. Select pharmaceutical agents can slow the progress of the disease (see later section on pharmaceuticals), however, HIV and the illnesses it brings are life threatening.

Table 6.6

Wellness and Illness Terms Relating to Immunity

Term	Meaning	Word Analysis	
acquired immunodeficiency syndrome (AIDS) ah-**kwIrd** im-myoo-nO-deh-**fish**-en-see **sin**-drOm	group of illnesses that occur as a result of infection with the HIV-1 virus	*immun/o* *deficiency*	immune to fail
anaphylaxis an-ah-fih-**lak**-sis	severe reaction caused by increased sensitivity to a substance;	*ana-* *phylaxis*	back; away protection
asthma **as**-mah	disorder in which airways are temporarily narrowed, resulting in difficulty in breathing, coughing, gasping, and wheezing	*asthma*	difficulty breathing
ataxia telangiectasia ah-**tak**-see-ah tel-**an**-jee-ek-tay-see-ah	progressive immunodeficiency disorder involving many systems, particularly the nervous system; it is hereditary, caused by immunoglobulin A (IgA) deficiency and decreased T helper cells	*a-* *taxia* *tel/o* *angi/o* *ect/o* *-ia*	absence order distance, end blood vessels outside condition

continued on next page

autoimmune aw-tO-ih-**myoon**	process in which the person's immune system turns against itself (relating to antibodies that attack the cells of the body producing them)	auto- immun/o	one: oneself free from catching a specific infectious disease
diabetes (type 1) dI-ah-**bee**-teez	metabolic disease caused by decreased production of insulin (normally produced in the pancreas); type 1 diabetes is thought to be autoimmune in nature	diabetes	siphon (perhaps because of the symptom of polyuria that occurs with diabetes)
glomerulonephritis glom-**er**-yoo-lO-neh-**frI**-tis	disease of cells in the kidneys (glomeruli) characterized by inflammatory changes resulting from an infection	glomerulo nephr/o -itis	a ball of yarn kidney inflammation
Graves' disease	autoimmune condition of the thyroid; a form of hyperthyroidism	Graves	Irish physician
Hashimoto's thyroiditis hah-shee-**mO**-tOz thI-roy-**dI**-tis	autoimmune condition of the thyroid whereby it is infiltrated with lymphocytes	Hashimoto thyr/o -itis	Japanese surgeon thyroid inflammation
hemolytic anemia **hee**-mO-**lit**-ik ah-**nee**-mee-ah	autoimmune disorder caused by antibodies directed against RBCs that results in increased destruction, leading to anemia	hem/o lys/o an- -emia	blood dissolution without blood
immune thrombocytopenic purpura ih-**myoon** throm-bO-sI-tO-**pee**-nik **per**-pyoo-rah	autoimmune disorder that produces platelet antibodies and results in the destruction of the body's own platelets	immun/o thromb/o cyt/o -penia -ic purpura	immune clot cell abnormal reduction pertaining to purple
immunodeficiency im-myoo-nO-deh-**fish**-en-see	state in which an individual has decreased immune function	immun/o deficiency	immune to fail
myasthenia gravis mI-as-**thee**-nee-ah **gra**-vis	immunologic disorder of neuromuscular transmission	my/o thenia gravis	muscle weakness grave
pernicious anemia per-**nish**-us ah-**nee**-mee-ah	vitamin B$_{12}$ deficiency that may be caused by an immunologic condition preventing absorption in the gastrointestinal tract; the erythrocytes are larger than normal and fewer are produced, causing the anemia	pernicious an- -emia	destructive without blood
retrovirus **ret**-rO-vI-rus	type of virus; a retrovirus causes HIV	retro- virus	backward poison
rheumatoid arthritis **roo**-mah-toyd ar-**thrI**-tis	painful condition affecting articulations; immunologic disorder causing pain and inflammation of the joints	rheuma arthr/o -itis	flux (a movement of fluid from a cavity) joint inflammation
scleroderma skler-O-**der**-mah	immunologic disorder characterized by thickening of the skin; can be systemic	scler/o derm/a	hardness skin
shotty **shot**-ee	rubbery, freely movable, normal-feeling lymph node	shot (pellet)	shotlike
systemic lupus erythematosus (SLE) sis-**tem**-ik **loo**-pus er-ih-them-ah-**tO**-sus	autoimmune disorder that causes inflammatory connective tissue disease in many areas of the body, including the kidneys, skin, and joints	systemic lupus erythem/a -osus (-osis)	affecting many parts of the body wolf redness condition

Wiskott-Aldrich syndrome **vis**-kot-**awl**-drik **sin**-drOm	hereditary immunodeficiency disorder characterized by ineffective antigen response; causes thrombocytopenia and frequent infections	*Wiskott* *Aldrich* *syn-* *drome*	German pediatrician U.S. pediatrician joined; together running

Word Analysis
Exercise 8

Identify the root in the following terms by drawing a box around it. Supply the definition for the root and a definition for the entire term.

Example [arthr]ography   joint   record of a joint

Term	Root Definition	Term Definition
1. toxicology	_____	_____
2. immunology	_____	_____
3. bacterial	_____	_____
4. anti-inflammatory	_____	_____
5. viral	_____	_____
6. hemolytic	_____	_____
7. rheumatoid	_____	_____
8. genetic	_____	_____
9. immunodeficiency	_____	_____
10. lymphoma	_____	_____

Comprehension Check
Exercise 9

Circle the correct term from each pair in the following sentences.

1. The examiner palpates/palpitations the lymph nodes.

2. As the immune/autoimmune system develops, the child begins to produce antibodies.

3. An enlarged/engrossed spleen may indicate an abnormality.

4. Lymphoid/Lymphosis tissue reaches adult size by about age 6.

5. Antigens/Antibodies are produced by the body.

6. Pernicious/Precious anemia is an autoimmune disorder found in older persons.

7. HIV/AIDS is the abbreviation for human immunodeficiency virus.

8. Lymphosis/Lymphoma is a malignancy of lymph tissue.

9. BT/TB is an infection caused by mycobacteria.

10. MTV/CMV refers to the cytomegalovirus.

Select a term from Column 1 to match a definition in Column 2. Write the number of the Column 1 term on the line beside the Column 2 definition.

Column 1		Column 2
1. scleroderma	_____	a. autoimmune disorder of the thyroid causing hyperthyroidism
2. retrovirus	_____	b. the immune system attacks its own body
3. Grave's disease	_____	c. infection with fungus (yeast) normally found in the gastrointestinal tract
4. hemolytic anemia	_____	d. malignancy of skin and lymph nodes often seen in persons with AIDS
5. anaphylaxis	_____	e. type of virus that causes HIV
6. candidiasis	_____	f. organism that causes tuberculosis
7. pernicious anemia	_____	g. Vitamin B_{12} deficiency caused by immunologic condition
8. Kaposi's sarcoma	_____	h. immunologic disorder characterized by thickening of the skin
9. *Mycobacterium tuberculosis*	_____	i. autoimmune disorder that results in destruction of RBCs
10. autoimmune	_____	j. severe allergic reaction

Use prefixes, roots, combining vowels, and suffixes to create medical terms for the definitions given. Write the term in the space beside the definition.

Definition	Term
1. pertaining to the system	_____
2. increased WBCs	_____
3. pertaining to lymph	_____
4. inflammation of the liver	_____
5. pertaining to the liver	_____
6. inflammation of a gland	_____
7. like or resembling lymph	_____
8. inflammation of the pharynx	_____
9. surgical removal of a lymph node	_____
10. study of diseases	_____

In the sentences that follow, incorrect prefixes or suffixes are used in the medical terms. Provide the correct prefix or suffix for each term by writing the corrected term on the line below the sentence.

1. Several immunitists have attempted to diagnose the problem.

   _____

2. Macrophils were observed ingesting bacteria in the tissue sample.

   _____

3. Avolution of the organ resulted in a smaller size.

   _____

4. Adenocytes is another term for tonsils in the back of the throat.

   _____

5. A progen can cause an individual to produce antibodies.

   _____

6. Adenopitis means disease of a gland.

   _____

7. A leukectomy is a white blood cell.

   _____

8. Eosinitis is the term meaning "attraction to eosin."

   _____

9. We observed thymophils under the microscope.

   _____

10. The thoracosis duct is a vessel of the lymphatic system.

   _____

Complete the concept map below depicting the disease process that occurs when AIDS develops.

Process by which HIV causes AIDS

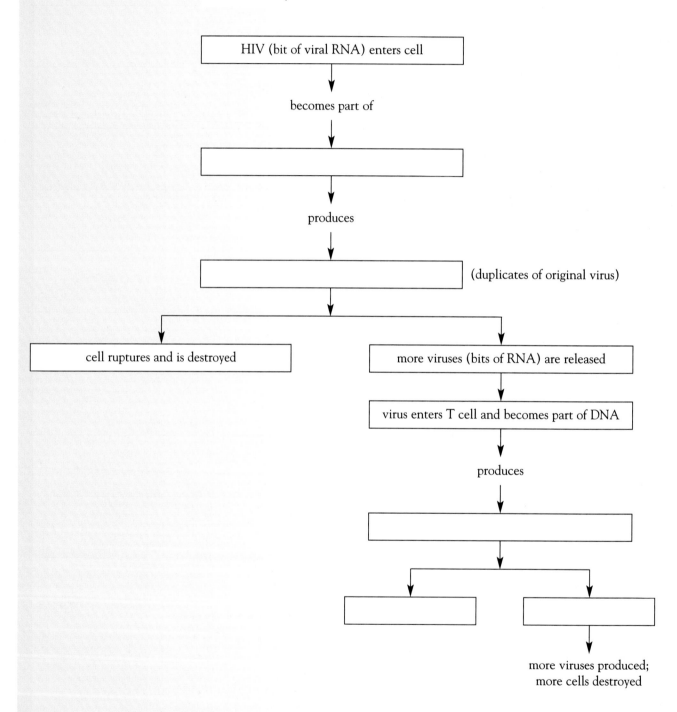

Diagnosing and Treating Problems

Tests, Procedures, and Pharmaceuticals

Laboratory tests are most important in diagnosing an immune disorder. A common test is the measurement of the immunoglobulins (Ig) IgM, IgG, IgA, IgD, and IgE. Table 6.7 shows the order (by the percentage found in the blood) and functions of immunoglobulins.

Table 6.7

Immunoglobulins and Their Functions

Ig	Percentage	Function
IgG	80	crosses the placenta and assists with passive and recall immunity
IgA	10-15	protects the gastrointestinal tract and eyes, since secretions may prevent antibody activity
IgM	5-10	first line of defense; formed first in response to an antigen
IgD	<0.1	lymphocyte receptor on activated B cells
IgE	<0.01	effects the release of agents from cells called mast cells that cause asthma, hay fever, and anaphylaxis

Other tests can determine T-cell numbers, T-cell subsets (such as T4 and T8), and their level of functioning. Antibodies from diseases such as polio and CMV can be detected in a blood test that measures B-cell function. The presence of HIV is assessed with one of the antibody-detection tests: the **enzyme-linked immunosorbent assay (ELISA)** or the **Western blot**.

Allergy testing is a common practice. Scratch tests (described in Chapter 5) can identify a person's specific allergies. The radioallergosorbent test (RAST) detects IgE-bound allergens that cause hypersensitivity (see Table 6.8).

Procedures

Lymphangiography is not performed often today, since it is possible to visualize the lymphoid tissue with an imaging process called a **gallium scan**. In this procedure, a radiopaque substance, gallium, is injected into the person; then the scan is performed to evaluate whether any lymph nodes are enlarged or affected.

Another procedure that is not being performed as commonly as a generation ago is **tonsillectomy and adenoidectomy (T&A)**. The operation is performed in children or adolescents who experience recurrent infections of the tonsils that cause morbidity such as frequent illness with fevers, recurrent documented bacterial infections, sinusitis as a result of these infections, and loss of school days. A specialist called an otolaryngologist, or an ear, nose, and throat (ENT) physician, usually performs this relatively short surgical procedure. Bleeding is the main complication.

Table 6.8

Tests Relating to the Immune System

Test	Description
antibody-detection tests	blood test that can detect specific antibodies
ELISA	very sensitive blood test used to detect infectious diseases including AIDS
gallium scan	imaging process in which radionuclide substance is injected into the patient to enhance the visibility of lymphoid tissue; abnormal uptake in the lymph tissues may indicate a malignancy or other process

continued on next page

lymphangiography	radiographic study that visualizes the lymphatic system after injection of a radiopaque substance
RAST	assay that detects IgE-bound allergens that cause hypersensitivity
Western blot	test that separates proteins; known as an immunoblot

Pharmaceutical Agents

Antibiotics are the mainstay of treatment for bacterial infections. The first antibiotics were produced from natural substances. Today, natural and semisynthetic substances are grouped into classes based on their mechanisms of action.

Many pharmacologic agents have been developed to treat HIV. Designed to interfere with replication of the virus, these **antiviral** agents include azidothymidine (AZT), or zidovudine; dideoxyinosine, or didanosine (DDI); and lamivudine (3TC). **Protease inhibitors** such as saquinavir are also used.

A trimethoprim-sulfamethoxazole combination (Bactrim) is the drug of choice for the prevention of *Pneumocystis carinii* pneumonia (PCP). Persons who are immunosuppressed may be given Bactrim to lower the risk of PCP. Herpes viruses can be treated with acyclovir, an **antiviral** agent.

Patients who have an immunodeficiency disorder may require administration of **intravenous immunoglobulin** infusions at least monthly. This product contains immunoglobulins that may be decreased or lacking in the patient's body. Numerous **antihistamines** are prescribed for allergies. These agents block the release of histamine, which causes the allergic symptoms.

Table 6.9

Pharmacologic Agents Relating to the Immune System

Drug Classes	Use	Generic Name	Brand Names
antibiotic (penicillin)	treat bacterial infections	penicillin V potassium amoxycillin	Veetids Amoxil
antibiotic (sulfonamide)	treat bacterial infections	sulfamethoxazole and trimethoprim	Bactrim
antifungal agents	treat local and/or systemic fungal infections	amphotericin B fluconazole nystatin	Fungizone, Amphotec Diflucan Mycostatin
antihistamines	block the release of histamine, which causes allergic reactions	diphenhydramine hydrochloride hydroxyzine hydrochloride	Benadryl Vistaril
antiviral agents	interfere with viral replication	acyclovir didanosine, DDI zidovudine, AZT foscarnet, PFA	Zovirax Videx Retrovir Foscavir
intravenous immune globulin (IVIG)	produced from the plasma of volunteers; plasma is heat-treated to kill pathogens that may be present	immune globulin, (intravenous), IVIG	Gamimune N; Gammagard S/D
protease inhibitors	inhibit the growth of HIV	indinavir sulfate	Crixivan

Table 6.10

Abbreviations

AIDS	acquired immunodeficiency syndrome
AZT	azidothymidine
CMV	cytomegalovirus
ELISA	enzyme-linked immunosorbent assay
HIV	human immunodeficiency virus
Ig	immunoglobulin
KS	Kaposi's sarcoma
MAI	*Mycobacterium avium–intracellulare* complex
PCP	*Pneumocystis carinii* pneumonia
SLE	systemic lupus erythematosus
STD	sexually transmitted disease
T&A	tonsillectomy and adenoidectomy
TB	tuberculosis

Word Building

Exercise 14

Use the root or combining form given and add other word parts to build a term that matches the definition. Write the term on the line provided.

Combining Form	Definition	
1. lymph/o	tumor of lymph	_____
2. splen/o	removal of the spleen	_____
3. aden/o	inflammation of a gland	_____
4. angi/o	repair of a vessel	_____
5. immun/o	specialist in the study of the immune system	_____
6. mono	single cell	_____
7. cyt/o	study of cells	_____
8. phag/o	condition of cell eating	_____
9. macro	large cell	_____
10. thym	pertaining to the thymus gland	_____

Read each sentence and determine which word best fits the sentence. Circle your choice.

1. Connie will have a tonsiloma/tonsilectomy this morning.

2. We will refer Tommy to a immunologist/lymphologist for his HIV.

3. Microscopy revealed several lymphocytes/lymphocytedema.

4. The pathophageology/pathophysiology laboratory will have the results in the morning.

5. The afferent/efferent vessel carries the fluid away from the node.

6. The spleen/splenectomy has ruptured.

7. Mrs. Wilson is an antilogous/autologous donor.

8. Involution/Evolution is the return of an organ or tissue from an enlarged to a smaller or normal size.

9. Mediaphages/Macrophages are phagocytic cells found in diseased or injured tissues.

10. Thymus/Thyroid is a gland in the mediastinum.

Matching

Exercise *16*

Match the list of procedures and treatments in Column 2 with the diagnosis or reason for the procedure in Column 1. Write the number of the diagnosis or problem in the space beside the name of the treatment or procedure. Note that some entries in Column 2 are diagnostic procedures.

Column 1		Column 2
1. suspicion of HIV	_____	a. lymphangiography
2. allergic reaction	_____	b. T&A
3. fungal infection	_____	c. scratch test
4. enlarged lymph nodes	_____	d. ELISA
5. viral infection	_____	e. Bactrim
6. recurrent infections of the tonsils	_____	f. gallium scan
7. specific allergies	_____	g. Benadryl
8. immunodeficiency disorder	_____	h. Mycostatin
9. bacterial infection	_____	i. Zovirax
	_____	j. intravenous immunoglobulin infusion

Find word parts in your text to construct medical terms for the definitions that follow. Write the term on the blank beside the definition. Then use the root or combining form to create a second word.

	Term	New Term
1. study of microbes	_____	_____
2. blood condition of decreased RBCs	_____	_____
3. against histamine	_____	_____
4. pertaining to a node	_____	_____
5. against (bacterial) life	_____	_____
6. pertaining to the thymus	_____	_____
7. like or resembling lymph	_____	_____
8. against a virus	_____	_____
9. pertaining to bacteria	_____	_____
10. surgical removal of adenoids	_____	_____

Read each term and determine whether it is spelled correctly. If the spelling is incorrect, write the correct spelling on the line provided.

1. monucyte   _____

2. tonsiles   _____

3. adenaid   _____

4. gland   _____

5. imunity   _____

6. aneamia   _____

7. retrovairus   _____

8. imunnodificencies   _____

9. infactions   _____

10. raedology   _____

The concept map below lists some common drug classifications with their actions and uses. Complete the map by filling in the blank spaces.

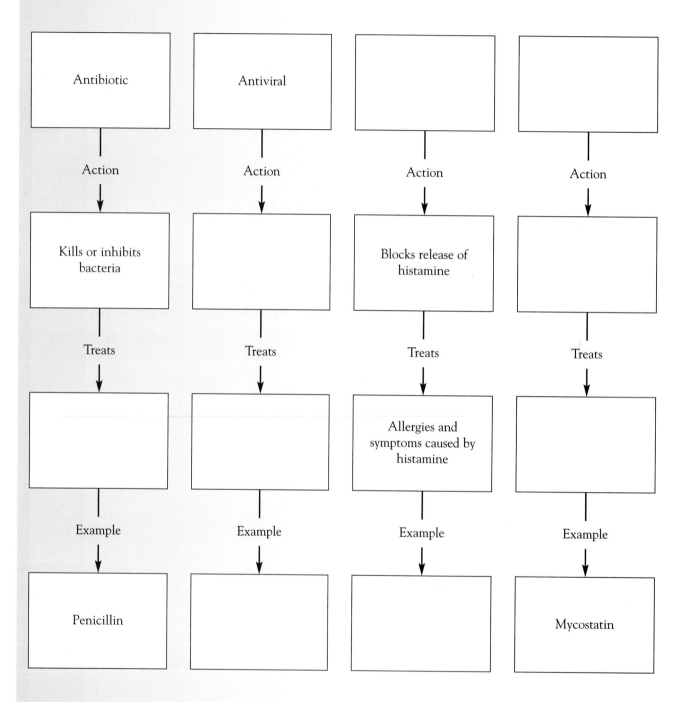

Performance Assessment 6

Crossword Puzzle

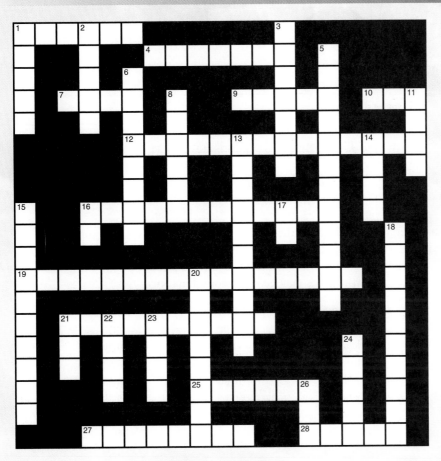

Across

1. local anaphylactic reaction in the respiratory system
4. diabetes antigen
7. suffix meaning study of
9. enzyme linked screening test
10. red blood cell
12. lymphoid tissue located on either side of the pharynx
16. specialist in the immune system
19. part of the lymphatic system, also called adenoids
21. glycoprotein that helps the body fight viruses
25. not susceptible
27. hormone of the thymus gland
28. number of sets of tonsils

Down

1. combining form for gland
2. watery fluid
3. causes the body to produce antibodies against it
5. "condition of cell eating"
6. "lymph tumor"
8. largest lymphiod structure, located in upper left quadrant of abdomen
11. cyt/o
13. organ or tissue returns to normal size
14. gallium _____
15. collection and filtration capsules of the lymphatic system
16. intravenous
17. immunoglobulin
18. "large eating cell"
20. means "like or resembling a gland"
21. abbreviation for Immunoglobulin E
22. combining form for poison
23. assay that detects IgE-bound allergens
24. taxia
26. abbreviation for otolaryngologist

What Do These Abbreviations Mean?

Write the definition of each abbreviation on the line provided.

1. AIDS   _____

2. Ig   _____

3. DPT   _____

4. ELISA   _____

5. T&A   _____

6. TB   _____

7. SLE   _____

8. STD   _____

9. KS   _____

10. CMV   _____

Build the Terms

In this exercise you will construct words from roots, prefixes, and suffixes.

    Select word parts from the lists to build a complete medical term for each definition given. Note that not all terms will have a root or combining form, prefix, and suffix. Some word parts may be used more than once.

Combining Forms	Prefixes	Suffixes
leuk/o	hyper-	-itis
splen/o	epi-	-logy
cyt/o	sub-	-logist
lymph/o	hypo-	-malacia
thymo/o	intra-	-pathy
morph/o	dis-	-penia
neutro/o	an-	-al
adeno/o	pre-	-oma
macr/o	de-	-ic
angi/o	anti-	-ular
immun/o	per-	-gram
chrom/o	bi-	-philic

1. study of structure and form of cells   _____

2. disease of the thymus   _____

3. softening of the spleen   _____

4. disease of a gland   _____

5. tumor of a gland   _____

6. inflammation of a gland   _____

7. specialist in the study of cells _____

8. decrease in the number of neutrophils _____

9. pertaining to the thymus _____

10. attraction to color _____

11. record (x-ray) of a lymphatic vessel _____

12. study of the immune system _____

Build the Terms

Provide the missing word parts to create the correct term for the definition provided.

1. _____osis means condition of cell eating.

2. _____itis refers to inflammation of cells.

3. _____ectomy is surgical removal of the spleen.

4. _____pathy refers to disease of the lymph gland.

5. _____ology is the study of bacteria.

6. _____logous means referring to the self.

7. _____atic means pertaining to lymph.

8. _____cyte means thymus cell.

9. Patho_____ is the study of disease.

10. _____toxic means poisonous to tissue.

What's Your Conclusion?

In this exercise you will practice selecting the correct explanation or logical next step. Read each mini medical record carefully, then select the correct response. Write the letter of your answer in the space provided.

1. Robin M., a 12-year-old female, is brought to the physician's office by her mother, who says that Robin has had a sore throat and fever for the past two days. The doctor's physical examination shows a very red pharynx, with yellowish exudate; the tonsils are enlarged and covered with the same exudate. Cervical and supraclavicular lymph nodes are distinctly palpable and shotty. The child has a temperature of 102° F. She is listless, and her skin, lips, and mucous membranes appear quite dry. Upon questioning, the mother states that Robin's appetite has been very poor. This is the third time in 6 months Robin has been seen for the same type of symptoms, and she had three such episodes in the past 12 months. You are a student nursing assistant, gaining clinical experience in the physician's office, and you understand that:

A. It is possible that Robin will need a T&A.
B. The condition in her throat is called parotitis, which is often treated with warm compresses to the submandibular area.

Your response: _____

2. Twenty-two year old Marian A. is the next patient. She comes with complaints of fatigue and weakness, loss of appetite, and weight loss. Examination shows lymphadenopathy and splenomegaly. She has a temperature of 101° F. Marian asks the doctor to explain what's wrong. What will he say?

A. The doctor will tell her she has enlarged lymph nodes and an enlarged spleen.
B. Marian will be told she probably has Hashimoto's thyroiditis.

Your response: _____

3. Henry Z. comes to the AIDS clinic with bluish-red skin nodules on various parts of his body. He was diagnosed with HIV infection four years ago and has recently stopped ZDV therapy.

A. Expect that the doctor will diagnose Kaposi's sarcoma, a malignant condition that arises from the lining of capillaries and is seen as bluish, reddish, or purplish skin lesions.
B. Anticipate that the physician will recognize the nodules as being bruises from some type of trauma to the tissue.

Your response: _____

Analyzing Medical Records

Read the clinic note on the next page and answer the questions below.

1. What does "general malaise" mean?

2. Describe three findings from the physical examination.

3. What is chronic cystitis?

4. What does the notation "D/C Triavil" mean?

5. What is Zoloft prescribed for? When will the patient take this medication?

Clinic Note

PATIENT: Daniel C.
DATE: July 13, xxxx

S: 36 y/o white male reports increasing night sweats, low back pain, headaches, persistent cough, lack of appetite, and general malaise. Denies polyuria, hematuria, and states he believes his longstanding cystitis may be better this week. He states that he easily becomes fatigued and often has difficulty sleeping. Patient states, "It is so hard to get up in the morning, most days I just stay in bed." He is unemployed and living with his parents following his diagnosis of HIV infection in 1994. He continues to be followed by Dr. H. Timmons in Chicago for treatment of his primary diagnosis and receives AZT; he reports taking that medication as directed. Patient states that in the past three months his CD4 count, which has been decreasing, seems to have stabilized. The count is still low, however, with an absolute value of 260. He acknowledges additional diagnoses of chronic active hepatitis, chronic cystitis, oral candidiasis, and depression. His depression is currently being treated with Triavil, and he reports taking that medication as directed. He states that he has stopped smoking, as of last month, and does not consume ETOH. He is seen in the clinic today for routine follow-up.

O: Patient is thin, pale, and appears somewhat fragile. Movements and speech are somewhat slow. Vital signs: T 98 F, P 88, R 24, BP 142/88. Supraclavicular lymph nodes are enlarged and shotty. Oral mucosa is slightly reddened, but appears otherwise normal. There is no leukoplakia. Mild bilateral wheezing on expiration. Left side of abdomen is soft and nontender; right side is mildly tender. No suprapubic tenderness. Liver margin is palpable approximately 2 cm below the costal margin; hepatomegaly is unchanged since last exam. Back is slightly tender to palpation throughout the lumbar area. Remainder of examination is unremarkable.

A: 1) HIV infection.
    2) Chronic hepatitis B.
    3) Chronic depression, not responding well to current therapy.
    4) Chronic cystitis.
    5) Chronic oral candidiasis infection.

P: 1) Patient will continue AZT therapy and will continue to be followed by Dr. Timmons.
    2) Zoloft, 50 mg, 1 q. a.m.
    3) Routine clinic labs.
    4) Social worker to discuss appropriate short- and long-term goals with patient and explore aspects of depression.

L. F. Cincaid, MD

Using Medical References

The following sentences contain medical terms that were not addressed on the tables in this chapter. Use medical reference books, your medical term analysis skills, and/or a medical dictionary to find the correct definition of each underlined word. Write the definition on the line below the sentence.

1. Dr. Kelly diagnosed <u>sarcoidosis</u> in the patient.

   _____

2. The professor explained the process of <u>lymphocytopoiesis</u> to a group of medical students.

   _____

3. The lab has received a grant to purchase new <u>cytometers</u>.

   _____

4. Mr. Thomas is an <u>autologous</u> donor.

   _____

5. Dr. Brown ordered a series of tests to confirm the diagnosis of <u>mononucleosis</u>.

   _____

6. This particular <u>cytomorphology</u> is not something we've seen before.

   _____

7. Intradermal skin testing reveals the patient to be <u>anergic</u>.

   _____

8. The microscopic examination showed <u>cytomegalic</u> changes consistent with the physician's diagnosis.

   _____

9. The <u>interstitial fluid</u> contained both bacteria and macrophages.

   _____

10. There was <u>purulent exudate</u> on the tonsils bilaterally.

    _____

11. The patient succumbed to <u>toxoplasmosis</u>.

    _____

12. The sigmoid colon and rectum revealed mucosal ulceration and <u>angioinvasion</u> by the fungus.

    _____

Short Answer

In your own words, describe the role of lymphocytes in the body's defense mechanism.

_____

_____

_____

_____

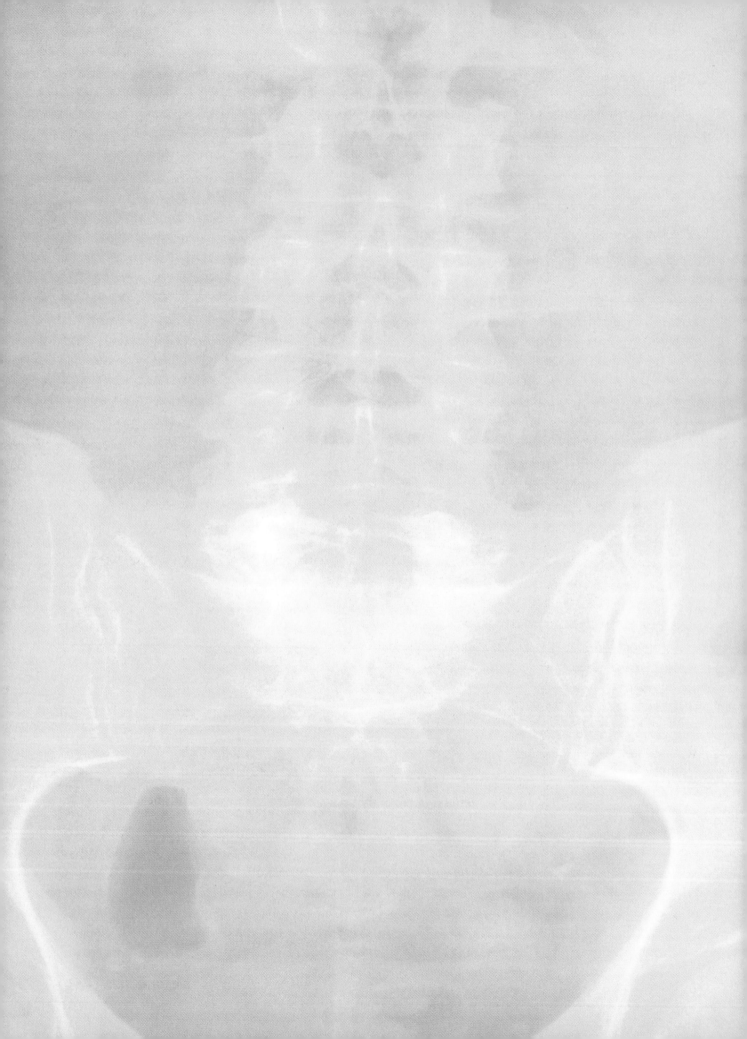

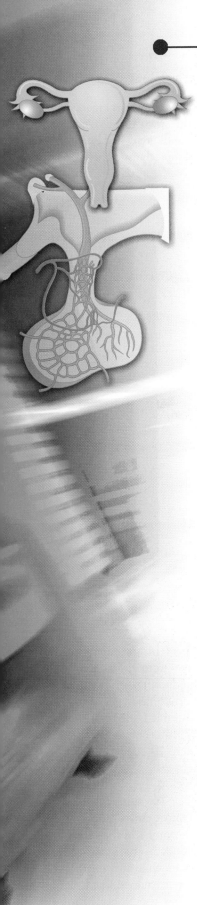

Chapter 7

The Endocrine System

Learning Outcomes

Students will be able to:

- Identify the major endocrine glands.
- Name the major hormones secreted by the endocrine glands and their function(s).
- Describe the role of negative feedback in maintaining homeostasis.
- List effects of hormonal abnormalities.
- Name tests and treatments for major hormonal abnormalities.
- Identify the life phases most commonly associated with various hormonal abnormalities.
- Correctly spell and pronounce endocrine system terminology.
- State the meaning of abbreviations related to the endocrine system.

Translation, Please? Translation, Please? Translation, Please?

Read this excerpt from a medical record and try to answer the questions that follow.

> HPI: Mrs. Smith presented with complaints of polydipsia, polyuria, and polyphagia. She reported a recent 5-pound weight loss.
> PE: On physical examination, she appeared tired and listless, with poor skin turgor. Mucous membranes appeared dry. Respiration deep and rapid. Temperature 100.8°F.
> Laboratory Data: Blood glucose level 350.
> Plan: FBS in the morning.

1. Does polydipsia mean she is very dizzy or very thirsty?
2. Does polyphagia mean that her symptoms have had many phases or is Mrs. Smith very hungry?
3. Does turgor refer to color or fullness?

Answers to "Translation Please?"

1. Polydipsia means thirsty. The root derives from the Greek word *dipsa*, which means thirst.
2. Polyphagia means hungry. The root derives from the Greek word *phagein*, meaning to eat.
3. Turgor is the normal tension produced by the fluid content of blood vessels, capillaries, and cells. The term comes from the Late Latin, *turgere*, which means swollen.

Identifying the Specialty

The System and Its Practitioners

The ductless glands that secrete substances called **hormones** into the blood make up the endocrine system. These hormones are chemical messengers that control many important life functions, including growth, reproduction, and metabolism. Some hormones released by the gland affect a target organ directly. Other hormones, known as **tropic hormones**, stimulate a target organ to secrete its own specific hormones.

The area of medicine concerned with the endocrine system is called **endocrinology**, and the specialized physician is an **endocrinologist**. Endocrinologists often work in concert with other specialists, depending on the system and hormones involved.

Anatomy and Physiology of the Endocrine System

The endocrine glands are located in several areas of the body, as shown in Figure 7.1. Recall from Chapter 3, "The Integumentary System," that the sweat glands contain ducts and their secretions move through these ducts. These glands are called **exocrine glands**. **Endocrine glands** are ductless and secrete their fluid directly into the blood, which carries it to specific organs.

Figure 7.1 - Endocrine Glands

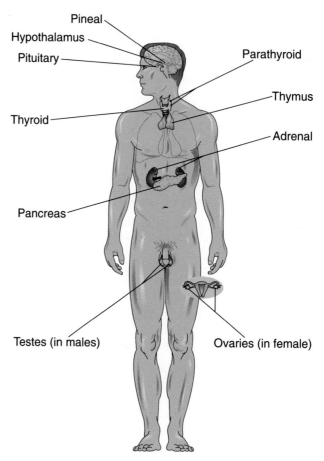

Pineal
Hypothalamus
Pituitary
Parathyroid
Thymus
Thyroid
Adrenal
Pancreas
Testes (in males)
Ovaries (in female)

The endocrine system produces two types of hormones, **protein hormones** and **steroid hormones**. Protein hormones are messengers that travel from an endocrine gland to a specific target organ and cause the target organ to produce its own hormone in a matter of seconds or minutes. Steroid hormones, on the other hand, pass directly into the cells of the target organ, and, because they are lipid-soluble (able to dissolve in a fatty substance), they pass into the nucleus of the cell. Within the nucleus, they form a composite or complex that produces a protein that exerts its effect on the target cell. This process requires several hours.

The body secretes hormones at a rate that keeps their level in the blood almost constant. It can do this because it receives continuous feedback. **Negative feedback** means that when the hormone level in the blood rises out of a target range, production of that hormone is stopped. When the concentration of the hormone in the blood decreases below the target range, more of the hormone is produced. This works to keep hormones at the right levels in the blood. This feedback mechanism controls many processes within the body and helps it maintain the proper balance within its internal environment, described as **homeostasis**. Figure 7.2 shows the process of negative feedback using the insulin hormone.

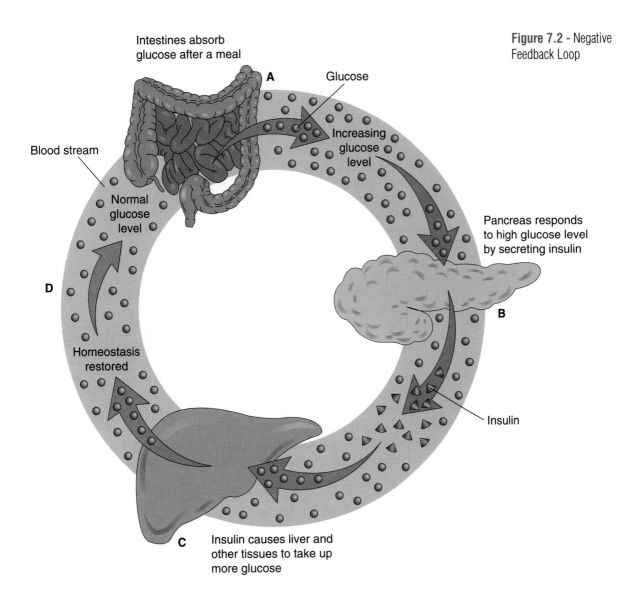

Figure 7.2 - Negative Feedback Loop

Intestines absorb glucose after a meal

A

Glucose

Increasing glucose level

Blood stream

Normal glucose level

D

Pancreas responds to high glucose level by secreting insulin

B

Insulin

Homeostasis restored

C

Insulin causes liver and other tissues to take up more glucose

The Endocrine Glands and Their Functions

In cephalocaudal (top to bottom) order, the endocrine glands include the **pineal body**, the **hypothalamus**, and the **pituitary**, all of which are located in the brain. In the neck and upper-chest area are the **thyroid**, the **parathyroid**, and **thymus glands**. The **adrenal** glands are located on top of the kidneys in the area of the back just above the waist. The **pancreas** is located in the upper abdomen, and completing this system are the **reproductive organs** in the lower abdomen.

PINEAL BODY   The **pineal body** is believed to control the body's internal clock. Although the complete role and all functions of the pineal gland are not fully understood, scientists do know that the pineal gland secretes the hormone **melatonin**. Melatonin is the substance that turns on the biological clock at puberty and also regulates circadian rhythms (day and night sleep patterns). Darkness stimulates production of melatonin; light inhibits it.

HYPOTHALAMUS   The **hypothalamus**, a structure of the brain, connects the endocrine system and the nervous system through a system of specialized capillaries and nerves. **Releasing factors (RF)** carry signals to the pituitary gland to stimulate or inhibit production and release of hormones:

- Thyrotropin-releasing hormone (TRH)
- Gonadotropin-releasing hormone (GnRH)
- Growth hormone-releasing hormone (GHRH)
- Corticotropin-releasing hormone (CRH)
- Somatostatin
- Dopamine
- Prolactin-releasing hormone
- Prolactin-inhibiting hormone

All of these are released into the blood and travel immediately to the anterior lobe of the pituitary, where they exert their effects. All of them are released in periodic spurts. In fact, replacement hormone therapy with these hormones does not work unless the replacements are also given in spurts.

PITUITARY GLAND   The **pituitary gland** is connected to the hypothalamus. Although it is small (the size of the tip of the little finger), it controls the release of most of the hormones in the body. The pituitary gland is divided into anterior and posterior lobes, the **adenohypophysis** and **neurohypophysis**, respectively, each of which secretes different hormones. The anterior pituitary controls seven hormones, and the posterior just two. The posterior pituitary releases both **antidiuretic hormone (ADH**, also known as **vasopressin)**, which exerts its influence on the kidneys by regulating the excretion of water by the kidney tubules, and **oxytocin**, which stimulates the flow of milk when the nursing baby sucks on the mother's breast. Oxytocin also increases the strength of uterine contractions during labor and delivery. In fact, it is often administered when women are experiencing **dystocia**, or decreased contractions during labor and delivery. Oxytocin is one of the few hormones released by a positive feedback mechanism—that is, the stronger the contractions are, the more oxytocin is released into the bloodstream.

Some of the pituitary hormones are **tropic hormones**, which stimulate specific target organs to produce their own hormones. Others exert their influence on body tissues rather than directly affecting specific endocrine glands. Table 7.1 lists the anterior pituitary hormones. Figure 7.3 depicts the relationship among the hypothalamus, the pituitary, and the hormones they produce.

Table 7.1

Pituitary Hormones

Anterior pituitary hormones	Action
Tropic hormones	
adrenocorticotropic hormone (ACTH)	stimulates the release of adrenocortical hormones (steroid hormones)
follicle-stimulating hormone (FSH)	in females, stimulates the ovaries to produce their hormones; in males, stimulates the testes to produce sperm
luteinizing hormone (LH)	in females, stimulates the ovarian follicle and ovum to mature and ovulate; in males, stimulates testosterone to be secreted by the testes
thyroid-stimulating hormone (TSH)	stimulates the thyroid gland to release its hormones
Nontropic hormones	
growth hormone (somatotropin) (GH)	increases protein production in many tissues, increases breakdown of fatty acids in fatty tissues (adipose tissue), and increases glucose level in blood
melanocyte-stimulating hormone (MSH)	stimulates production and release of the melanin pigment in skin (see Chapter 3, "The Integumentary System"); not technically an anterior pituitary hormone—it can be extracted from all parts of the pituitary
prolactin	acts on breast tissue to stimulate milk production

continued on next page

Posterior pituitary hormones (both are non-tropic)	Action
antidiuretic hormone	decreases the amount of water lost through the kidneys
oxytocin	causes uterine contractions and promotes milk release

Figure 7.3 - Pituitary Hormones

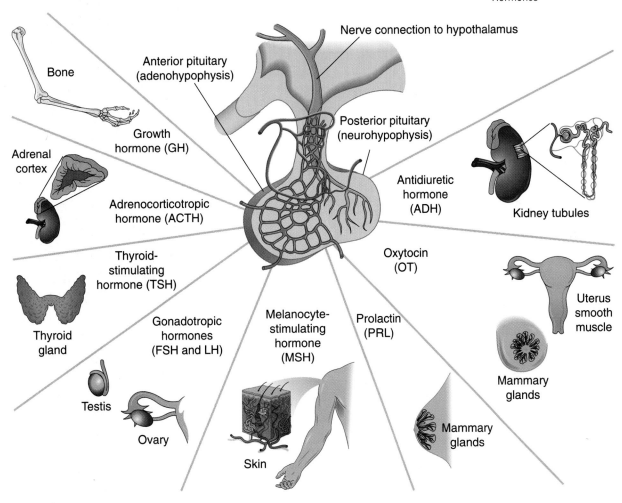

THYROID GLAND   The **thyroid gland** is located in the lower portion of the neck, below the larynx (see Figures 7.1 and 7.4). It is butterfly shaped, with two lobes connected by a small, thin **isthmus**. The thyroid gland houses **follicles**, whose cavities are lined with cuboidal epithelium cells. The cavities store two thyroid hormones, **triiodothyronine (T_3)** and **thyroxine (T_4)**. T_3 and T_4 are stored as a **colloid**, a gluelike substance, until needed by the body. When stimulated by TSH, the thyroid releases them (see Table 7.1).

T_3 and T_4 are named for the number of atoms of iodine contained in each molecule, and iodine must be ingested in the diet to ensure adequate production of these two hormones. The thyroid hormones influence every cell in the body: they direct **metabolism** (the use of cellular energy), cellular replication and brain development.

The thyroid gland also secretes **calcitonin**, or **thyrocalcitonin**. Calcitonin is not released as a result of TSH stimulation but rather in response to high levels of calcium in the blood. When the level of calcium is high, the blood deposits it in bone. In other words, an increased concentration of calcium in the blood causes calcitonin secretion, which leads to resorption of calcium into the bone. Note that this balancing process is another example of homeostasis and a negative feedback loop.

PARATHYROID GLANDS Embedded behind the thyroid gland are two sets of **parathyroid glands,** two in each of the lobes of the thyroid gland (Figure 7.4). The parathyroid glands secrete **parathyroid hormone, or parathormone (PTH).** When the concentration of calcium in the blood is decreased, PTH causes osteoclasts in the bone to break down bone, freeing calcium, which then moves into the bloodstream. This process, in turn, increases the calcium level in the blood.

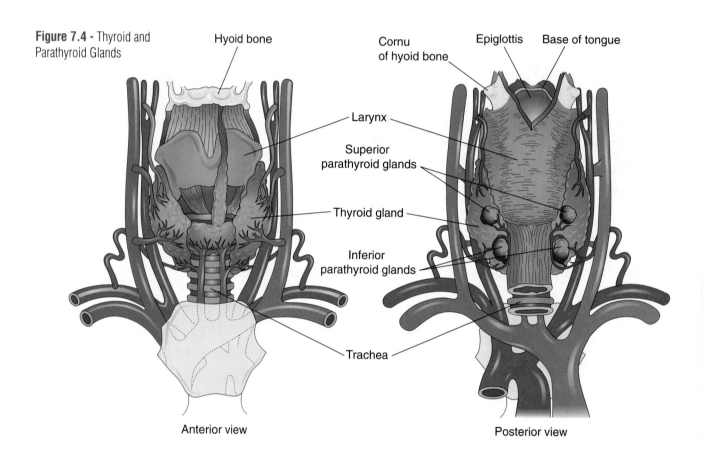

Figure 7.4 - Thyroid and Parathyroid Glands

Hyoid bone

Cornu of hyoid bone

Epiglottis

Base of tongue

Larynx

Superior parathyroid glands

Thyroid gland

Inferior parathyroid glands

Trachea

Anterior view

Posterior view

PTH works in concert with calcitonin to ensure the correct amount of calcium in the blood; however, the two hormones perform opposite functions, called an **antagonistic** effect. When the calcium concentration is increased, calcitonin is secreted; when the calcium level is decreased, PTH is secreted. Figure 7.5 illustrates this antagonistic process.

Figure 7.5 - Antagonistic Feedback Effect

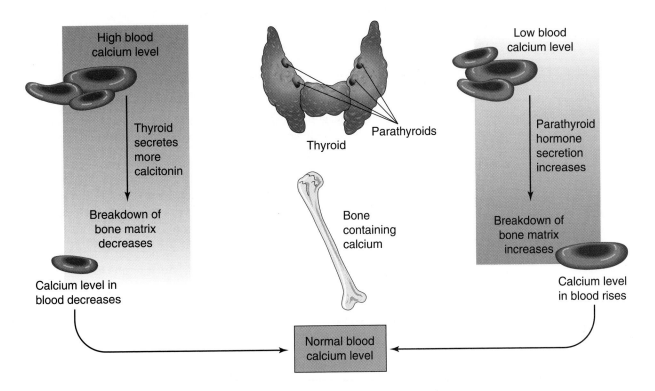

THYMUS GLAND The **thymus gland**, located in the **mediastinum** in the chest, secretes the hormone **thymosin** and plays an important role in immune function. (Refer to Chapter 6, "The Immune System," for a further discussion of the thymus and its function.)

ADRENAL GLANDS The **adrenal glands** are triangular-shaped glands located on the top of each kidney (refer to Figure 7.1). They consist of an outer portion, the **cortex**, and an inner portion, the **medulla**. Each area synthesizes and secretes different hormones with different functions. The cortex secretes three types of **corticosteroid** hormones. The medulla secretes hormones known as **catecholamines**.

The three types of hormones produced by the adrenal cortex are **glucocorticoids**, **mineralocorticoids**, and sex hormones. As a group, the corticosteroids produced by the adrenal cortex influence glucose metabolism, regulate sodium and potassium use in the kidney, and play a role in metabolism, antibody production, and the development of secondary sex characteristics. The adrenal medulla functions as part of the autonomic nervous system, which is fully described in Chapter 8, "The Nervous System." The adrenal medulla secretes the catecholamines **epinephrine** and **norepinephrine**. Epinephrine, or **adrenalin**, is the primary hormone, accounting for about 80 percent of the adrenal medulla's secretion. Epinephrine causes the "fight or flight" response, the body's physical preparation either to escape or do battle when faced with a dangerous or challenging situation. This reaction is also known as the stress response. Consider what occurs when you are scared:

- Blood flow is decreased to the tissues that need it least, such as the gastrointestinal tract and the kidneys.
- Blood flow is increased to the areas that need to perform in an emergency situation, including the heart, skeletal muscles, and brain.
- The adrenal medulla secretes catecholamines, which increase metabolism and elevate the level of blood glucose (to provide increased energy).

PANCREATIC GLANDS The **pancreas**, an organ located in the upper abdomen, contains clumps of cells scattered throughout its structure. These cells are called **pancreatic islets**, or **islets of Langerhans**, and are actually microscopic hormone-secreting endocrine glands. The pancreas has both exocrine function, in the form of digestive enzymes (discussed in Chapter 12, "The Gastrointestinal System"), and endocrine function.

Within the pancreatic islets are three kinds of cells, each of which produces a different hormone: alpha cells, beta cells, and delta cells.

1. **Alpha cells** secrete **glucagon**, which raises the blood glucose concentration by converting glycogen in the liver to glucose. When the blood glucose level falls, glucagon is released to increase it.

2. **Beta cells** secrete **insulin**, perhaps the best-known hormone and one that is essential for proper body functioning. Insulin, which is regulated by the level of glucose in the blood, decreases blood glucose levels by storing it as fat in adipose tissue. Therefore, insulin is an antagonist to glucagon.

3. **Delta cells** secrete a hormone called **somatostatin**. Somatostatin interferes with the release of growth hormone and glucagons, which results in decreased blood glucose level. In other words, somatostatin generates a **hypoglycemic** effect. Release of growth hormone and glucagons causes the opposite effect, **hyperglycemia**, or elevated blood glucose concentration.

REPRODUCTIVE ORGANS The organs of reproduction are also endocrine glands. **Ovaries** in the female secrete **estrogen**, which promotes the development of female sex characteristics. They also secrete **progesterone**, which, after egg fertilization, works to prevent miscarriage and prepares the mammary glands for milk production. The **placenta** is also an endocrine structure, secreting human chorionic gonadotropin (hCG), estrogen, and progesterone . A placenta forms and functions only temporarily, during gestation. In the male, **testes** secrete **testosterone**, the hormone that promotes male sex characteristics. The structure and function of these glands and hormones are discussed further in Chapter 14, "The Male Reproductive System" and Chapter 15, "The Female Reproductive System." Table 7.2 lists combining forms used in reference to the endocrine system, and Table 7.3 lists endocrine anatomy and physiology terms.

Table 7.2

Combining Forms Relating to the Endocrine System

Combining form	Meaning	Example
aden/o	glands	adenocarcinoma
adren/o	adrenals	adrenocorticoids
andr/o	masculine	androgen
estr/o	female	estrogen
gluc/o	glucose (sugar)	glucocorticoid
gonad/o	sex organs	gonadotropin
melan/o	skin pigment	melanocyte
pancreat/o	pancreas	pancrelipase
somat/o	relationship to the body	psychosomatic
thyr/o	thyroid	thyroxin
-tropic (tropin)	turning toward, changing	somatotropin

Table 7.3

Anatomy and Physiology Terms Relating to the Endocrine System

Term	Meaning	Word Analysis	
adrenal cortex ah-**dree**-nal **kor**-teks	outer portion of the adrenal glands	ad- renal cortex	to kidney bark (of a tree)
adrenal medulla ah-**dree**-nal med-**ul**-ah	inner portion of the adrenal glands	ad- renal medulla	to kidney middle
androgen **an**-drO-jen	adrenocortical hormone (e.g., testosterone) that stimulates secondary male sex characteristics	andr/o -gen	male to produce
antagonist an-**tag**-ah-nist	one process or agent that works against another	anti- agon	against fight
calcitonin kal-sih-**tO**-nin	hormone that increases calcium in bone and lowers the calcium in blood	calci tonos	lime stretching
catecholamine **kat**-eh-kol-**am**-een	hormones secreted in times of stress: epinephrine, norepinephrine, and dopamine	catechol amine	chemical component compound derived from ammonia
colloid **kol**-oyd	yellowish, translucent substance that resembles glue	colloid	appearance of glue
endocrine gland **en**-dO-krin	type of gland that secretes hormones directly into ductless glands	endo- -crine	within secrete
estrogen **es**-trO-jen	hormone that stimulates secondary sex characteristics; controls the menstrual cycle	estrus -gen	mad desire (the time that female animals are most fertile) to produce
exocrine gland **eks**-O-krin	gland that secretes outwardly through ducts	exo- -crine	outside, outward secrete
glucagon **gloo**-kah-gon	hormone secreted by the islet cells of the pancreas to cause the increase in blood glucose	gluc/o -ago	pertaining to glucose (sweetness) to lead
glucocorticoid **gloo**-kO-kor-tih-koyd	steroid hormones	gluc/o corticoid	pertaining to glucose (sweetness) hormone of the adrenal cortex
homeostasis hO-mee-O-**stay**-sis	state of having all body functions in balance	home/o -stasis	alike stop, standing
hormone **hor**-mOn	chemical substance secreted by specific organs and/or glands and carried into the bloodstream to stimulate another organ	hormon	setting in motion
hyperglycemia **hI**-per-glI-**see**-mee-ah	increased glucose concentration in the blood	hyper- glykys -emia	increased sweet blood condition
hypoglycemia **hI**-pO-glI-**see**-mee-ah	decreased glucose concentration in the blood	hypo- glykys -emia	low, decreased sweet blood condition
hypothalamus **hI**-pO-**thal**-ah-mus	area of the brain that stimulates target organs to secrete hormones; located inferior to the thalamus	hypo- thalam/o	low, decreased thalamus

continued on next page

insulin **in**-suh-lin	hormone secreted by the islets of Langerhans of the pancreas; promotes the use of glucose in the body, protein synthesis, and fat utilization	*insulin*	island
islets of Langerhans I-lets uv **Lang**-er-hahns	little masses of cells resembling islands in the pancreas that secrete the hormone insulin	*islet* *Langerhans*	small island nineteenth-century German anatomist
isthmus **is**-mus	narrow area that connects two larger parts	*isthmos*	narrow passage
melatonin mel-ah-**tO**-nin	hormone, secreted by the pineal gland, concerned with circadian rhythm (the body's mechanism to differentiate day and night)	*melanophore* *tonos* *-in*	dermal pigment cell that changes colors quickly stretching in, on
metabolism meh-**tab**-ah-liz-em	process that causes chemical change in the body	*metabole* *-ism*	change state, condition, process
mineralocorticoid **min**-er-al-O-**kor**-tih- koyd	steroid hormone secreted by the adrenal cortex; influences sodium (salt) metabolism	*mineral* *corticoid*	mines hormone secreted by the adrenal cortex
negative feedback	process that controls hormone production in response to the hormone level in the blood	*nego*	to deny
ovary **O**-vah-ree	female reproductive gland (paired)	*ovari/o*	ovary
pancreas **pan**-kree-as	gland that extends from the duodenum to the spleen; exocrine portion secretes pancreatic juices directly into the intestine; endocrine portion secretes insulin and glucagon	*pancreas*	all flesh
parathyroid par-ah-**thI**-royd	gland adjacent to the thyroid that secretes parathormone, the hormone that regulates calcium level in the blood	*para-* *thyroid*	alongside, near thyroid gland
pineal body **pin**-ee-al	pinecone-shaped gland located in the center of the brain that secretes melatonin	*pineal*	pine
placenta plah-**sen**-tah	organ that provides transfer of substances between the fetus and the mother	*placenta*	cake (perhaps because of its shape)
progesterone prO-**jes**-ter-On	steroid hormone secreted by the ovary and placenta; available as synthetic agent	*pro-* *gesto*	before to bear
prototype **prO**-tO-tIp	the first form or type from which others are copied	*proto-* *typos*	the highest rank type
somatostatin sO-mah-tO-**stat**-in	hormone secreted by the hypothalamus that inhibits growth hormone release	*somat/o* *-stasis* *-in*	body standing still not; in, within
testis **tes**-tis	male reproductive glands located within the scrotum; male gonads; testicles	*testis*	testicle
testosterone tes-**tos**-ter-On	androgen hormone secreted by the testes and to a lesser degree by the ovaries and adrenal cortex	*test/o*	testicle
thymosin **thI**-mO-sin	hormone (of the thymus gland) that stimulates the thymus to release its hormones	*thym/o*	thymus

thymus **thI**-mus	lymphoid organ located behind the mediastinum; functions in the development of the immune system until puberty	*thym/o*	thymus
thyroid **thI**-royd	gland in the neck that secretes thyroxine and triiodothyronine	*thyr/o*	thyroid
thyroxine (T_4) thI-**rok**-sin	hormone secreted by the thyroid gland	*thyr/o*	thyroid
triiodothyronine (T_3) trI-I-O-dO-**thI**-rO-nee	hormone secreted by the thyroid gland	*tri- iodo- thyronine*	three iodine amino acid related to thyroxine
tropic hormones	pituitary hormones that affect growth or function of other glands	*troph/o*	turning toward

Word Analysis

Exercise 1

Separate the terms into their word parts and give a definition for each term. Use a root or combining form from each term to create a new, related term.

1. adenitis _____

2. adrenal _____

3. pancreatitis _____

4. android _____

5. glucometer _____

6. melanocarcinoma _____

7. thyroidectomy _____

8. androgenous _____

9. hyperglycemic _____

10. thymic _____

Comprehension Check

Exercise 2

Circle the correct word from each pair to fit the following sentences.

1. A portion of the placenta/placebo was retained.

2. The adrenal humors/hormones affect the nervous system.

3. The patient was found to be deficient in calcitonin/calcaneus.

4. The hypoglycemia/hypothalamic area of the brain was affected.

5. The testes/ovaries produce male sex hormones.

6. In the female, the testes/ovaries are sometimes the site of malignancies.

7. Correction of the hormonal abnormalities will return the body to a state of flux/homeostasis.

8. The thymus/isthmus gland was dissected.

9. Glucagon is secreted by the feedback/islet cells of the pancreas.

10. Glucocorticoids are hormones of the adrenal loop/cortex.

Matching

Match the term or abbreviation in Column 1 with the correct definition in Column 2. Write the number of the term on the line before the definition.

Column 1

1. endocrine glands

2. negative feedback

3. hormones

4. hypothalamus

5. thymus

6. pituitary gland

7. neurohypophysis

8. growth hormone

9. thyroid gland

10. follicles

11. metabolism

12. prolactin

Column 2

_____ a. gland of the endocrine system that secretes thymosin and plays a role in immune function

_____ b. posterior lobe of the pituitary gland

_____ c. lined with cells

_____ d. another name for somatotropin; secreted by the anterior pituitary

_____ e. process by which secretion of almost all hormones in the body is controlled

_____ f. process by which cells produce energy

_____ g. ductless glands that secrete their products directly into the bloodstream

_____ h. connected to the hypothalamus

_____ i. substances secreted by the ductless glands of the endocrine system

_____ j. acts on breast tissue to stimulate milk production

_____ k. butterfly-shaped gland in the lower portion of the neck; contains follicles that store thyroxine and triiodothyronine

_____ l. area of the brain that provides a connection between the nervous system and the endocrine system

Word Building

In the sentences that follow, the correct combining form is used in each underlined term, but the prefix or suffix does not match the definition. Rewrite the word, supplying the correct word part.

1. The <u>postdiuretic hormone</u> is a hormone of the pituitary that exerts its influence on the kidneys.

_____

2. The <u>hyperthalamus</u> provides a connection between the nervous system and the endocrine system.

_____

3. An <u>endocrinal</u> is a specialist in the study of the endocrine system.

_____

4. The <u>melanous-stimulating hormone</u> stimulates production and release of the melanin pigment in skin.

_____

5. The <u>hyporenal gland</u> is located atop each kidney and has a cortex and a medulla that secrete different hormones.

_____

6. The <u>pancreaticle islets</u> are also called islets of Langerhans.

_____

7. <u>Preglycemia</u> means elevated blood glucose concentration.

_____

8. <u>Subcalcemia</u> means elevated calcium level.

_____

9. A <u>melanostatic</u> is a cell that produces dark skin pigment.

_____

10. <u>Peribolism</u> is a process that causes chemical change in the body; cellular energy.

_____

Spelling Check

Correct the misspelled words in each sentence by writing the correct spelling on the blank provided.

1. Progusterone is one of the stoeroid hormones.

_____

2. The ovarys are part of the female reprdouctive system.

_____

3. The minerialcorticoids influence sodium metaboluism.

_____

4. Melatoninun is secreted by the pinal gland.

_____

5. The ilsets of Langerhands are found in the pancreaus.

_____

6. Many metobolic processes are influenced by hormenes.

_____

7. Inulsin production was found to be normal.

_____

8. The mensutral cycle is influenced by esrtrogen.

_____

9. The decreased clacium level in the blood is the result of an increase in caclitonin.

_____

10. Both adreneal cortixes were damaged.

_____

The accompanying concept map depicts the endocrine functions of the pancreas. Fill in the missing information.

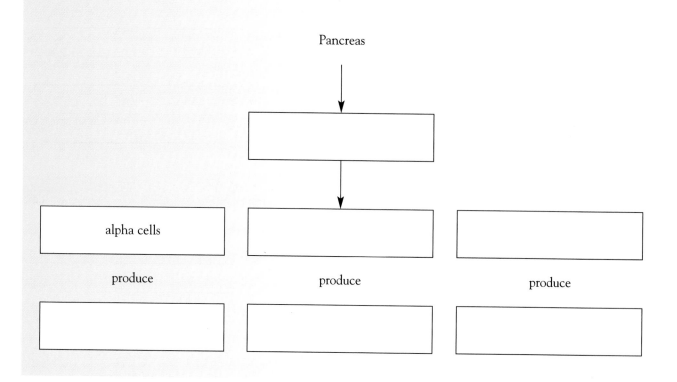

Assessing Patient Health

Wellness and Illness through the Life Span

Any malfunction in the endocrine glands and the hormones they secrete can cause problems in almost every body system. Observation of the patient's physical size, body shape, and physical and developmental milestones can provide important clues in diagnosing abnormal hormone secretion. Visual signs of possible endocrine imbalance include abnormal hair distribution, patchy hair loss, spotty skin pigmentation, and tremors.

A patient's medical history can also reveal information about endocrine health and potential problems. For example, a patient with a family history of endocrine diseases such as diabetes or thyroid disease may be at higher risk of certain disorders. The family history may contain information about diabetes symptoms: **polyuria** (increased urinary output), **polydipsia** (increased thirst), and **polyphagia** (increased appetite). The history may also contain information about other symptoms of endocrine disorders, such as changes in skin pigmentation or texture, intolerance to heat or cold, excessive sweating, and an abnormal relationship between appetite and weight. Beyond the physical examination and a complete history, the most important assessment of hormonal function comes from laboratory testing.

Hormonal abnormalities occur because of too little or too much secretion. These abnormalities are named with the prefixes *hypo-* (too little) and *hyper-* (too much) plus the particular organ or hormone name. Table 7.4 lists hormonal abnormalities and the manifestations associated with them.

Table 7.4

Hormonal Abnormalities and Their Manifestations

Gland and hormone	*Hypo-* manifestation	*Hyper-* manifestation
adrenal glands—corticosteroids and mineralocorticoids	Addison's disease (decreased glucocorticoid): weakness, fatigue, anorexia (decreased appetite), weight loss, hyper pigmentation, and hypotension (decreased blood pressure)	Cushing's syndrome (excessive glucocorticoid): obesity, moon face, osteoporosis, thin skin, striae, muscle weakness, hypertension (increased blood pressure), and mood swings
testes—testosterone	hypogonadism in males (eunuchism): testes and penis are abnormally small at birth; later, lack of development in secondary sex characteristics, i.e., facial, pubic, and axillary hair is scant or absent; voice remains high pitched; increased fat in hip area, buttocks, and breasts; and long arms	precocious puberty: early development of signs of puberty, i.e., facial, pubic, and axillary hair; enlargement of penis and scrotum; early voice change; and some breast development
hypothalamus—antidiuretic hormone	diabetes insipidus (DI): polyuria, polydipsia,	syndrome of inappropriate secretion of antidiuretic hormone (SIADH): water intoxication, loss of appetite, irritability, personality changes, stupor, and seizures
ovaries—estrogen	Turner's syndrome: absence of ovaries, short stature, webbing of neck, prominent ears, broad chest giving appearance of wide-spaced nipples	precocious puberty: early development of signs of puberty, i.e., facial, pubic, and axillary hair; early voice change; breast development; and enlarged clitoris
parathyroid glands—parathyroid hormone (parathormone)	hypoparathyroidism: symptoms of hypocalcemia (i.e., weakness, muscle cramps, paresthesia of hands and feet, and tetany [prolonged muscle spasm])	hyperparathyroidism: symptoms of hypercalcemia (i.e., weakness, fatigue, decreased concentration, polyuria, anorexia, nausea, vomiting, and constipation)
pituitary—growth hormone	hypopituitarism: congenital defects, optic nerve hypoplasia, delay in linear growth, hypogammaglobulinemia, and short stature	hyperpituitarism: gigantism and acromegaly
thyroid—thyroid hormone	hypothyroidism: cold intolerance, weakness, tiredness, muscle cramps, stiffness, hoarseness, decreased hearing, paresthesias, myxedema, weight gain, constipation, dry skin, decreased perspiration, and somnolence	hyperthyroidism: nervousness, irritability, mood changes, increased perspiration, heat intolerance, palpitations, weight loss, dyspnea, fatigue, weakness, frequent bowel movements, and menstrual dysfunction

Fetuses

The endocrine system begins to develop in fetal life. Abnormal organ development, abnormal secretion of tropic hormones, or abnormal chromosome arrangements can cause defects in the fetus.

Congenital **hypothyroidism** occurs in about 1 in 4,000 infants worldwide. In 90 percent of these infants, the thyroid is missing (see Table 7.4 for symptoms). Extreme hypothyroidism results in a condition called **cretinism**, in which the child may be obese, short, and learning disabled. Because the symptoms of hypothyroidism are so serious, even life threatening, all infants are screened for it at birth. Early identification and intervention with thyroid hormone replacement therapy can reverse some of the effects.

A chromosomal abnormality or insufficient hormonal stimulation of gonad tissue *in utero* can cause **hermaphroditism**. In this condition, the genitals are neither clearly female nor clearly male; they are **ambiguous genitalia**. Determining the hermaphroditic baby's gender requires tests to identify the actual chromosomal makeup and ultrasound to determine whether a uterus and ovaries are present. In some cases, surgery is performed to construct female genitalia or testosterone is injected to stimulate penile growth.

Newborns and Infants

Assessment of the infant at birth can identify potential endocrine abnormalities. Hormonal dysfunction may be present if a baby's weight and length and their relationship differ from the normal ranges on a growth chart (Figure 7.6); if the limbs' overall size, shape, and relationship to the body are abnormal; or if the size and shape of the sex organs are abnormal.

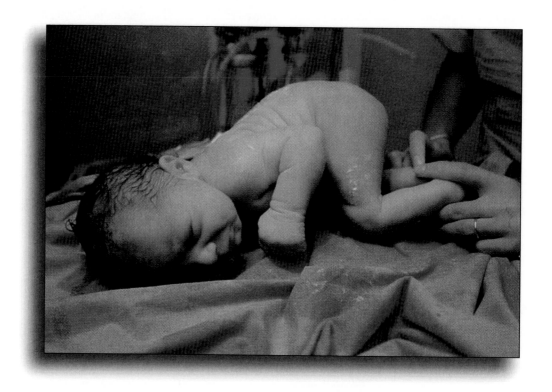

Aplasia (absence or defective development) of the parathyroid glands (known as DiGeorge syndrome) is associated with aplasia or hypoplasia of the thymus gland and cardiac defects. Some infants with this condition may have **tetany** (severe and prolonged muscle spasms), which requires emergency management. Other infants may not display signs and symptoms until days or weeks after birth.

There is a risk that infants of diabetic mothers will be unusually large, with an abnormally large body **(macrosomia)**. Hypoglycemia develops in about 75 percent of these infants. If the mother's diabetes was well controlled during gestation, the infant may not manifest symptoms of hypoglycemia for hours or days after birth. Within the first three days of life, the hypoglycemic infant may become irritable and lethargic and suck poorly. These infants do have a greater-than-normal risk of developing diabetes later in life.

Figure 7.6 - Girls Growth Chart

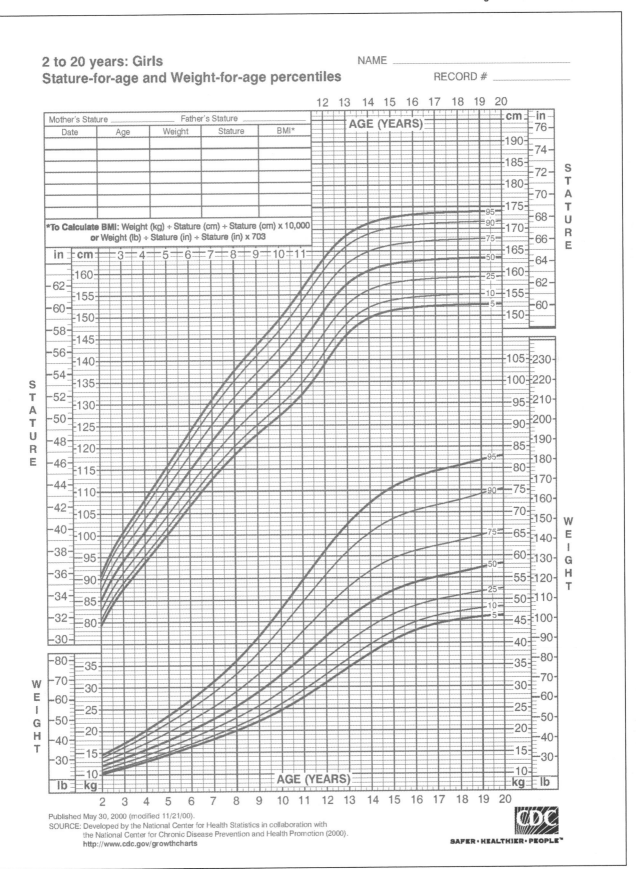

2 to 20 years: Girls
Stature-for-age and Weight-for-age percentiles

NAME _____

RECORD # _____

Published May 30, 2000 (modified 11/21/00).
SOURCE: Developed by the National Center for Health Statistics in collaboration with
the National Center for Chronic Disease Prevention and Health Promotion (2000).
http://www.cdc.gov/growthcharts

Source: **U.S. DEPARTMENT OF HEALTH AND HUMAN SERVICES Centers for Disease Control and Prevention** National Center for Health Statistics Hyattsville, MD

The Endocrine System 269

Children and Adolescents

Juvenile-onset diabetes mellitus (type 1 diabetes) is a syndrome caused by insulin deficiency. This deficiency causes abnormal metabolism of carbohydrates, proteins, and fats. Type 1 diabetes is the most common endocrine disorder of childhood and adolescence, with an incidence of about 1 in 1,430 5-year-olds to 1 in 360 16-year-olds. Persons with type 1 diabetes always need exogenous (from the outside) insulin to maintain homeostasis. Therefore, this type of diabetes is known as insulin-dependent diabetes mellitus (IDDM). Persons with type 2 diabetes mellitus, formerly known as adult-onset diabetes, usually do not require exogenous insulin. The classic symptoms of diabetes are polyuria, polydipsia, polyphagia, and weight loss. The Centers for Disease Control and Prevention (CDC) states "Type 2 diabetes, a disease usually diagnosed in adults aged 40 years or older, is now becoming more common among children and adolescents, particularly in American Indians, African Americans, and Hispanic/Latinos. Among youth, obesity, physical inactivity, and prenatal exposure to diabetes in the mother have become widespread, and may contribute to the increased development of type 2 diabetes during childhood and adolescence." (Source: http://www.cdc.gov/diabetes/faq/groups.htm#9, accessed 6-28-05.)

The insulin deficiency of type 1 diabetes creates an increased blood glucose concentration, known as **hyperglycemia**. A high blood sugar level results in **glucosuria**, or increased glucose in the urine. Glucosuria, in turn, causes the kidneys to produce more urine, a condition called polyuria. An increased urine output, **diuresis**, results in a loss of electrolytes, and dehydration ensues. Dehydration then stimulates the body's thirst (polydipsia). The loss of glucose and electrolytes from the urine causes a daily loss of about 1,000 calories, approximately half of the calories needed by a child. Therefore, weight loss ensues, in spite of the increased appetite that occurs as a compensatory mechanism.

The abnormal breakdown of carbohydrates, proteins, and fats that results from insulin deficiency also produces problems. Other hormones attempt to correct the situation, but **lipolysis**, or breakdown of fats, increases and lipid synthesis (production) decreases. This leads to increased concentrations of lipids in the blood and free fatty acids. These fatty acids form **ketone bodies**, which accumulate and eventually result in **metabolic acidosis**, or **ketoacidosis**, a situation in which excessive carbon dioxide builds up in the body. When this happens, the affected person breathes very deeply **(Kussmaul respirations)** to get rid of the extra carbon dioxide. In contrast, the immediate effects of type 2 diabetes is much more subtle. The hyperglycemia is frequently discovered during the routine testing of a physical exam.

The long-term effects of uncontrolled or poorly controlled hyperglycemia are sinister. Damage to delicate nerves and blood vessels leads to a much higher incidence of heart disease, blindness (retinopathy), kidney failure (nephropathy), and amputations of limbs (peripheral vascular disease).

Each term in the list is part of the type 1 diabetes process. Put them in the order in which they happen by numbering them from 1 to 7.

_____ polyuria

___1___ hyperglycemia

_____ dehydration

_____ weight loss

_____ glucosuria

_____ diuresis

_____ polydipsia

Word Maps: Hyperglycemia

Exercise 8

Each term in the list is part of the type 1 diabetes process. Put them in the order in which they happen by numbering them from 1 to 7.

_____ ketoacidosis/metabolic acidosis

_____ Kussmaul respirations

_____ inability to properly metabolize nutrients

_____ excessive CO_2

_____ lipolysis increase

_____ insulin deficiency

_____ ketone bodies

Adults and Seniors

When the thyroid gland becomes hyperplastic, containing an overabundance of cells, it produces excessive hormone, which can result in **Graves' disease**, or **thyrotoxicosis**, believed to be an autoimmune disease. The increase of thyroid cells produces a **goiter**—a nodular growth or enlargement of the thyroid gland. Another symptom of hyperthyroidism is exophthalmos, or protrusion of the eyeballs, which results from swollen tissue behind the eye sockets.

Myxedema is a form of hypothyroidism that occurs in older adults as a result of thyroid atrophy. The skin and subcutaneous tissue become edematous (swollen), causing a firm pouch under the eyes. Myxedema also results in decreased mental capacity, loss of hair, and accumulation of fluid around the heart. These symptoms can be reversed by the administration of thyroid replacement therapy.

General Illnesses

Hypoglycemia can occur during any stage of life, from birth to old age. Persons with type 1 diabetes are at a higher risk, and may experience hypoglycemia or "insulin reaction" if they do not balance diet, exercise and insulin. The term literally means decreased glucose in the blood. A low blood sugar level stimulates hormones, including epinephrine, norepinephrine, glucagon, cortisol, and growth hormone, to raise the blood glucose concentration (refer to Figure 7.2). This hormone response causes the symptoms that appear with hypoglycemia: sweating, palpitations, hunger, tachycardia, tremors, confusion, headache, speech difficulties, and anxiety. The symptoms are usually sporadic (except in diabetes) and are relieved by eating or drinking a sugar-containing substance. Severe and prolonged hypoglycemia can result in seizures, stupor, coma, and even death.

Pheochromocytoma is a tumor, usually benign, that secretes increased amounts of epinephrine and norepinephrine, which lead to symptoms of hypertension, palpitations, headaches, facial flushing, and increased perspiration. Treatment consists of surgical removal of the tumor and treatment with antihypertensives to control symptoms.

Thyroid carcinoma is treated by thyroidectomy, radio-ablation, and sometimes chemotherapy. Thyroid suppression with thyroid hormone can prevent tumor recurrence. Adrenocortical carcinoma, pituitary adenoma, and craniopharyngioma are other endocrine cancers.

Other illnesses associated with hormone dysfunction are shown in Table 7.4 according to their *hypo-* or *hyper-* state.

Word Building

Supply a term to match the definition provided. Then create a new term using one or more word parts from the original term. Define the new term.

1. _____: manifested by gigantism and/or acromegaly

   New term: _____

   Definition: _____

2. _____: excessive thirst

   New term: _____

   Definition: _____

3. _____: excessive eating

   New term: _____

   Definition: _____

4. _____: abnormal sensation; numbness and/or tingling

   New term: _____

   Definition: _____

5. _____: excessive pigmentation

New term: _____

Definition: _____

6. _____: decreased blood pressure

New term: _____

Definition: _____

7. _____: excessive thyroid gland activity

New term: _____

Definition: _____

8. _____: difficulty breathing

New term: _____

Definition: _____

9. _____: eunichism

New term: _____

Definition: _____

10. _____: abnormally large body

New term: _____

Definition: _____

Comprehension Check

Select the correct medical term from the list to substitute for the underlined definition in each sentence.

axillary	diuresis	hermaphroditism	seizure
bradypnea	dysfunction	hyperglycemia	tachycardia
chromosomal	edematous	ketoacidosis	Turner's syndrome
dehydration	glycosuria		

1. <u>Pertaining to chromosomes</u> derangements can produce various abnormalities in the fetus. _____

2. <u>Pertaining to the axilla</u> hair is scant. _____

3. <u>Chromosomal abnormality of insufficient hormonal stimulation of gonadal tissue *in utero*</u> is characterized by the presence of ambiguous genitalia.

4. The problem is a result of thyroid <u>difficult, abnormal, or faulty function</u>.

_____

5. Urinalysis revealed a marked <u>condition of sugar in the urine</u>.

_____

6. Upon arrival in the emergency room, the patient was severely <u>in a condition without water</u>.

_____

7. The condition of loss of fluid from the tissues resulting from <u>increased or large-volume urine output</u> has resulted in a loss of electrolytes.

_____

8. Laboratory studies revealed that the patient was in a state of <u>accumulation of ketone bodies</u>.

_____

9. The patient had a <u>rapid heart rate</u>.

_____

10. Tissues of the leg were <u>swollen</u>.

_____

Matching

Match the term in Column 1 with the definition in Column 2. Write the number of the term in the space beside the definition.

Column 1		Column 2
1. endocrinologist	_____	a. literally, "on the kidneys (renal)"
2. polydipsia	_____	b. antidiuretic hormone
3. polyphagia	_____	c. has two lobes
4. adrenal	_____	d. posterior lobe of the pituitary gland
5. ADH	_____	e. specialist in the endocrine system
6. pituitary gland	_____	f. hormone secreted by the thyroid gland
7. neurohypophysis	_____	g. excessive thirst
8. TSH	_____	h. hormone secreted by the pancreas
9. calcitonin	_____	i. thyroid-stimulating hormone
10. insulin	_____	j. excessive hunger

Word Building

Supply word parts to complete the terms that follow, using the context of the sentences as a guide.

1. A_____ refers to decreased development or shrinkage.

2. Lipo_____ is the breakdown of fats.

3. Thyro_____ is a condition of thyroid poisoning (destructive excess of thyroid hormone).

4. Somato_____ refers to changes in the body.

5. _____renal _____ is the inner portion of the adrenal gland.

6. _____plasia means excessive formation (enlargement).

7. _____cyte is a thymus cell.

8. _____oma means tumor of the thymus.

9. Adeno_____ is cancer or malignancy of a gland.

10. Coll_____ means gluelike.

Spelling Check

Write the correct spelling of each term or abbreviation on the blank provided.

1. glucagun   _____

2. seccretion   _____

3. metabloic   _____

4. antagontism   _____

5. parthromone   _____

6. glucocrotorticoid _____

7. panceras   _____

8. medulae   _____

9. ovarys   _____

10. progsterone   _____

11. ATCH   _____

12. IDMD   _____

Word Maps

Complete the concept map by filling in the missing labels.

Tests, Procedures, and Pharmaceuticals

Most endocrine testing measures hormone levels in the blood (Table 7.5). However, some testing checks the tropic hormones to determine their proper functioning. Thyroid testing can be performed by measuring the serum T_3 and T_4 levels. T_4 is tested using a radioimmunoassay technique, and T_3 is measured directly. A T_3 resin uptake test measures the amount of thyroid hormone bound to thyroxine-binding globulin (TBG).

Tests of thyroid-stimulating hormone (TSH) include a radioimmunoassay, an assay with labeled monoclonal antibody to TSH, and a thyrotropin-releasing hormone (TRH) test. This test involves injecting TRH and then drawing blood samples to measure TSH levels. Blood measurements of thyroglobulin, which are only produced by thyroid tissue, are made following thyroidectomy for thyroid cancer. Iodine uptake by the thyroid is measured by injecting radioactive iodine, ^{131}I, and following up with a thyroid scan. The scintiscan also measures radioactive iodine uptake by identifying "hot" and "cold" areas, that is, those areas with increased and decreased iodine uptake, respectively.

The parathyroid hormone level is measured directly in the blood. A persistent hypercalcemic state may indicate a defect in parathormone function. Measurements of catecholamines are used to assess adrenal function by determining norepinephrine and epinephrine concentrations in the blood. Also, urinary measurements of the metabolites of catecholamines (i.e., metanephrines [MN], homovanillic acid [HVA], and vanillylmandelic acid [VMA]) assess adrenal dysfunction.

Some tests help evaluate adrenocortical activity. A 24-hour collection of urine measures free cortisol levels, metabolites of cortisol, and androgen metabolites. Stimulation tests determine ACTH production.

Pancreatic islet functioning can be checked with a fasting blood sugar (FBS) test, in which the patient's blood glucose level is tested after a 12-hour fast. Another test, the glucose tolerance test (GTT), is performed in the morning, after a 12-hour fast. After the patient is given a portion of glucose, blood tests are performed over several hours to determine the blood glucose levels over time. The postprandial (PP) test measures blood glucose concentration after a meal.

Table 7.5

Tests and Procedures Relating to the Endocrine System

Test	Description
fasting blood sugar (FBS)	blood test performed after a 12-hour fast; measures the glucose concentration in the blood
glucose tolerance test (GTT)	blood test performed after a 12-hour fast; a glucose drink is taken and the blood is tested several times to determine the glucose level over time
homovanillic acid (HVA)	a chemical substance found in urine that is a metabolite of catecholamines secretion; elevated in the presence of certain tumors
metanephrine (MN)	a product of the breakdown of epinephrine; found in the urine
postprandial (PP) test	blood test performed after eating to determine the blood glucose level
radioactive iodine, ^{131}I	a radioactive substance that is taken up by the thyroid gland; used to determine thyroid pathology; can also be used to treat thyroid disease
scintiscan	scanning machine used to measure radioactive iodine uptake in the thyroid
vanillylmandelic acid (VMA)	metabolite of catecholamine secretion found in the urine; increases when certain tumors are present

Surgical Procedures

Treating dysfunctional or diseased endocrine glands often involves surgery to remove part of or the entire gland. Table 7.6 lists some of the common procedures involving the endocrine system.

Table 7.6

Surgical Procedures Relating to the Endocrine System

Term	Meaning	Word Analysis	
adrenalectomy	removal of the adrenal gland	adren/o	pertaining to the adrenal glands
		-ectomy	surgical removal
hypophysectomy	removal of the pituitary gland; hormone replacement is necessary	hypo/	under, less
		phys/o	swell (under the hypothalamus)
		-ectomy	surgical removal
lobectomy	removal of lobe of an organ or gland, i.e., lobe of the pituitary	lobe/	portion (lobe) of organ, gland
		-ectomy	surgical removal
parathyroidectomy	removal of the parathyroid gland(s)	para/	alongside; pair
		thyr/o	pertaining to the thyroid
		-ectomy	surgical removal
pinealectomy	removal of the pineal gland	pineal/	pertaining to the pineal gland
		-ectomy	surgical removal
thyroidectomy	removal of the thyroid gland	thyr/o	pertaining to the thyroid gland
		-ectomy	surgical removal

Pharmaceutical Agents

Physicians prescribe various pharmaceutical agents to augment decreased or absent function of a particular hormone or to suppress hormone secretion. The exception is the use of adrenal corticosteroids, such as prednisone and hydrocortisone, which are used for many disorders and conditions. Their anti-inflammatory and anti-allergic properties make them particularly valuable. Table 7.7 lists commonly used corticosteroids.

Table 7.7

Commonly Used Corticosteroids

Generic name	Trade name
beclomethasone	Beconase AQ, Vancenase
cortisone	Cortisone AC
dexamethasone	Decadron, Dexasone, Hexadrol
hydrocortisone	Cortef, Solu-Cortef
methylprednisolone	Medrol, Solu-Medrol
prednisolone	Prelone
prednisone	Deltasone, Prednicot
triamcinolone	Aristocort, Kenalog, Azmacort

A variety of insulin replacement agents are used to treat diabetes mellitus. They are often prescribed in combination because they act in differing time frames. Treating diabetes is a complex process, involving proper diet, exercise, monitoring of blood glucose levels, medication as needed, and patient education. Table 7.8 lists the insulin preparations available for the treatment of diabetes mellitus.

Table 7.8

Insulin Preparations and Categories

Category	Type	Onset of action and duration	Brand names
Short-acting	Regular (R)	½-1 hr, 4-6 hrs	Regular Iletin II Humulin R Novolin R
Intermediate-acting	NPH	3-4 hr, 16-20 hrs	NPH Iletin II Humulin N Novolin N
	Lente (L)	1-3 hr, 18-28	Lente Iletin II Humulin
Long-acting	Ultralente (UL) Glargine	6-8 hrs, 20-30 hrs	Humulin U Lantus
Mixed	Combination by percent of R and NPH insulins	½ hr, 24 hr	Humulin 70/30 Humulin 50/50 Novolin 70/30

Table 7.9

Abbreviations

Abbreviation	Meaning
ACTH	adrenocorticotropic hormone
ADH	antidiuretic hormone (vasopressin)
Ca	calcium
CRF	corticotropin-releasing factor
DI	diabetes insipidus
DKA	diabetic ketoacidosis
DM	diabetes mellitus
FBS	fasting blood sugar
FSH	follicle-stimulating hormone
GH	growth hormone
GHRH	growth hormone–releasing hormone
GTT	glucose tolerance test
HGH	human growth hormone
HVA	homovanillic acid
IDDM	insulin-dependent diabetes mellitus
K	potassium
LH	luteinizing hormone
MSH	melanocyte-stimulating hormone
Na	sodium
OT	oxytocin
PIH	prolactin-inhibiting hormone
PP	postprandial

PRH	prolactin-releasing hormone
PRL	prolactin
PTH	parathyroid hormone (parathormone)
RIA	radioimmunoassay
SIADH	syndrome of inappropriate antidiuretic hormone
T_3	triiodothyronine
T_4	thyroxine
TFT	thyroid function test
TRH	thyrotropin-releasing hormone
TSH	thyroid-stimulating hormone
VMA	vanillylmandelic acid

Word Building

Exercise 15

Write the definition of each combining form in the Definition column. Then write a term using that combining form in the Term column.

Combining Form	Definition	Term
1. adren/o	_____	_____
2. aden/o	_____	_____
3. thyr/o	_____	_____
4. cortic/o	_____	_____
5. ket/o	_____	_____
6. gluc/o	_____	_____
7. somat/o	_____	_____
8. gonad/o	_____	_____
9. ton/o	_____	_____

Comprehension Check

Exercise 16

Write the meaning of the underlined term on the line below the sentence. You may need to use a medical dictionary for this exercise. Keep your answers brief.

1. Endemic goiter can result from an inadequate diet.

_____

2. Hyponatremia is frequently a result of overactivity of the adrenal cortex.

_____

3. Hypokalemia can produce cardiac arrhythmias.

_____

4. The patient was admitted to the hospital with an <u>electrolyte</u> imbalance.

_____

5. We will identify the <u>sella turcica</u> and locate the pituitary gland.

_____

6. The laboratory tests will show increased production of <u>estradiol</u>.

_____

7. We will also test for <u>TSH</u>.

_____

8. Upon examination, the <u>thyroid cartilage</u> was noted to be quite prominent.

_____

9. <u>Cholesystokinin</u> was identified by laboratory analysis.

_____

10. <u>Gastrin</u> is necessary for proper digestive function.

_____

Matching

Match the abbreviations in Column 1 with the definitions in Column 2. Write the number of the abbreviation in the space beside the definition.

Column 1		Column 2
1. IDDM	_____	a. follicle-stimulating hormone
2. TSH	_____	b. antidiuretic hormone
3. FSH	_____	c. melanocyte-stimulating hormone
4. Na	_____	d. parathyroid hormone
5. Ca	_____	e. insulin dependent diabetes mellitus
6. ADH	_____	f. growth hormone
7. GH	_____	g. homovanillic acid
8. PTH	_____	h. sodium
9. MSH	_____	i. calcium
10. HVA	_____	j. thyroid-stimulating hormone

Supply the word parts to complete each term, according to the definition provided.

1. endocrino_____ = disorder of an endocrine gland

2. melano_____ = black cell

3. _____lysis = breakdown of fats

4. _____ic = pertaining to the pancreas

5. _____thyroid_____ = decreased secretion of thyroid hormones

6. _____calcem_____ = condition of excessive calcium in the blood

7. _____diabetic agent = substance used to treat diabetes

8. _____thyroid = around or near the thyroid

9. _____pnea = difficulty breathing

10. _____pnea = rapid breathing

11. _____kalemia = excessive amount of potassium in the blood

12. _____uria = increased glucose in the urine

Supply the correct definition for each abbreviation given by writing the definition on the line beside the abbreviation.

1. TRH _____

2. RIA _____

3. T_3 _____

4. T_4 _____

5. PIH _____

6. K _____

7. LH _____

8. PP _____

9. FBS _____

10. GTT _____

The concept map below shows the sequence of events in the development and treatment of hyperglycemia (diabetes mellitus) and hypoglycemia. Label the blank areas of the map to complete the information.

excessive blood glucose:

insufficient blood glucose:

produces symptoms of

produces symptoms of

treatment:

treatment:

Crossword Puzzle

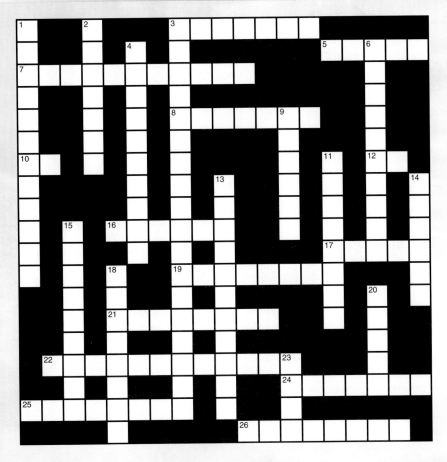

Across

3. narrow portion that connects two larger parts
5. endocrine gland that is part of the female reproductive system
7. responsible for the body's "internal clock"
8. literally meaning "like or resembling a shield"
10. abbreviation for sodium
12. abbreviation for oxytocin
16. severe and prolonged muscle spasms
17. combining form that means female
19. hormone secreted by alpha cells in the pancreas
21. promotes development of secondary sex characteristics in the female
22. gland whose name means "below the thalamus"
24. yellowish, translucent substance resembling glue
25. inflammation of a gland
26. endocrine gland located in the upper abdomen, behind the stomach

Down

1. causes abnormally small testes and penis
2. tumor of a gland
3. hormone-secreting endocrine glands in the pancreas
4. instrument for measuring glucose (sugar) in the blood
6. process or agent that works against another
9. _____ of Langerhans
11. organ that provides transfer of substances between fetus and mother
13. endocrine gland located in the mediastinum
14. suffix meaning surgical removal
15. first form or type from which others are copied
18. any disease or condition of a gland
20. combining form meaning sugar
23. scinti _____; process that measures radioactive uptake

Build the Terms

Select word parts from the lists to build a complete medical term for each definition given. Note that not all terms will have a root or combining form, prefix, and suffix. Some word parts may be used more than once.

Combining Forms	Prefixes	Suffixes
glyc/o	hyper-	-ia
natr/o	a-	-logy
thym/o	sub-	-logist
kal/i	hypo-	-oma
pancreat/o	pre-	-tomy
thyr/o	dys-	-ism
o/o	an-	-al
phag/o	pre-	-emia
tax/o	de-	-ic
endocrin/o	anti-	-uria
lip/o	per-	-genesis
calc/i	bi-	-lysis

1. glucose (sugar) in the urine _____

2. cutting operation on the thyroid _____

3. breakdown of fats _____

4. difficulty swallowing (eating) _____

5. specialist in the study of the endocrine system _____

6. lack of coordination _____

7. tumor of the pancreas _____

8. pertaining to the thymus _____

9. excessive calcium in the blood _____

10. excessive potassium in the blood _____

11. excessive sodium (salt) in the blood _____

12. origin or creation of an egg _____

Using Medical References

The following sentences contain medical terms that may not have been addressed on the charts in this chapter. Use medical reference books, your medical term analysis skills, and/or a medical dictionary to find the correct definition of each underlined word. Write the definition on the line below the sentence.

1. When Dr. Morrison saw the lab results, he diagnosed <u>hyperkalemia</u>.

   _____

2. Mrs. Tindal is scheduled for an <u>oophorectomy</u> next week.

   _____

3. The <u>testicular carcinoma</u> was diagnosed early.

   _____

4. Laboratory testing will identify <u>metabolites</u> of the drug.

   _____

5. Damage to the kidneys has resulted in a decrease in <u>erythropoietin</u>.

   _____

6. His <u>cortisol</u> levels remained high.

   _____

7. The <u>mammae</u> are rapidly affected by prolactin.

   _____

8. She will carry <u>epinephrine</u> in a sealed bag.

   _____

9. There appears to be an excess of <u>thyrocalcitonin</u>.

   _____

10. Mr. Taber was found to be <u>euthyroid</u>.

    _____

11. Dr. Hattern will perform the <u>hypophysectomy</u> today.

    _____

12. We've found these tumor cells to be <u>estrogenic</u>.

    _____

Read each mini medical record or scenario carefully; and then select A or B as the most likely response. Write the letter of your answer in the space provided.

1. A 66 y/o female is seen in the physician's office with periorbital edema, hair loss, weakness, fatigue, muscle cramps, hoarseness, weight gain, and dry skin. What will the physician diagnose?

   A. Hypothyroidism or myxedema
   B. IDDM

   Physician's response: _____

2. A 27 y/o pregnant female comes to the office with symptoms that include sweating, palpitations, tremor, mental confusion, and headache. She has had no prior health problems. Her lab results include serum glucose of 50. You expect that the diagnosis will be:

   A. TIA
   B. Hypoglycemia

   Physician's response: _____

3. As you transcribe the doctor's notes on a 79 y/o male patient, you have difficulty hearing the diagnosis clearly, but you are able to decipher a "rule out" diagnosis consisting of two distinctly separate words. The first word begins with a "D." You notice that the physician has ordered a GTT. You would:

   A. Transcribe as much of the report as possible and leave it on the doctor's desk with a note asking her to clarify the diagnosis. Tell her that you believe she said "diabetes mellitus," but you aren't certain.
   B. Type "dyspnea" for the diagnosis and file the report in the patient's chart.

   Your response: _____

Analyzing Medical Records

Read the physician's progress note on the next page. Then answer the following questions.

1. What brought this patient to the doctor's office?

2. What is the patient's prior diagnosis?

3. What kind of test did the patient have in the office? Was the patient's blood sugar checked?

4. What was the condition of the patient's skin?

5. Was any medication prescribed? When is it to be given?

6. List two tests that are to be performed. When are they to be done?

7. Why is it necessary to hospitalize the patient?

Physician's Progress Note

PATIENT: Deborah P
DATE: August 13, xxxx

S: This 18 y/o female is seen in the office, c/o nausea and vomiting for the past six hours. She is
accompanied by her sister, who provides much of the history. Pt. reports a severe headache, and states
she feels like she has in the past when she was on the verge of coma. She was diagnosed with IDDM at
the age of 10 and has taken insulin ever since. She is on an 1800 cal. ADA diet. She uses an Accu-
Chek at home and evaluates her glucose levels b.i.d. She reports that her levels have been around 60 to
70 for the past four days. Two days ago she had an episode where she felt shaky, anxious, and confused.
She had palpitations, was sweating, and felt weak. She has not taken her insulin since that time.

O: T 96, P 105, R 22, B/P 120/66. Skin is warm and dry. Xerosis of hands, arms, and perioral area. Odor of
ketones is detectable in the breath. Biochem results: sodium 125, potassium 4.2, chloride 101, CO2 10,
glucose 412.

A: Diabetic ketoacidosis.

P: 10 units regular insulin stat.; check BS in 1h., then q.4h.; urine checks for sugar, acetone, and volume q
voiding; admit to Lakeshore Memorial Hospital, unit L400.

K. Mahoney, MD

Short Answer

Describe the role of negative feedback in maintaining homeostasis.

_____

_____

_____

_____

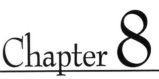

Chapter 8

The Nervous System

Learning Outcomes

Students will be able to:
- Label the organs of the nervous system shown on a drawing.
- Distinguish between the central nervous system and the peripheral nervous system.
- Name the function(s) of the major areas of the brain.
- Describe the mechanisms of innervation and neurotransmitters.
- Correctly use the terminology of the nervous system in written and oral communication.
- List nervous system abnormalities and their effects.
- Correctly spell and pronounce nervous system terminology.
- State the meaning of abbreviations related to the nervous system.
- Name tests and treatments for major nervous system abnormalities.

Translation, Please?Translation, Please?Translation, Please?

Read this excerpt from a medical record and try to answer the questions that follow.

The patient suffers from ataxia, paresthesias, and a progressive aphasia. There have been reports of mild TIAs without loss of consciousness. The diagnosis is consistent with cerebrovascular accident.

1. Was this patient in a work-related accident or did she have a stroke?
2. Is this patient having difficulty with speech and walking, or sights and sounds?
3. Is a TIA a total internal arrest or transient ischemic attack?

Answers to "Translation, Please?"
1. She had a mild stroke. We know this from the symptoms and because she had experienced previous mild TIAs.
2. She is having difficulty with speech and walking. Ataxia is motor difficulty. Aphasia refers to impaired speech.
3. A TIA is a transient ischemic attack.

Identifying the Specialty

The System and Its Practitioners

The nervous system serves as the body's electrical "wiring system" by sending the impulses and signals that drive all functions. The study of the nervous system is called **neurology**, and the physician specialist is a **neurologist**.

Examining the Patient ♂♀

Anatomy and Physiology of the Nervous System

The nervous system has two parts: the **central nervous system (CNS)**, consisting of the **brain** and **spinal cord**, and the **peripheral nervous system (PNS)**, which includes the twelve pairs of **cranial nerves** and the thirty-one pairs of **spinal nerves** plus their branches. The CNS receives its messages from the PNS by way of sensory receptors. The CNS sends messages to the muscles and glands. Table 8.1 lists the cranial nerves, the body area each controls, and the specific functions associated with each area. Figure 8.1 shows the network of nerves that make up the CNS and the PNS.

Table 8.1

The Cranial Nerves: Areas of Innervation and Functions

Cranial nerve	Area of innervation	Function
olfactory (I)	nose	smell
optic (II)	eye	visual acuity and visual fields
oculomotor (III)	eye muscles	eyeball movements; pupil size
trochlear (IV)	external eye muscles	eye movements
trigeminal—ophthalmic branch (V)	skin and corneal reflex	blinking
trigeminal—maxillary branch (V)	lower eyelid, upper lip, cheek and nose	sensations of face and eye
trigeminal—mandibular branch (V)	muscles of mastication (chewing)	chewing muscles
abducens (VI)	external eye muscles	outward-turning eye movements
facial (VII)	taste; facial expressions	movement of facial muscles and taste
vestibulocochlear—cochlear branch (VIII)	ear	hearing
vestibulocochlear—vestibular branch (VIII)	ear	balance
glossopharyngeal (IX)	throat muscles and salivary glands	movement of back of throat and taste
vagus (X)	throat, larynx, chest, and abdominal organs	gag reflex, swallowing, voice, heartbeat, and peristalsis
spinal accessory (XI)	muscles of lower neck and shoulders	head turning and shrug; voice production
hypoglossal (XII)	muscles of tongue	movement of tongue and proper speech (enunciation)

Brain

The brain, housed in the cranial cavity of the skull, and the spinal cord, surrounded by the vertebrae of the back, are protected by the bones that encase them. The brain and spinal cord are covered by fluid-containing membranes called **meninges**, which provides further protection. Three layers of meninges cover the CNS: the outer layer is the **dura mater**, the middle layer is the **arachnoid**, and the inner layer that is closest to the brain is the **pia mater**. A cushioning and nourishing fluid called **cerebrospinal fluid (CSF)** fills the subarachnoid space of the CNS and the **ventricles** (spaces) in the brain.

The largest structure of the brain is called the **cerebrum**, and its outer layer, the **cerebral cortex**, is composed of nerve cells called gray matter. This area controls higher functions, such as thought, memory, reasoning, sensation, and voluntary movement. Folds, or gyri, on the surface of the brain increase the amount of gray matter that can fit inside the skull. The cerebrum is divided into two hemispheres: the left hemisphere, which controls muscles on the right side of the body, reasoning, language, and skills necessary for math and science; and the right hemisphere, which controls the muscles on the left side of the body, imagination, insight, and artistic and musical abilities.

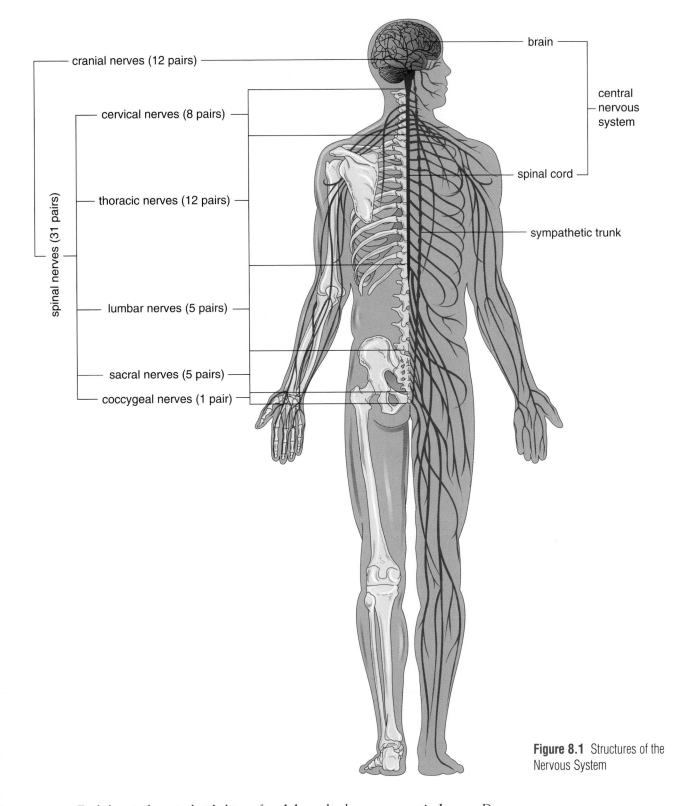

cranial nerves (12 pairs)

brain

central
nervous
system

spinal nerves (31 pairs)

cervical nerves (8 pairs)

thoracic nerves (12 pairs)

spinal cord

sympathetic trunk

lumbar nerves (5 pairs)

sacral nerves (5 pairs)

coccygeal nerves (1 pair)

Figure 8.1 Structures of the Nervous System

Each hemisphere is divided into four **lobes,** also known as **cortical areas**. Deep fissures or crevices called **sulci** separate the lobes. Figure 8.2 shows the cerebral lobes and their specific functions. The **frontal lobe** is located in the front of the brain and is separated from the **temporal lobe** on the lateral aspect of the brain by the **lateral fissure**. The **parietal lobe** is found on the top of the brain and is separated from the frontal lobe by the **central sulcus**. The **occipital lobe** is located in the back of the brain and is contiguous with (touching) the temporal and parietal lobes.

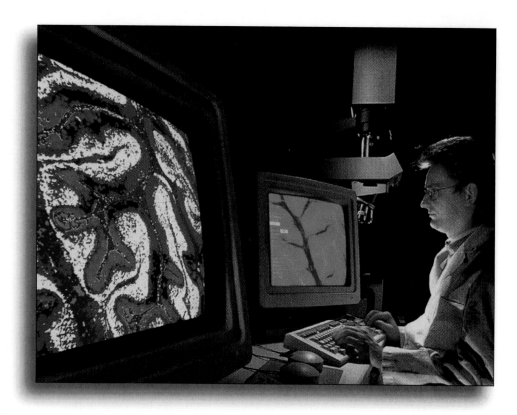

Computer analysis of brain tissue.

Figure 8.2 - Lobes of the Brain
8.2A: The Cerebrum

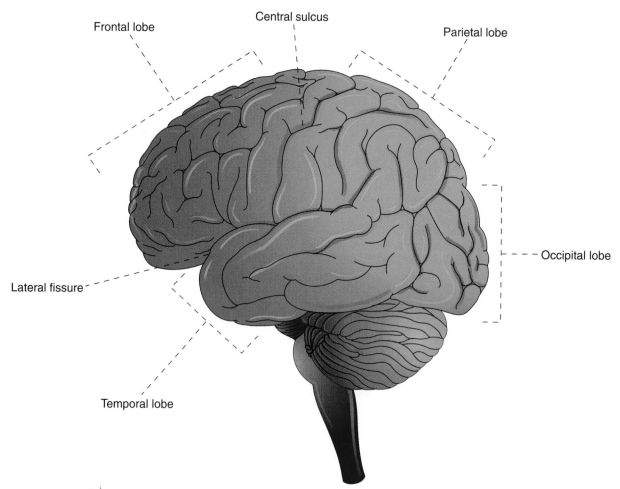

Frontal lobe

Central sulcus

Parietal lobe

Occipital lobe

Lateral fissure

Temporal lobe

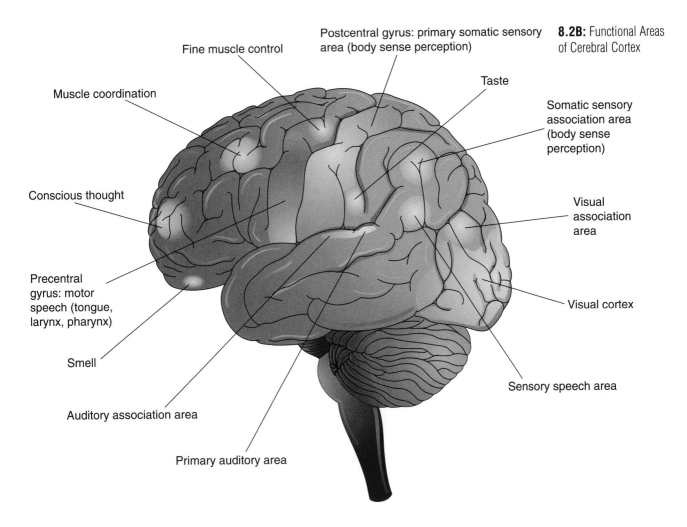

Fine muscle control

Muscle coordination

Postcentral gyrus: primary somatic sensory area (body sense perception)

Taste

8.2B: Functional Areas of Cerebral Cortex

Somatic sensory association area (body sense perception)

Visual association area

Conscious thought

Visual cortex

Precentral gyrus: motor speech (tongue, larynx, pharynx)

Smell

Sensory speech area

Auditory association area

Primary auditory area

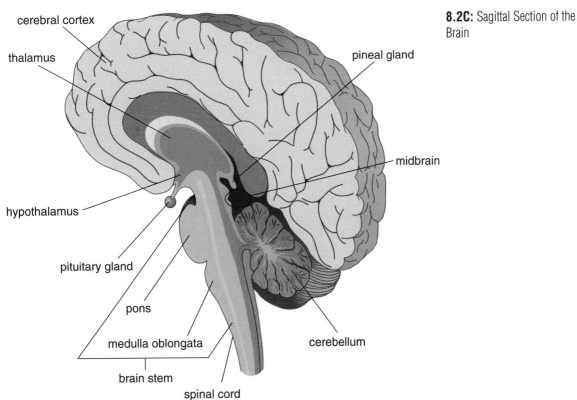

cerebral cortex

thalamus

8.2C: Sagittal Section of the Brain

pineal gland

midbrain

hypothalamus

pituitary gland

pons

medulla oblongata

brain stem

spinal cord

cerebellum

The brain is subdivided into areas responsible for specific functions. Inferior to the cerebrum is the **diencephalon**, an area that contains the **thalamus** and the **hypothalamus**. The thalamus, which is dumbbell-shaped and lies within the third ventricle, enables the body to experience sensations by relaying impulses from the sense organs to the cerebral cortex. It is also responsible for emotions and feelings.

The hypothalamus sits directly inferior to the thalamus, and despite the fact that it is small, it is one of the most important areas of the brain. Attached to the hypothalamus is the pituitary gland. Impulses from the hypothalamus travel to the spinal cord and are sent to muscles throughout the body. The hypothalamus controls all of the internal organs, including the heart and blood vessels, and serves as the main regulator of body temperature. It is also involved in regulating sleep, water balance, appetite, and some emotions and pain.

The **brainstem** is located deep to the cerebrum and consists of the **midbrain**, the **pons**, and the **medulla oblongata**. The brainstem conducts impulses to and from the spinal cord, and is responsible for running many of the reflex centers of the body, including respiration and heartbeat.

Spinal Cord

The brainstem is connected to the spinal cord. The spinal cord extends from the brainstem down to the bottom of the first lumbar vertebra. Depending on the individual's height, the spinal cord is about 17 to 18 inches long. It is composed of gray matter and white matter, or **myelinated** nerve fibers or **spinal tracts**. These tracts are actually pathways that conduct impulses to and from the brain. Ascending tracts that travel up to the brain transmit pain, touch, and temperature sensations. Motor impulses travel down the descending tracts from the brain. In other words, the spinal cord transmits sensory impulses *to* the brain and motor impulses *from* the brain.

Peripheral Nervous System (PNS)

The PNS is composed of the **cranial** and **spinal nerves** and is divided into the **somatic nervous system (SNS)** and the **autonomic nervous system (ANS)**. The somatic nerve fibers **innervate** (send nerve impulses) to the skeletal muscles, which are under the voluntary control of the individual. The autonomic fibers innervate involuntary action, the actions not consciously controlled, such as those in smooth muscle, cardiac muscle, glandular tissue, and body parts involved in digestion.

The autonomic nervous system is further subdivided in two sections: the **sympathetic** and **parasympathetic nervous systems**. The sympathetic nervous system is the body's emergency system that sends messages to the adrenal medulla, causing the release of **catecholamines**, which are hormones released in response to stress (described in Chapter 7, "The Endocrine System"). The parasympathetic system has neurons located in the gray matter of the brainstem and the sacral area of the spinal cord. This system functions as the control for the sympathetic system by slowing the heartbeat and increasing the muscle movements of the digestive system. Figure 8.3 shows the pathways of the sympathetic and parasympathetic nervous systems as well as the body functions they involve.

Neurons

The cells of the nervous system are the structures that pass information from one area to another. The **neuron** is the basic structural and functional cell of the nervous system. Figure 8.4 shows the structures of the neuron: the main portion is the **cell body**, with its **nucleus**; the **dendrites** receive information from other neurons or

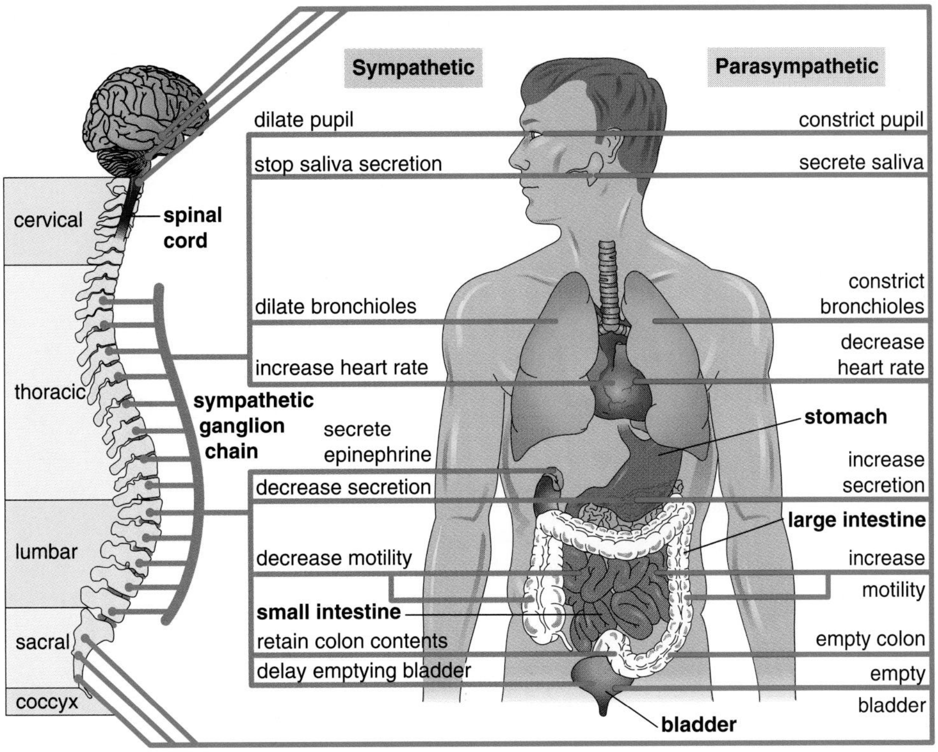

Figure 8.3 - Autonomic Nervous System

from sensory cells; and the **axon**, or long branch, extends from the neuron to other neurons or to muscles or glands.

The axons outside of the CNS are surrounded by a white, fatty sheath called **myelin**, which is made up of **Schwann cells**. The **nodes of Ranvier** are the indentations between each adjoining Schwann cell. The Schwann cells of the PNS are covered by an outer cell layer called the **neurilemma** that allows these axons to regenerate when injured. The axons within the CNS do not have this layer, so it's extremely difficult for these cells to self-repair when they are injured.

For neurons to transmit their signal, or impulse, they must be connected to one another. This connection is called a **synapse**. The nerve impulse causes the release of **neurotransmitters**, chemicals that carry the signal across the synapse to the next neuron. Table 8.2 shows the neurotransmitters released at the synapses.

Table 8.2

Neurotransmitters and their Locations

Neurotransmitter	Location
acetylcholine	released at synapses in the spinal cord and at neuromuscular junctions
dopamine	type of catecholamine released from the CNS and basal ganglia
endorphin	released from spinal cord and brain synapses in the pain conduction pathway; acts as an opioid or internal morphine
enkephalin	type of endorphin released from parts of brain and other receptor sites
serotonin	highly concentrated in hypothalamus and basal ganglia; acts as a vasoconstrictor

Types of Neurons

The three types of neurons are classified according to the direction in which they transmit their impulses. The **sensory neurons**, called **afferent neurons**, transmit

Figure 8.4 - Neuron (Nerve Cell)

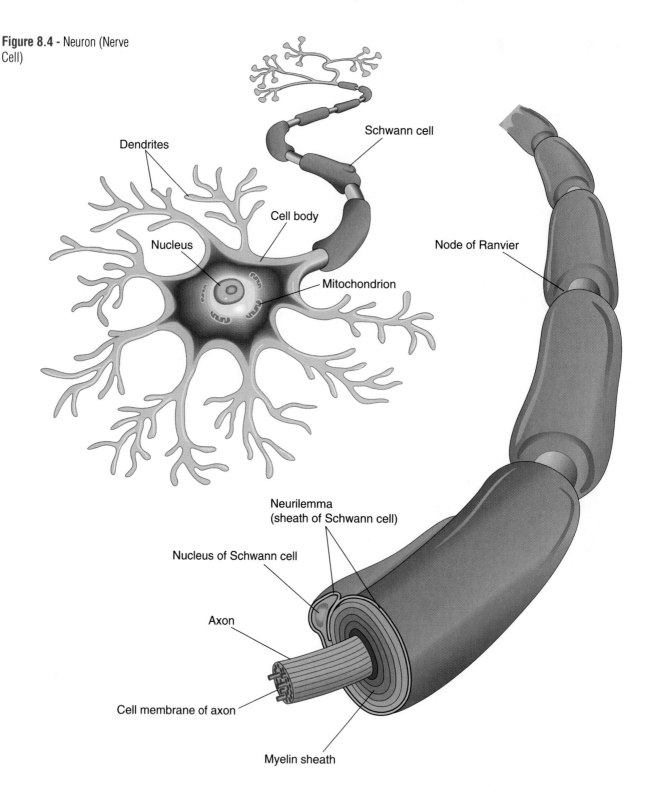

Dendrites

Schwann cell

Cell body

Nucleus

Node of Ranvier

Mitochondrion

Neurilemma
(sheath of Schwann cell)

Nucleus of Schwann cell

Axon

Cell membrane of axon

Myelin sheath

impulses to the spinal cord and brain from all over the body. The **motor neurons**, called **efferent neurons**, transmit impulses away from the brain and spinal cord to muscles and glandular tissue. Connecting neurons called **interneurons** conduct impulses from sensory neurons to motor neurons.

Special supportive cells called **glia**, or **neuroglia**, hold and protect the neurons. One type of glia called **astrocytes** (meaning star-shaped) have threadlike protrusions from their surfaces that hold the neurons close to small blood vessels. Together, this compound structure forms the **blood-brain barrier**, which protects brain tissue from almost all harmful substances that may be carried in the blood. Small astrocytes, called **microglia**, are phagocytic cells that surround degenerating or inflamed brain cells and ingest them. **Oligodendroglia** are the glial cells that produce the myelin sheath and help to hold the neurons together.

Nerve Impulse Pathways

Nerves are constantly sending messages from one part of the body to another, from the outside in and vice versa. Nerve impulses travel over billions of routes or pathways, called **reflex arcs**. The direction of the impulse is one-way, beginning with sensory neurons located at a distance from the spinal cord. One type of reflex arc is demonstrated when the doctor hits a small rubber hammer against the patellar tendon below the knee. This action elicits a reflex response that causes the knee jerk, in which the lower leg moves outward. The movement is caused by the stimulation of the stretch receptors in the muscle, whose signal travels along the length of the sensory neuron to the group of nerve cell bodies in the PNS, called **posterior** or **dorsal root ganglion**. The impulse continues along the dendrites, cell body, and axon of the motor neuron to the effector organ, in this case a muscle. Figure 8.5 shows the reflex arc and the patellar reflex. Table 8.3 lists combining forms and Table 8.4 lists anatomy and physiology terms related to the nervous system.

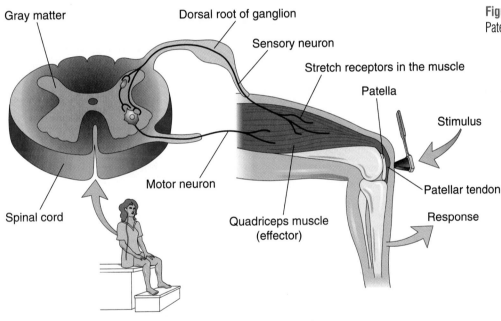

Figure 8.5 - The Reflex Arc: Patellar Reflex

Gray matter
Dorsal root of ganglion
Sensory neuron
Stretch receptors in the muscle
Patella
Stimulus
Motor neuron
Patellar tendon
Spinal cord
Response
Quadriceps muscle (effector)

Table 8.3

Combining Forms Relating to the Nervous System

Combining form	Meaning	Example
astr/o	star-shaped	astrocytoma
-blast/o	young cells or tissue	medulloblastoma
cephal/o	head	diencephalon
cerebell/o	cerebellum	cerebellar
cerebr/o	cerebrum	cerebral
crani/o	cranium	cranial
cyt/o	cell	astrocytoma
electr/o	electricity	electroencephalogram

continued on next page

encephal/o	related to the brain	encephalopathy
gangli/o	swelling, collection	ganglioneuroma
gli/o	gluey substance	neuroglia
kinesi/o	movement	dyskinesia
medull/o	medulla	medulloblastoma
mening/o	membrane covering brain and spinal column	meningitis
myel/o	spinal cord	myelocele
neur/o	nerve	neuritic
occipit/o	occiput (back of the head)	occipital lobe
-oma	pertaining to a tumor	glioblastoma
pariet/o	relationship to a wall	parietal
phas/o	speech	dysphasia
psych/o	mental, the mind	psychiatrist
rachi/o	spine	rachiotomy
sacr/o	sacrum	sacroiliac
somat/o	body	somatic
tempor/o	temporal	temporal lobe

Table 8.4

Anatomy and Physiology Terms Relating to the Nervous System

Term	Meaning	Word Analysis	
afferent neurons **af**-er-ent **noor**-ons	nerves that conduct sensory impulses	afferent neuron	to bring to nerve
arachnoid ar-**ak**-noyd	delicate, spiderweblike membrane forming the middle of the three coverings of the CNS	arachne -oid	spider, cobweb appearance, resemblance
astrocyte **as**-trO-sIt	large neuroglial cell of the nerve tissue	astron -cyte	star cell
autonomic nervous system aw-tO-**nom**-ik **ner**-vus **sis**-tem	part of the nervous system that innervates smooth muscle, cardiac muscle, and gland cells	auto- nomos	self law
axon **ak**-son	area of the nerve cell that conducts impulses away from the cell body	axon	axis
brain	portion of the anatomy (part of the CNS) housed within the cranium	braegen	brain
brainstem	portion of the brain	braegen stem	brain structure resembling a stalk
catecholamine kat-eh-**kol**-am-een	hormones secreted in times of stress: epinephrine, norepinephrine, and dopamine	catecholamine	chemical name
cell body	body of a nerve from which dendrites and an axon arise	cella bodig	cell body
central nervous system	composed of the brain and spinal cord		
cerebral cortex **ser**-eh-bral **kor**-teks	area of the brain located in the outer portion of the cerebrum and responsible for voluntary motor functions	cerebr/o cortic/o	brain outer layer, cortex
cerebrospinal fluid **ser**-eh-brO-**spI**-nal **floo**-id	fluid that surrounds the brain and spinal cord	cerebr/o spin/o -al fluo	brain spinal cord pertaining to flow

cerebrum se-**ree**-brum	portion of the brain that includes the cerebral hemispheres	cerebr/o	brain
dendrite **den**-drIt	treelike structure branching out of the nerve cell body	dendrite	tree
diencephalon dI-en-**sef**-ah-lon	part of the brain that contains the hypothalamus and thalamus	dia- en- cephal/o	through inside head
dorsal root	sensory nerve cell located in the PNS	dorsal	pertaining to the back
dura mater **doo**-rah **may**-ter	outer layer of the meninges	dura mater	hard, tough mother
efferent neurons **ef**-er-ent **noo**-rons	neurons that carry motor impulses	efferent neuron	to bring out nerve
frontal lobe	area in the anterior portion of the brain	frontal lobe	front part, subdivision
ganglion **gang**-lee-on	collection of nerve cell bodies in the PNS	ganglion	a swelling
glia **glI**-ah	supportive cells, also known as neuroglia, that hold and protect neurons	glia	glue
gyri **jI**-rl	elevations that form the cerebral hemispheres	gyros	circle
hemisphere **hem**-is-feer	a lateral half of the cerebrum or cerebellum	hemi- spher/o	half globe
hypothalamus **hI**-pO-**thal**-ah-mus	area of the brain that stimulates target organs to secret hormones; located inferior to the thalamus	hypo- thalam/o	under thalamus
innervate (v) **in**-er-vayt	to stimulate by nerve fibers	in- nervus	within nerve
interneurons in-ter-**noo**-ons	groups of neurons between sensory and motor neurons	inter- neuron	between nerve
medulla oblongata med-**ul**-ah ob-long-**gah**-tah	central structure of the brain	medulla oblongata	marrow long
meninges (pl) men-**in**-jeez	membranes covering the brain and spinal cord	mening/o	membrane
microglia mI-**krog**-glee-ah	phagocytic nerve cells	micro- glia	small glue
midbrain	area in the central portion of the brain	mid- brain	middle brain
myelin **mI**-el-lin	fatty substance that covers components of the PNS	myel/o	the sheath of nerve fibers
neuroglia noo-**rog**-lee-ah	cellular components of the CNS and PNS; nonneural tissue	neur/o glia	nerve glue
neurology noo-**rol**-ah-jee	study of the nervous system and its components	neur/o -logy	nerve study of
neuron **noo**-ron	cellular component of the nervous system; passes electrical messages from one part of the body to another	neuron	nerve
neurotransmitter noo-rO-**trans**-mit-er	chemical released at synapses that passes the electrical impulse from one neuron to another	neur/o transmission	nerve to send across

continued on next page

node of Ranvier ron-vee-**ay**	area between two segments of the axon of a nerve cell	*node* *Ranvier*	resembling a knot nineteenth-century French pathologist
occipital lobe ok-**sip**-ih-tal	area of the brain located posteriorly	*occipit/o* *-al* *lobe*	the back of the head pertaining to part; subdivision
oligodendroglia ol-ig-O-den-**drog**-lee-ah	type of glia cell that forms myelin in the CNS	*olig/o* *dendron* *glia*	a few, a little tree glue
parasympathetic nervous system **par**-ah-sim-pah-**thet**-ik	part of the ANS located in the brain stem and sacral area of the spinal cord that slows the heartbeat and increases muscle movement of the digestive system	*para-* *sympathetic/o*	alongside, near; departure from normal relating to the sympathetic (autonomic) nervous system
parietal lobes pah-**rI**-eh-tal	areas of the brain located on either side of the skull	*pariet/o* *lobe*	denoting any relationship to a wall part; subdivision
peripheral nervous system per-**if**-er-al	system that includes the 12 pairs of cranial nerves, the 31 pairs of spinal nerves, and their branches	*peri-* *phero*	around, about to carry
pia mater **pI**-ah **may**-ter	innermost membrane of the meninges, covers the brain and spinal cord	*pia* *mater*	affectionate mother
pons ponz	portion of the brain located in the brainstem	*pons*	bridge
reflex arc **ree**-fleks ark	transmission of nerve impulses and neurotransmitters that causes an involuntary movement in muscles	*reflex* *arc*	to bend back bow
Schwann cells shvahn	cells that make up the white, fatty myelin sheath that covers the axons outside of the CNS	*Schwann*	nineteenth-century German histologist and physiologist
somatic nervous system sO-**mat**-ik	system that involves skeletal (voluntary) muscle innervation	*somat/o*	body
sulci (pl) **sul**-sI	grooves on the surface of the brain	*sulcus*	ditch
sympathetic nervous system sim-pah-**thet**-ik	body's emergency system that sends a message to the adrenal medulla causing the release of stress hormones	*sympath/o*	refers to the sympathetic nervous system (part of the autonomic nervous system)
synapse **sin**-aps	area of the nerve cells where neurotransmitters are released from one nerve cell to the next	*syn-* *hapto*	together, with clasp
temporal lobe **tem**-por-al	area of the brain located at the temples	*tempor/o* *-al* *lobos*	temples (of the head) pertaining to lobe
thalamus **thal**-ah-mus	area of the brain located in the center	*thalam/o*	bedroom
ventricle **ven**-trih-kl	cavity of the brain	*ventricle*	belly

On the line provided, write a combining form for each definition in the first column; then use the combining form to create a medical term that matches the definition in the second column.

Definition	Combining form	Definition	Term
pain	_____	pain in the head	_____
electricity	_____	record of electrical activity in the brain	_____
movement	_____	pertaining to movement	_____
spinal cord	_____	inflammation of the spinal cord	_____
nerve	_____	related to a nerve	_____
brain	_____	inflammation of the brain	_____
head	_____	incision in the head	_____
glue or gluey substance	_____	nerve glue	_____
cell	_____	nerve cell	_____
body	_____	pertaining to the body	_____

Circle the correct term from the pair in each sentence.

1. Mr. Taber was referred to a neurologist/neuroma.

2. The patient's neurologist ordered an electrocardiogram/electroencephalogram.

3. Several patients in this hospital have been diagnosed with meningitis/meninges.

4. Ms. Murphy has a diagnosis of ganglioneuroma/ganglioplasty of the brachial nerve.

5. Astrocytes/Astrocytosis in the area were found to be abnormal.

6. This disease has affected the automatic/autonomic nervous system.

7. The nerve impulse is interrupted by the damage to the dendrites/denturites.

8. Cerebrospinal/Cerebrosacral fluid was obtained for laboratory analysis.

9. The axon/axis conducts impulses away from the cell body.

10. The area is innervated/unnerved by a branch of the popliteal nerve.

Match the correct term <u>and</u> its correct spelling with the definition provided. Note that multiple spellings are given, so you will need to make sure you select the correct one. Read each choice very carefully and write the answer you select in the space beside the definition.

1. star cell
   astracyte/astracel/astronomical/astrocyte

   _____

2. cranial nerve involved in the sense of smell
   olpactory/offactory/olfactory/olfactorie

   _____

3. brain
   cerabral/cerebrul/cerebrum/cerebrospinal

   _____

4. specialist in the nervous system
   neonatologist/nephrologist/neuralogist/neurologist

   _____

5. partial paralysis of one side of the body
   hemiplegia/hemisphere/hemineurologist/hemiplagia

   _____

6. lobe of the brain located to the side, or lateral aspect, of the skull
   temploral/temporal/temparal/tempora

   _____

7. term referring to the brain and spinal cord
   cerebralspinal/cerebrum/cerebral/cerebrospinal

   _____

9. division of the peripheral nervous system, abbreviated ANS
       automatic nervous system
       autologous nervous system
       autonomic nervous system

   _____

10. membrane covering the brain and spinal cord
    menininges/menninges/meninges/meaninges

    _____

Create a medical term for each of the ten definitions. For each term, use one of the combining forms listed and a prefix and/or suffix from the list. Use each combining form once. A prefix or suffix may be used more than once.

Combining forms		Prefixes		Suffixes	
neur/o	crani/o	hemi-	dys-	-itis	-al
cephal/o	mening/o	intra-	di-	-oma	-ic
kinesi/o	somat/o	pre-	para-	-cyte	-gram
astro	gangli/o	epi-	epi-	-plasty	-logy
myel/o	gli/o	en-	intra-	-otomy	-algia

Definition   **Term**

1. difficult movement   _____

2. large neuroglial cell   _____

3. incision into a nerve   _____

4. within the head   _____

5. pertaining to the brain _____

6. inflammation of the membranes covering the brain _____

7. tumor of glue (type of nerve cell) _____

8. pertaining to the body _____

9. collection of nerve tumor _____

10. repair of the spinal cord _____

Spelling Check

Find the misspelled words in the following sentences and write the correct spelling and define the term on the blanks provided.

1. The myielin has been damaged, resulting in impaired function. _____

_____

2. This patient's cerebelar area was damaged in a motor vehicle accident. _____

_____

3. Dr. Houston performed a creniotomy in an effort to relieve the pressure. _____

_____

4. The axions were unable to conduct nerve impulses. _____

_____

5. A type of ancephalopethy causes the disturbances. _____

_____

6. Dendrits of the affected cells were unable to receive the impulses. _____

_____

7. The neuratransmiter substances are not being properly reabsorbed. _____

_____

8. Acetylcoholin is one of the substances we are studying. _____

_____

9. These are neurons of the parosympiathetic nervous system. _____

_____

10. The medula obolongota was intact and its gross appearance was normal. _____

_____

Complete the concept map below showing the divisions of the nervous system.

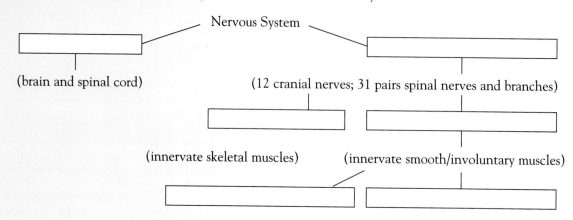

Assessing Patient Health

Wellness and Illness throughout the Life Span

Neurological disorders can present with a variety of symptoms, including paralysis, numbness, twitching, weakness, headaches, seizures, and gait disturbances. Also, cognitive impairments such as forgetfulness and problems with word recognition, word retrieval, behavior, and ability to perform activities of daily living are indications of possible neurological dysfunction. The examiner may be able to determine the neurological source of an abnormality (e.g., the cerebrum, cerebellum, cranial nerves, or sensory-motor neurons) by the symptom displayed.

The assessment begins when the examiner observes the patient's mobility, speech, knowledge of current events, orientation to time and place, and ability to move parts of the body. The level of consciousness, affect (or mood), intellect, and memory are determined by reviewing the patient's history. This procedure is known as the mental status assessment. The neurologic examination proceeds in the following sequence: mental status, cranial nerves, motor function, sensory function, and reflexes.

The examiner next attempts to determine if the cranial nerves, which are part of the peripheral nervous system, are functioning properly. Twelve pairs of cranial nerves connect the brain to the sensory organs of the skin and the skeletal muscles in the head, neck, thorax, and abdominal cavity (Figure 8.6).

The 31 pairs of spinal nerves attach to the spinal cord in segments that correspond to the areas of the spine (Figure 8.7A), and emerge from the spinal cord to form the peripheral nerves of the trunk and limbs (areas not innervated by the cranial nerves). Different areas of the skin's surface, called **dermatomes**, are supplied by specific spinal nerves (Figure 8.7B). Spinal cord lesions can be identified and located by abnormalities in sensation on particular areas of the skin.

Reflexes

The **deep tendon reflexes (DTRs)** are assessed by hitting a rubber-tipped hammer against the various tendons: biceps, triceps, brachioradialis, quadriceps (knee jerk),

Figure 8.6 - Cranial Nerve Attachment

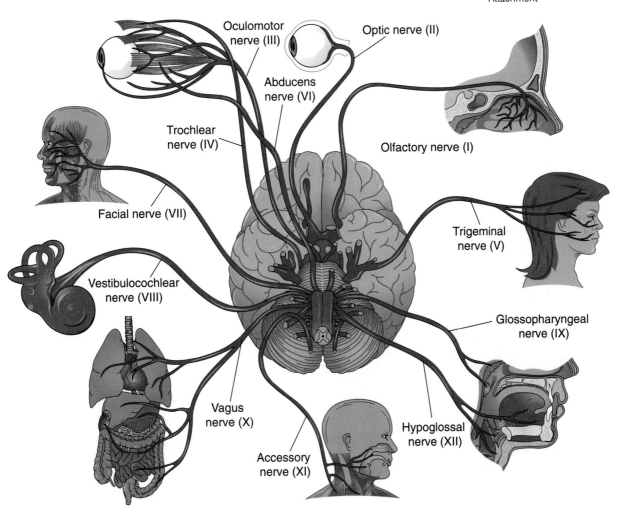

Oculomotor nerve (III)

Optic nerve (II)

Abducens nerve (VI)

Trochlear nerve (IV)

Olfactory nerve (I)

Facial nerve (VII)

Trigeminal nerve (V)

Vestibulocochlear nerve (VIII)

Glossopharyngeal nerve (IX)

Vagus nerve (X)

Hypoglossal nerve (XII)

Accessory nerve (XI)

and Achilles (ankle jerk). Nerve conduction from the muscle causes the connected muscle to react. Table 8.5 shows the way in which the DTR assessment is recorded in the medical record.

Table 8.5

Deep Tendon Reflex Assessment

Test result	Meaning
0	No response
1+	Diminished response
2+	Normal response
3+	More brisk than average response
4+	Hyperactive response (hyperreflexia)

Some reflexes are superficial, because they have receptors in the skin rather than the muscles. Table 8.6 lists the types of superficial reflexes. One set of these reflexes, the abdominal reflexes, is shown in Figure 8.8.

Figure 8.7A - Spinal Nerves

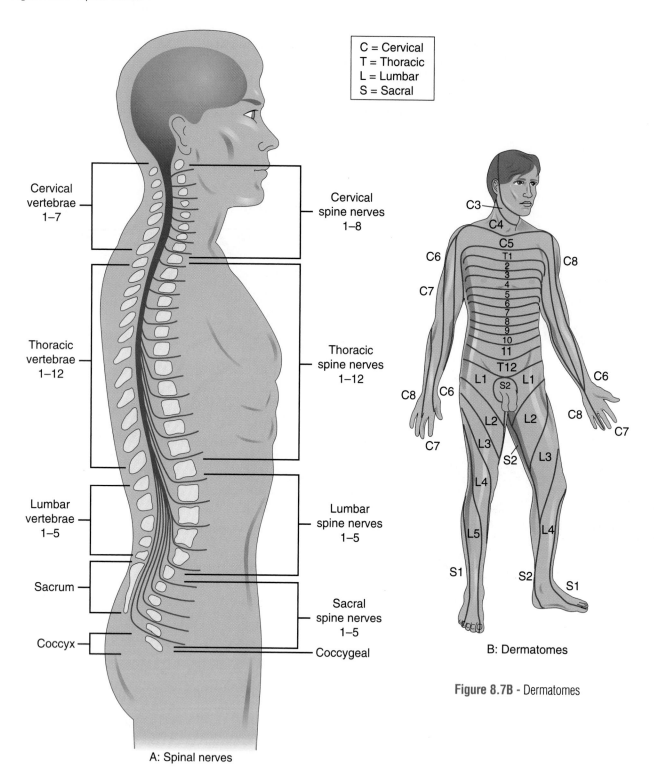

C = Cervical
T = Thoracic
L = Lumbar
S = Sacral

Cervical
vertebrae
1–7

Cervical
spine nerves
1–8

Thoracic
vertebrae
1–12

Thoracic
spine nerves
1–12

Lumbar
vertebrae
1–5

Lumbar
spine nerves
1–5

Sacrum

Sacral
spine nerves
1–5

Coccyx

Coccygeal

A: Spinal nerves

C3
C4
C5
C6
C7
C8
T1
2
3
4
5
6
7
8
9
10
11
T12
L1
S2
L1
C8
C6
L2
L2
C8
C7
L3
C7
L3
S2
L4
L4
L5
S1
S2
S1

B: Dermatomes

Figure 8.7B - Dermatomes

Table 8.6

Superficial Reflexes

Reflex	Description
abdominal reflex	back of hammer is moved from the side of the abdomen toward the midline; normal response is contraction of abdominal muscle on ipsilateral side and deviation of umbilicus toward the motion
cremasteric reflex	on the male, the inner aspect of the thigh is stroked and elevation of the ipsilateral testicle noted
plantar reflex	back of hammer is stroked up the lateral side of the sole of the foot and across the ball of the foot to elicit plantar flexion of the toe

Certain reflexes are abnormal, indicating illness or an abnormal lesion within the brain or spinal cord. Because these reflexes are abnormal findings, the notation on the patient's chart indicates a positive finding. Table 8.7 describes these pathologic reflexes.

Figure 8.8 - Abdominal Reflexes

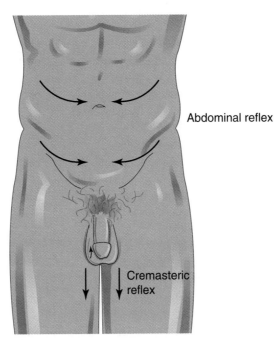

Abdominal reflex

Cremasteric reflex

Table 8.7

Abnormal Reflexes

Reflex	Description	Word analysis	
Babinski bah-**bin**-skee	stroking on the lateral aspect and across the ball of the foot causes extension of the great toe and fanning of the toes	Babinski	19th-century French neurologist
Brudzinski broo-**jin**-skee	flexing chin to the chest elicits resistance and pain	Brudzinski	19th-century Polish physician
Kernig **ker**-nig	when leg is raised straight, resistance and pain occur down the posterior thigh	Kernig	19th-century Russian physician

Infants

The infant's neurological system is not completely developed at birth. The neurons are not yet myelinated (completed by about five years of age), motor activity is not coordinated, and movement is primarily under the control of primitive reflexes, called **infantile automatisms** (Table 8.8). The cerebral cortex develops during the first year of life, causing these reflexes to disappear in a predictable timetable. Their retention may be an indication of CNS disturbance.

Table 8.8

Infantile Automatisms

Reflex	Description	Age at appearance	Age at disappearance
Babinski's sign bah-**bin**-skeez	stroke infant's foot up the lateral edge and across the ball of the foot; note fanning of toes (positive Babinski's sign)	birth	by 24 months
Moro's reflex **mO**-rOz	startle infant to note a symmetric abduction and extension of the arms and legs, fanning fingers, and curling of index finger and thumb to C position; then infant will bring arms and legs inward	birth	1-4 months
palmar grasp **pahl**-mer	offer your finger to the infant from the ulnar side (away from the thumb); grasp should be tight	birth (strongest at 1-2 months)	3-4 months
placing reflex	hold infant upright under arms, near a table; touch top of foot to underside of table; note flexion of hip and knee to attempt to place foot on table	birth	4 days
plantar grasp **plan**-ter	toes curl down tightly with firm touch at ball of foot	birth	8-10 months
rooting reflex	brush side of face near mouth and infant turns the head toward that side and opens mouth	birth	3-4 months
stepping reflex	hold infant upright under arms with feet on flat surface; note regular alternating steps	birth	before walking
sucking reflex	touch lips and offer finger to suck (examiner notes strength of suck)	birth	10-12 months
tonic neck reflex **ton**-ik	with infant supine and relaxed, turn head to one side; ipsilateral arm and leg should extend, and opposite arm and leg should flex; known as "fencing" position	2-3 months	4-6 months

Sensory and motor development gradually proceeds as the infant's neural tracts become myelinated, because myelin is needed to conduct most impulses. Myelinization follows a cephalocaudal and proximodistal order, so the infant will develop movement from head to toe and from trunk to extremities. Motor milestones are noted in the following order: lifts head, lifts head and shoulders, rolls over, moves whole arm, uses hands, walks. Milestones are measured as a means of assessing the infant through childhood.

Several congenital anomalies involve defects in the nervous system. The absence of the brain is known as **anencephaly**, a quickly fatal and relatively rare condition. **Microcephaly** refers to an abnormally small brain and head. **Hydrocephalus** relates to abnormally enlarged ventricles from the accumulation of CSF; this condition can be present at birth or occur at any time. **Meningomyelocele** is the condition caused by the protrusion of part of the spinal cord through a defect in the spinal column that necessitates surgical intervention shortly after birth. Depending on the extent of each of these anomalies, the infant may be mildly to severely learning-disabled, have motor function disabilities, or be relatively unaffected. **Spina bifida** is also caused by a defect in the spinal canal's formation that allows the cord to protrude.

Cerebral palsy is a paralytic neuromuscular disorder of infancy and childhood usually caused by an intrauterine event, birth trauma, or lack of oxygen at birth. Affected infants may manifest mild to severe abnormalities.

Toddlers and School-Aged Children

Children's milestones, including play activities, reaction to parents, and cooperation, are observed and noted during the first ten years. To determine motor activities, the examiner watches the child walk, get dressed, color, cut, ride a tricycle, and balance on one foot.

Muscular dystrophy, a hereditary, progressive, degenerative group of disorders, primarily affects skeletal muscle and can be seen in this age group.

Attention deficit hyperactivity disorder (ADHD) is usually diagnosed in this age group. It is characterized by symptoms that can include such problems as underachievement in school, hyperactivity with a short attention span, obsessive-compulsive behaviors, and tics. Stimulant drugs are used to control the hyperactivity (see the section on pharmacologic agents).

Tourette's syndrome begins in childhood and is characterized by facial and/or vocal tics. It is caused by a defect in the basal ganglia resulting in excessive dopamine excretion, which may be controlled by dopamine-blocking agents.

Young Adults

Multiple sclerosis (MS) is a demyelinating disorder of the CNS that affects young adults. Clearly defined areas that have been demyelinated (plaques) are found in the brain and spinal cord and cause symptoms consisting of weakness, visual loss, paresthesias, and mood changes. Remissions and exacerbations of the symptoms are characteristic.

Middle-Aged Adults

Parkinsonism usually begins in middle age. It is a defect of the **extrapyramidal tract**, especially in the basal ganglia. Classic motor disturbances include flat facial expression, immobility, excessive salivation, stooped posture, and balance and walking disturbances.

Seniors

Because the aging process causes loss of neurons, particularly in the brain and spinal cord, the aging adult shows slower response to requests during the history interview, and motor response may also be slow. The ability to taste and smell declines in this age group. While grip remains relatively strong, the muscles may appear wasted. **Senile tremors** may be noted, including an **intention tremor** that occurs when the person attempts to move, particularly the head, hand, and tongue. Touch and pain sensation may be decreased because of the slowing of message transmission at the synapses, and deep tendon reflexes are less brisk.

The **cerebrovascular accident (CVA)**, commonly known as a **stroke**, is caused by mild to severe interruption of blood flow to the brain; a mild form is a **transient ischemic attack (TIA)**. A stroke or TIA can cause difficulties such as: **aphasia**, inability or difficulty with speaking or writing; **dysphasia**, difficulty with language; **dysphagia**, difficulty swallowing; and **ataxia**, difficulty with motor coordination and muscle movement and gait. Table 8.9 describes more of these terms.

Alzheimer's disease is the primary cause of senile dementia in persons over age 65, and the risk of getting Alzheimer's disease doubles every five additional years. Researchers project that by the year 2050, more than 14 million Americans will have dementia. It is the third most expensive disease in the U.S. and costs over $100 billion annually. Average lifetime expenses are $174,000 per patient. The disease results from structural changes in the brain. Cognitive function gradually declines and usually ends with total disability and ultimately death. Some of the criteria to diagnose Alzheimer's disease include acquired memory impairment, aphasia, **apraxia** (impairment in the performance of skilled or purposeful movements), **agnosia** (impairment in the ability to recognize or comprehend the meaning of various sensory stimuli), and a decline from prior baseline in functional abilities. The cause of Alzheimer's disease is still unknown, and extensive research is currently being conducted in this area. Recent research has indicated that low activity in the hippocampus area of the brain can be seen in Alzheimer's patients up to nine years before onset of symptoms.

Amyotrophic lateral sclerosis (ALS) is also known as Lou Gehrig's disease because of the famous baseball player who died of this disease. It is a chronic, progressive disease characterized by atrophy of the muscles and hardening of the lateral columns of the spinal cord.

GENERAL NERVOUS SYSTEM ILLNESSES

Seizures can occur at any age and involve different muscles and areas of the body. Table 8.10 describes several types of seizures. An **aura**, or particular smell or feeling, often occurs before the seizure (the **preictal** phase) that can allow the individual to anticipate the actual seizure. The person may or may not lose consciousness, but loss of bowel and bladder control during the seizure is common. The period during the seizure is known as the **ictal** phase. The **postictal** phase occurs after the seizure and is characterized by tiredness or sleep.

Table 8.9

Wellness and Illness Terms Relating to the Nervous System

Term	Meaning	Word Analysis	
agnosia	impaired ability to recognize or comprehend the meaning of various sensory stimuli	a- gnosis -ia	without knowledge condition of
Alzheimer's disease **ahltz**-hI-merz	neurologic disease involving the progressive loss of intellectual and cognitive functions	Alzheimer	19th-century German neurologist
amyotrophic lateral sclerosis ay-mI-O-**trO**-fik **lat**-er-al skler-**O**-sis amyotrophia ay-**mI**-O-**trO**-fee-ah	progressive neuromuscular disorder of the lateral columns and anterior horns of the spinal cord characterized by atrophy, hyperreflexia, spasticity, and twitching; known as Lou Gehrig's disease	a- my/o troph/o scler/o -osis	without muscle relating to nutrition; food hard condition

Term	Definition	Word Parts	Meaning
anencephaly **an**-en-**sef**-al-ee	fatal disorder in which the newborn is without a brain	an- -en cephal/o -y	without within brain condition
aphasia ah-**fay**-zha	impaired ability to speak or write due to a lesion in the brain	a- phas/o -ia	without speech condition of
apraxia	impairment in the performance of skilled or purposeful movements	a- pratto -ia	without to do condition
ataxia ah-**taks**-ee-ah	difficulty with motor coordination causing abnormal gait (walking)	a- taxis -ia	away order condition of
aura **aw**-rah	symptoms that occur before a seizure	aura	breeze, odor, and light
Bell's palsy **pahl**-zee	paralysis of the face (cranial nerve VII) brought on by a virus	Bell palsy	18th-century Scottish surgeon paralysis
cerebral palsy **ser**-eh-bral **pahl**-zee	paralytic neuromuscular disorder usually caused by an intrauterine event, birth trauma, or lack of oxygen at birth	cerebr/o palsy	brain, cerebrum paralysis
cerebrovascular accident **ser**-eh-**brO**-vas-kyoo-lar **aks**-sih-dent	event that causes a decreased blood supply to the brain	cerebr/o vascul/o accident	brain vessels (blood supply) refers to an event
decerebrate dee-**ser**-eh-brayt	implies being without a brain; an abnormal position or posture indicating brainstem dysfunction	de- cerebr/o -ate	away, cessation brain pertaining to
decorticate dee-**kor**-tih-kayt	removal of the cortex; an abnormal posture indicating a lesion of the cerebral cortex	de- cortic/o -ate	away, cessation outer layer; cortex pertaining to
dementia dee-**men**-shee-ah	progressive loss of cognitive and intellectual function	de- mens -ia	away, cessation mind condition of
dermatome **der**-mah-tOm	sections of the skin innervated by the spinal nerves	derm/a -tome	skin segment
dysphagia dis-**fay**-jee-ah	difficulty swallowing	dys- phag/o -ia	difficult, bad, painful eat, swallow condition of
dysphasia dis-**fay**-zee-ah	difficulty speaking	dys- phas/o -ia	difficult, bad, painful speech condition of
extrapyramidal tract eks-trah-pih-**ram**-ih-dal	pathways that innervate the large muscles involved in walking, running, and so forth	extra- pyramid	other than, beyond, outside pyramid-shaped
hydrocephalus hI-drO-**sef**-ah-lus	increased fluid in the brain	hydr/o cephal/o	water brain
ictal **ik**-tal	relating to a seizure; the actual period of time when the seizure occurs	ictus -al	stroke or seizure pertaining to

continued on next page

W The Nervous System **3*11***

infantile automatisms **in**-fan-tIl aw-**tom**-ah-tiz-ems	reflexes that are normal for the newborn (automatisms are involuntary actions)	infans auto- matos	not speaking referring to self moving
intention tremor in-**ten**-shun **trem**-er	fine motor movement that occurs during precise actions	intentio tremor	intention shaking
meningomyelocele men-**in**-gO-**mI**-el-O-seel	protrusion of the spinal cord through the vertebrae	mening/o myel/o -cele	refers to brain and/or meninges (spinal cord) spinal cord swelling, hernia (protrusion)
microcephaly mI-krO-**sef**-ah-lee	having a small head	micro- cephal/o -y	small, tiny head condition of
multiple sclerosis skler-**O**-sis	disorder of the CNS in which the brain and spinal cord nerves are demyelinated, causing hard plaques	multi- scler/o -is	many, much hard condition
muscular dystrophy **mus**-kyoo-lar **dis**-trah-fee	hereditary, progressive, degenerative group of disorders affecting skeletal muscles	muscul/o -ar dys- troph/o -y	muscle pertaining to bad, difficult, painful nutrition condition
opisthotonos O-pis-**thot**-ah-nus	abnormal posture characterized by arching of the back, with head and heels bent backward	opisth/o tonos	backward, behind tone
paralysis par-**al**-ih-sis	loss of voluntary movement	para- lys/o -is	near; abnormal; referring to both parts of a pair lysis, dissolution condition
paresis pah-**ree**-sis	partial paralysis	paresis	letting go
paresthesia par-es-**thee**-zee-ah	abnormal sensation	para- aisthesis	near; abnormal; referring to both parts of a pair sensation
Parkinson's disease	defect in extrapyramidal tract displaying various motor disturbances	Parkinson	18th-century British physician
poliomyelitis **pO**-lee-O-mI-el-I-tis	inflammation of the gray matter of the spinal cord caused by infectious process	poli/o myel/o -itis	gray matter referring to marrow; spinal cord inflammation
seizure **see**-zher	sudden convulsion	seizure	grasp
spina bifida **spI**-nah **bif**-ih-dah	congenital abnormality caused by a failure of one or more of the spinal arches to fuse	spin/o bifed	vertebral column separated into two parts
Tourette syndrome too-**ret**	syndrome characterized by facial and/or vocal tics caused by a defect in the basal ganglia resulting in excessive dopamine excretion	Tourette	19th-century French physician

| transient ischemic attack **tran**-see-ent is-**kee**-mik ah-**tak** | brief period in which blood supply to the brain is decreased | transient
ischo
-heme
-ic | short-lived
to keep back
blood
pertaining to |

Table 8.10

Types of Seizures

Term	Meaning	Word Analysis	
grand mal grahn mahl	sudden onset of generalized contraction of the muscles, causing the individual to fall (also called tonic-clonic)	grand mal	large illness
jacksonian jak-**sO**-nee-an	progressive spread of the seizure usually occurring on one side of the body	Jackson	19th-century English neurologist
myoclonic mI-O-**klon**-ik	single or repetitive muscle jerks	my/o klonos	muscle tumult
petit mal peh-**tee** mahl	brief pause in activity without loss of consciousness (also called absence)	petit mal	small illness
tonic-clonic **ton**-ik **klon**-ik	sudden onset of generalized contraction of the muscles causing the individual to fall	tonos klonos	tone tumult

Abnormalities in muscle movement include **paresis** or **paralysis** of any body part (see Table 8.11). These aberrations refer to decreased and complete loss of motor ability, respectively, caused by a problem with either motor nerves or muscle fibers. Possible causes of paralysis include **poliomyelitis,** an infectious disease involving inflammation of the gray matter of the spinal cord; **Bell's palsy**, a type of unilateral paralysis of the face brought on by a virus; and malignant or nonmalignant lesions or tumors of the brain or spinal cord. Table 8.12 summarizes some common abnormal muscle movements, and Figures 8.9-8.15 illustrate these movements. Several neuromuscular abnormalities involve the position of the body and are usually caused by lesions in the brain (Figures 8.16-8.19).

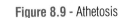

Figure 8.9 - Athetosis

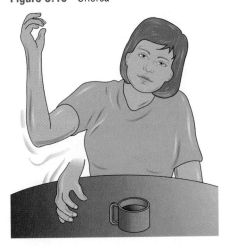

Figure 8.10 - Chorea

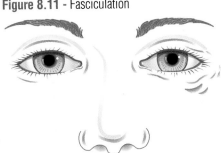

Figure 8.11 - Fasciculation

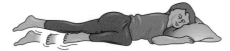
Figure 8.12 - Myoclonus

Figure 8.13 - Tic
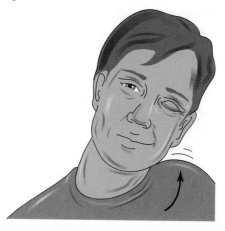

Figure 8.14 - Tremor
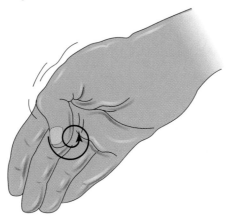

Figure 8.15 - Twitch
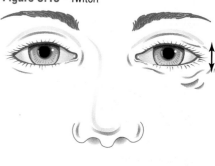

Table 8.11

Types of Paralyses

Term	Description	Word analysis	
hemiplegia **hem**-ih-**plee**-jee-ah	paralysis of one side of the body	*hemi-* *-plegia*	half paralysis
paraplegia par-ah-**plee**-jee-ah	paralysis of the lower extremities	*para-* *-plegia*	denoting both parts of a pair paralysis
quadriplegia kwod-rih-**plee**-jee-ah	paralysis of all four extremities	*quadri-* *-plegia*	four paralysis
spastic paraplegia **spas**-tik par-ah-**plee**-jee-ah	type of paresis (partial paralysis) of the lower extremities in which there are spasms of muscle contractions	*spastic* *para-* *-plegia*	drawing in denoting both parts of a pair paralysis

Table 8.12

Types of Abnormal Muscle Movements

Term	Description	Word analysis	
athetosis **ath**-eh-**tO**-sis	constant, slow, involuntary movement of fingers and hands in all directions	*athetosis*	without position
chorea kO-**ree**-ah	involuntary, irregular, spasmodic movement of limbs	*chorea*	dance
fasciculation fah-sik-yoo-**lay**-shun	involuntary contraction of groups of muscle fibers	*fascis*	bundle
myoclonus mI-**ok**-lO-nus myoclonic (adj) mI-O-**klon**-ik	involuntary, rapid contraction of a muscle group	*my/o* *klonos* *-ic*	muscle tumult pertaining to
tic tik	habitual and usually voluntary contraction of certain muscles	*tic*	French term
tremor **trem**-er	involuntary repetitive, irregular contraction	*tremor*	shaking
twitch	very quick spasmodic contraction of a muscle group	*twiccian*	to pluck

Decorticate rigidity indicates a lesion of the cerebral cortex. The upper extremities are flexed and adducted; the lower extremities are extended, with internal rotation and plantar flexion (Figure 8.16).

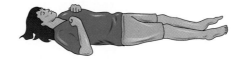

Figure 8.16 - Decorticate Rigidity

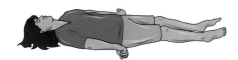

Figure 8.17 - Decerebrate Rigidity

Decerebrate rigidity indicates a lesion in the brainstem, usually at the midbrain or upper pons. The upper extremities are stiff, extended, and adducted, with internal rotation and flexed palms (Figure 8.17). The teeth are clenched.

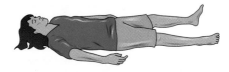

Figure 8.18 - Flaccid Quadriplegia

Flaccid quadriplegia indicates complete loss of muscle tone and a nonfunctional brainstem (Figure 8.18).

Figure 8.19 - Opisthotonos

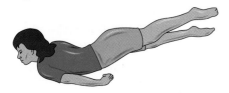

Opisthotonos indicates meningeal irritation and is characterized by arching of the back, with head and heels bent backward (Figure 8.19).

Neuro-Oncology is a field of practice that involves oncologic diseases of the nervous system. Brain tumors are abnormal growths of brain tissue with or without involvement of the meninges. They may be malignant or benign, and may be classified as primary or secondary. Brain tumors are usually named for the tissue from which they arise. Symptoms of a brain tumor occur as a result of the expansion of the tumor into the brain tissue, which may cause many neurological dysfunctions such as headaches, dizziness, vomiting, ataxia, personality changes, and other symptoms depending upon the area of the brain that is affected.

Surgical removal and/or debulking of the tumor, important treatment modalities, are not always possible because of potential damage to the involved and surrounding tissues. Radiation and chemotherapy may also be used, although many chemotherapeutic agents are not effective because they do not cross the blood-brain barrier. Intracranial radiotherapy (radiation therapy that is given during the surgical excision) and chemotherapeutic implants (chemical-soaked wafers that slowly dissolve within the tumor or brain tissue) are among the newer treatments used to treat and try to control the growth of brain tumors.

Astrocytoma

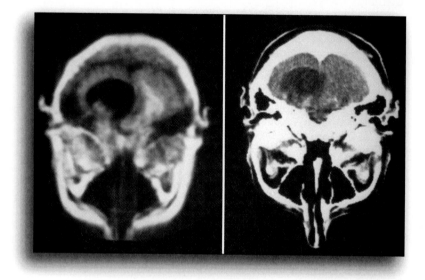

Glioma

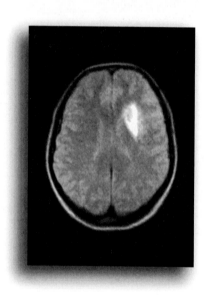

Meningioma

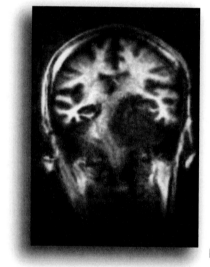

Table 8.13

Types of Brain Tumors

Name	Approximate incidence	Characteristics
astrocytoma	10% of all brain tumors	slow-growing
brain stem gliomas	10% of all pediatric brain tumors	occurs most often in children
ependymomas	6% of all brain tumors	usually within 4th ventricle and extend into spinal cord
glioblastoma multiforme	20% of all brain tumors	arise in the cerebral hemisphere
oligodendrogliomas	5% of all brain tumors	occur usually in the frontal lobe
medulloblastoma	4% of all brain tumors	occurs most often in children
meningiomas	15% of all brain tumors	slow-growing, vascular tumors occurring in adults

MENTAL HEALTH AND PSYCHIATRIC DISORDERS

The field of mental health encompasses several types of practitioners. A physician who practices in the field of psychiatry, diagnosing and treating mental disorders, is called a **psychiatrist**. Another type of practitioner is a **psychologist**, a nonmedical person who may have a doctoral or a master's degree in methods of psychotherapy, analysis, and research. **Social workers** and **counselors** also care for persons with mental disorders.

Disruptive Behavior Disorders

The most common disorder in the DSM (Diagnostic and Statistical Manual of Mental Disorders) classification is **attention-deficit hyperactivity disorder** (ADHD), characterized by inattentiveness and impulsivity. It is usually diagnosed when a child first starts school. ADHD children are unable to concentrate and complete tasks. They may be disruptive and become a discipline problem in the classroom and at home. This disorder is ten times more common in boys, is usually familial, and may be helped by the administration of stimulant drugs. ADHD is thought to be caused by a neurological impairment. **Tics**, or motor or vocal movements and/or sounds, may be associated with ADHD. Often the child will require psychological intervention to help gain control and mastery over actions and the feelings associated with them.

Eating Disorders

Anorexia nervosa and **bulimia nervosa** are disorders most common in teenage girls, and are associated with poor self-image and an obsession with weight and being "fat." Decreased eating, increased exercise, and the use of diuretics and laxatives characterize anorexia nervosa. Bulimia nervosa involves eating (often gorging on food), followed by vomiting (called purging), and the use of diuretics and/or laxatives.

Affective Disorders

Affective disorders are disorders of the person's **affect**, a term for mood or emotions. They can range from abnormal and/or prolonged grief to mild or severe depression. Thinking of emotions as a continuum, it may be difficult to determine when a person is adapting to normal situations. However, prolonged affective disorders, or situations that prevent a person from functioning personally or in society, are abnormal. Any emotion that is suppressed may eventually become an affective disorder.

    Depressive disorders may be considered depression that is outside the bounds of normal "feeling down" as a result of bereavement grief or other loss. Persons with depression lose interest in life or social contacts and may feel overwhelming hopelessness, helplessness, and suicidal ideation. **Manic-depressive disorders,** also called **bipolar disorders**, consist of episodes of depression and mania (excitement).

Anxiety Disorders and Neuroses

Certain disorders that affect the individual may be associated with moderate to severe levels of anxiety. A **neurosis** is a mental disorder characterized by anxiety that does not include any reality distortion.

Post-traumatic stress syndrome is a fairly new diagnosis involving feelings of anxiety and stress following (even years later) a life stress or traumatic event. Combat veterans and victims of violent crime face a higher risk of this disorder than the general population.

Panic attacks are sudden episodes in which the person may feel like they are about to faint, have a heart attack, choke, go insane or die. The attack passes, and the person may never experience another one. Panic disorder is characterized by recurrent panic attacks, and may be treated by psychotherapy and/or drugs.

Phobias (from the Greek, *phobos*, for fear) are actually panic disorders; the individual cannot cope with certain situations and has an intense fear of them. Specific phobias are listed in Table 8.14.

Table 8.14

Common Phobias

Phobia	Fear of	Word analysis	
acrophobia	heights	*acr/o*	tip, peak
agoraphobia	being in a crowd or public place; leaving a familiar place	*agora*	marketplace
allodoxaphobia	others' opinions	*allo*	other
		doxa	concept, theory, opinion
astraphobia	lightning	*astro/a*	star
claustrophobia	being in a closed-in place	*claustrum*	enclosed space
entomophobia	insects	*entomo*	insects
hemophobia	blood	*hemo*	blood
hydrophobia	water	*hydro/a*	water
radiophobia	x-rays	*radio*	energy
social phobia (also called social anxiety disorder)	public scrutiny	*socius*	partner, companion
thermophobia	heat	*therm/o*	heat
xenophobia	foreigners	*xen/o*	strange, foreign

Obsessive-compulsive neurosis is an anxiety disorder that presents with symptoms of recurring thoughts and repetitive acts that are performed ritualistically. Elimination of any step of the ritual causes severe anxiety.

Schizophrenia

A **psychosis** is differentiated from a neurosis in terms of the person's ability to cope with everyday living. Psychotic symptoms include hallucinations (seeing things that are not there), delusions (ideas for which there is no basis in reality), and bizarre behavior. **Schizophrenia** (there are a number of subtypes) is a type of disorder in which psychotic symptoms may be observed. The individual withdraws from reality and slips into a private world of the mind. Some terms of mental health and psychiatry are described in Table 8.15.

Table 8.15

Mental Health and Psychiatric Terms

Terms	Meaning	Word analysis	
affect **a**-fect	apparent mood or feelings	*affectus*	state of mind
anorexia-nervosa ann-Oh-**rex**-e-ah ner-**vO**-sah	decreased eating, increased exercise and abuse of laxatives and diuretics	*an-* *orexis* *nervosa*	without appetite nerves
bulimia nervosa bull-**e**-me-ah ner-**vO**-sah	binge eating followed by purging and abuse of laxatives and diuretics	*bous* *limos* *nervosa*	ox hunger nerves
catatonic schizophrenia cat-a-**tonic** skitz-Oh-**free**-knee-ah	person does not speak, move, or relate to the outside world	*cat/a* *ton/o* *schizo-* *phren*	down, lower tone split mind
delusion	idea or belief with no basis in reality	*de* *ludo*	from play
disorganized schizophrenia dis-**organ**-eye-zed skitz-Oh-**free**-knee-ah	ideas change from one to another with total disassociation; language may be incoherent	*dis* *organum* *schizo-* *phren*	not organ split mind
hallucinations	person hears voices or sees visions that do not exist	*alucinor*	for wander in mind
mania **may**-knee-ah	increased activity and speech, and loss of good judgement	*mania*	frenzy
paranoid schizophrenia **pair**-a noid skitz-Oh-**free**-knee-ah	delusions of persecution and grandeur	*par/a* *-oid* *schizo-* *phren*	departure from normal resemblance to split mind

Table 8.16

Abbreviations

ADHD	attention-deficit hyperactivity disorder
CA	chronological age
GAF Scale	Global Assessment of Functioning is a subjective assessment tool used to rate ability to function on a scale of 1–100, where 1 = poor mental health and inability to function and 100 = good mental health and ability to function well
IQ	intelligence quotient (normal = 90–110)
MA	mental age
OCD	obsessive compulsive disorder
PDDNOS	pervasive developmental disorder not otherwise specified
SAD	seasonal affective disorder
WAIS	Wechsler Adult Intelligence Scale
WISC	Wechsler Intelligence Scale for Children

Identify the root of each term by drawing a box around it, and then write the definition for the term on the line provided.

Term	Definition
1. neurological	
2. cephalocaudal	
3. meningomyelocele	
4. cerebrovascular	
5. demyelinating	
6. ataxia	
7. anencephaly	
8. dystrophy	
9. paresthesia	
10. neuronal	

Comprehension Check

Circle the correct term from the pair in each sentence.

1. The cranial nerve/nerves are intact.

2. The ventricles/ventricle are enlarged.

3. This patient's reflex/reflexes are abnormal.

4. This laboratory has studied the cerebral cortex/cortices of several species of mammals.

5. The muscular dystrophy/dystrophies constitute a group of neurological disorders that affect skeletal muscles.

6. Some of the older patients exhibit an intention tremors/tremor.

7. These patients perceive various types of aurae/aura before seizure activity.

8. Mrs. Anderson suffered a transient ischemic attack/attacks.

9. The message transmission fails at the various synapse/synapses.

10. Mary has had several seizure/seizures in the past week.

Matching

Match the correct spelling of a term in Column 1 with the term's definition in Column 2. Write the number of the correctly spelled term in the space beside the definition.

Column 1

1. preicical
2. preictal
3. parietal
4. hydrocefalus
5. hydrocephalus
6. neuronal
7. neural
8. neutral
9. ventricles
10. ventricular
11. cortec
12. cortex
13. kortex
14. cefalocaudal
15. cephalic
16. cephalocaudal
17. quadraplegia
18. paraplegia
19. transient ischemic attack
20. transiten ischimic attack
21. cerebrovascular accident
22. siezure
23. seizure
24. seizural
25. parisis
26. paresis
27. parasthesia

Column 2

_____ a. fluid-filled spaces within the brain

_____ b. outer layer of the brain

_____ c. pertaining to a neuron or neurons

_____ d. "head-to-toe"

_____ e. brief period of decreased blood supply to the brain

_____ f. sudden convulsion

_____ g. phase of a seizure preceding the actual convulsion

_____ h. partial paralysis

_____ i. paralysis of the lower extremities

_____ j. literally meaning "water on the brain"

Word Building

Use word parts or entire words to complete a term matching the definition. Write the part you supply on the blank provided.

1. different areas on the surface of the skin that are served by different nerves: _____tomes

2. one of the cranial nerves that serves the throat muscles and salivary glands: glosso_____

3. superficial reflex that involves plantar flexion of the toes when the lateral side of the sole of the foot and ball of the foot are stroked: _____ar reflex

4. primitive reflexes in the infant: infantile _____

5. infantile reflex in which baby grasps object placed in the hand: _____grasp reflex

6. fluid that bathes and helps to protect the brain and spinal column: cerebro_____ fluid

7. tremors in older adults resulting from loss of neurons due to the aging process: _____ile tremors

8. absence seizure in which there is a brief stoppage of activity without loss of consciousness: _____
   seizure

9. type of paresis (partial paralysis) of the lower extremities in which there are spasms of muscle contraction:
   spastic _____

10. condition of constant, slow, involuntary movement of fingers and hands in all directions: athet_____

Spelling Check

Circle the misspelled word or words in each sentence, then write the correct spelling of the word(s) on the line provided.

1. The child displayed flacid quadroplegia following the accident.

   _____

2. Larry developed Bell's palasy after a mild illness.

   _____

3. The patient displayed decorticuate posturing in the emergency room.

   _____

4. This 87-year-old female demonstrates atexia, aphiasia, and tremors.

   _____

5. The speech impairment is a result of an old cerebrevascluar acident.

   _____

6. The patient had previously been diagnosed with epileipsy and went into cardiac arrest during a posticital
   period.

   _____

7. An elderly patient is unable to swallow tablets because of disphagia secondary to a CNA.

   _____

8. James was diagnosed with muiltiple scllerosis at age 23.

   _____

9. The child had surgery a few days after birth to correct spinus bifada.

   _____

10. The Kellys' child was anecphalic at birth and survived only a few hours.

   _____

Word Maps

Complete the concept map below showing the stages of a seizure.

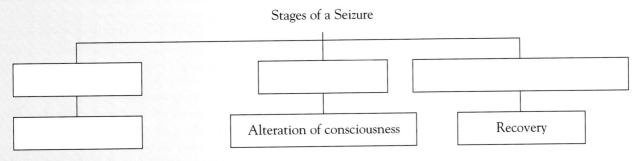

Characterized by: abnormal smell, feeling, taste, sound   Characterized by: fatigue, lethargy, sleep, confusion

Name That Term: Phobias

On the line provided, write the name of the phobia described.

1. fear of heights   _____

2. fear of leaving a familiar place   _____

3. fear of being in a closed-in place   _____

4. fear of blood   _____

5. fear of others' opinions   _____

6. fear of foreigners   _____

7. fear of heat   _____

8. fear of insects   _____

9. fear of lightning   _____

10. fear of x-rays   _____

Comprehension Check

Draw a circle around the correct term from each pair.

1. Joel, who is 10, is disruptive and unable to concentrate. He might have ADHD/DSM.

2. A person who is severely fearful of heights might be said to have acromania/acrophobia.

3. A general term for disorders of emotions is affective disorders/emotophobias.

4. Bipolar disorders consist of manias and phobias/mania and depression.

5. A mental disorder characterized by anxiety without any reality distortion is a neurosis/nervosis.

6. Phobia/psychosis is from the Greek word for fear.

7. Persons affected with bulimia nervosa/bipolar disorder engage in overeating followed by vomiting.

8. A physician who diagnoses and treats mental disorders is a psychiatrist/psychologist.

9. Fear of closed spaces is called kleptomania/claustrophobia.

10. Anxiety and stress following a catastrophic or dramatic, emotional event is obsessive-compulsive disorder/post-traumatic stress syndrome.

11. A term with parts that mean "split" and "the mind" is paranoia/schizophrenia.

12. Catatonic schizophrenia is a type of psychosis/phrenosis.

Diagnosing and Treating Problems

Tests, Procedures, and Pharmaceuticals

Most testing of nervous system function involves evaluation of the cranial nerves; muscle movement, strength and tone; and reflexes as described previously (see Table 8.13). Other tests can determine neuromuscular and neurosensory function and are performed during the physical examination.

Cerebellar function evaluation includes gait and balance tests. Observation of the person's walk can reveal abnormalities such as **ataxia** and uncoordinated or unsteady gait. The ability to walk a straight line and heel-to-toe walking are also assessed. The **Romberg test** is performed as part of the assessment. The patient stands with feet together and arms at sides; with the eyes closed, the person should be able to maintain this position without sway or position change.

Tests for coordination involve the patient performing rapid alternating movements with the feet and fingers. The sensory system is assessed in several ways. Touch, vibration, temperature, discrimination, and position (kinesthesia) are elicited sensations.

The **electroencephalogram (EEG)** is a diagnostic tool used to measure the electrical impulses of the brain. If there are abnormalities, they may be identified with this test.

A **lumbar puncture**, or **spinal tap**, is performed by inserting a small-gauge needle between the vertebrae at level L2-L3. The CSF is collected and tested to determine whether organisms or tumor cells are present. When intracranial pressure is increased, drainage of fluid may relieve some of the pressure. **Intrathecal** (*intra*: within; *thecal*: relating to a sheath) refers to the subarachnoid or subdural space. When medications are injected into the CSF, it is known as intrathecal administration.

A **brain scan** calls for an injection of a radioactive substance into a vein, after which the brain is scanned to find any lesions. **Computerized axial tomography**, called a **CAT** scan, is used to visualize the brain using x-ray images taken from many angles and then a three-dimensional image is constructed from that data. **Magnetic resonance imaging (MRI)** is a method of scanning the brain using an electromagnetic field and radio waves to produce the image. **Positron emission tomography (PET)** uses a thin x-ray beam to visualize a cross-section of the brain after injection of a radioactive isotope. **Single photon emission computed tomography (SPECT)** involves the injection of a radioactive sugar substance that is metabolized by the brain. The brain is then scanned to identify any abnormalities.

Surgical Procedures

Any procedure involving a surgical opening into the skull is known as a **craniotomy**. A **lobectomy** is the excision of a lobe of the brain. A **ventriculotomy** is a surgical incision into a ventricle of the brain to relieve fluid pressure in patients with hydrocephalus or swelling from head trauma.

A **rhizotomy**, or **radicotomy**, is a surgical procedure to dissect nerve roots of the spine in order to relieve pain. A **chordotomy** is performed to interrupt the pain impulses to the brain by making an incision in the spinal cord. **Neuroplasty** is the repair of a nerve.

Table 8.17

Tests and Procedures Relating to the Nervous System

Test or procedure	Description
brain scan	nuclear image with an injection of radioactive dye to scan and view the brain
chordotomy	procedure performed by an incision in the spinal cord to stop pain
craniotomy	incision into the brain
electroencephalogram	measurement of the electrical activity of the brain
lobectomy	removal of a lobe of the brain
lumbar puncture	procedure performed by inserting a needle between the vertebrae at level L2-L3 to obtain CSF for examination
magnetic resonance imaging (MRI)	method of scanning the brain using an electromagnetic field and radio waves to produce the image
neuroplasty	repair of a nerve
positron emission tomography (PET)	thin x-ray beam is used to visualize a cross-section of the brain after injection of a radioactive isotope
radicotomy	surgical procedure to dissect a nerve root of the spine
rhizotomy	surgical procedure to dissect a nerve root of the spine
Romberg test	test to determine cerebellar function; measures balance
single photon emission computed tomography (SPECT)	scan using the injection of a radioactive sugar substance, metabolized by the brain; brain is then imaged
spinal tap	procedure performed by inserting a needle between the vertebrae at level L2-L3 to obtain CSF for examination
ventriculotomy	surgical incision into a ventricle of the brain

Pharmaceutical Agents

Anticonvulsants are agents used to control seizures (see Table 8.14). The most common agents are classified as **hydantoins, benzodiazepines, dicarbamates**, and **barbiturates**. Many agents are used to help with hyperactivity, and ironically they are classified as CNS stimulant agents; the most common are **amphetamines** and **methylphenidates**. Although the mechanism of action is not fully understood, they may act by blocking the reuptake of dopaminergic neurons. They must be used with great caution.

Persons with Parkinson's disease often take several medications known as **anti-Parkinson agents.** The focus for treatment is the replacement of missing neurotransmitters; therefore, agents such as levodopa are used. Other drugs are often needed to control the debilitating symptoms of the disease.

Immunologic agents such as interferon and new biopharmaceuticals are being used for diseases that are thought to be autoimmune, such as multiple sclerosis.

Various muscle relaxants and nonsteroidal anti-inflammatory agents are used for neuromuscular aches and pains. They decrease the inflammation and relax the spasms often associated with pain, particularly in the spinal area of the back and neck.

Table 8.18

Pharmacologic Agents Relating to the Nervous System

Drug classes	Use	Generic name	Brand names
anti-Alzheimer's (dementia)	inhibit acetylcholinesterase	donepezil galantamine tacrine	Aricept Reminyl Cognex
antianxiety		nefazodone venlafaxine	Serzone Effexor
anticonvulsants (e.g., barbiturates, benzodiazepines, dicorbamates, hydantoins)	interfere with the mechanisms that cause seizures	clonazepam clorazepate diazepam felbamate phenobarbital phenytoin sodium	Klonopin Tranxene Valium Felbatol Bellergal, Donnatal Dilantin
antidepressants	selective serotonin reuptake inhibitors monoamine oxidase inhibitors miscellaneous	fluoxetine sertraline paroxetine phenelzine tranylcypromine bupropion methylphenidate	Prozac Zoloft Paxil Nardil Parnate Wellbutrin, Zyban Ritalin
anti-mania		lithium carbamazepine	Lithobid Tegretol
anti-Parkinson agents	treat debilitating symptoms of Parkinson's disease	benztropine biperiden carbidopa-levodopa levodopa phenobarbital	Cogentin Akineton Sinemet Larodopa Bellergal, Donnatal
antipsychotics		chlorpromazine mirtazapine	Thorazine Remeron
central nervous system stimulants (e.g., amphetamines)	stimulate the nervous system	dextroamphetamine methylphenidate	Dexedrine Ritalin

Table 8.19

Abbreviations

ADHD	attention deficit hyperactivity disorder
ALS	amyotrophic lateral sclerosis
ANS	autonomic nervous system
CAT	computerized axial tomography
CNS	central nervous system
CP	cerebral palsy
CSF	cerebrospinal fluid
CT	computed tomography
CVA	cerebrovascular accident
DTR	deep tendon reflex
EEG	electroencephalogram or electroencephalography
LP	lumbar puncture

MRI	magnetic resonance imaging
MS	multiple sclerosis
PD	Parkinson's disease
PET	positron emission tomography
PNS	peripheral nervous system
SPECT	single photon emission computed tomography
SNS	somatic nervous system
TIA	transient ischemic attack

Word Analysis

Write the combining forms in each term. Give the meaning of the combining form.

Term	Combining form	Meaning
1. Craniotomy	_____	_____
2. Neuroplasty	_____	_____
3. Rhizotomy	_____	_____
4. Lobectomy	_____	_____
5. Ventriculotomy	_____	_____
6. Radicotomy	_____	_____
7. Tomography	_____	_____
8. Chordotomy	_____	_____

Comprehension Check

Circle the correct term from the pair in each sentence. You may need to use a medical dictionary.

1. The doctor will order a <u>CAT/MAT</u> scan for this patient today.

2. During the neurological examination, the patient was unable to perform the <u>Romberg/Romaine</u> test without falling.

3. A lumbar puncture was performed; a sample of <u>cerebrospinal/cerebral</u> fluid was obtained and sent to the laboratory.

4. Please prepare Mrs. Martin for an <u>EEG/GTT</u>.

5. A <u>brain scan/bran scan</u>, performed after the accident, showed no abnormalities.

6. The patient's physician performed a <u>chordotomy/craniectomy</u> to relieve the intractable pain.

7. Dr. Williams recommends a <u>ventriculotomy/ventricular</u> for the child.

8. The hand reconstruction included <u>neuroplasty/necroplasty</u> of the metacarpal nerves.

9. Mr. Marks was treated with <u>anticonvulsants/antibiotics</u> for his epilepsy.

10. Some physicians prescribe central nervous system <u>stimulants/steroids</u> for ADHD patients.

What Do These Abbreviations Mean?

Provide a definition for each abbreviation.

1. ALS _____

2. CNS _____

3. DTR _____

4. CSF _____

5. MS _____

6. PNS _____

7. MRI _____

8. LP _____

9. EEG _____

10. TIA _____

Word Building

Supply the word parts to complete each term, according to the definition provided.

1. A _____vascul_____ accident is a mild stroke.

2. An electro _____ is a record of electrical activity in the brain.

3. _____ al means pertaining to the lumbar and sacral area of the spine.

4. _____ ar means pertaining to the nerves and muscles.

5. _____ y means pertaining to the nerves and senses.

6. A _____ refers to without coordination; unsteady or uncoordinated gait.

7. _____ ology is the study of movement.

8. _____ cranial means inside the cranium (skull).

9. En _____ pathy refers to disease related to the brain.

10. _____ oma refers to tumor of a nerve ganglion.

11. _____ ar means pertaining to the cerebellum.

12. _____ al means pertaining to the sacrum.

Read the terms that follow and then indicate whether the term is singular or plural by writing an *S* or a *P* after the term. Supply the other form (either singular or plural) of the term.

	P/S	Opposite term
1. seizures	_____	_____
2. palsy	_____	_____
3. dermatome	_____	_____
4. neuroplasties	_____	_____
5. ventriculotomy	_____	_____
6. barbiturate	_____	_____
7. amphetamines	_____	_____
8. anticonvulsant	_____	_____
9. neurotransmitters	_____	_____
10. neurologists	_____	_____

Mark the body illustrations to indicate the affected limbs and the degree of impairment in each classification. Place a star (*) over each limb that would be paralyzed and an X over each limb that would be only slightly or partially paralyzed.

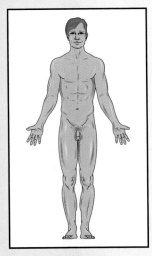

Hemiplegia

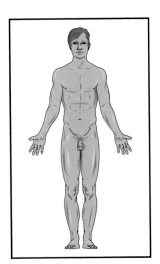

Paraplegia

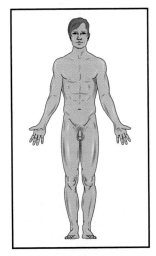

Spastic Paraplegia

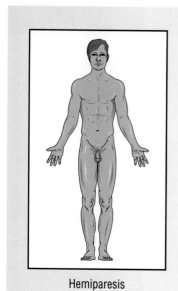

Hemiparesis

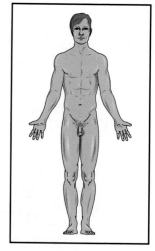

Quadriplegia

Paraparesis

Performance Assessment 8

Crossword Puzzle

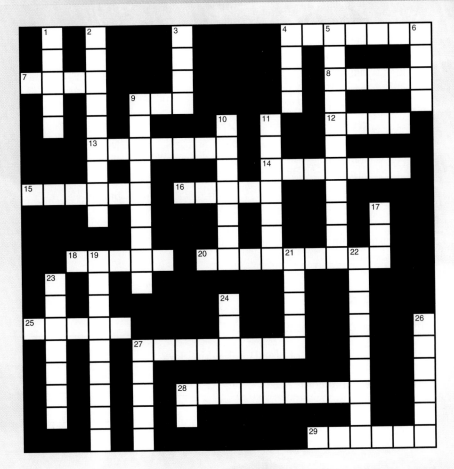

Across

4. inability to properly use language
7. special cells that protect neurons
8. combining form for speech
9. prefix meaning difficulty
12. folds on the surface of the brain
13. neurons that transmit nerve impulses to the spinal cord
14. impaired ability to recognize the meaning of various sensory stimuli
15. combining form for cerebrum
16. part of the CNS in the cranium
18. cortical areas
20. special cells that hold and protect the neurons
25. _____ neck reflex
27. cranial nerve involved in hearing
28. cells that eat inflamed brain cells
29. sheeth around axons outside the CNS; made up of Schwann cells

Down

1. French term meaning paralysis
2. composed of the pons, midbrain, and medulla oblongata
3. one of the structures that make up the brainstem
4. Latin for breeze or light
5. nerve that controls muscles of the tongue
6. long branch from neuron to muscles
9. structures of a nerve cell; receive information from other neurons
10. neuron connections
11. toe flexion reflex
17. transient ischemic attack
19. lobe of the brain located at the back of the head
21. cranial nerve involved in vision and visual fields
22. send nerve impulses
23. lobe in the front of the skull
24. central nervous system
26. basic structural cell
27. combining form for star-shaped
28. multiple sclerosis

Build the Terms

Select word parts from the lists to build a complete medical term for each definition given. Note that not all terms will have a root or combining form, prefix, and suffix. Some word parts may be used more than once. This exercise may require use of a medical dictionary.

Combining Forms	Prefixes	Suffixes
astr/o	hyper-	-ia
blast/o	a-	-logy
neur/o	sub-	-esthesia
medull/o	hypo-	-oma
myel/o	pre-	-ous
phag/o	dys-	-pathy
hemat/o	an-	-al
dur/o	pre-	-lepsy
narco/o	de-	-ic
hydro/o	hydro-	-rrhaphy
cephal/o	per-	-genesis
astr/o	bi-	-lysis
esthesi/o	sub-	-ary
blast/o	en-	-cele
cyt/o	quadri-	-otomy

1. tumor arising from immature nerve cells _____

2. pertaining to the medulla _____

3. breakdown of myelin _____

4. difficulty swallowing (eating) _____

5. blood tumor (collection of blood) below the dura _____

6. hernia of the spinal cord _____

7. seizure with numbness or drowsiness _____

8. pertaining to water in the brain _____

9. tumor arising from an astral cell _____

10. excess sensation _____

11. suture of a nerve _____

12. disease of the brain _____

Word Analysis

Read each sentence carefully, noting each underlined word. Separate the underlined word into its word parts, using hyphens. Then write the definition of the term on the line provided.

1. Myelinization follows a <u>cephalocaudal</u> order. _____

   _____

2. The infant was born <u>anencephalic</u>. _____

   _____

3. Following a traumatic head injury, the patient developed <u>hemiplegia</u>.

   _____

   _____

4. The <u>cerebrovascular</u> accident was sudden and massive.

   _____

   _____

5. The patient was noted to have <u>aphasia</u> following the CVA.

   _____

   _____

6. The child's <u>microcephaly</u> was evident, even to a layperson.

   _____

   _____

7. <u>Muscular</u> wasting was most evident in the lower extremities.

   _____

   _____

8. <u>Hemiplegia</u> was the primary diagnosis. _____

   _____

9. Mr. Jackson has been a <u>paraplegic</u> since age five. _____

   _____

10. The <u>optic</u> nerve is essential for vision. _____

    _____

What Do These Abbreviations Mean?

Write the definition of the abbreviation in the space provided.

1. ANS _____

2. MS _____

3. TIA _____

4. PET _____

5. LP _____

6. CVA _____

7. CNS _____

8. CAT _____

9. CSF _____

10. ADHD _____

Word Building

Read each word part in the Word Parts list and supply a definition. Then select a word part (or parts) from the list below to create a term that matches each definition. Write the entire term in the blank. The first one has been done for you.

Word Parts

hemi-	_____	-ectomy	_____
-ar	_____	-ic	_____
e-	_____	-ology	_____
-itis	_____	-otomy	_incision_
-al	_____	a-	_____
-ia	_____	hydro-	_____
-oma	_____	-ostomy	_____

Combining form	Definition	Term
1. crani/o	incision into the skull (head)	_craniotomy_
2. neur/o	study of nerves	_____
3. cerebr/o	pertaining to the brain	_____
4. tax/o	pertaining to without coordination	_____
5. cephal/o	pertaining to water on the brain	_____
6. ventricul/o	pertaining to the ventricle	_____

7. chord/o   incision into the spinal cord   _____

8. spher/o   half sphere or globe   _____

9. my/o   removal of a muscle   _____

10. mening/o   tumor of meninges   _____

What's Your Conclusion?

Read each mini medical record or scenario carefully; then select the correct response. Write the letter of your answer in the space provided.

1. A 16-year-old male is seen in the emergency room following a motor vehicle accident. He has contusions and lacerations of the head and face, and the police officer who investigated the accident reports that the patient was not wearing a seatbelt. His vital signs are within normal limits, but his apical pulse is borderline tachycardiac. While being questioned about his health history and current symptoms, he becomes agitated and verbally aggressive, then combative. His behavior captivates the attention of the entire emergency staff and chaos ensues. Three male ER staff members are required to subdue the patient. You recognize that:

   A. The teenager is misbehaving, making it difficult for the staff to care for his scrapes and bruises. The nursing staff may need to call hospital security.
   B. The teenager may have a head injury, internal bleeding, or both. His heartbeat is rapid, and he has become restless and tried to fight off the staff.

   Your response: _____

2. You are shopping in the supermarket when your son stops in the aisle and says, "I smell something funny." He falls to the floor. His muscles are contracted, his teeth are clenched, and he does not respond when you speak to him. You observe a loss of bladder function. You are aware that:

   A. He may have had an aura during a preictal phase.
   B. He has suffered a preictal ischemic attack.

   Your response: _____

3. A 19-year-old female is brought to the emergency room after her parents were unable to awaken her from a nap. They report that she has been mildly ill for several days, but has started to feel worse in the past 24 hours. There is no recent history of sore throat or respiratory infection. She has complained of headaches and feeling very tired and has missed several days of school because of fatigue. She is sleepy most of the time and, when awake, has been increasingly irritable. She has a temperature of 101° F and a rapid pulse. Upon questioning during her neurological exam, she is uncertain of the date or day of the week. She is unable to state the names of any of her teachers or what subjects she is studying. She states that her head and neck hurt and her neck is stiff. There is no hemiparesis. The patient begins vomiting during the examination. You anticipate that the doctor will diagnose:

   A. Acute viral encephalitis or meningitis
   B. CVA

   Your response: _____

Analyzing Medical Records

Read the physician's progress note, and then answer the following questions.

1. What is the patient's mental status?

2. Briefly describe the findings from the physical examination.

3. What is the analysis? Is this an infectious disease?

4. Was any medication prescribed?

5. What radiologic studies will be done? Will further laboratory studies be done?

6. Why will the patient see another physician?

Physician's Progress Note

PATIENT: Mary B
DATE: November 16, xxxx

<u>S</u>: Mary B, a 69 y/o female patient of this clinic, was seen in the clinic, accompanied by her sister, Mabel R. The sister states that she went to Mary's home to pick her up and bring her to the clinic for a routine visit, related to Mary's previous diagnosis of hypertension. She found Mary in an agitated, confused state. The sister was somewhat alarmed, since this represents a dramatic change from Mary's condition of just two days ago. She decided to go ahead and bring Mary in for her regular appointment and an evaluation. She does not know of any illnesses or other diagnoses, aside from those we have been following Mary for. She is not aware of any accidents, falls, or injuries. Mabel states that she believes Mary has been taking her medication as prescribed. The patient is unable to provide adequate history or description of current problems due to aphasia and mental confusion.

O: T 98.4, P 88, R 20, BP 148/90.
Previous diagnoses: hypertension, mild peripheral vascular disease, status one year post-mastectomy secondary to diagnosis of breast malignancy.
Neurological exam reveals several deficiencies in functioning; otherwise, examination is unchanged from clinic visit of three weeks ago. Patient is aphasic and appears anxious. She is somewhat able to answer "yes" or "no" to questions by moving her head, but this is not a consistent ability. She is mentally confused. There is diminished sensation of the right arm, thorax, and leg. There is a steady stream of tears from the right eye and ptosis of the right lid. Vision is blurred, but actual visual status is difficult to ascertain because of patient's current mental status. Patient is ataxic, with some hemiparesis on the right side; motor reflexes are intact on the left and slightly exaggerated on the right. Preliminary laboratory studies of blood and urine are unremarkable.

A: R/O cerebral lesion of unknown etiology.
R/O endocrine disorder.

P: 1) Admit to West Madison Memorial Hospital, Unit 3 East.
2) Obtain brain scan, EEG, and skull x-rays ASAP.
3) Laboratory studies for liver, renal, and thyroid function.
4) Neurological consult with Dr. Montgomery.

L. Martinson, MD

Using Medical References

The following sentences contain medical terms that may not have been addressed on the charts in this chapter. Use medical reference books, your medical term analysis skills, and/or a medical dictionary to find the correct definition of each underlined word. Write the definition on the line below the sentence.

1. Pathology reports showed degeneration of the <u>Schwann cells</u> and the <u>neurilemma</u>.

_____

2. There was a great deal of <u>microglial</u> activity in this area.

_____

3. Researchers speculate about the potential of <u>oligodendroglia</u> to regenerate myelin.

_____

4. The <u>subarachnoid</u> space was filled with blood.

_____

5. The <u>brachial plexus</u> has been damaged, resulting in loss of function of the arm.

_____

6. The area of the <u>central sulcus</u> was sclerotic and discolored.

_____

7. The <u>cauda equina</u> was damaged when the coccyx was fractured.

_____

8. <u>Myasthenia gravis</u> was diagnosed after the muscle weakness developed.

_____

9. Attempts to reduce the <u>cerebral edema</u> were unsuccessful.

_____

10. The patient failed to respond to painful <u>stimuli</u>.

_____

11. Sharon's limp is a result of <u>poliomyelitis</u>.

_____

12. The <u>pons</u> was completely destroyed by the malignancy.

_____

13. The patient lost his driving privilege because of a history of <u>syncope</u>.

_____

Short Answer

Explain the cause and describe the symptoms of multiple sclerosis.

_____

_____

_____

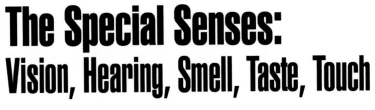

Chapter 9

The Special Senses:
Vision, Hearing, Smell, Taste, Touch

Learning Outcomes

Students will be able to:
- Identify the structures of the five special senses.
- Describe the physiology of vision, hearing, smell, taste, and touch.
- List and define the combining forms most commonly used to create terms related to the senses.
- Use the language of the special senses correctly in oral and written communications.
- Correctly spell and pronounce terminology related to the five special senses.
- State the meaning of abbreviations related to the five special senses.

Translation, Please?Translation, Please?Translation, Please?

Read this excerpt from a physician's report of an eye examination and try to answer the questions that follow it.

OBJECTIVE: On examination, visual acuity at distance was 20/20 in both eyes. The intraocular pressure was 20 OU. There was good motility, and the pupils were normal. External exam revealed a chalazion on the lateral aspect of the upper lid OS. Slit-lamp examination revealed a white conjunctiva and clear cornea. Dilated funduscopic examination revealed normal macula, blood vessels, and retina.

1. What does OU stand for?
2. What could a chalazion be?
3. In your own words, identify the location of the chalazion.

Answers to "Translation, Please?"
1. OU stands for the Latin "*oculus uterque*" and means both eyes.
2. A chalazion is a little cyst on the eyelid. The word "chalazion" is Greek for small pimple.
3. The patient's chalazion is located on the outside corner of the left upper eyelid.

OVERVIEW OF THE SENSES

The five special senses are vision, hearing, smell, taste, and touch. They connect us with our environment, seeking and receiving information that is communicated via the nervous system to the body's intelligence center, the brain. The senses can tell us when to be scared, when we are in danger, and when we are secure. We take our sensory organs for granted when they are working properly, but a malfunction of any of the senses can disrupt many other body functions.

Because the senses work together closely, this chapter deals with the anatomy, physiology, pathology, and vocabulary of all five senses together. The primary focus is the terminology associated with the eyes and ears; the important relationships with smell, taste, and touch are highlighted in a final section, along with the essential associated terms.

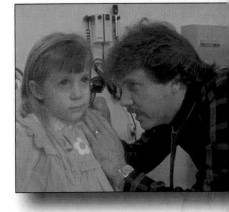

The Vision System and Its Practitioners

Vision is the sense that permits us to view our surroundings and provides the brain with detailed information about what the eyes see. The study of the eye and its diseases is called **ophthalmology.** The professionals within this specialty include the **ophthalmologist,** a medical doctor (MD) who diagnoses and treats eye disorders; the **optometrist,** a doctor of optometry (OD) who specializes in refraction of the eyes to determine the extent of vision and prescribes glasses to assure optimal sight; and the **optician,** who takes the prescription from the MD or OD and cuts the glass or plastic to fill the prescription. During the past decade, subspecialties focusing on new eye surgeries have burgeoned. The increased longevity of people has expanded the need for the correction and treatment of eye disorders, and researchers have responded with new products and procedures that make it possible to surgically correct abnormalities that previously were accepted as an unchangeable fact of growing older.

Examining the Patient ♂♀

Anatomy and Physiology of the Eye

The eye is the body's camera, scanning its surroundings and capturing complex visual data. Although this body organ is relatively small, it consists of numerous components, each of which plays an important role in achieving vision.

Eye Structure from the Outside In

The two eye sockets are located on the anterior plane of the skull in the orbital cavity, surrounded by the bones of the skull. Six muscles attach the eyeball to the orbit, allowing the eye to move in several directions. The outer structures of the eye serve to encase and protect the eyeball. The eyelids, or **palpebrae,** are composed of a thin protective layer of skin that shields the eye from the outside elements and from extreme light and injury. In fact, this layer is the thinnest skin in the human body.

Figure 9.1 - External Eye Structure

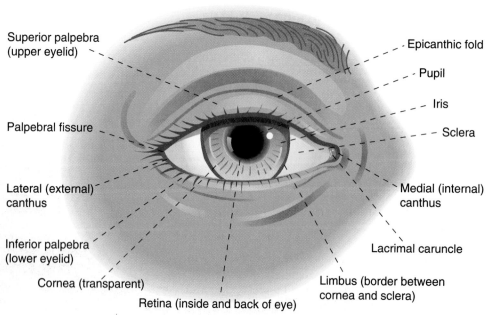

Superior palpebra (upper eyelid)

Palpebral fissure

Lateral (external) canthus

Inferior palpebra (lower eyelid)

Cornea (transparent)

Retina (inside and back of eye)

Epicanthic fold

Pupil

Iris

Sclera

Medial (internal) canthus

Lacrimal caruncle

Limbus (border between cornea and sclera)

The superior (upper) **palpebra** is divided into the **epicanthic fold** and the **canthus.** The superior and inferior (lower) palpebrae join on each side to form the internal and external canthi. At the medial canthus is the **lacrimal caruncle,** the area that contains sebaceous glands. Within the upper and lower canthi are **meibomian glands,** which excrete an oily lubricating substance into the eye. The opening of the canthi, the **palpebral fissure**, is surrounded by eyelashes, which further protect the eye from environmental dangers.

The **sclera** is a white covering continuous with the **cornea**. The cornea is the clear tissue bubble at the front of the eye where a contact lens may rest. The cornea covers the **iris** (the colored portion of the eye) and **pupil** (the black center). The iris contains muscles that constrict and dilate the pupil to allow the appropriate amount of light onto the **retina**, the nerve tissue that conducts impulses to the brain.

The retina is composed of 10 layers containing about 120 million **rods**, 6 million **cones**, and neurons. Rods are extremely sensitive to light and are responsible for night vision, called **scotopic** vision. **Photopic** vision, or vision in bright light, and color vision are the function of the cones. The point of greatest visual acuity is the **fovea centralis,** a rod-free, cone-packed area of the retina. The axons of the neurons leave the eye as the optic nerve.

The **lens** is an elastic, highly movable disk located behind the pupil. It has a **ciliary body**, a muscle that causes the lens to bulge for focusing on near objects and to flatten for focusing on distant objects. This process is called **accommodation**. When the ciliary muscle is relaxed, the eye is considered to be in normal position, or **emmetropic**.

The **conjunctiva** is the area visualized when the physician looks at the eye. The lower eyelid should appear just at the **limbus**, the border between the sclera and cornea. The **lacrimal gland** is located in the upper outer corner over the eye. It secretes tears, which wash across the eye and drain into the **puncta**, tiny openings visible in the corners of the upper and lower inner canthi (Figure 9.2). The tears empty into the **nasolacrimal sac**, through the nasolacrimal duct, and then into an opening within the nose.

Figure 9.2 - Flow of Tears

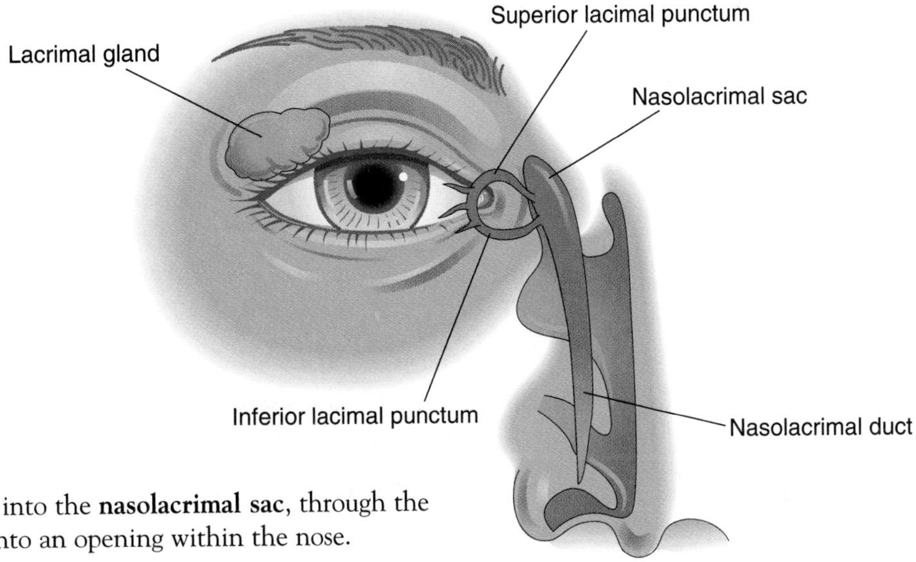

- Lacrimal gland
- Superior lacimal punctum
- Nasolacrimal sac
- Inferior lacimal punctum
- Nasolacrimal duct

Vision and Other Functions of the Eye

Among the sense organs, the eye has one of the most complicated physiologic mechanisms. Think of the eye as five interrelated systems:

1. Its protective casing, the sclera, is composed of tough collagen fibers.
2. A lens system, composed of the cornea and crystalline lens, focuses light on the retina's receptors.
3. A system of blood vessels, the **choroid**, nourishes the structures of the eyeball.
4. The **fovea centralis**, a small area within the **macula lutea** at the back of the eye, is where visual acuity is greatest.
5. The nerve tissue, or retina, conducts impulses from the receptors to the brain.

The process of vision occurs when light rays are refracted first through the lens system, consisting of the cornea and the crystalline lens, then to the retina (Figure 9.3A–B). The retina transforms this stimulus into nerve impulses that move through the optic nerve to the visual cortex of the brain. The image formed on the retina is upside down and reversed from the real image. As the image passes through the optic chiasm of the brain, it is transposed so that the right side of the brain sees the left side of the outside view and the left side of the brain sees the right side. Both eyes send pictures to the brain, which then merges the information into one image.

Figure 9.3 - Internal Eye Structure

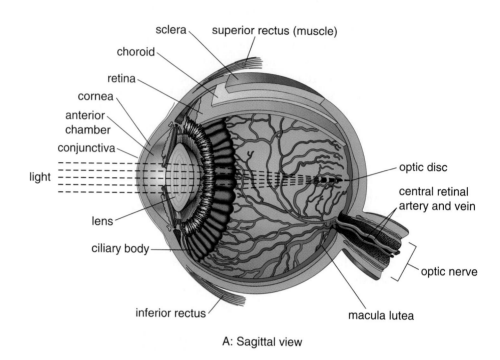

A: Sagittal view

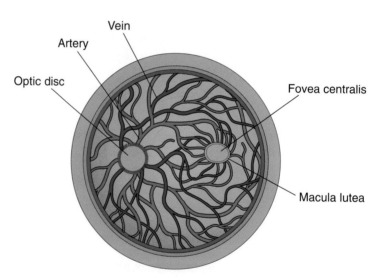

B: Fundus (Interior of eye)

Table 9.1 lists the meanings of some common combining forms related to the eye. Anatomy and physiology terms relating to the eye are found in Table 9.2.

Table 9.1

Combining Forms Relating to the Eye

Combining form	Meaning	Example
ambly/o	dull	amblyopia
aque/o	water	aqueous humor
blephar/o	eyelid	blepharitis
conjunctiv/o	conjunctiva	conjunctivitis
corne/o	cornea	corneal
dacry/o	tear	dacryoadenitis
dipl/o	double	diplopia
emmetr/o	correct measure	emmetropia
glauc/o	blue-gray	glaucoma
irid/o	iris	iridectomy
kerat/o	cornea	keratitis
lacrim/o	tears	lacrimal
mi/o	less	miotic
mydr/o	widen	mydriasis
ocul/o	eye	ocular
ophthalm/o	eye	ophthalmology
opt/o	eye/vision	optometrist
palpebr/o	eyelid	palpebral
phac/o	lens of the eye	phacoemulsification
phot/o	light	photophobia
presby/o	old age	presbyopia
pupill/o	pupil	pupillary
retin/o	retina	retinitis
scler/o	sclera (outer membrane)	scleritis
scot/o	dark	scotoma
uve/o	uvea	uveitis
vitre/o	glassy	vitreous humor

Table 9.2

Anatomy and Physiology Terms Relating to the Eye

Term	Meaning	Word Analysis	
accommodation ah-kom-ah-**day**-shun	the ability to focus and see	accommod/o	to adapt
aqueous humor **ay**-kwee-us **hyoo**-mer	watery fluid in front of the lens	aqueous humor	water-like clear liquid
canthus **kan**-thus	angle formed where upper and lower eyelids meet	kanthos	corner
choroid **kO**-royd	highly vascular membrane between retina and sclera	chori/o	membrane
conjunctiva kon-junk-**tI**-vah	clear mucous membrane lining the inner eyelids and anterior of the eye	conjunctus	joining
cornea **kor**-nee-ah	the outer portion of the eye through which light passes to the retina	corneus	horny membrane

continued on next page

epicanthic fold ep-ih-**kan**-thic	extension of a skin fold over the inner angle or both angles of the eye	*epi-* *kanthos* *-ic*	upon corner pertaining to
fundus **fun**-dus	part farthest away from the opening	*fundus*	bottom
intraocular in-trah-**ok**-yoo-ler	within the eye	*intra-* *ocul/o* *-ar*	inside eye pertaining to
iris **I**-ris irides (pl) **ir**-ih-deez	the colored portion of the eye	*irid/o*	iris
lacrimal **lak**-rih-mal	pertaining to tears	*lacrim/o* *-al*	tears pertaining to
lacrimal caruncle **lak**-rih-mal **kar**-ung-kl	small follicular area at the eye's medial angle	*lacrim/o* *-al* *carnuncle*	tears pertaining to small, protruding mass of flesh
lacrimal punctum **lak**-rih-mal **punk**-tum	point or opening within the upper and lower canthi to drain tears	*lacrim/o* *-al* *punctum*	tears pertaining to point
limbus **lim**-bus	edge, border	*limbus*	border
lens	structure to focus light	*lens*	lentil
macula lutea **mak**-yoo-lah **loo**-tee-ah maculae **mak**-yoo-lee	small yellowish spot of the retina	*macula* *luteus*	spot yellow
nasolacrimal nay-zO-**lak**-rih-mal	pertaining to the nasal and lacrimal bones or ducts	*nas/o* *lacrim/o* *-al*	nose tears pertaining to
ophthalmologist of-thal-**mol**-ah-jist ophthalmology of-thal-**mol**-ah-jee	physician specializing in diseases of the eye	*ophthalm/o* *-logist*	eye one who studies
ophthalmoscope of-**thal**-mah-skOp	instrument to view the eye	*ophthalm/o* *-scope*	eye instrument for visualizing an area
ophthalmus of-**thal**-mus	eye	*ophthalm/o*	eye
optic **op**-tik	pertaining to the eye or sight	*opt/o* *-ic*	vision relating to
optometrist op-**tom**-eh-trist	professional who tests visual acuity and prescribes corrective lenses	*opt/o* *-metrist*	vision one who measures
palpebra pal-**pee**-brah	eyelid	*pebra*	eyelid
pupil pew-pil	central opening of the iris	*pupa*	doll
sclera **sklee**-rah	outer, dense, fibrous, opaque white layer of the eye	*scler/o*	sclera
vitreous humor **vit**-ree-us **hyoo**-mer	jelly-like fluid behind the lens	*vitre/o* *humor*	glassy clear liquid

Supply a combining form for each definition; then use the combining form to create the term that matches the definition.

Definition	Combining Form	Term
1. study of the eye	_____	_____
2. inflammation of the eyelid	_____	_____
3. tumor of tears (produces obstruction of the lacrimal duct)	_____	_____
4. repair of the cornea	_____	_____
5. inflammation of the conjunctiva	_____	_____
6. removal of the iris	_____	_____
7. pertaining to the cornea	_____	_____
8. pertaining to the eyelid	_____	_____
9. fear (aversion) of light	_____	_____
10. inflammation of the retina	_____	_____

Comprehension Check *Exercise 2*

Using the context of the following sentences, circle the correct term from each pair.

1. The palpations/palpebrae protect the eye from bright lights and injury.

2. The nasolacrimal/nasopharyngeal duct drains tears from the eye.

3. Extraocular/Extraorbital muscles attach the eyeball to the orbit.

4. The retinue/retina is a structure essential for vision.

5. Light rays are refracted/retracted through the lens to the retina.

6. Hilarious/Vitreous humor fills the inside of the eyeball.

7. The tough, white tissue of the eyeball is the sclera/scar.

8. The ophthalmologist /optometrist prescribes corrective lens.

9. The limbus/limbo is a border between two important structures.

10. The colored portion of the eye is the fundus/iris.

Name the Term

Provide the missing word parts to create the correct term for the definition given.

1. _____ocular means beyond, or outside, the eye.

2. _____orbital means around the eye socket.

3. _____itis is an inflammation of the membrane that lines the lids and covers the front of the eye.

4. _____ocular means inside the eye.

5. _____l means pertaining to the transparent membrane that is part of the outer portion of the eye.

6. _____itis is an inflammation of the multilayered membrane of nervous tissue that includes rods, cones, and neurons.

7. The _____canthic fold is a skin flap over the angle of the eye.

8. Pupill_____ is the recording of the reactions of the pupil.

9. A fundu____ is used to look at the fundus of the eyeball.

10. Ophthalm____ describes pain of the eyeball.

Word Building

Use root words, combining forms, prefixes, and suffixes to construct a medical term to match each definition provided.

1. instrument used to examine the eye   _____

2. field of medicine concerned with the eye   _____

3. pertaining to the cornea   _____

4. pertaining to the orbit   _____

5. pertaining to the pupil   _____

6. inflammation of the iris   _____

7. inflammation of the eyelid   _____

8. pertaining to the yellow spot on the retina   _____

9. pertaining to the eyelid   _____

10. removal of the lens   _____

Find the misspelled words in the following sentences. Write the correct spelling on the blank provided.

1. Vishion is the sense that permits a person to view his or her surroundings.   _____

2. Many people wear disposable contact lenzes.   _____

3. Dr. Wharton is the clinic's opthalamologist.   _____

4. Lazer surgery can correct many eye problems.   _____

5. An opthician can fill a prescription for eyeglasses.   _____

Word Maps

Exercise 6

In the accompanying illustration of the eye, label the following structures.

1. palpebrae

2. medial canthus

3. cornea

4. lens

5. sclera

6. iris

7. pupil

8. retina

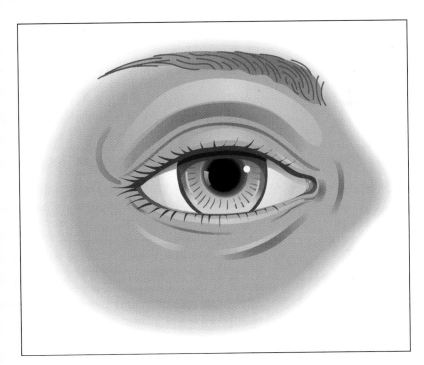

Assessing Patient Health

Wellness and Illness through the Life Span

When examining the eyes, the physician first observes the areas around them, looking for symmetry of the eyes, placement on the face, and the ability of the person to move the external eye muscles, eyebrows, and eyelids. This procedure screens for neuromuscular function. Figure 9.4 shows the eye muscles, the direction of their movements, and the cranial nerves that control them.

Figure 9.4 - Movement of Eyes with Cranial Nerves

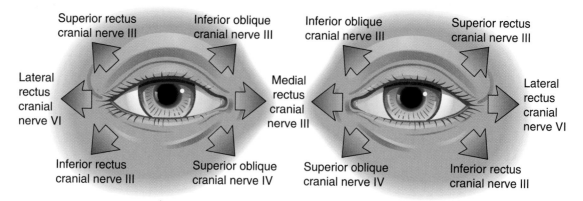

The sclerae should appear white; the cornea should be clear and round. The pupils are checked for size, equal appearance, and reaction to light, an assessment that—if normal—appears in medical records as PERRLA (pupils equal, round, reactive to light and accommodation). In a darkened room and using an instrument called the ophthalmoscope, the physician looks straight into the eye and notes the light being reflected back, called a light reflex. It is normally red. Also visible are the retinal blood vessels entering a point at the posterior area of the globe. This area is called the optic disk, which is also known as the blind spot because it has no visual receptors. Also visible is the yellowish spot of the macula lutea.

Infants and Toddlers

Within an hour of birth, and preferably immediately after birth, the newborn is administered silver nitrate drops in the conjunctival sac of each eye to protect against gonococcal infection. Gonococcus is transmitted from an infected mother during the baby's passage through the birth canal. Immediate prophylactic treatment has all but eradicated the problem.

Infants have limited eye function. While peripheral vision is present in the newborn, the macula lutea is absent. It develops by about four months and matures by eight months. Eye movements are poorly coordinated until about three to four months. About 80 percent of infants are born farsighted, but this condition corrects itself after about eight months. Eyeball structure reaches adult size by about age eight.

Retinopathy of prematurity (ROP) is a type of blindness that occurs when an infant is born three or more months prematurely. In ROP, the retina is not fully developed, and the blood vessels can become leaky, causing irreversible blindness. Oxygen use in the newborn's care has been implicated, and is therefore carefully controlled. Current research is examining whether the fluorescent lighting of the intensive care unit plays a role in retinopathy.

Examination of the eye is difficult from infancy to young school age. Frequently, the physician must sedate the young patient in order to complete the examination. Deviations of eye control should be diagnosed early in childhood. **Strabismus** (nonparallel orientation of the eyes) is typically the result of a weakness in one of the muscles controlling eye movement. Diagnosis of this condition is usually made in childhood. **Diplopia** (double vision) is common and can lead to **amblyopia** (decreased vision), which is reversible if diagnosed before the age of about seven years. Other deviations of eye control include **esotropia** (inward turning of the eyes), **exotropia** (outward turning of the eyes), and **hypertropia** (upward squinting). Treatment options include drugs, eye exercises, special lenses, and surgery.

Retinoblastoma is a type of eye cancer most commonly seen in infants and toddlers. It is often diagnosed when **leukocoria** (white-appearing pupil caused by the reflection of a white mass) is first noted in the child's eye. Retinoblastoma can affect one or both eyes; when presenting bilaterally it is usually hereditary. Treatment includes enucleation (removal) of the entire affected eye and as much optic nerve as possible. For bilateral occurrence, a number of other treatments are available to attempt to preserve vision in one eye.

Adolescents

Keratoconus is a progressive thinning of the cornea that becomes evident in puberty and most often affects females. In keratoconus, vision is distorted, leading to astigmatism and myopia that are difficult to correct even with eyeglasses or contact lenses. Surgery may be necessary to treat this condition.

Middle-Aged Adults

Problems with accommodation, or shifting focus, begin to occur after the age of forty. The lens becomes increasingly hard, decreasing its ability to curve as needed. This inflexibility makes reading difficult, a condition called **presbyopia**, or farsightedness associated with aging.

Glaucoma is one of the leading causes of blindness in the Western world, although most cases can be prevented with early diagnosis and management. All persons over the age of thirty-five are at risk. Between 0.5 and 1 percent of the adult population over the age of forty has glaucoma. Glaucoma is characterized by a progressive optic neuropathy frequently associated with elevated intraocular pressure. Peripheral vision is typically affected first, but complete blindness can result from untreated or poorly controlled glaucoma. The treatment for glaucoma usually includes pharmaceutical agents that relieve the intraocular pressure (IOP) and restore the normal flow of aqueous humor. Primary glaucoma is thought to be hereditary and is usually bilateral. Secondary glaucoma, or open-angle glaucoma, is often unilateral and is due to an increased resistance to aqueous humor outflow through the trabecular meshwork, a supporting tissue of the eye. Laser surgery seeks to create holes in this meshwork.

A **cataract** is a clouding of the crystalline lens. While usually associated with aging, cataracts can be caused by systemic diseases such as diabetes mellitus, as well as by radiation exposure, or some medications. The opaque lens scatters the entering light and vision becomes blurred and distorted. The pupil appears cloudy. Surgical replacement of the lens with a plastic prosthetic lens helps many.

Retinal detachment is a separation of the neurosensory retina from the epithelial layer of the retina. Loss of sight occurs because the detached rods and cones no longer receive nourishment. The most common type of detachment is rhegmatogenous, or tear-induced, detachments, which occur in one of every 10,000 persons between 40 and 70 years. Laser surgery, diathermy, or cryotherapy can be employed for reattachment.

Seniors

Diabetic **retinopathy** (degeneration of the retina without inflammation) is a common complication of diabetes mellitus. The longer a person has diabetes, the greater the risk. Early detection and treatment, including tight control of blood glucose and blood pressure, can usually prevent the loss of vision. Laser photocoagulation may be used to seal minute hemorrhages. **Macular degeneration** is caused by damage to the photoreceptor cells in the area of the macula. It may be hereditary and is the leading cause of severe visual impairment for people over sixty-five years old.

General Diseases and Conditions of the Eye

Nearsightedness, or **myopia**, results when the eyeball is too long, causing light rays to focus in front of the retina instead of on it. Concave glass lenses, which are thicker at the sides than in the middle, are prescribed to focus the light correctly. Farsightedness, or **hyperopia**, results from a shorter-than-normal eyeball, causing light rays to focus behind the retina. This condition is corrected with convex lenses, which are thicker in the middle than at the sides.

Because the eyelids play an important role in protecting the eyeball from injury and disease, it is important to seek medical attention whenever abnormalities of the eyelid become apparent. Irritation, inflammation, or infection of the eyelid, including **blepharitis**, an inflammation of the margins of the lid, or **chalazion**, a sterile granuloma (node or mass) from inflammation of the **meibomian gland** (lubricating glands), can be present. A **sty** (hordeolum) is an infection of the eyelid usually caused by *Staphylococcus aureus*.

Conjunctivitis is an inflammation of the conjunctiva (the lining of the eye and eyelid) and can be caused by bacterial, viral, fungal, or parasitic organisms. Symptoms include hyperemia (the red appearance gives it the nickname "pinkeye"), discharge (called "matter"), tearing, itching or burning, and a feeling of having a foreign body in the eye.

Corneal abrasions occur from trauma, foreign bodies (including contact lenses), or any defect to the flow of protective tears. Examining the cornea requires use of a slit lamp to provide magnification and light. The nerve fibers in the cornea make it extremely sensitive to pain, so a local anesthetic is used to relieve discomfort during the examination. Sometimes fluorescein (a dye) staining is used to outline any epithelial defects.

Keratitis is an infection of the cornea and can be caused by any organism that has entered the cornea through an abrasion. Because the eye allows infectious agents easy entry into the body, patients with severe infectious keratitis are hospitalized and placed on antibiotic therapy. Table 9.3 lists common conditions and diseases of the eye.

Table 9.3

Wellness and Illness Terms Relating to the Eye

Term	Meaning	Word Analysis	
amblyopia am-blee-**O**-pee-ah	poor vision in one eye	ambly/o -opia	dullness, dimness relating to vision
aphakia ah-**fAk**-e-ah	absence of the lens of the eye	a- phak/o; phac/o -ia	absence of lens-shaped; lens condition of
astigmatism ah-**stig**-mah-tiz-em	condition of unequal curvatures	a- stigma -ism	absence of identifying mark condition of; state of
cataract **cat**-ah-ract	loss of transparency of the lens of the eye, or its capsule	cataracta	a waterfall
chalazion ka-**lays**-E-on	inflammatory cyst or granuloma of the meibomian gland	chalaza	a sty

conjunctivitis kon-junk-**tI**-vI-tis	inflammation of the lining of the eye	*conjunctus*	joining
diplopia dih-**plO**-pee-ah	double vision	*-itis* *-opia*	inflammation relating to vision
esophoria es-O-**fO**-ree-ah	inward turning of the eye without double vision	*eso-* *phor/o* *-ia*	inward; within carrying; bearing condition of
esotropia es-O-**trO**-pee-ah	inward turning of the eye with double vision	*eso-* *trope* *-opia*	inward; within turn relating to vision
exophoria eks-O-**fO**-ree-ah	outward turning of the eye without double vision	*ex/o* *phor/o* *-ia*	outward carrying; bearing condition of
exotropia eks-O-**trO**-pee-ah	outward turning of the eye with double vision	*ex/o* *trope* *-opia*	outward turn relating to vision
glaucoma glaw-**cO**-ma	condition of increased intraocular pressure	*glaukos*	blue gray color
hyperopia hI-per-**O**-pee-ah	farsightedness	*hyper-* *-opia*	above, beyond pertaining to vision
hypertropia hI-per-**trO**-pee-ah	condition in which one eye is higher than the other	*hyper-* *trope* *-ia*	greater; above turn condition of
keratitis ker-ah-**tI**-tis	infection of the cornea	*kerat/o* *-itis*	cornea inflammation
keratoconus **ker**-at-O-kO-nus	progressive thinning of the cornea, causing a protrusion	*kerat/o* *conus*	cornea conelike
leukocoria loo-kO-**kor**-ee-ah	white reflection from a mass in the eye	*leuk/o* *core/o* *-ia*	white pupil condition of
microphthalmia mI-krof-**thal**-mee-ah	abnormally small eye	*micro-* *ophthalm/o* *-ia*	small eye condition
myopia mI-**O**-pee-ah	nearsightedness	*my/o* *-opia*	muscle pertaining to vision
presbyopia prez-bee-**O**-pee-ah	farsightedness due to aging	*presby/o* *-opia*	aging pertaining to vision
retinoblastoma ret-ih-nO-blas-**tO**-mah	cancer of the retina	*retin/o* *-blast* *-oma*	retina pertaining to budding of cells; immature cells pertaining to cancer
retinopathy ret-ih-**nop**-ah-thee	disease of the retina	*retin/o* *-pathy*	retina denoting disease
strabismus strah-**biz**-mus	misalignment of the axis of the eyes because of weakness of the ocular muscles; crossed eyes	*strabismus*	squint

Each of the following sentences contains an underlined medical term. Identify the root in the term by drawing a box around it and then supply the definition. Make a new, related term using the root or its combining form. Give a definition for the related term you have supplied.

Example: The diagnosis is bilateral retin|oblastoma, a cancer of the eye.

Root definition: pertaining to the retina.

Related term and definition: retinopathy. Retinopathy means disease of the retina.

1. It will be necessary to perform an <u>iridectomy</u> because of damage to the left eye.

   Root definition: _____

   Related term and definition: _____

2. Curtis was referred by Dr. Pedigo for evaluation and possible radial <u>keratotomy</u>.

   Root definition: _____

   Related term and definition: _____

3. Elaine is an 86-year-old female, post CVA, whose vision is impaired due to severe <u>blepharoptosis</u>.

   Root definition: _____

   Related term and definition: _____

4. The instrument through which the inner eye is viewed is called the <u>ophthalmoscope</u>.

   Root definition: _____

   Related term and definition: _____

5. The patient is a 36-year-old male who recently experienced abrasion of the cornea during his work as a welder; more recently he has developed <u>keratitis</u> and is being treated for that condition.

   Root definition: _____

   Related term and definition: _____

6. <u>Cataracts</u> were observed upon initial examination, and it was explained to the parents that the infant requires corrective surgery.

   Root definition: _____

   Related term and definition: _____

7. The patient was scheduled for a <u>lacrimotomy</u>.

   Root definition: _____

   Related term and definition: _____

8. The lens was removed by phacoerysis.

   Root definition: _____

   Related term and definition: _____

9. The patient received laser treatment for macular degeneration.

   Root definition: _____

   Related term and definition: _____

10. The pain in the patient's eye was diagnosed as scleritis.

   Root definition: _____

   Related term and definition: _____

Comprehension Check   Exercise 8

Select the correct medical term from the list to substitute for the underlined definition in each sentence.

astigmatism	esotropia	presbyopia	strabismus
chalazion	ophthalmologists	retinoblastoma	glaucoma
esophoria	exophoria	hyperopia	sty

1. During routine process of measuring increased intraocular pressure screening, Gail was found to have an early stage of the disease.   _____

2. Imp: inflammatory growth of the meibomian gland   _____

3. Procedures involving the eye are performed by medical specialists in examination and treatment of the eye.   _____

4. The patient had surgery last week for a tumor of the retina.   _____

5. The patient's eye condition was described as deviating inward without double vision.   _____

6. Ms. Olsson had never needed a vision correction until she experienced farsightedness due to aging.   _____

7. The doctor prescribed a hot compress applied directly on the localized, painful infection on the eyelid.   _____

8. Safe driving was impossible for the man with double vision because the axis of his eyes converged.   _____

9. Prescription lenses were carefully ground to correct the condition of different focal distances because of unequal curvatures.   _____

10. The child had difficulty reading classroom materials because of her vision clear and focused only for distant objects.   _____

Select a term from Column 1 to match each definition in Column 2. Write your choice on the line beside the definition.

Column 1

1. accommodation
2. cornea
3. macula
4. conjunctiva
5. canthus
6. iris
7. presbyopia
8. strabismus
9. myopia
10. keratoconus

Column 2

_____ a. nearsightedness

_____ b. angle where upper and lower eyelids meet

_____ c. cross-eyes

_____ d. small yellowish spot in back of the retina

_____ e. ability to focus and see

_____ f. thinning of the cornea

_____ g. farsightedness due to aging

_____ h. colored portion of the eye

_____ i. mucous membrane lining the inner eyelids

_____ j. outer portion of eye through which light passes to the retina

Use prefixes, root words, combining vowels, and suffixes to create medical terms for the definitions given. Write the term in the space beside the definition. Separate the word parts with hyphens.

1. surgical repair of the eyelids _____

2. drooping of the eyelid _____

3. pertaining to the eye _____

4. inflammation of the iris _____

5. surgical incision into the cornea _____

Find the misspelled medical term in each sentence, circle it, and then rewrite the term correctly and define it.

1. The patient underwent a kerratoplasty several years ago.

_____

2. I will refer the patient to an opthalamologist in his geographic area.

_____

3. This 4-year-old child has been diagnosed with miopya and requires vision correction.

_____

4. There is an outbreak of canjunctivittis at the local day care center.

_____

5. Shrinkage of the vetrious caused traction on the retina and resulted in a posterior tear.

_____

6. Imp: retinatis

_____

7. The patient was experiencing dyplopia upon examination in the emergency department.

_____

8. Mrs. Miller will require preoperative teaching prior to her caterect surgery next week.

_____

Word Maps

Complete the diagram below to illustrate the process of vision.

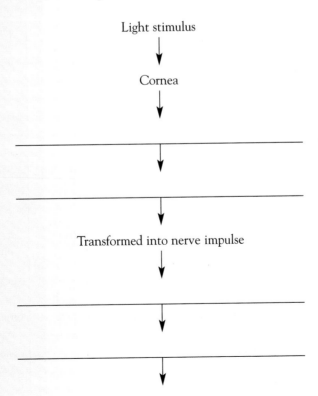

Light stimulus

↓

Cornea

↓

_____

↓

_____

↓

Transformed into nerve impulse

↓

_____

↓

_____

↓

Diagnosing and Treating Problems

Tests, Procedures, and Pharmaceuticals Relating to the Eye

A number of procedures to correct certain visual defects can now be done on an outpatient basis in the physician's office. These procedures typically require exacting measurement and delicate manipulation of the eye structures. The highly technical apparatus includes computerized sensing devices and high magnification viewing devices. Some procedures to detect and correct eye problems are described in Table 9.4.

Surgical procedures to correct refractive problems by reshaping the cornea are called keratotomy. There are specific procedures for specific situations. One eye procedure that has received a great deal of exposure because of marketing and publicity is LASIK (laser assisted *in situ* keratomileusis), whereby the surface of the cornea is cut to form a flap. The underlying tissue is sculpted to the precise shape needed to correct the refractive error, and then the flap is replaced. Healing of the cut edge occurs quickly without stitches.

Severely diseased or damaged corneas can be replaced with full-thickness corneas and surrounding tissue taken from deceased donors. Using a circular blade called a trephine, the surgeon cuts out the damaged cornea and sutures a new cornea into place. Healing may be slow because of the decreased blood supply to the cornea, which has few blood vessels. A transplant eye bank makes donated corneas available nationwide.

Lens replacement procedures to correct cataracts are now commonplace. The procedure may use ultrasound energy to dissolve and then extract the natural lens.

Table 9.4

Tests and Procedures Relating to the Eye

Term	Meaning	Word Analysis	
blepharectomy **blef**-ar-**ek**-tO-mee	excision of a lesion of the eyelid	*blephar/o* -ectomy	eyelid surgical removal
gonioplasty **gO**-nee-O-plas-tee	contraction of the peripheral iris to eliminate contact with the trabecular meshwork	*gonia* -plasty	angle surgical repair
gonioscopy **gO**-nee-**os**-kah-pee	procedure to visualize the anterior chamber angle to determine whether the angle is open or closed in glaucoma	*gonia* -scopy	angle use of instrument to visualize an area
laser surgery **lay**-zer	primary treatment of glaucoma and other eye disorders	*laser*	device that produces amplified light beam
ophthalmoscopy **of**-thal-**mos**-kah-pee	procedure to visualize the retina, retinal blood vessels, and the optic disk (the point where the optic nerve leaves the eye)	*ophthalm/o* -scopy	eye use of an instrument to visualize an area
perimetry per-**im**-eh-tree	test that measures the scope of the visual fields	*peri-* -metry	around process of measuring
peripheral iridectomy peh-**rif**-er-al ir-ih-**dek**-tah-mee	procedure that creates a hole in the iris, allowing the aqueous humor to flow from the posterior chamber to the anterior chamber	*periphereia* -al *irid/o* -ectomy	outer part pertaining to iris surgical removal
phacoemulsification **fak**-O-ee-mul-sih-fih-**kay**-shun	method of using ultrasonic waves to disintegrate a cataract, which is then aspirated and removed	*phac/o* emulsification	lens process of breaking up

sclerotomy skleh-**rot**-ah-mee	surgical formation of an opening in the sclera	scler/o -tomy	sclera incision
sphincterotomy sfink-ter-**ot**-ah-mee	procedure to make cuts in the iris sphincter muscle to allow pupillary enlargement	sphincter/o -tomy	band incision
tonometry tO-**nom**-ah-tree	test that measures for increased intraocular pressure (IOP)	ton/o -metry	a stretching process of measuring
trabeculoplasty trah-**bek**-yoo-lO-**plas**-tee	procedure to increase aqueous humor outflow to control IOP in open-angle glaucoma	trabecul/a -plasty	bundles of fibers surgical repair

Pharmaceutical Agents

Ophthalmic agents can be divided into groups based on therapeutic use. Conjunctivitis is treated with topical antibiotics or corticosteroids. Miscellaneous agents include ocular lubricants, which act as artificial tears, and silver nitrate, which is administered to prevent gonococcal ophthalmic infections.

Miotic agents constrict the eye muscles during cataract surgery, keratoplasty, and iridectomy. Most commonly, miotic agents are used in the treatment of glaucoma to lower intraocular pressure.

Table 9.5

Abbreviations

ACC	accommodation
D	diopter
DCR	dacryocystorhinostomy
ECCE	extracapsular cataract extraction
Em	emmetropia
EOM	extraocular movements
ERG	electroretinography
ICCE	intracapsular cataract extraction
IOL	intraocular lens
IOP	intraocular pressure
L&A	light and accommodation
LASIK	laser-assisted *in situ* keratomileusis
my	myopia
OD	right eye (*oculus dexter*); doctor of optometry
OS	left eye (*oculus sinister*)
OU	both eyes (*oculus uterque*)
PAN	periodic alternating nystagmus
PERLA	pupils equal, reactive to light and accommodation
PERRLA	pupils equal, round, reactive to light and accommodation
PRK	photorefractive keratectomy
REM	rapid eye movement
ROP	retinopathy of prematurity
ST	esotropia
VA	visual acuity
VF	visual field
XT	exotropia

Draw a box around the combining form in each term and provide a definition for the combining form. Then, provide a definition for the entire term.

	Combining form definition	**Term definition**
1. blepharoplasty		
2. palpebral		
3. retinitis		
4. ophthalmoscope		
5. lacrimal		
6. ophthalmologist		
7. intraocular		
8. iridoplegia		
9. choroiditis		
10. vitrectomy		

Comprehension Check

Read each sentence carefully noting the two terms provided. Select the term that best fits the sentence, then circle your answer.

1. This patient is being referred to an otolaryngologist/ophthalmologist for an eye exam.

2. Examination of the retina/presbyopia revealed several aneurysms.

3. We will attempt a keratitis/keratoplasty.

4. During routine tonometry/palpebral screening, Ms. Freeman was found to have early-stage glaucoma.

5. The vitreous humor/inner canthus was removed as part of the retinoplasty.

6. Eleven-year-old Timmy's optic nerve/presbyopia was damaged by the tumor.

7. She was sent home from school because of conjunctivitis/blepharitis—the dreaded "pinkeye."

8. Hemorrhages of the retinal/lacrimal blood vessels are an important finding.

9. The border between the sclera and the cornea is the lutea/limbus.

10. The ophthalmoscope was necessary to examine the fundus/canthus.

Matching

Match the list of procedures and treatments in Column 2 with the diagnosis or reason for the procedure in Column 1. Write the number of the diagnosis or problem in the space beside the name of the treatment or procedure. Note that some entries in Column 2 are diagnostic procedures. Also, some Column 1 entries are used more than once.

Column 1

1. irreversible injury to the cornea
2. myopia
3. glaucoma
4. lesion of the eyelid
5. phacoemulsification
6. blepharoptosis
7. retinal detachment
8. contagious conjunctivitis

Column 2

_____ a. nearsightedness

_____ b. antibiotic

_____ c. blepharopexy

_____ d. laser surgery to reattach retina

_____ e. vision correction lenses

_____ f. corneal transplant

_____ g. blepharectomy

_____ h. use of ultrasonic waves to disintegrate

_____ i. pharmaceutical agent to relieve intraocular pressure

_____ j. tonometry

Word Building

Exercise 16

Write the term for each definition on the blank provided. Separate the parts of the term with hyphens.

1. pertaining to the eye

2. within the eye

3. inflammation of the conjunctiva

4. pertaining to the sclera

5. around the orbit

6. disease of the retina

7. process of tears

8. inflammation of the cornea

9. test to measure for IOP

10. laser sculpting of corneal tissue

The Special Senses 359

Provide the plural term for each singular term given.

1. cataract   _____

2. palpebra   _____

3. sclera   _____

4. sty   _____

5. retinopathy   _____

6. macula   _____

7. iris   _____

8. limbus   _____

9. canthus   _____

10. chalazia   _____

Word Maps

Exercise 18

Complete the diagram by providing medical terms or translations for each type of abnormality.

Abnormality:	nearsightedness	_____	farsightedness
Medical term:	_____	diplopia	_____
Abnormality:	turning inward of eye	turning outward of eye	poor vision in one eye
Medical term:	_____	_____	_____

Identifying the Specialty

The Hearing System and Its Practitioners

The specialist in the diagnosis and treatment of ear diseases and hearing problems is the **otorhinolaryngologist** (*ot/o* means ear, *rhin/o* refers to nose, and *laryn/o* means larynx), also called an otolaryngologist or ENT (ear/nose/throat) specialist. These physicians also treat nose and throat problems. An audiologist is an allied health professional who tests a patient's hearing and recommends an appropriate type of hearing aid, if necessary.

Anatomy and Physiology of the Ear

Ears have the structures for both hearing and maintaining balance. When both ears are working properly, we can hear the sounds around us and determine the direction of the source. When only one ear is working, it may be difficult to distinguish the direction of the source of sounds. Equilibrium is a complex mechanism that depends on normal fluid levels within the inner ear and on proper coordination of visual signals with the nervous system.

External Ear

The ear is divided into three parts: the external ear, the middle ear, and the inner ear (Figure 9.5). The visible portion of the external ear is called the **auricle**, or **pinna**. The auricle collects sound waves and passes them through the **external auditory meatus**, a canal leading to the eardrum. Glands within the auditory canal secrete **cerumen**, the brownish substance (earwax) that discourages microorganism growth and provides protection for the ear.

The eardrum, or **tympanic membrane**, separates the external canal from the air-filled middle ear, a cavity that opens via the **eustachian** tube into the nasopharynx (see Figure 9.5). The tube is usually closed, but it opens during swallowing, chewing, and yawning to equalize the air pressure on both sides of the membrane.

Beyond the tympanic membrane lies a series of three bones called the **ossicular chain (auditory ossicles)**, consisting of the **malleus** (hammer), the **incus** (anvil),

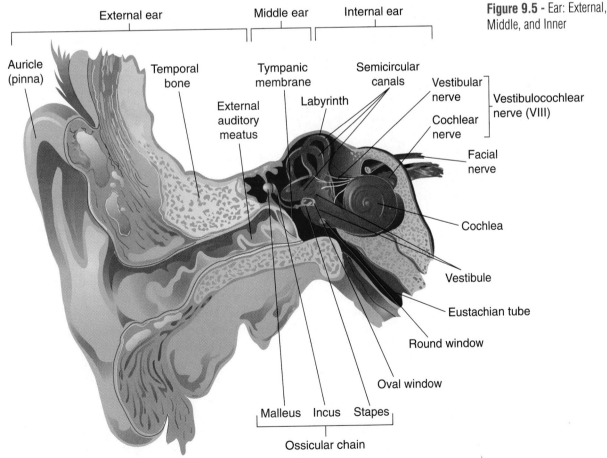

Figure 9.5 - Ear: External, Middle, and Inner

External ear   Middle ear   Internal ear

Auricle (pinna)
Temporal bone
External auditory meatus
Tympanic membrane
Labyrinth
Semicircular canals
Vestibular nerve
Cochlear nerve
Vestibulocochlear nerve (VIII)
Facial nerve
Cochlea
Vestibule
Eustachian tube
Round window
Oval window
Malleus   Incus   Stapes
Ossicular chain

and the **stapes** (stirrup). Named for the objects they resemble, these tiny bones conduct sound vibrations to a membrane called the **oval window**, or **fenestra ovalis**, which amplifies the sound and transmits it into the inner ear.

Internal Ear

The inner ear is called the **labyrinth**, from the Greek word that means "maze," a term that describes the two types of channels that wind through the inner ear (see Figure 9.6). One channel is the bony labyrinth, which is filled with fluid called **perilymph**. Also found within the bony labyrinth is the membranous labyrinth, a flexible tube filled with fluid called **endolymph**.

Figure 9.6 - Inner Ear

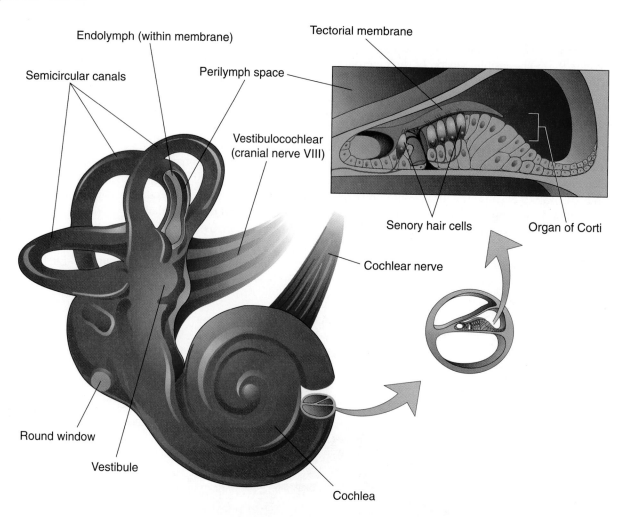

Special names exist for various sections of the bony labyrinth: vestibule, semicircular canals, cochlea, and the auditory and vestibular receptors of the eighth cranial nerve (vestibulocochlear nerve). The vestibule communicates with the base of the stapes. Contained within the vestibule are saclike structures called the **utricle** and **saccule**; the semicircular canals are found behind the vestibule. The utricle, saccule, and semicircular canals work together to maintain the body's sense of balance. The **round window** at the base of the vestibule acts as a secondary tympanic membrane.

The cochlea is considered the main organ of hearing. Moving fluid within the cochlea stimulates receptor hair cells within the **organ of Corti**, and the auditory nerve transmits the neural stimulation to the brain, where it is interpreted as sound.

The Process of Hearing

The outer, middle, and inner ear structures are all involved in the process of hearing (Figure 9.7). The outer ear acts like a satellite dish antenna that "catches" sound waves and funnels them through the auditory canal until they strike against the tympanic membrane, causing vibrations. The middle ear structures pass the vibrations from one bone to another and on into the inner ear, where they are received and converted into nerve impulses by the cochlea. Finally, the nerve impulses travel through the auditory nerve to the brain, which translates them into sounds. The complicated process of hearing seems all the more remarkable when you consider that this chain of events occurs instantaneously.

Figure 9.7 - Movement of Sound Waves

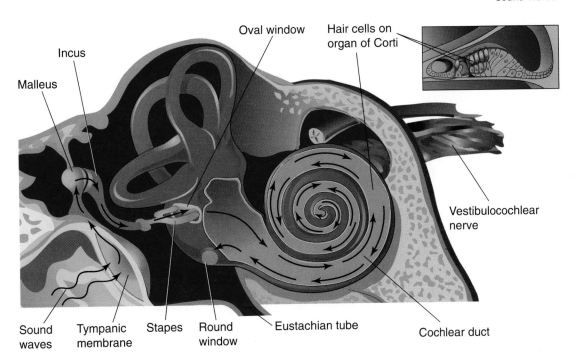

Table 9.6

Combining Forms Relating to the Ear

Combining form	Meaning	Example
acous/o	hearing	acoustic
audi/o	hearing, sound	audiology
aur/o	ear	aural forceps
auricul/o	ear	auricular
myring/o	tympanic membrane	myringotomy
ot/o	ear	otic
tympan/o	drum	tympanic membrane

Table 9.7

Anatomy and Physiology Terms Relating to the Ear

Term	Meaning	Word Analysis	
acoustic ah-**koos**-tik	sound	acoust/o -ic	hearing pertaining to
amplitude **am**-plih-tood	range or extent (of sound)	ampli- -tude	width quality or state
auditory **aw**-dih-tO-ree	hearing	audi/o -ory	hearing pertaining to
aural **aw**-rel	relating to the ear	aur/o -al	ear pertaining to
auricle **aw**-rih-kl	external ear	auricul/o	ear
cerumen she-**roo**-men	earwax	cera	wax
cochlea **kok**-lee-ah	spiral-shaped structure within the ear	cochlea	snail
concha **kon**-kah	the shell-shaped structure of the outer ear	concha	shell
endolymph **en**-dO-limf	lymphatic fluid within the labyrinth	endo- lymph	within clear fluid
eustachian tube yoo-**stay**-kee-an toob	passageway leading from the middle ear to the nasopharynx	Eustachio	16th-century Italian anatomist
fenestra ovalis feh-**nes**-trah O-**vay**-lis	oval opening between the middle ear and the vestibule	fenestra ovalis	opening oval-shaped
helix **hee**-liks	folded edge of the external ear	helix	coil
incus **in**-kus	anvil-shaped bone in the middle ear	incus	anvil
labyrinth **lab**-ir-inth	structure of the inner ear	labyrinth	maze
malleus **mal**-lee-us	bone of the middle ear	malleus	hammer
meatus mee-**ay**-tus	opening	meatus	passage
organ of Corti **kor**-tee	organ within the inner ear	Corti	19th-century Italian anatomist
ossicle **os**-sih-kl	bone of the middle ear	os/i -icle	bone small
periauricular per-ee-aw-**rik**-yoo-ler	surrounding the ear	peri- auricul/o -ar	around ear pertaining to
perilymph **per**-ih-limf	fluid surrounding the labyrinth	peri- lymph	around clear fluid
pinna **pin**-ah	the external ear	pinna	wing
saccule **sak**-yool	membranous sac within the vestibule	sac -ule	sac or bag small
semicircular canal sem-ih-**ser**-kyoo-ler kan-**al**	fluid-filled loops in the labyrinth	semi- circul/o canal	half round passageway

stapes **stay**-peez	small bone of the middle ear	*stapes*	stirrup	
tragus **tray**-gus tragi (pl)	small, goatee-shaped projection of cartilage on the outer ear	*tragos*	goat (refers to the goat's beard)	
tympanic membrane tim-**pan**-ik **mem**-brayn	eardrum	*tympan/o* *-ic*	drum pertaining to	
utricle **yoo**-trih-kl	membranous pouch in the vestibule	*uter*	leather bag	
vestibule **ves**-tih-byool	the central cavity of the labyrinth	*vestibul/o*	space	

Word Analysis

Separate each term into its individual word parts, using slashes. Identify each part by type, using the following letters: P = prefix, S = suffix, R = root word, CV = combining vowel. Then provide a definition for the whole term. Remember that all word parts may not be found in any one term. Some terms will have only two word parts.

Word analysis   **Definition**

1. tympanosclerosis _____

2. periauricular _____

3. otoscope _____

4. biaural _____

5. endolymphatic _____

6. ossicle _____

7. myringotomy _____

8. tubotympanic _____

9. labyrinthitis _____

10. postauricular _____

Matching

Select a term from Column 1 to match each definition in Column 2. Write the number of your selection on the line beside the definition.

Column 1	Column 2
1. pinna	_____ a. goat's beard
2. stapes	_____ b. shell-shaped structure of the outer ear
3. meatus	_____ c. anvil
4. amplitude	_____ d. opening
5. concha	_____ e. hammer
6. acoustic	_____ f. range or extent of sound
7. helix	_____ g. stirrup
8. malleus	_____ h. folded edge of the outer ear
9. incus	_____ i. external ear
10. tragus	_____ j. pertaining to sound

Word Building

Use root words, combining forms, prefixes, and suffixes to construct a medical term to match each definition provided.

1. instrument used to examine the ear   _____

2. little sac (structure within the vestibule) _____

3. pertaining to a drum (hearing)   _____

4. around the ear   _____

5. pertaining to the vestibule   _____

6. fluid of the bony labyrinth   _____

7. oval window   _____

8. superior segment of the pharynx   _____

9. ear, nose, and throat doctor   _____

10. dissolves earwax   _____

Find the misspelled words. Write the correct spelling on the blanks provided.

1. The precrisption was written by Dr. Martino. _____

2. The membranous labaryrinth contains a fluid called entolymph. _____

3. The autidiotory receptors are contained within the organ of Corti. _____

4. The semicircular cannals are located behind the vestibular. _____

5. The cocchulea is a spiral-shaped structure. _____

6. Dr. Yates performed the miriengotomy on Jason yesterday. _____

In the accompanying illustration of the ear, label the following structures.

1. auricle or pinna

2. external auditory meatus

3. tympanic membrane

4. eustachian tube

5. ossicular chain

6. cochlea

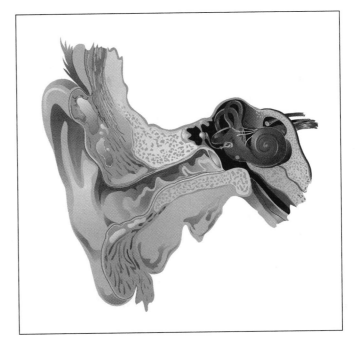

Assessing Patient Health

Wellness and Illness through the Life Span

The most frequently used terms describing wellness and illness of the ear are provided in Table 9.8.

Infants and Children

Infants can be born with malformed ears, absent ears (or **anotia**), or more than two ears (called **polyotia**). Congenital disorders occur during development and include deformities of the pinna, large ears (called **macrotia**), and small ears (called **microtia**).

Physicians screen for congenital deafness by clapping loudly next to the infant's ears during the first neonatal assessment; the noise should startle the child. Cochlear implant technology has revolutionized the rehabilitation of hearing-impaired children, enabling them to have marked gains in speech and understanding of spoken language.

One of the most common ear problems is **otitis media**, an inflammation of the middle ear. An upper respiratory infection can provide a trigger for this process. Children are plagued by otitis media because the eustachian tube is shorter, narrower, and more curved than in an adult. Together, these factors allow bacteria from the nasopharynx to enter the middle ear easily, cause inflammation, and impair the drainage of the resulting fluid. Clinical signs of otitis media include redness (called **injection**), bulging, retraction, perforation of the tympanic membrane, and the production of exudates. Ear pain, or **otalgia**, results from the increase in fluid and pressure. Pressure from the increased fluid can perforate the eardrum, or a deliberate perforation called a **myringotomy** may be performed. Perforation is accompanied by a bloody discharge, called **otorrhagia. Otopyorrhea**, a discharge of pus, may be present when the child has a serious ear infection.

Adults

Various ear illnesses are more common to adults than infants and children. **Labyrinthitis** is an inflammation of the inner ear resulting in vertigo, the sensation of spinning or dizziness. **Ménière's disease** is a disturbance of the labyrinth characterized by various manifestations, such as vertigo with or without tinnitus (ringing in the ears), hearing loss, nausea, and vomiting. Balance may also be affected. **Cholesteatomas** are a type of benign mass within the middle ear that appear in adults who have had chronic otitis media and rupture of the tympanic membrane.

Seniors

As the body ages, bone loses its calcium, becoming weak and porous, including the bone in and around the ear. **Otosclerosis** is the hardening of the spongy bone surrounding the oval window. Hardening of the tympanic membrane is called **tympanosclerosis**. Both of these processes result in hearing loss. **Presbycusis** is an aging-related hearing loss that involves inner ear and nerve deterioration.

Table 9.8

Wellness and Illness Terms Relating to the Ear			
Term	**Meaning**	**Word Analysis**	
anotia an-**O**-shyah	absent ears	*an/* *ot/o* *-ia*	without ear condition
cholesteatoma kol-es-tee-at-**O**-mah	tumor-like mass of scaly epithelial tissue and cholesterol in the middle ear	*choleste/a* *-oma*	cholesterol mass
labyrinthitis lab-ih-rin-**thI**-tis	inflammation of the inner ear	*labyrinth* *-itis*	maze inflammation
macrotia mak-**rO**-shee-ah	large ears	*-ia* *macr/o* *ot/o*	condition large ear
Ménière's disease main-y**airz**	condition characterized by vertigo	*Ménière*	French physician

microtia mI-**krO**-shee-ah	small ears	*micr/o* *ot/o* *-ia*	small ear condition
myringitis mir-in-**jI**-tis	inflammation of the tympanic membrane	*myring/o* *-itis*	tympanic membrane inflammation
otalgia o-**tal**-jee-ah	earache	*ot/o* *alg/o* *-ia*	ear pain condition
otitis externa O-**tI**-tis eks-**ter**-nah	inflammation of the external ear (swimmer's ear)	*ot/o* *-itis* *externa*	ear inflammation pertaining to the outside
otitis media O-**tI**-tis **mee**-dee-ah	inflammation of the middle ear	*ot/o* *-itis* *media*	ear inflammation pertaining to the middle
otorrhea Oh-**toe**-ree-ah	drainage from the ear	*ot/o* *-rrhea*	ear drainage
otosclerosis **O**-tO-sklah-**rO**-sis	hardening of the bone surrounding the oval window	*ot/o* *scler/o* *-sis*	ear hard condition
polyotia pol-ee-**O**-shee-ah	more than one ear on one side of the face	*poly-* *ot/o* *-ia*	many ear condition
presbycusis pres-bee-**kyoo**-sis	the inability to hear sounds due to aging	*presby/o* *acusis*	old age hearing
tinnitus tih-**nI**-tus/**tin**-ih-tus	ringing in the ears	*tinnio* *-tus*	jingling condition
tympanosclerosis tim-pah-nO-sklah-**rO**-sis	hardening of the tympanic membrane	*tympan/o* *scler/o*	tympanic membrane hardening
vertigo **ver**-tih-gO/ver-**tI**-gO	sensation of spinning, dizziness	*verto*	turn

Diagnosing and Treating Problems

Tests, Procedures, and Pharmaceuticals Relating to the Ear

Performing procedures involving the ear is challenging because the interior of the ear is small and difficult to access. Nonetheless, the procedures are often performed in an outpatient surgical area, and the patient is released shortly after recovering from the anesthesia (see Table 9.9).

Table 9.9

Tests and Procedures Relating to the Ear

Term	Meaning	Word Analysis	
audiometry au-dee-**om**-eh-tree audiology au-dee-**ol**-ah-jee audiometer au-dee-**om**-eh-ter	tests for determining the intensity of sound a person can hear; various tests can be done to determine hearing threshold and hearing frequencies; evoked potential measures electrical stimulation from the cortex of the brain; localization measures a person's ability to locate the source of a sound	*audi/o* *-metry*	hearing process of measuring
cochlear implant **kok**-lee-er	hearing device implanted under the skin behind the ear; it sends electrical signals to electrodes implanted within the cochlea to stimulate nerves	*cochlea* *im-* *plant*	snail into place or put
fenestration fen-es-**tray**-shun	formation of an opening into the labyrinth of the ear	*fenestra*	window-like opening
labyrinthectomy lab-ih-rin-**thek**-tO-mee	surgical removal of the labyrinth	*labyrinth* *-ectomy*	maze surgical removal
labyrinthotomy lab-ih-rin-**thot**-O-mee	incision into the labyrinth	*labyrinth* *-tomy*	maze incision
myringectomy mir-in-**jek**-tO-mee	excision of the tympanic membrane	*myring/o* *-ectomy*	tympanic membrane surgical removal
myringoplasty mir-**ing**-gO-plas-tee	surgical repair of the tympanic membrane	*myring/o* *-plasty*	tympanic membrane surgical repair
myringotomy mir-in-**got**-O-mee	surgical incision into the tympanic membrane, usually done to relieve fluid pressure; myringotomy tubes are placed through the incision to keep the fluid drained and pressure equalized, especially in children with chronic otitis media	*myring/o* *-tomy*	tympanic membrane incision
otoscope **O**-tO-skOp	medical instrument used to visualize the external ear canal and the tympanic membrane; when a bulb tube is attached to the otoscope, air is pushed in by squeezing the bulb, making it possible to determine whether the membrane is moving in and out appropriately	*ot/o* *-scope*	ear instrument to visualize area
Rinne's test **rin**-ez	test that uses a tuning fork to compare the perception of air conduction with bone conduction in each ear; the person should hear air vibration longer than bone vibration	*Rinne*	German otologist
stapedectomy sta-pee-**dek**-tO-mee	surgical removal of the stapes in the middle ear, and insertion of a prosthesis	*staped/o* *-ectomy*	stirrup surgical removal
tympanectomy tim-pah-**nek**-tah-mee	excision of the tympanic membrane	*tympan/o* *-ectomy*	tympanic membrane surgical removal
tympanotomy tim-pah-**not**-ah-mee	surgical puncture of the tympanic membrane	*tympan/o* *-tomy*	tympanic membrane incision
Weber's test **vay**-berz	test that uses a tuning fork to determine whether sound is heard equally in both ears	*Weber*	German otologist

Table 9.10

Abbreviations

ABR	auditory brainstem response
AC	air conduction
AD	right ear (*auris dexter*)
AOM	acute otitis media
AS	left ear (*auris sinister*)
AU	both ears (*auris uterque*)
BC	bone conduction
dB	decibel
EAC	external ear canal
EENT	eyes, ears, nose, and throat
ENT	ears, nose, and throat
PE tubes	pressure-equalizing tubes
TM	tympanic membrane

Word Analysis and Building

Exercise 24

For each of the underlined medical terms in the following sentences, identify the root by drawing a box around it. Supply the definition of the root, then supply the definition of the whole term.

1. The patient is a 6-month-old female, currently being treated with amoxicillin for bilateral <u>otitis media</u>.

   Root definition: _____

   Term definition: _____

2. Dr. Harmon will perform Timmy's <u>myringotomy</u> this afternoon.

   Root definition: _____

   Term definition: _____

3. Initial impression is abnormality of the <u>ossicular</u> chain, although further studies will be required to confirm this diagnosis.

   Root definition: _____

   Term definition: _____

4. Please schedule Mrs. Kelly for a <u>labyrinthectomy</u> at 10 A.M. tomorrow.

   Root definition: _____

   Term definition: _____

5. The persistence of fluid indicated the need for insertion of a <u>tympanostomy</u> tube in the left ear.

   Root definition: _____

   Term definition: _____

6. Mr. Louis has arrived for his scheduled excision of a <u>preauricular</u> appendage.

   Root definition: _____

   Term definition: _____

7. The plastic surgeon harvested skin grafts to perform the <u>canaloplasty</u>.

   Root definition: _____

   Term definition: _____

8. The patient had to travel to another state to have the <u>electrocochleography</u> performed.

   Root definition: _____

   Term definition: _____

9. To correct the defect, the surgeon performed a <u>fenestration</u> of the labyrinth.

   Root definition: _____

   Term definition: _____

10. The prognosis was guarded following the <u>stapediolysis</u>.

    Root definition: _____

    Term definition: _____

Comprehension Check

Exercise 25

Read each sentence, noting the pair of terms provided. Select the term that best fits the sentence and circle your choice.

1. Mr. Osborne is scheduled for a tympanectomy/amplitude this afternoon.

2. Sig: 3 gtt AD/ABR b.i.d.

3. Vestibular/Stapedectomy tumor was located and excised.

4. Ossicular/Neuroplasty was performed in an attempt to partially restore the patient's hearing.

5. While he was hospitalized Mr. Myer reported tinnitus/polyotia.

6. The myringectomy/myringotomy was performed followed by insertion of a ventilation tube.

7. The examination using the otoscope/ophthalmoscope revealed the tympanic membrane appeared injected.

8. The patient's perception of hearing by bone conduction and air vibration was evaluated by Rinne's/Weber's test.

9. Sounds were muffled because of the patient's bilateral otitis media/externa.

10. The otologist's objective was to establish sensitivity to sounds by using a cochlear/labyrinth implant.

Name the Term

Write the medical term that matches the underlined definition in each sentence. Write the term on the blank provided.

1. The patient is a 60-year-old male who was diagnosed with <u>a disturbance of the labyrinth characterized by vertigo, hearing loss, nausea, and vomiting</u> by Dr. Presley. _____

2. Suspect hearing loss due to <u>a mass composed of cholesterol within the middle ear</u>. _____

3. Grace has come to the clinic today because of an increase in severity of her chronic <u>ringing in the ears</u>. _____

4. Plan: <u>hearing test</u> to determine extent of hearing loss. _____

5. <u>Viewing with medical instrument used to examine the external ear canal and the tympanic membrane</u> reveals heavy cerumen accumulation; unable to visualize TM. _____

6. Plan: <u>excision of the tympanic membrane</u>. _____

Word Building
Exercise 27

Use prefixes, root words, combining vowels, and suffixes to create medical terms for the definitions given. Write the term on the blank provided. Separate the word parts with hyphens.

1. study of the ears _____

2. without ears _____

3. inflammation of the labyrinth _____

4. surgical removal of the mastoid cells _____

5. discharge or hemorrhage of the ear _____

Spelling Check
Exercise 28

Correct the spelling of each term. Write your answer on the line provided.

1. auriclle _____   5. ossiccle _____

2. cochalea _____   6. sacule _____

3. endalymph _____   7. tragas _____

4. meateaus _____   8. vestibuel _____

Complete the diagram below to illustrate the process of hearing.

Sound → Auricle → _____ → Auditory canal → _____

_____ → _____ → Inner ear → Auditory receptor cells

_____ → _____

Examining the Patient ♂♀

Anatomy, Physiology, and Pathology of Taste, Smell, and Touch

When we see food, we can smell it and even taste it without taking a bite. The senses of smell and taste are nearly inseparable. The sense of sight also is highly integrated with smell and taste. Working together, the three can stimulate the flow of saliva in the mouth. If one of these senses is not working correctly, such as during an upper respiratory infection, taste can be diminished.

The sense of touch is widely distributed, with high concentrations of receptors in a few critical areas, such as the pads of the fingertips. Because the nervous system is central to the sense of touch, problems are referred to a neurologist.

Taste

Figure 9.8 - Tongue Structure

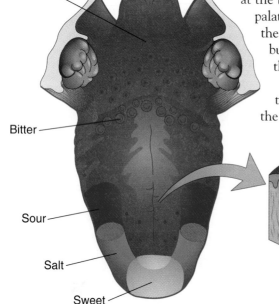

Root of tongue

Bitter

Sour

Salt

Sweet

Taste buds

The sense of taste occurs on the tongue (Figure 9.8), which contains more than 10,000 taste buds in the **fungiform** (the mushroom-shaped area near the tip of the tongue), in the **vallate papillae** (rows of tiny, pimplelike projections at the back and along the sides of the tongue), and on the soft palate arranged in a "V" shape. Other taste buds are located in the mucosa of the epiglottis, palate, and pharynx. Each taste bud is made up of supporting cells and hair cells known as the **gustatory receptors**.

The four basic tastes are sensed by different parts of the tongue: (1) sweet—tip of the tongue, (2) sourness—along the edges, (3) bitter—on the back, and (4) saltiness—on the anterior dorsum. Figure 9.8 shows the areas where the basic tastes are sensed.

Smell

The sense of smell depends on hair cells within the nose that act as **olfactory** (smell-sensing) receptors. They lie at the roof of the nasal cavity and in the upper portion of the septum. These olfactory receptors merge into the olfactory nerve (cranial nerve I). From there, the signals are transmitted to the **rhinencephalon** regions in the temporal lobe of the brain, where they are translated as smells. Animals rely on their sense of smell for survival in various ways, including food, danger, and reproduction. Humans can use the smell of noxious odors to protect them from harm, as well. Some odors may stimulate sexual arousal; others may trigger memory. The sense of smell also enhances the enjoyment and taste of foods, thereby improving health and nutrition.

Touch

Receptors all over the body can sense touch, although the receptors are most numerous in the skin of the fingers and lips and less abundant in the skin of the trunk. Touch includes the sensations of itch and tickle, light and deep pain, temperature discrimination, and **proprioception**, an awareness of the position of one's body parts in relation to the whole body.

Comprehension Check   Exercise 30

Using the context of the following sentences, circle the correct term from each pair.

1. The lacrimal duct/olfactory bulb contains nerve cells that provide the sense of smell.

2. The gustatory/nasopharyngeal cells are part of the taste buds.

3. Dysgeusia/Hypogeusia is an abnormal sense of taste.

4. Osmesis/Osmosis is the act of smelling.

5. Papillae/Anosmia refers to an absence of the sense of smell.

6. Proprioception/Reception is a sense of knowing the location of your own body parts.

7. Meissner's corpuscle/Olfaction is a receptor for light touch.

8. The olfactory/temporal nerve transmits nerve impulses to the temporal lobe of the brain, where olfaction takes place.

Performance Assessment 9

Crossword Puzzle

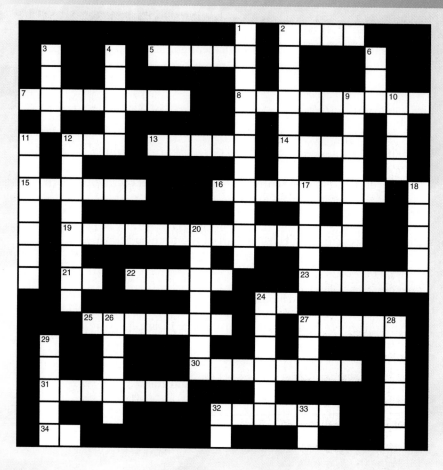

Across
2. disk behind the pupil
5. black center of the eye
7. little ears
8. visual field test
12. combining form meaning ear
13. point of greatest visual acuity
14. labyrinth
15. eye nerve tissue
16. double vision
19. inflammation of eye lining
21. abbreviation for left ear
22. combining form for nose
23. clear iris covering
24. abbreviation for right ear
25. otalgia
27. ear bone with anvil shape
30. night vision
31. absence of eye lens
32. ear bone with stirrup shape
34. doctor of optometry

Down
1. eyelid infection
2. pertaining to tears
3. colored portion of the eye
4. combining form meaning light
6. abbreviation for otolaryngologist
9. palpebrae
10. responsible for night vision
11. visible portion of the ear
12. fills glasses prescriptions
17. pertaining to the eye
18. Greek for angle
20. eyelid part
24. lacking ears
26. relating to the ear
27. symptom of glaucoma (abbreviation)
28. white eye covering
29. combining form meaning eye lens
32. abbreviation for esotropia
33. abbreviation for emmetropia

What Do These Abbreviations Mean?

Write the meaning of the abbreviation on the line provided.

1. AC _____

2. AOM _____

3. EAC _____

4. ENT _____

5. TM _____

6. EENT _____

7. AU _____

8. EOM _____

9. IOP _____

10. PERRLA _____

11. OU _____

12. OD _____

Analyze the Terms

Separate each term into its individual word parts, using slashes. Identify each part by type, using a letter (P = prefix, S = suffix, R = root, CV = combining vowel). Finally, provide a definition for the entire term.

1. tonometry

_____

2. sphincterotomy

_____

3. ophthalmoscopy

_____

4. retinoblastoma

_____

5. anotia

_____

6. sclerotomy

_____

7. tympanic

_____

8. otitis

_____

9. aural

_____

10. retinopathy

_____

Build the Terms

Select word parts from the lists to build a complete medical term for each definition given. Note that not all terms will have a root or combining form, prefix, and suffix. Some word parts may be used more than once.

Combining Forms	Prefixes	Suffixes
ophthalm/o	hyper-	-itis
ot/o	epi-	-logy
audi/o	sub-	-logist
aque/o	hypo-	-otomy
ocul/o	intra-	-ous
aur/o	dis-	-sis
tympan/o	an-	-al
myring/o	pre-	-ar
corne/o	de-	-ic
dacry/o	anti-	-lysis
scler/o	per-	-phobia
phot/o	bi-	-lytic

1. study of the eye   _____

2. pertaining to water   _____

3. breakdown of tears   _____

4. inflammation of   _____

5. pertaining to the ear   _____

6. condition of   _____

7. inflammation of the sclera   _____

8. pertaining to inside the eye   _____

9. fear of light   _____

10. incision into the tympanic membrane   _____

What's Your Conclusion?

In this exercise you will practice selecting the correct explanation or logical next step. Read each mini medical record carefully, then select the correct response. Write the letter of your answer in the space provided.

1. Richard L. is a 5 y/o male with recurrent otitis media for one year. In a recent development, his parents report that his speech patterns have changed and his preschool teacher says that he sometimes fails to respond when his name is called. He will be evaluated today by Dr. Martin, an EENT specialist.

   A. Dr. Martin will refer Richard to an audiologist for testing.
   B. Dr. Martin will call the surgery department and request that Richard be scheduled for a rhinoplasty with tube placement.

Your response: _____

2. Diagnosis: chronic otitis media with purulent exudate bilaterally and nasal hypertrophy with chronic adenitis and adenoid hypertrophy.

   A. The physician has diagnosed an ear infection and swollen auditory tubes with drainage from the nose.
   B. The physician has diagnosed a recurring ear infection and infected and swollen adenoids.

Your response: _____

3. S: Pt. c/o a clogged left ear and tinnitus. O: TMs are dull and nonmobile bilaterally. Serosanguineous discharge was noted. You understand that:

   A. The patient has ringing in the ear and possible OM.
   B. This is an emergency, and transfusion is necessary.

Your response: _____

Analyzing Medical Records

Read the operative report on the next page, then answer the questions below.

1. What is the name of the procedure?

2. Where was the procedure performed?

3. Why was the procedure performed? Is an infectious disease involved?

4. Was any medication prescribed?

5. What two procedures were performed immediately following intubation?

6. What two things were removed from the right ear before it was examined?

7. What was the condition of the right tympanic membrane prior to incision?

8. What was the condition of the left tympanic membrane prior to incision?

9. Where was the tube placed in the left ear? In the right ear?

10. What kind of dressings were used?

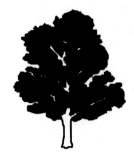

Hayes-Oakwood General Hospital
Department of Ophthalmology

407 S. Parkway
phone (333) 555-1234

Accord City, KS 77709-4321
fax (333) 555-1235

Operative Report

PATIENT: Lucinda C.
DATE: January 5, xxxx
DATE OF OPERATION: January 5, xxxx
PREOPERATIVE DIAGNOSIS: Chronic bilateral otitis media with effusion
POSTOPERATIVE DIAGNOSIS: Chronic bilateral otitis media with effusion
OPERATION PERFORMED: Bilateral myringotomy with tubes
SURGEON: L. L. Ball, MD
ANESTHESIOLOGIST: M. Modamusi, MD

Procedure and Findings: The patient was brought to the surgical suite following the usual preoperative preparation. Following intubation, general anesthesia was induced and the ears were prepped and draped for microscopic myringotomy. After debridement and removal of cerumen and debris from the right ear, the TM was examined and found to be dull and immobile. A myringotomy was carried out in the right ear. The inferior anterior quadrant circumference was incised and mucoid material was aspirated. A Shepard tube was positioned without incident and cotton dressing applied. The TM of the left ear was found to be similarly dull and immobile, and an inferior anterior myringotomy was performed. Mucoid material was aspirated, and a Shepard tube placed. A sterile cotton dressing was applied to the ear canal. No adenoiditis or adenoid hypertrophy was noted. The patient tolerated the procedure well and was extubated without complications. She was sent to the recovery room in satisfactory postoperative condition.

L. L. Ball, MD

Using Medical References

The following sentences contain medical terms that may not have been addressed on the tables in this chapter. Use medical reference books, your medical term analysis skills, and/or a medical dictionary to find the correct definition of each underlined word. Write the definition on the line below the sentence.

1. The patient has a considerable corneal abrasion due to bilateral <u>entropion</u>.

2. The patient is an 18 y/o male with a large <u>hordeolum</u>.

3. Mrs. Clarke's <u>nystagmus</u> has become progressively worse over the past two weeks.

_____

4. Examination reveals <u>dacryocystitis</u> of the left eye.

_____

5. Imp: marked <u>asthenopia</u>.

_____

6. The patient's <u>ocular prosthesis</u> will have to be removed prior to surgery.

_____

7. Mr. Tomes will undergo surgery for <u>enucleation</u> tomorrow and will be fitted with a prosthesis next week.

_____

8. Dr. Horton ordered ear irrigation for <u>ceruminolysis</u>.

_____

9. The patient presents with a marked <u>otopyorrhea</u>.

_____

10. Mr. Hunter will require an excision of the stapes to correct his <u>otosclerosis</u> and resultant hearing loss.

_____

11. The patient presented in the emergency room with <u>otorrhagia</u> following the MVA.

_____

12. This patient came to the clinic with symptoms of <u>aerotitis media</u> following a flight from Buenos Aires.

_____

Short Answer

In your own words, describe the work of a otolaryngologist, an ophthalmologist, and an optometrist.

_____

_____

_____

_____

Chapter 10

The Respiratory System

Learning Outcomes

Students will be able to:

- Name the structures of the respiratory tract and label them.
- Explain the breathing process.
- Describe the role of the lungs in respiration.
- Explain the function of oxygen and carbon dioxide in the maintenance of homeostasis in the body.
- List and describe abnormalities and pathologies of the respiratory system.
- Distinguish among tests, procedures, and pharmaceuticals related to the respiratory system.
- Correctly use the terminology of the respiratory system in oral and written communication.
- State the meaning of abbreviations related to the respiratory system.
- List and define the combining forms most commonly used to create terms related to the respiratory system.
- Name tests and treatments for respiratory system abnormalities and pathologies.

Translation, Please? Translation, Please? Translation, Please?

Read this excerpt from a physician's report and try to answer the questions that follow.

The patient was observed in orthopneic position having respirations at 30 per minute. The color was noted to be cyanotic. The eyes were edematous, as well as the feet. There was obvious SOB with dyspnea on lying down. During the examination, sputum was produced on several occasions. Bilateral wheezes were noted in all lung fields.

1. This patient was lying in the bed. True or false?
2. The color of the patient was normal. True or false?
3. How is sputum produced?
4. When lying down, the patient had difficulty with urine production. True or false?

Translation Please: Answers
1. False. The orthopneic position is sitting.
2. False. Cyanotic means the patient was bluish.
3. Sputum is produced by coughing.
4. False. SOB with dyspnea refers to shortness of breath with difficulty breathing.

Identifying the Specialty

The System and Its Practitioners

The respiratory system is composed of the nose, mouth, pharynx, epiglottis, esophagus, trachea, lungs, bronchi, bronchioles, and alveoli (Figure 10.1). These all function together, along with the circulatory system, to transport oxygen and carbon dioxide between the lungs and tissues of the body.

The field of medicine concerned with the respiratory system is **pulmonology**, from the Latin term for lung, *pulmo*. A physician who specializes in the respiratory system is called a **pulmonologist**.

Before birth, the fetus is in the protective fluid of the amniotic sac, and all of its needs are passed from the mother through the placenta. After the first gasp of air at birth, the body must breathe to survive. With each **inspiration** (inward breath) through the nose or mouth, we inhale oxygen, use it, and convert it into carbon dioxide, a waste product that is expelled with each **expiration** (outward breath). Humans cannot live for more than a few minutes without oxygen coming into and carbon dioxide going out of the body. The respiratory system is responsible for this process.

Examining the Patient ♂♀

Anatomy and Physiology of the Respiratory System

The respiratory system is divided into the upper and lower tracts, as shown in Figure 10.1. The upper respiratory tract includes the upper airways that are outside of the thoracic cavity (the chest), consisting of the nose, pharynx, and larynx. The lower respiratory tract consists of the structures within the **thorax**: the **trachea**, the entire **bronchial tree**, and the **lungs**.

Figure 10.1 - Organs of the Respiratory System

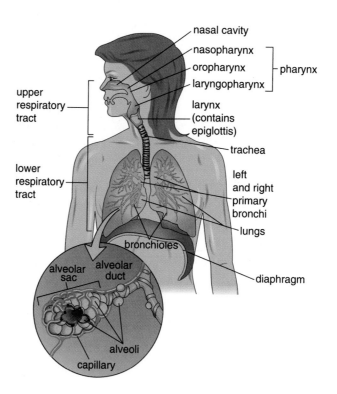

Pathway of Oxygen from Inhalation through Exhalation

The **nose** is the uppermost structure of the upper respiratory tract and the entry point for oxygen and other elements from the outside. Air enters through the **nares**, or nostrils, and passes into the two nasal cavities, which are lined with tiny hairs and respiratory **mucosa**. This lining, found throughout the respiratory tract, consists of a layer of mucus that covers **cilia**, hairlike structures that filter and protect the inside of the body from outside elements. The mucosal layer secretes about one-half cup of mucus daily. The cilia cover the epithelial cells of the respiratory tract and cause the mucus to move from the lower respiratory tract up toward the pharynx.

As air enters the nares, it is separated by the **nasal septum**, which forms the two nasal cavities. The air is warmed by the nasal hairs and mucus. The **olfactory** receptors are found in the nasal cavities; their nerve endings provide the sense of smell.

The other structures of the upper respiratory tract include the four **paranasal sinuses**—frontal, maxillary, sphenoid, and ethmoid—named for the bones in which they lie (Figure 10.2). Sinuses are hollow spaces in the head that help produce mucus, lighten the weight of the skull, and amplify sound.

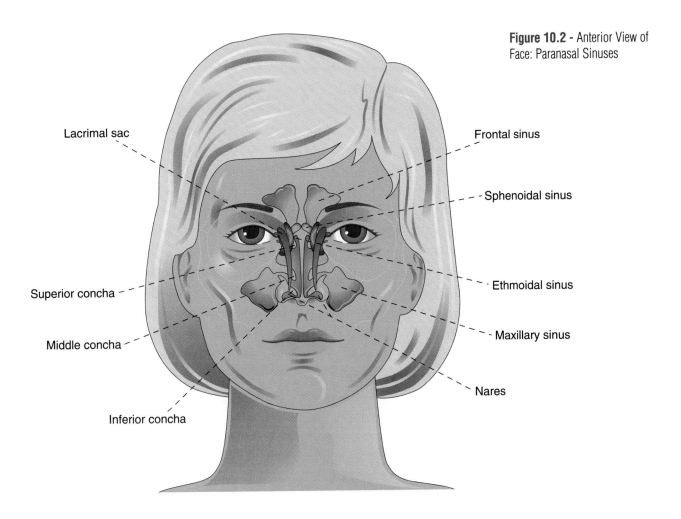

Figure 10.2 - Anterior View of Face: Paranasal Sinuses

Lacrimal sac

Superior concha

Middle concha

Inferior concha

Frontal sinus

Sphenoidal sinus

Ethmoidal sinus

Maxillary sinus

Nares

Two ducts within the nasal cavity that lead from the lacrimal sacs drain tears into the nasal cavity. On each side of the nasal cavity are **conchae** (superior, middle, and inferior), which also help to warm, humidify, and filter the air. From the nasal cavity, air moves to the **pharynx**, or throat.

The pharynx is a tubelike structure, about 5 inches long, extending from the nose into the upper chest (see Figure 10.3). It consists of three sections, the **nasopharynx**, located behind the nose; the **oropharynx**, located behind the mouth; and the **laryngopharynx**, located at the lower end immediately above the larynx. The pharynx further filters air as it passes into the body. The back of the oral cavity meets the pharynx, and food passes through it on its way to the stomach. The eustachian tubes from the ears open into the nasopharynx and equalize pressure in the ears. The tonsils and adenoids are also found within the pharynx. (See Chapter 6 for a complete description of the tonsils and adenoids.)

Below the laryngopharynx is the **larynx**, also known as the voice box (see Figure 10.4). It is composed of cartilaginous areas, the largest of which is the thyroid cartilage or **Adam's apple**. The vocal cords are two fibrous bands stretched across the larynx. High-pitched sound is produced when air is passed between the bands as they are tensed; the sound is lower when they are relaxed. The **glottis** is the area between the vocal cords. The **epiglottis** is a cartilaginous structure that covers the larynx during swallowing to prevent food from entering the **trachea**, or windpipe.

Figure 10.3 - Sagittal Views of Head and Neck

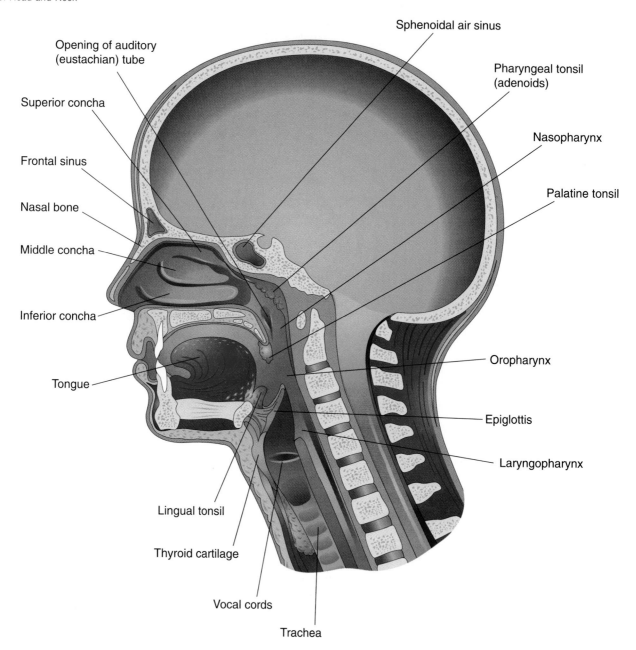

Opening of auditory (eustachian) tube

Superior concha

Frontal sinus

Nasal bone

Middle concha

Inferior concha

Tongue

Lingual tonsil

Thyroid cartilage

Vocal cords

Trachea

Sphenoidal air sinus

Pharyngeal tonsil (adenoids)

Nasopharynx

Palatine tonsil

Oropharynx

Epiglottis

Laryngopharynx

Figure 10.4 - Trachea

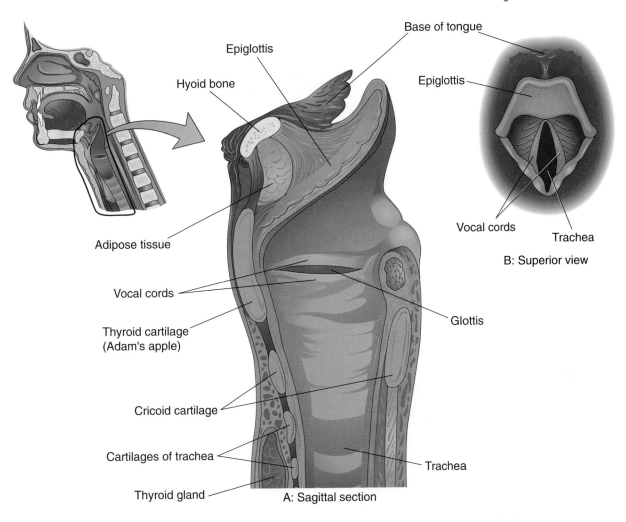

Epiglottis

Base of tongue

Hyoid bone

Epiglottis

Adipose tissue

Vocal cords

Trachea

B: Superior view

Vocal cords

Thyroid cartilage
(Adam's apple)

Glottis

Cricoid cartilage

Cartilages of trachea

Trachea

Thyroid gland

A: Sagittal section

The trachea is a tubelike structure, which extends about 4 to 5 inches into the lower respiratory tract (i.e., the bronchi in the chest). Horseshoe-shaped cartilage rings form the trachea and they protect it from collapsing. Inside the trachea, cilia wave continuously toward the mouth to capture and expel invading matter.

The next structure encountered on the journey within the respiratory tract is the **bronchial tree** (Figure 10.5). The bronchial tree consists of the right main bronchus and the left main bronchus, which form the trunks of the tree; the **bronchioles**, which resemble branches; and the **alveoli**, which are comparable to leaves. The left main bronchus is approximately 1.5 to 2 inches long and leads into the left lung, which consists of superior and inferior lobes. The right bronchus is about 1 inch long and leads into the right lung, which consists of three lobes: the superior, middle, and inferior. The bronchi bifurcate, or divide further, until they reach the bronchioles. The bronchioles end in alveoli, which are the areas where gas exchange takes place.

Figure 10.5 - Bronchial Tree

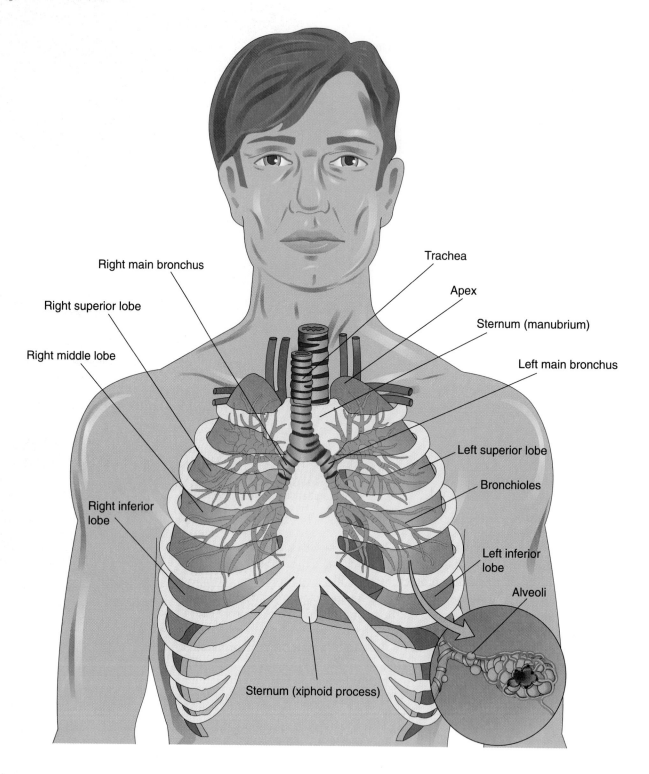

Right main bronchus

Right superior lobe

Right middle lobe

Right inferior lobe

Trachea

Apex

Sternum (manubrium)

Left main bronchus

Left superior lobe

Bronchioles

Left inferior lobe

Alveoli

Sternum (xiphoid process)

The **alveoli** are berrylike clusters located around the **alveolar duct** in an **alveolar sac** (Figure 10.6). The average adult body has about 600 million alveoli. A substance called **surfactant** covers the insides of the alveoli and helps reduce the surface tension, keeping the alveoli from collapsing during gas exchange. A network of **capillaries**, tiny blood vessels responsible for exchanging oxygen and carbon dioxide, cover about 75 percent of the alveolar surface.

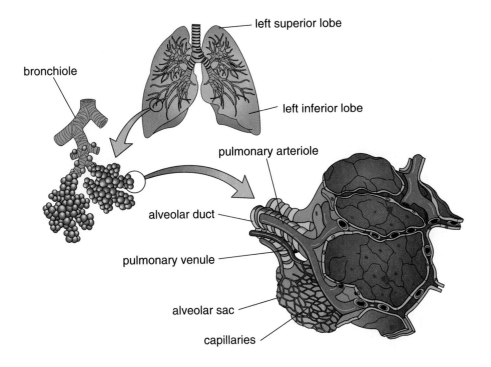

Figure 10.6 - Alveoli

The **lungs** lie within the rib cage and consist of the right lung (which has three **lobes**, or sections) and the left lung (which has two lobes), as shown in Figure 10.5. The superior, narrow portion, or **apex**, of each lung is found under the collarbone. The inferior portion, called the base, is wider and rests on the diaphragm. Covering the outer surfaces of the lungs and the inner surfaces of the ribs is the **pleura**, a thin, moist membrane that allows the lungs and ribs to move smoothly against each other during respiration.

Respiration

Respiration consists of inspiration, in which oxygen is **inhaled**, or brought into the body through the nose or mouth, and expiration, in which carbon dioxide is **exhaled**. Key players in the respiration process are the **diaphragm**, a muscle located within the thoracic cavity, behind the ribs and under the lungs, and the **intercostal muscles**, which are attached to the ribs.

During inspiration, the chest cavity enlarges as the diaphragm contracts and the intercostal muscles cause the ribs to elevate. This movement increases the volume of the thoracic cavity but decreases the pressure within the cavity, which allows air to enter. The lungs expand, and air moves into the lungs and alveoli. During expiration the diaphragm relaxes, which reduces the thoracic cavity volume. Air pressure increases and forces the air out of the lungs. Figure 10.7 illustrates the mechanics of respiration.

Figure 10.7 - Respiration

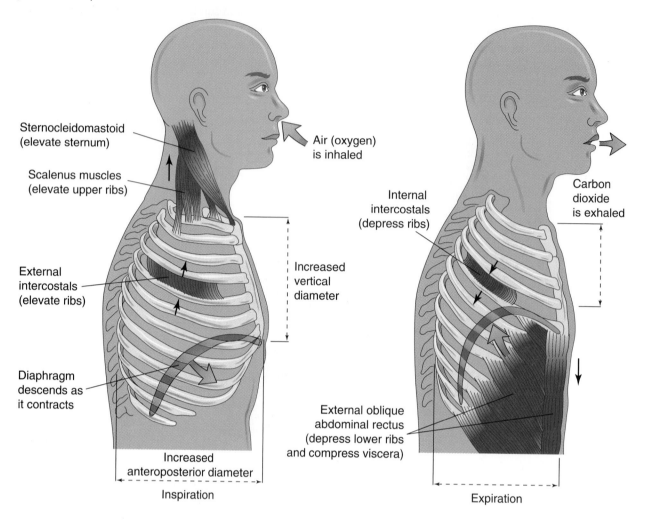

Sternocleidomastoid
(elevate sternum)

Scalenus muscles
(elevate upper ribs)

External
intercostals
(elevate ribs)

Diaphragm
descends as
it contracts

Air (oxygen)
is inhaled

Increased
vertical
diameter

Increased
anteroposterior diameter

Inspiration

Internal
intercostals
(depress ribs)

Carbon
dioxide
is exhaled

External oblique
abdominal rectus
(depress lower ribs
and compress viscera)

Expiration

Gas Exchange

Gas exchange refers to the exchange of oxygen between the alveoli and the lung's capillaries and to the exchange of carbon dioxide between the circulatory blood and the lung's capillaries. The process is handled jointly by the respiratory system and the circulatory system—the system that moves blood through the body via the blood vessels (veins and arteries). Blood is pumped from the right ventricle of the heart into the pulmonary artery, which leads to the lungs, filling the capillaries that are near the alveoli.

Through the process of **diffusion**, the high concentration of oxygen in the alveoli is exchanged for the low oxygen concentration in the capillaries of the lungs. Carbon dioxide, a waste product, is also present in blood within the lung capillaries, because this blood has traveled through the body. The carbon dioxide is exchanged between the circulatory blood and the lung capillaries. During expiration, the air is forced out of the alveoli, through the lungs, and out of the nose or mouth, taking the carbon dioxide with it (Figure 10.8).

Table 10.1 lists common combining forms related to the respiratory system, and Table 10.2 lists the essential anatomy and physiology terms for this system.

Figure 10.8 - Exchange of Oxygen and Carbon Dioxide

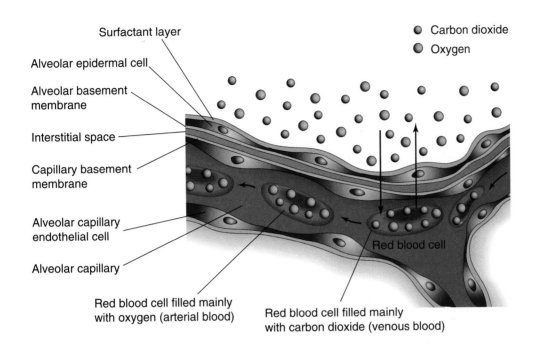

- Carbon dioxide
- Oxygen

Surfactant layer

Alveolar epidermal cell

Alveolar basement membrane

Interstitial space

Capillary basement membrane

Alveolar capillary endothelial cell

Alveolar capillary

Red blood cell

Red blood cell filled mainly with oxygen (arterial blood)

Red blood cell filled mainly with carbon dioxide (venous blood)

Table 10.1

Combining Forms Relating to the Respiratory System

Combining form	Meaning	Example
aer/o	air	aerobic
alveol/o	hollow sac	alveoli
bronch/o	airway	bronchial
bronchiol/o	bronchiole	bronchiolitis
laryng/o	larynx	laryngoscope
nas/o	nose	nasopharynx
ox/o	oxygen molecule	oxygenation
pharyng/o	throat	pharyngeal
phon/o	sound	dysphonia
phren/o	diaphragm	diaphragmatic
pleur/o	rib area	pleural space
pne/o	breath	apnea
pneum/o	lung, air	pneumonitis
pulmon/o	lung	pulmonary
rhin/o	nose	rhinorrhea
thorac/o	chest	thoracic
trache/o	windpipe	tracheal

Table 10.2

Anatomy and Physiology Terms Relating to the Respiratory System

Term	Meaning	Word Analysis	
Adam's apple	projection on the anterior neck formed by the thyroid cartilage of the larynx	N/A	
alveolus al-**vee**-ah-lus	grapelike portion at the terminal end of the bronchial tree; the area where oxygen and carbon dioxide are exchanged	*alveol/o*	hollow sac (from alveus, bowl)
apex **ay**-peks	top portion of the lung located beneath the upper ribs	*apex*	tip
bronchial tree **bron**-kee-el tree	portion of the lower respiratory tract that looks like a tree, consisting of the two primary bronchi, like the trunk of the tree; the bronchioles, like the branches; and the alveoli, like the leaves	*bronch/o* *-al*	windpipe pertaining to
bronchiole **bron**-kee-Ol	subdivision of the bronchi (less than 1 mm in diameter); part of the bronchial tree	*bronchiol/o*	bronchiole
bronchus **bron**-kus	section of the respiratory tract formed from the trachea; it branches into right and left sections	*bronch/o*	windpipe
capillary **kap**-ih-lar-ee	smallest unit of the vascular system; location of oxygen and carbon dioxide exchange	*capillaris*	relating to hair
carbon dioxide **kar**-bon dI-**ok**-sId	gas molecule removed from the body by the process of respiration	*carbon* *dioxide*	charcoal two atoms of oxygen
cilia **sil**-ee-ah	hairlike structures that line certain structures within the body to move substances; the cilia in the respiratory tract move foreign substances up and toward the outside world	*cilia*	eyelid
epiglottis ep-ih-**glot**-is	elastic cartilage that acts as a valve over the glottis to prevent food from being aspirated into the trachea during swallowing	*epi-* *glottis*	upon, following mouth of the windpipe
esophagus ee-**sof**-ah-gus	structure between the pharynx and the stomach	*oisophagos*	gullet
expiration eks-pih-**ray**-shun	process of breathing out; exhalation	*exspirare*	breathing out
inspiration in-spih-**ray**-shun	process of breathing in; inhalation	*inspirare*	breathing in
intercostal muscles in-ter-**kos**-tel	muscles between the ribs	*inter-* *cost/o* *-al*	between rib pertaining to
laryngopharynx lah-**rin**-gO-**far**-enks	area of the pharynx above the opening of the larynx	*laryng/o* *pharyng/o*	larynx pharynx
larynx **lar**-inks	area of the respiratory tract between the pharynx and trachea; contains the vocal cords	*laryng/o*	larynx
lobes	sections of an organ or body part	*lobus*	lobe, part
lungs	organs within the chest cavity in which respiration and gas exchange take place	*lungen*	lung
mouth	oral cavity	*muth*	opening, orifice

mucosa myoo-**kO**-sah	mucous tissue that lines many structures in the body	*muc/o*	mucous
naris **nay**-ris	opening of the nose; nostril	*nasus*	nose
nasal septum **nay**-zel **sep**-tum	separation of the nasal cavity	*nas/o* *-al* *septum*	nose pertaining to partition
nasopharynx nay-zO-**far**-inks	part of the pharynx located above the soft palate that opens into the nasal cavity and connects with the oropharynx	*nas/o* *pharyng/o*	nose pharynx
nose	opening of the body that provides air entry	*nosu*	nose
olfactory ol-**fak**-tah-ree	relating to smell	*olfactorius*	smell
oropharynx **or**-O-**far**-inks	area of the pharynx behind the mouth that joins the nasopharynx	*or/o* *pharyng/o*	mouth pharynx
oxygen **ok**-sih-jen	gaseous element	*ox/o* *-gen*	oxygen producer
paranasal sinuses par-ah-**nay**-zel **sI**-nus-es	cavities in the head that surround the nose; they lighten the weight of the skull	*para-* *nas/o* *-al* *sinus*	surrounding nose pertaining to cavity
pharynx **far**-inks	area between the mouth and nasal cavities and the esophagus; the throat	*pharyng/o*	pharynx
pleura (general use and sing n) **ploor**-ah	membrane surrounding the lungs	*pleur/o*	rib
pulmonology pool-mO-**nol**-ah-jee	relating to the lungs; the area of medical practice concerned with the lungs	*pulmon/o* *-logy*	lungs study of
respiration res-pih-**ray**-shun respiratory res-**pI**-rah-tor-ee	process of breathing	*respiration*	breath
surfactant ser-**fak**-tent	substance secreted into the alveoli to decrease surface tension	*surfactant*	from *surface active agent*
trachea **tray**-kee-ah	air tube that leads from the larynx into the chest	*trache/o*	trachea

Word Analysis

Separate the terms into their word parts, using slashes, then provide a definition for the term.

	Word Parts	Definition
1. pulmonary	_____	_____
2. aerophagia	_____	_____
3. pneumonitis	_____	_____
4. bronchiole	_____	_____
5. tracheostomy	_____	_____

6. rhinorrhea   _____   _____

7. dysphonia   _____   _____

8. pharyngeal   _____   _____

9. thoracotomy   _____   _____

10. laryngoscope   _____   _____

11. oxygenation   _____   _____

12. alveolar   _____   _____

Comprehension Check

Exercise 2

Circle the appropriate term from the pair in each sentence.

1. Upon examination of the patient's throat, it was noted that the epiglottis/epidermis was swollen and inflammed.

2. The nasal/natal passages are patent.

3. Thomas was diagnosed with pleuritis/arthritis, following a pulmonary examination and chest x-rays.

4. When the EMTs arrived, the patient was experiencing an episode of oxonea/apnea.

5. Mark has successfully completed the board exams to become a pulmonologist/entomologist.

6. The workers developed osteitis/alveolitis after inhaling toxic fumes.

7. The needle was inserted through the seventh intercostal/coastal space.

8. Carbon dioxide is inhaled/exhaled.

9. The upper portion of the lung is called the napex/apex.

10. Detergent/Surfactant covers the inside of the alveoli.

Name the Term

Exercise 3

Supply a term for each definition. Write the term in the space provided.

1. process by which substances move from an area of higher concentration to an area of lower concentration

_____

2. gas molecule removed from the body by the process of respiration

_____

3. Latin for tip; the top portion of the lungs, located beneath the upper ribs

_____

4. air tube that leads from the pharynx into the chest

_____

5. separation of the nasal cavity

_____

6. area of the respiratory tract between the pharynx and trachea; contains the vocal cords

_____

7. muscles between the ribs

_____

8. opening of the body that provides air entry

_____

9. membrane that surrounds the lungs

_____

10. chest cavity

_____

Word Building   Exercise 4

Supply the missing word part to complete each term, using the definition provided.

1. Hyper_____ia means excess carbon dioxide.

2. _____itis refers to inflammation of the bronchioles.

3. Naso_____ means nose and pharynx.

4. The _____ tree is a portion of the lower respiratory tract that looks like a tree; it consists of the two primary bronchi, the bronchioles, and the alveoli.

5. Para_____ sinuses are sinuses located around the nose: frontal, maxillary, sphenoidal, and ethmoidal sinuses.

6. _____ous means pertaining to cartilage.

7. Epi_____ refers to above the glottis.

8. _____al means pertaining to the bronchus or bronchi.

9. _____ means breathing in, inspiration.

10. Hyp_____ia is a condition of deficient oxygen.

Spelling Check

Circle the correctly spelled word from each pair in the following sentences.

1. The cilia/scilia line the respiratory/inspiratory tract.

2. The pharnyx/pharynx is a tubelike structure extending from the nose into the upper chest.

3. The larynx/lynx is composed of cartilage/carnage.

4. The broccoli/bronchi are structures in the respiratory/repairatory system.

5. The apox/apex of each lung lies just under the collarbone.

6. Carbon dioxide is exhaled/exhailed through expiration/expariation.

7. The intercostal/intracosticl muscles are important in the respiratory process.

8. When the diaphragm/diaghram relaxes, it reduces the volume of the thoracic/theoretic cavity.

9. A substance called surfactent/surfactant covers the inside of the alveoli/alimentary canal.

10. The process of diffusion/difusion occurs when substances move from an area of higher concentration to an area of lower concentration.

Word Map

The diagram below traces air flow through the respiratory system during inhalation. Complete the diagram by labeling each area.

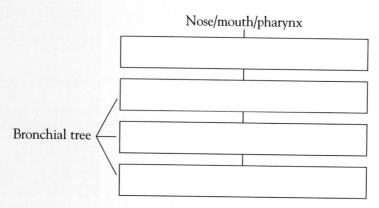

Nose/mouth/pharynx

Bronchial tree

Word Map

Group the following terms into three categories:

alveoli, astrocyte, bronchioles, myelin sheath, nares, neurilemma, oropharynx, superior concha, trachea

Upper Respiratory Tract	Lower Respiratory Tract	Not in the Respiratory Tract
_____	_____	_____
_____	_____	_____
_____	_____	_____

Assessing Patient Health

Wellness and Illness through the Life Span

The physician's assessment of the respiratory system begins with looking at the nose, observing for a deviated septum or other abnormalities that might decrease the amount of air entering the body. The chest is inspected for size, shape, and symmetry. Respirations are counted as movements of the chest during inspiration and expiration. Posture, contour, and movement are important elements in proper air exchange. Infants and children normally breathe with the diaphragm muscle, while most adults use the chest muscles.

Palpation of the back includes feeling for **fremitus**, the vibrations caused by breathing. A resonant sound should be produced when **percussing**, or tapping, on the chest over the area of the lungs. The ribs and sternum produce a dull sound. On **auscultation** with the stethoscope, the examiner listens for breath sounds on inspiration and expiration.

Abnormal sounds, or **adventitious** sounds, on auscultation indicate the type of abnormality present. These sounds are usually described as discontinuous, discrete sounds, called **crackles** or **rales**; or continuous, coarse, or musical sounds, which include **wheezes** and **rhonchi**. Table 10.3 lists the sounds heard during auscultation of the chest.

Table 10.3

Chest Sounds

Term	Description
bronchophony	while patient is speaking, the examiner listens through the stethoscope and the sounds should not be understood
egophony	nasal quality heard through stethoscope
pleural rub	sounds loudest at the end of inspiration; caused by the lung wall scraping against the pleura
rales	heard during forced respiration usually at the end of inspiration; caused by air rushing through mucus
rhonchi	continuous sounds, usually more prominent during expiration and cleared with coughing; loud gurgling noises transmitted from secretions in the pharynx
stridor	high-pitched, like wind blowing, indicating obstruction of the larynx or trachea
wheeze	whistling, squeaking, musical sound made by air passing through narrowed airways

Table 10.4 lists terms describing abnormalities in the physical examination of the respiratory system.

Table 10.4

Abnormalities in the Physical Examination of the Respiratory System

Term	Meaning	Word Analysis	
cyanosis sI-ah-**nO**-sis	bluish color associated with decreased oxygen	cyan/o -osis	blue condition
dyspnea **disp**-nee-ah	difficulty breathing	dys- -pnea	difficult, painful relating to breath
fremitus **frem**-ih-tus	vibration transmitted to the hand lying on the chest	fremitus	a dull roaring sound
hypercapnia hI-per-**kap**-nee-ah	having too much carbon dioxide	hyper- kapnos -pnea	increased smoke, vapor breath

continued on next page

hypoxia hI-**pok**-see-ah	having too little oxygen	hypo- ox/o -ia	decreased oxygen condition
orthopnea or-thop-**nee**-ah orthopnea position	difficulty breathing when lying down position in which a person sits up and leans forward in order to breathe	orth/o -pnea	straight breath
stridor **strI**-der	high-pitched, noisy breath indicating a tracheal obstruction	stridere	a creaking sound
tachypnea tak-ip-**nee**-ah	rapid breathing	tachy- -pnea	rapid breath

Fetuses, Infants, and Children

Lung tissue develops during the first five weeks of fetal life. By sixteen weeks the pathways for respiration are the same as in the adult. Surfactant appears by about thirty-two weeks to help during inflation of the alveolus. In utero, the respiratory system is the only nonfunctional system. At birth, the infant produces the cry that brings in air, and the first breath is taken. When the umbilical cord is cut, the placental blood supply is cut off, and the newborn begins to use his or her pulmonary and systemic circulation.

Premature infants who are born before surfactant has been produced are at risk for **infant respiratory distress syndrome (IRDS)**, a life-threatening condition and major cause of death of premature infants. An inability of the alveoli to inflate completely causes them to collapse, a condition known as **atelectasis.** A synthetic drug is now available to replace the missing surfactant, with the result that many lives have been saved.

The infant breathes through the nose rather than the mouth until about three months of age. The chest is rounded, and there is little thoracic expansion. Normally, the newborn takes thirty to forty breaths per minute.

Infants and young children are especially vulnerable to **respiratory syncytial virus (RSV)**, a type of virus that causes cells to mesh rather than remain singular. In adults, the virus produces only coldlike symptoms, but children can become extremely ill with **pneumonia,** an inflammation of lung tissue.

Cystic fibrosis (CF) is usually diagnosed in infancy. An inherited disease, it causes airway obstruction and pancreatic insufficiency. Children with CF must take pancreatic enzymes to replace those missing so that their systems can absorb food properly. The patient has frequent episodes of pneumonia. Careful **pulmonary toilet,** or deep breathing and percussion, is necessary to loosen the thick, sticky secretions associated with this disease.

Young children tend to suffer from frequent **upper respiratory infections (URIs)**. Several factors cause this phenomenon. First, as described in Chapter 9, "The Special Senses," the eustachian tubes are shorter and more curved in children than they are in adults, providing an easy entryway for bacteria. Second, each time a child is exposed to an outside organism he or she becomes sick with the associated disease; many of these organisms cause URIs. On the positive side, however, the child then develops immunity against these organisms.

Croup is a type of laryngotracheobronchitis that occurs in infants and young children. Caused by certain viruses, it produces difficult and noisy respiration and a barklike cough. **Bronchiolitis** is caused by a viral pathogen and is characterized by difficulty breathing, respiratory distress, and pneumonia.

Acute epiglottitis is a life-threatening condition that is rare, but dangerous, in the young child. It is frequently caused by the *Haemophilus influenzae* type b organism and may cause respiratory obstruction.

Asthma (see Chapter 6, "The Immune System") often is first diagnosed in childhood. It may be caused by allergy to the environment, food, or other substances.

Young Adults

Active young adults may be exposed to the potential for injury, including trauma to the respiratory system, from motor vehicle collisions, occupational injuries, and sports or household mishaps. One of the more serious conditions is pneumothorax (sometimes called "collapsed lung"), which is air collecting in the pleural space—where the lung tissue is normally "inflated." The air (blood or pus can also collect there) in that space prevents the lung tissue from fully expanding, inhibiting gas exchange and, if severe enough, can lead to a disruption of both pulmonary and cardiac function and death.

Seniors

Through the aging process, the costal cartilages become calcified, and chest expansion may be decreased. This decreased expansion prevents good air entry and makes the older person especially susceptible to respiratory diseases. The most common is **emphysema,** in which loss of alveolar elasticity prevents movement of air from the air sacs. Associated with emphysema is chronic **bronchitis,** a continual inflammation of the bronchi.

Another chronic illness of the respiratory tract is **chronic obstructive pulmonary disease (COPD),** also known as **chronic obstructive lung disease (COLD).** This disease occurs when there is difficulty with oxygenation over a long period of time. In late stages, the affected person becomes very debilitated and requires continuous delivery of oxygen.

Tuberculosis is a contagious, opportunistic infection, caused by the organism *Mycobacterium tuberculosis,* in which a tubercle is formed, usually within the lung tissues, that then becomes fibrotic. The disease is commonly found in areas where people live very close together, have poor nutrition, and are therefore susceptible. The spread of tuberculosis was decreasing in the United States until the outbreak of AIDS, in which opportunistic infections are common.

Pneumonia is an inflammatory process affecting lung tissue. It is usually caused by infectious organisms but may also result from inhaling or aspirating chemicals. The examiner may hear adventitious chest sounds, including rattling breath sounds, increased tactile fremitus, and dullness on percussion.

Lung cancer, also known as **bronchogenic carcinoma,** is the leading cause of cancer deaths in men and women. This is a group of malignant tumors usually associated with cigarette smoking. Lung cancer is divided into two categories: non-small-cell lung cancer (NSCLC) and small-cell lung cancer (SCLC). In early-stage disease, NSCLC is treated with surgery. In more advanced disease, surgery and/or radiation therapy, with or without chemotherapy, may be used. Small-cell lung cancer is highly malignant and is usually advanced at diagnosis. It is treated with surgery, chemotherapy, and radiation therapy, although treatment is considered palliative.

Mesothelioma is a rare malignant tumor arising from the lining of the pleural surface of the lungs. It is associated with exposure to asbestos.

Table 10.5 lists other major wellness and illness terms relating to the respiratory system.

Table 10.5

Wellness and Illness Terms Relating to the Respiratory System

Term	Meaning	Word Analysis	
asthma **as**-mah	disorder in which airways are temporarily narrowed, resulting in difficulty in breathing, coughing, gasping, and wheezing	*asthma*	difficulty breathing
atelectasis at-ah-**lek**-tah-sis	absence of gases from the lungs because of the inability of the alveoli to expand	*atelectasis*	incomplete expansion
bronchiectasis bron-kee-**ek**-tay-sis	dilation of the bronchi or bronchioles as a result of inflammatory disease or obstruction	*bronch/o* *ect/o* *-esis*	bronchus, windpipe outer condition
bronchiolitis bron-kee-O-**II**-tis	inflammation of the bronchioles	*bronchiol/o* *-itis*	bronchiole inflammation
bronchogenic carcinoma **bron**-kee-O-jen-ick car-sin-**O**-ma	lung cancer	*bronch/o* *-genic* *carcin/o* *-oma*	bronchus, windpipe beginning, production cancer tumor
croup kroop	laryngotracheobronchitis caused by a parainfluenza virus in infants and young children	*Croup*	cry aloud
cystic fibrosis **sis**-tik fI-**brO**-sis	hereditary disorder characterized by respiratory difficulties and frequent, mushy, foul-smelling stools because of missing pancreatic enzymes	*cystic* *fibr/o* *-osis*	refers to cysts fiber (fibrous) condition
emphysema em-fih-**see**-mah	chronic condition of increased air in the alveoli that cannot be exhaled	*emphysema*	bellows
epiglottitis ep-ih-glot-**I**-tis	usually an acute illness caused by the *Haemophilus influenzae* type b organism; may cause respiratory obstruction	*epi-* *glottis* *-itis*	over, on mouth of the windpipe inflammation
mesothelioma mez-o-thee-lee-**O**-ma	type of lung cancer of the pleura	*meso-* *thel/o* *-oma*	middle a nipple-like structure; a cellular layer tumor
pleural effusion **ploor**-el ef-**yoo**-zhun	condition in which fluid from the body accumulates in the pleural cavity	*pleur/o* *-al* *effusio*	lungs pertaining to pouring out
pleurisy **ploo**-rih-see	inflammation of the pleura (membrane around the lungs)	*pleur/o* *-y*	rib condition
pneumonia noo-**mO**-nee-ah	inflammation of the lung tissue	*pneum/o* *-ia*	lungs, air, gas condition
pneumothorax noo-mO-**thO**-raks	condition in which air is present in the pleural cavity	*pneum/o* *thorac/o*	lungs, air, gas chest
sinusitis sI-nah-**sI**-tis	inflammation of one of the paranasal sinuses	*sinus* *-itis*	cavity inflammation
tuberculosis too-ber-kyoo-**IO**-sis	disease caused by the organism *Mycobacterium tuberculosis*; forms infectious tubercles	*tubercul/o* *-osis*	tubercle condition

Draw a box around the root in each term. Write the definition for the root word and then write the definition for the entire term

Term	Root Word Definition	Whole Term Definition
1. stethoscope	_____	_____
2. cyanosis	_____	_____
3. orthopnea	_____	_____
4. tachypnea	_____	_____
5. epiglottitis	_____	_____
6. pulmonary	_____	_____
7. pneumothorax	_____	_____
8. sinusitis	_____	_____
9. tuberculosis	_____	_____
10. bronchiolitis	_____	_____

Circle the appropriate term from each pair in the following sentences.

1. Cystic fibrosis/fibrositis is usually diagnosed in infancy.

2. Infants and young children are especially vulnerable to RSV/RSVP.

3. UIR/URI is a common diagnosis in children.

4. Emphysema/Empathy is often associated with chronic bronchitis.

5. CORD/COPD is a chronic respiratory illness.

6. Asthma/Anathema may be caused by allergies.

7. RIDS/IRDS is a life-threatening condition of premature infants.

8. Aspiration/Assumption pneumonia can result from inhaling chemical fumes.

9. Atolitis/Atelectasis is a Greek term meaning incomplete expansion.

10. Pleurisy/Purist is an inflammation of the membrane around the lungs.

Match a term from the first column with a definition from the second column. Write the number of the term on the line beside the definition.

Terms   **Definitions**

1. thoracotomy   _____   a. discharge from the nose (runny nose)

2. thoracentesis   _____   b. condition of blueness (blue color of skin and mucous membranes)

3. pharyngitis   _____   c. visual examination of the bronchi with a lighted instrument

4. lobectomy   _____   d. incision into the chest

5. rhinorrhea   _____   e. excessive breathing

6. hemothorax   _____   f. puncture of the chest to remove fluid

7. cyanotic   _____   g. inflammation of the pharynx

8. laryngospasm   _____   h. removal of a lobe (of the lung)

9. hyperventilation   _____   i. collection of blood in the chest

10. bronchoscopy   _____   j. spasm of the larynx

Use prefixes, root words, combining forms, and suffixes to create medical terms for the definitions given. Write the term on the blank provided.

1. inflammation of the nose   _____

2. surgical incision into the trachea   _____

3. surgical repair of the thorax   _____

4. examination of the thorax using an instrument   _____

5. pertaining to the larynx   _____

6. inflammation of the pleura   _____

7. lack of breathing or respiration   _____

8. inflammation of the bronchi   _____

9. removal of a lung   _____

10. hernia of the bronchus   _____

Identify each term as singular or plural by writing a *P* or *S* beside the term; then give the opposite form (i.e., either plural or singular).

1. bronchi   _____   _____

2. alveoli   _____   _____

3. lung   _____   _____

4. pulmonectomy   _____   _____

5. diaphragm   _____   _____

6. cilia   _____   _____

7. pleura   _____   _____

8. capillary   _____   _____

9. sinus   _____   _____

10. tonsils   _____   _____

The following list has seven terms that describe respiration, all using the same suffix. Supply the terms to match the definitions. What does the suffix mean?

Definition	Suffix
difficult breathing	_____/pnea
easy or normal breathing	_____/pnea
rapid breathing	_____/pnea
slow breathing	_____/pnea
positional (in proper order) breathing	_____/pnea
deep and/or rapid breathing	_____/pnea
shallow and/or slow breathing	_____/pnea

Categorize the following wellness and illness terms according to the life stage in which they usually appear.

Terms

cystic fibrosis	emphysema	IRDS
respiratory syncytial virus	croup	chronic obstructive lung disease
bronchogenic carcinoma	acute epiglottitis	bronchitis

Fetus/Infant/Children   **Seniors**

_____   _____

_____   _____

_____   _____

_____   _____

_____   _____

Diagnosing and Treating Problems

Tests, Procedures, and Pharmaceuticals

One of the most common procedures performed to assess the respiratory system is the chest x-ray. This procedure can help the examiner determine the presence of an abnormality such as infection or increased fluid. When a malignancy is suspected, or if further detail of the respiratory structures is indicated, the physician orders a chest computed tomography (CT) or magnetic resonance imaging (MRI) scan.

A **bronchogram**, or lung scan, is an x-ray procedure that uses a contrast medium to view the bronchial tree. Bronchoscopy is an examination of the bronchi using a flexible instrument called an endoscope, which is inserted through the mouth. **Endoscopy** and **laryngoscopy** use the same instrument to view the larynx, trachea, and esophagus.

Pulmonary function tests help in diagnosing chronic obstructive pulmonary diseases and other lung disorders. These breathing tests include measurement of lung volume and the distribution of gases as they are diffused within the respiratory system.

A **spirometer** measures the amount of air exchanged during each breath. The normal person can take in about 500 ml (about a pint) of air during inspiration and expel it with expiration. The **tidal volume (TV),** named for the flow of the tides, measures the air inhaled and exhaled. The **vital capacity (VC)** measures the largest amount of air breathed out in one expiration after a maximal inhalation. Other measurements include the **expiratory reserve volume (ERV),** the largest amount of air that can be forced out after expiring the tidal volume; **inspiratory reserve volume (IRV)** represents the opposite measurement. The **residual volume (RV)** is the air that remains in the lungs after forceful expiration. Table 10.6 lists pulmonary function test abbreviations.

Table 10.6

Pulmonary Function Test Abbreviations

Abbreviation	Meaning
ERV	expiratory reserve volume
FEF	forced expiratory flow
FEF_{25-75}	forced midexpiratory flow during the middle half of the FVC
FEV	forced expiratory volume
FEV_1	forced expiratory volume in 1 second
FEV_3	forced expiratory volume in 3 seconds
FVC	forced vital capacity
FVL	flow volume loop
IRV	inspiratory reserve volume
PEF	peak expiratory flow
RV	residual volume
TV	tidal volume
VC	vital capacity

The surgical procedure to correct defects in the nose is known as **rhinoplasty** (sometimes called a "nose job"); it can be performed for functional or cosmetic reasons. Table 10.7 summarizes the tests and procedures commonly used in assessing and treating problems of the respiratory system.

Table 10.7

Tests and Procedures Relating to the Respiratory System

Term	Meaning	Word Analysis	
bronchoscopy bron-**kos**-kO-pee	examination of the bronchi	bronch/o -scopy	bronchus use of instrument to examine an area
endoscopy en-**dos**-kO-pee	examination of interior structures of the body with an endoscope	endo- -scopy	within use of instrument to examine an area
intubation in-too-**bay**-shun	insertion of a tube into the nose or mouth to provide for artificial breathing	in- tubus	within tube
laryngectomy lar-in-**jek**-tah-mee	surgical removal of the larynx	laryng/o -ectomy	larynx surgical removal
laryngoscopy lar-in-**gos**-kah-pee	procedure to view the larynx using an endoscope	laryng/o -scopy	larynx use of instrument to examine an area
laryngotomy lar-in-**got**-ah-mee	surgical incision of the larynx	laryng/o -tomy	larynx incision
lobectomy lO-**bek**-tah-mee	surgical removal of a lobe of the lung	lobos -ectomy	lobe surgical removal
pulmonary function tests **pul**-mah-nar-ee **funk**-shun	tests using a special instrument called a spirometer to measure the function of the lungs	pulmon/o -ary	lungs pertaining to

rhinoplasty **rI**-nO-plas-tee	procedure to correct the nose for either physiologic or cosmetic reasons	*rhin/o* *-plasty*	nose surgical repair or reconstruction
spirometry spI-**rom**-ah-tree	pulmonary function test	*spir/o* *-metry*	breath process of measuring
thoracentesis thor-ah-sen-**tee**-sis	procedure to place a hole in the pleural space to remove fluid	*thorac/o* *centesis*	chest surgical puncture
thoracotomy thor-ah-**kot**-ah-mee	incision into the chest wall	*thorac/o* *-tomy*	chest incision
tracheostomy tray-kee-**os**-tah-mee tracheotomy tray-kee-**ot**-ah-mee	surgical procedure to make an opening into the trachea (throat)	*trache/o* *os* *-tomy*	trachea orifice incision

Pharmacologic Agents

Many of the agents used to correct problems in the respiratory system are antibiotics, which are important in fighting infections. Cough and cold preparations can be purchased over the counter or with a prescription. Allergy medications are given to suppress the symptoms of allergies and colds. Table 10.8 lists pharmacologic agents pertinent to the respiratory system.

Table 10.8

Pharmacologic Agents Relating to the Respiratory System

Description	Use	Drug class	Generic name	Brand names
allergy preparations	decrease the symptoms of allergies (see Chapter 6, "Immunology," for further discussion)		loratadine	Claritin
antibiotics, antibacterials, antimicrobials	treat bacterial infections	aminoglycosides cephalosporins penicillins miscellaneous	gentamicin tobramycin cefaclor cefazolin ceftazidime clarithromycin amoxicillin vancomycin	Garamycin Tobrex Ceclor Ancef Fortaz Biaxin Amoxil Vancocin
antifungals	treat fungal infections		amphotericin B fluconazole nystatin	Fungizone Diflucan Mycostatin
antimycobacterial (antituberculosis)	treat *mycobacterium* infections		ethambutol isoniazid rifampin	Myambutol Nydrazid Rifadin
antivirals	treat viral disease		acyclovir zidovudine	Zovirax Retrovir
antipyretics	decrease fever		acetaminophen aspirin (not to be used for infants and children) ibuprofen	Tylenol Genuine Bayer Advil, Motrin

antitussives	suppress cough		benzonatate codeine guaifenesin and dextromethorphan	Tessalon Perles (various brands) Robitussin-DM
asthma preparations	open the respiratory airways and prevent further constriction		albuterol sulfate theophylline beclomethasone dipropionate ipratropium bromide	Proventil, Ventolin Theochron Beconase Atrovent
decongestants	decrease the stuffy nose and congested sinus cavities associated with URI		pseudoephedrine sulfate	Sudafed

Table 10.9

Abbreviations

Abbreviation	Meaning
ABG	arterial blood gas
AFB	acid-fast bacilli
AP	anterior posterior (used with x-ray views)
ARDS	acute respiratory distress syndrome
BiPAP	bilevel positive airway pressure
CO_2	carbon dioxide
COLD	chronic obstructive lung disease
COPD	chronic obstructive pulmonary disease
CPAP	continuous positive airway pressure
CPR	cardiopulmonary resuscitation
CXR	chest x-ray
DNR	do not resuscitate
IRDS	infant respiratory distress syndrome
IPPB	intermittent positive pressure breathing
IS	incentive spirometry
MDI	metered-dose inhaler
O_2	oxygen
PA	posterior anterior (used with x-ray views)
PAP	positive airway pressure
PEEP	positive end-expiratory pressure
PFT	pulmonary function test
RDS	respiratory distress syndrome
SOB	shortness of breath
TB	tuberculosis
URI	upper respiratory infection
VC	vital capacity

Divide each term into its individual word parts, then write a definition of the term. Use hyphens to separate the word parts.

1. bronchioles _____

2. laryngoscope _____

3. nasal _____

4. pulmonologist _____

5. spirometry _____

6. rhinitis _____

7. thoracostomy _____

8. tracheobronchitis _____

9. tubercular _____

10. pleuritis _____

Comprehension Check

Exercise 16

Circle the correct term from the pair in each sentence.

1. Mr. Tyson has an order for home O_2 for his <u>COPD/DOD</u>.

2. The doctor prescribed codeine as an <u>antitussive/antiemetic</u> for Tara's cough.

3. The patient's temperature was 102° F; the physician ordered ASA as an <u>antipyretic/antitussive</u>.

4. <u>Intubation/Mediation</u> was achieved without difficulty, and inhalation anesthesia was started at 8:05 A.M.

5. The patient was on assisted <u>ventilation/application</u> for three weeks following the accident.

6. <u>Antibiotic/antineoplastic</u> ointment will be applied to the wound twice daily, at each dressing change.

7. The patient was given a prescription for a <u>decongestant/debridement</u> and an antibiotic and was instructed to RTC in 1 week.

8. The patient's <u>tidal volume/tidal income</u> was measured during the test.

9. Plan: <u>Ibuprofen/Coumadin</u> every four hours, elevate leg, and apply moist heat to affected joint for thirty minutes four times daily.

10. The patient's chart is flagged for <u>DNR/MVA</u>, at his own request.

Match the term to the definition.

1. stridor _____ a. difficulty breathing

2. hypoxia _____ b. incision into the trachea

3. hypercapnia _____ c. inflammation of the pleura

4. dyspnea _____ d. noisy breathing indicating a tracheal obstruction

5. bronchiolitis _____ e. disease caused by the organism Mycobacterium tuberculosis

6. pharyngitis _____ f. inflammation of the pharynx

7. pleurisy _____ g. inflammation of the bronchioles

8. pneumonia _____ h. having too much carbon dioxide

9. tuberculosis _____ i. inflammation of the lung tissue

10. tracheostomy _____ j. having too little oxygen

Word Building

Supply the word parts to complete each term, according to the definition provided.

1. Fibro_____ is a condition of fiber.

2. Laryngo_____ means inflammation of the larynx, trachea, and bronchi.

3. Dys_____ refers to difficulty breathing.

4. _____y means pertaining to respiration or breathing.

5. Bronchi_____ means chronic dilation of the bronchi and bronchioles due to obstruction or disease.

6. Cyst___ means pertaining to a cyst.

7. A laryngo_____ is an instrument to examine the larynx.

8. A lob_____ is a removal of a lobe of the lung.

9. _____otomy refers to incision into the larynx.

10. ___tub_____ means insertion of a tube into the nose or mouth for assisted ventilation.

11. _____eal means pertaining to the pharynx.

12. Thora_____ refers to puncture of the thorax to remove fluid.

Read each term and decide if it is spelled correctly. If not, write the correct spelling on the line. Otherwise write "correct."

1. organusm _____

2. x-ray _____

3. aerway _____

4. gasseous _____

5. virusses _____

6. tisseu _____

7. imhalation _____

8. pneumonogram _____

9. infection _____

10. pathogem _____

Word Maps

Exercise 20

The terms listed below are names for diagnostic and therapeutic procedures. Create a chart by organizing the terms under the correct category.

laryngotomy   lobectomy   tracheostomy   pulmonary function tests

laryngectomy   endoscopy   spirometry   thoracentesis

bronchoscopy   intubation   laryngoscopy

lobotomy   thoracotomy   rhinoplasty

Diagnostic Procedures

_____

_____

_____

_____

_____

_____

_____

_____

_____

Therapeutic Procedures

_____

_____

_____

_____

_____

_____

_____

_____

Performance Assessment 10

Crossword Puzzle

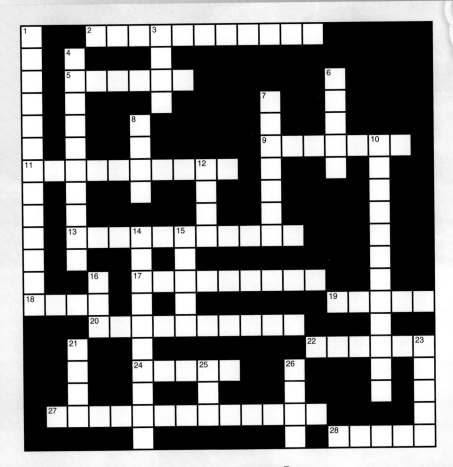

Across
2. separates the nasal cavity
5. membrane surrounding the lungs
9. tiny hollow sacs containing air
11. area of pharynx behind the mouth
13. muscles between and attached to the ribs, used in respiration
17. pertaining to the lungs
18. suffix meaning incision
19. pertaining to the nose
20. substance in the alveoli; decreases surface tension
22. name for type of membrane that lines respiratory system
24. Latin for tube
27. waste gas exhaled by humans
28. nostrils

Down
1. physician specializing in the respiratory system
3. a combining form meaning air
4. elastic cartilage that acts as valve on top of larynx
6. sections of the lungs
7. windpipe
8. root meaning blue
10. instrument used to examine the larynx
12. a combining form meaning nose
14. breathing out
15. hairlike structures that propel mucus and invading matter toward the mouth
16. prefix meaning difficult or painful
21. suffix meaning breath
23. Latin for cavity
25. abbreviation for infection of the upper respiratory tract
26. prefix meaning within

Build the Terms

Select word parts from the lists to build a complete medical term for each definition given. Note that not all terms will have a root or combining form, prefix, and suffix. Some word parts may be used more than once. This exercise may require use of a medical dictionary.

Combining Forms	Prefixes	Suffixes
pneumo/o	hyper-	-ia
aer/o	dys-	-itis
pharyng/o	sub-	-genic
thorac/o	hypo-	-pnea
pleur/o	pre-	-ology
sinus/o	para-	-pathy
ox/y	an-	-al
bronch/o	pre-	-cele
alveol/o	de-	-ic
phon/o	hydro-	-centesis
rhin/o	per-	-lithiasis
trache/o	bi-	-ia
pneumon/o	sub-	-ary
py/o	-en	-cele
pulmon/o	quadra-	-otomy

1. pouch filled with air   _____

2. puncture of the lung to withdraw fluid   _____

3. formation of stones (calculi) in the lungs   _____

4. difficulty speaking   _____

5. inflammation in the lungs   _____

6. iflammation of the bronchioles   _____

7. incision into the lung   _____

8. pertaining to the thorax   _____

9. inflammation of the sinuses   _____

10. deficient oxygen   _____

11. study of the organs of respiration   _____

12. originating or arising in the bronchi   _____

Analyze the Terms

Circle the root (or roots) of each term. Write a definition for the root (or roots) and a definition for the entire term.

1. pulmonary _____

_____

2. edematous _____

_____

3. dyspnea _____

_____

4. bilateral _____

_____

5. mesothelioma _____

_____

6. epiglottis _____

_____

7. nasopharynx _____

_____

8. alveolar _____

_____

9. lobectomy _____

_____

10. paranasal _____

_____

What Do These Abbreviations Mean?

Provide a definition for each of the abbreviations listed.

1. ARDS _____

2. BiPAP _____

3. CPAP _____

4. CXR _____

5. IRDS _____

6. MDI _____

7. PA _____

8. PEEP _____

9. PFT _____

10. TB _____

What's Your Conclusion?

Read each mini medical record or scenario carefully; then select the physician's likely response. Write the letter of your answer in the space provided.

1. A 10-year-old male patient presents in the Family Practice Residency clinic with symptoms of coryza, malaise, muscle pain, and productive cough of forty-eight hours duration. Auscultation reveals rales and wheezing following coughing. Temperature is 101° F; other VS are WNL. He is accompanied by his grandmother who reports that he has no chronic illnesses, and aside from an occasional ear infection as an infant, he has always been well. You expect:

   A. That the doctor will diagnose COPD and order a CXR.
   B. The child has flulike symptoms and Tylenol will be prescribed. The doctor may want to recheck the patient in five to seven days, and will prescribe an antibiotic only if the child's condition becomes worse as evidenced by increased fever, increased sputum production, or purulent sputum.

   Your response: _____

2. On the same day, a 49-year-old male comes to the clinic. He lists his occupation as "foundry worker." He reports a dry cough and mild dyspnea. He states he has come to the clinic to satisfy his wife, who believes "there is something wrong." He reports that he was a smoker for twenty-five years, but quit about six years ago. VS: T 98.6° F, P 84, R 38, BP 140/88. You expect the doctor will:

   A. Auscultate all lung fields and order a CXR and initial pulmonary function tests to rule out silicosis.
   B. Tell the patient that his lungs have not yet recovered from his smoking, and his current illness reflects that. She will prescribe an antibiotic.

   Your response: _____

3. A 19-year-old male is the last patient of the day. He comes in just as the clinic is closing. He is accompanied by both his mother and father, and the family states that he was involved in a motorcycle accident about two hours ago. His injuries did not initially appear to be serious, but since the accident he has begun to experience sharp, stabbing pain in the area of his right shoulder and a lesser pain in his chest. He is slightly dyspneic and has various abnormalities in his breath sounds. Respirations are 28. PE reveals a small puncture wound on the right lateral chest, in the 5th intercostal space. You expect the physician will:

   A. Call the x-ray department and tell them there is a patient with a suspected pneumothorax and order a stat. CXR.
   B. Tape the patient's ribs and prescribe rest and Tylenol.

   Your response: _____

Analyzing Medical Records

Read the physician's clinic note on the next page, then answer the following questions.

1. What is the patient's occupation? Might this be a factor in the illness?

2. What are two findings with regard to the patient's health history?

3. Briefly describe the findings from the physical examination.

4. What is the analysis? Is this a chronic illness?

5. Which medications were prescribed? How often will the patient take the medications and for how long?

6. What radiologic studies will be done?

7. Will further laboratory studies be done? If so, what are they?

8. What additional action is the patient to take?

Hayes-Oakwood Clinic, Inc.

407 S. Parkway, Accord City, KS 77709-4321
phone (333) 555-1122 fax (333) 555-1234

Physician's Clinic Note

PATIENT: Brenda M
DATE: January 20, xxxx

S: This is a 24 y/o female, in no obvious respiratory distress. Patient c/o sudden onset of chest pain, beginning two days ago. This is a vague, generalized discomfort that is aggravated by breathing and coughing. She states that she often becomes fatigued and must stop to rest when doing even simple activities. She reports no other symptoms, and states she has no chronic illnesses and has not been involved in any accidents recently. She has a history of childhood asthma, but no attacks in several years. She is a medical office worker, and has no known exposure to toxic substances. She was ill about a month ago with pneumonia, which was treated with antibiotics. She did not keep her follow-up appointment to recheck the pneumonia following therapy.

O: VS: T 102° F, P 70, R 30 and shallow, BP 120/68.
Breath sounds are diminished; no wheezes, rales, or crackles are noted. Coughing is minimal and nonproductive. A few fine crackles are auscultated over the right lateral chest. No cyanosis; motion of the chest wall is symmetrical. No other remarkable findings.

A: Pleurisy.

P: 1) Obtain CXR to R/O fluid accumulation in the pleural space.
2) Oral penicillin G, 400,000 U, q.6h., for 10 days.
3) Ibuprofen, 800 mg, q.4h.
4) Pt. to phone the clinic tomorrow for results of CXR and follow-up instructions.

_____
C. McCann, MD

Using Medical References

The following sentences contain medical terms, which may not have been addressed on the charts in this chapter. Use medical reference books, your medical term analysis skills, and/or a medical dictionary to find the correct definition of each underlined word. Write the definition on the line below the sentence.

1. The patient was admitted to Crone Medical Center with a diagnosis of <u>pulmonary embolism</u>.

   _____

2. Mrs. Gates is being treated for <u>pulmonary edema</u>, secondary to cardiovascular disease.

   _____

3. P: Obtain <u>sputum</u> specimen for C&S.

_____

4. The <u>mediastinum</u> was shifted toward the area of atelectasis.

_____

5. The patient's atelectasis developed slowly and was <u>asymptomatic</u>.

_____

6. <u>Postmortem</u> examination revealed pulmonary embolism.

_____

7. With a diagnosis of pneumonia, the <u>prognosis</u> for a healthy adult is good.

_____

8. Second-year residents will describe the <u>pathogenesis</u> of each illness.

_____

9. Sharp pain was present in the involved <u>hemithorax</u>.

_____

10. Dr. Halliston performed the <u>pulmonary embolectomy</u>.

_____

11. As the illness evolves, <u>expectoration</u> typically increases.

_____

12. <u>Hemorrhagic</u> areas were observed throughout the lungs.

_____

Short Answer

Answer one of the following questions in plain language.

Why can humans not live for more than a few minutes without oxygen coming into and carbon dioxide going out of the body?

    OR

Describe the process of gas exchange.

_____

_____

_____

_____

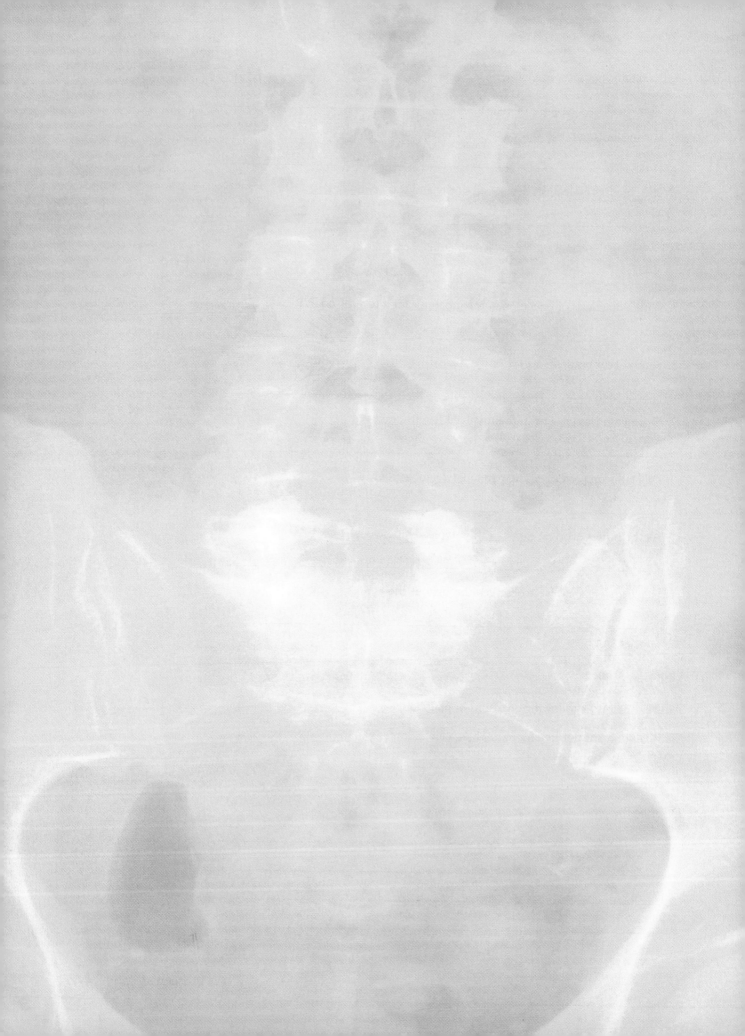

Chapter 11

The Cardiovascular System

Learning Outcomes

Students will be able to:
- Identify the structures of the heart.
- Trace the elements of the cardiac cycle.
- Describe the function of the heart and major vessels.
- Explain how blood flows through the body.
- Use correctly the terminology of the cardiovascular system in written and oral communication.
- Correctly spell and pronounce cardiovascular system terminology.
- State the meaning of abbreviations related to the cardiovascular system.
- List and define the combining forms most commonly used to create terms related to the cardiovascular system.
- Name tests and treatments for major cardiovascular abnormalities.

Translation, Please?Translation, Please?Translation, Please?

Read this excerpt from a physician's report and try to answer the questions that follow it.

The patient was taken to the CCU after the cardiac catheterization with balloon angioplasty. Following the procedure, there was no evidence of ischemia, and the patient was released to the post-CCU without incident.

1. Did this patient go to an intensive care unit?
2. A balloon was placed into the patient's heart. True or false?
3. Is ischemia part of the ischium or a term to describe blood flow?

Answers to "Translation Please?"
1. Yes, to an intensive care unit called the coronary care unit.
2. False. Angio- means vessel, not heart. The suffix -plasty means repair.
3. Ischemia is a term used to describe decreased blood flow.

Identifying the Specialty

The System and Its Practitioners

Some say that the heart is the most important organ in the body, a perspective clearly reflected in the original meaning of its Indo-European root *kerd*: the physical blood-pumping organ and the residence of life, soul, or spirit. Kerd became *kardia* in Greek, *cor* in Latin, *heorte* in Old English, and *heart* in modern English.

By practical measures, the heart ranks as one of the hardest-working organs, providing the pumping system for all of the vital fluids of the body and working 24 hours every day of our lives. Besides the heart, the cardiovascular

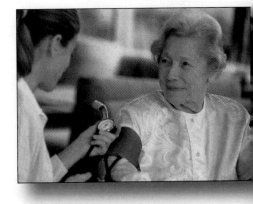

system includes the intricate system of blood vessels throughout the body. The heart is the pump that moves blood, nutrients, lymph, chemical gases, electrolytes, and other components from one area to another. The vessels provide the miles of "roadway" for this transportation system.

The medical specialty is known as **cardiology** (root is *cardi* from the Greek *kardia* for heart). The physicians who treat problems of the cardiovascular system include the **cardiologist**, the **interventional cardiologist**, and the **cardiac surgeon**. The vessels are treated by **vascular surgeons** (often called **cardiovascular surgeons**).

Examining the Patient ♂♀

Anatomy and Physiology of the Cardiovascular System

The **heart** is located in the center of the thoracic cavity, between the lungs and behind the sternum (Figure 11.1A). Two-thirds of the heart is located in the left side of the chest, with the pointed portion, the **apex**, facing downward and to the right, and the base facing upward on the left side. This fist-sized organ has a three-layer wall, as shown in Figure 11.1B:

- An outer membrane called the **pericardium**, a fibrous tissue that itself is layered into a **parietal pericardium** (an outer layer lining the pericardium) and a **visceral pericardium**, or **epicardium** (an inner layer covering the heart); between the layers is a tiny space, called the **pericardial cavity**, which is filled with a moist serous fluid that prevents friction.

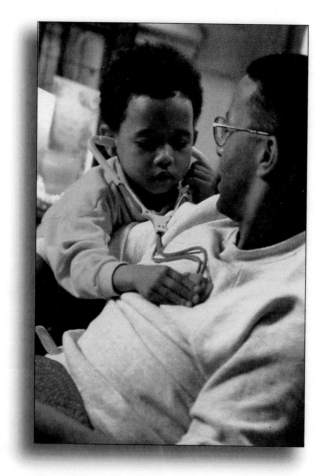

- A middle layer of thick muscle tissue called the **myocardium**.

- An inner layer of epithelial tissue called the **endocardium**.

- An outer pericardial sac completely surrounds the heart and bathes it in pericardial fluid to prevent further rubbing during each heartbeat.

The heart is hollow, consisting of two halves separated lengthwise by a wall called the **septum**. The right half pumps oxygen-depleted blood to the lungs, where it is resupplied with oxygen. The left half pumps oxygen-rich blood to the body's tissues. Each half has an upper and lower chamber. The upper chambers, or **atria,** are the blood-receiving chambers and thus are less muscular than the lower chambers, the **ventricles**, which are the actual pumps. The chambers are named for their location within the heart: right and left atria and right and left ventricles (Figure 11.1B).

Valves connect the upper and lower chambers within each half of the heart, serving as floodgates for the blood flow. The two atrial valves that open into the ventricles are known as **atrioventricular (AV) valves**. The **bicuspid valve** is located between the left atrium and ventricle. It is also known as the **mitral valve** because its shape resembles that of a bishop's hat with two corners (*mitra* is Latin for headband or turban; the term evolved to *miter*, meaning the headdress worn by bishops). The **tricuspid valve** is located between the right atrium and ventricle. The AV valves prevent blood from flowing back into the atria. The mitral

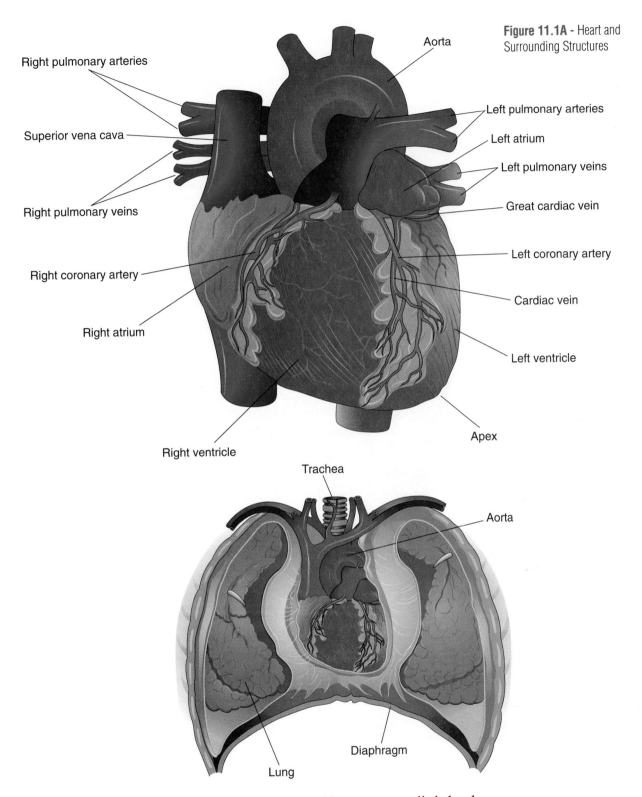

Figure 11.1A - Heart and Surrounding Structures

Right pulmonary arteries

Superior vena cava

Right pulmonary veins

Right coronary artery

Right atrium

Right ventricle

Aorta

Left pulmonary arteries

Left atrium

Left pulmonary veins

Great cardiac vein

Left coronary artery

Cardiac vein

Left ventricle

Apex

Trachea

Aorta

Diaphragm

Lung

and tricuspid valves open and close together. Stringlike structures called **chordae tendineae** attach the valves to the heart walls.

Additional valves located within the ventricular chambers are known as **semilunar valves**. They lead into the large vessels of the body that carry blood to and from the heart. The **pulmonary semilunar valve** is located at the opening of the pulmonary artery, and the **aortic semilunar valve** is located at the opening of the aorta. The semilunar valves also work at the same time. They are closed when the AV valves are open, and they are open when the AV valves are closed.

Figure 11.1B - Internal View of the Heart

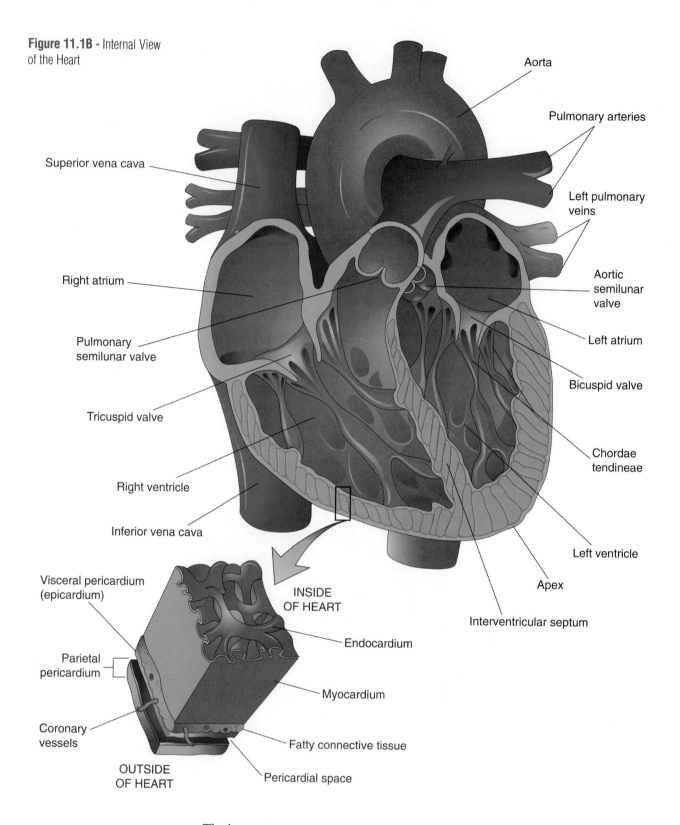

Aorta

Pulmonary arteries

Superior vena cava

Left pulmonary veins

Aortic semilunar valve

Right atrium

Left atrium

Pulmonary semilunar valve

Bicuspid valve

Tricuspid valve

Chordae tendineae

Right ventricle

Left ventricle

Inferior vena cava

Apex

Interventricular septum

INSIDE OF HEART

Visceral pericardium (epicardium)

Endocardium

Parietal pericardium

Myocardium

Coronary vessels

Fatty connective tissue

OUTSIDE OF HEART

Pericardial space

The heart is a strong, muscular structure that contracts to pump blood through the body. Each contraction, called **systole**, is followed by a relaxation phase called **diastole**. Each heartbeat is a contraction, first by the atria and then by the ventricles. The systole and diastole paired together represent the **cardiac cycle**, which takes about 0.8 second to complete if a person has a heart rate of about 72 beats per minute. A patient's **cardiac output** is the volume of blood pumped by the ventricle in 1 minute.

ATRIAL SYSTOLE

Figure 11.2A - Blood Flow through the Heart.
A: Atrial Systole

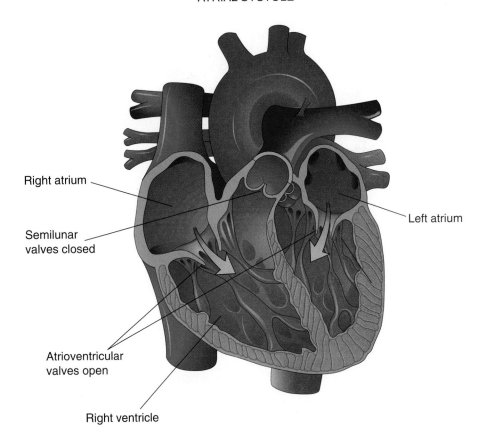

Right atrium

Semilunar
valves closed

Left atrium

Atrioventricular
valves open

Right ventricle

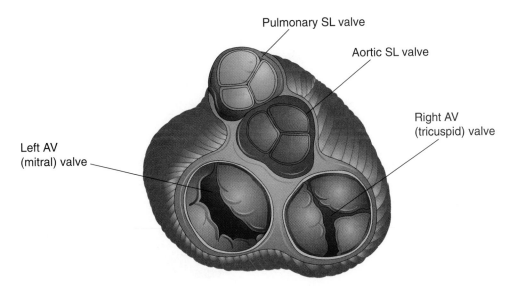

Pulmonary SL valve

Aortic SL valve

Right AV
(tricuspid) valve

Left AV
(mitral) valve

Blood Flow through the Heart

The pumping of blood through the heart begins with the atrial systole (Figure 11.2A). Blood enters the right atrium through the large vessels known as the **superior** and **inferior venae cavae**. This blood arrives from all over the body and thus has a low oxygen and high carbon dioxide content. It passively flows through the tricuspid valve into the right ventricle. On the next contraction, the blood is forced into pulmonary circulation—through the pulmonary semilunar valve, into the pulmonary artery, and

Figure 11.2B - Blood Flow through the Heart.
B: Ventricular Systole

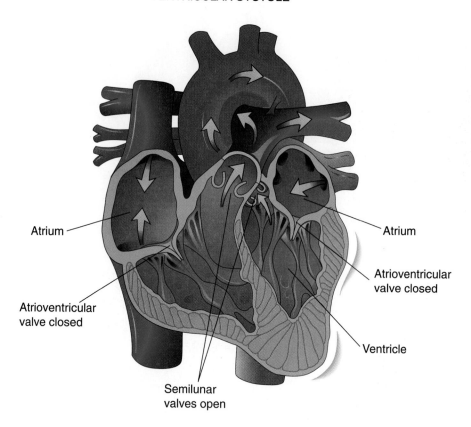

Atrium

Atrioventricular valve closed

Atrioventricular valve closed

Ventricle

Semilunar valves open

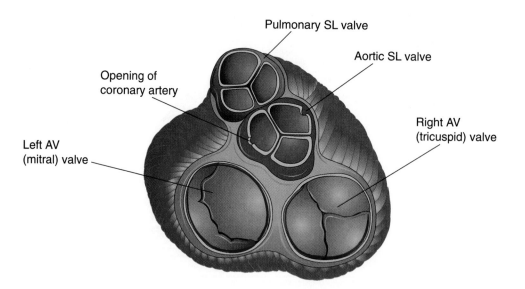

Pulmonary SL valve

Aortic SL valve

Opening of coronary artery

Right AV (tricuspid) valve

Left AV (mitral) valve

eventually to the lungs. Gas exchange occurs in these organs (recall Chapter 10, The Respiratory System), the blood is replenished with oxygen, and the carbon dioxide is removed (exhaled). Figure 11.3 depicts this cycle.

The left ventricle pumps reoxygenated blood into the blood vessel network for circulation throughout the body. This blood is the source of oxygen and nourishment for each of the approximately 75 trillion cells in the human body.

Blood flows from the liver to the inferior vena cava and from the head and upper extremities to the superior vena cava. The blood continues into the right atrium to

Figure 11.3 - Gas Exchange

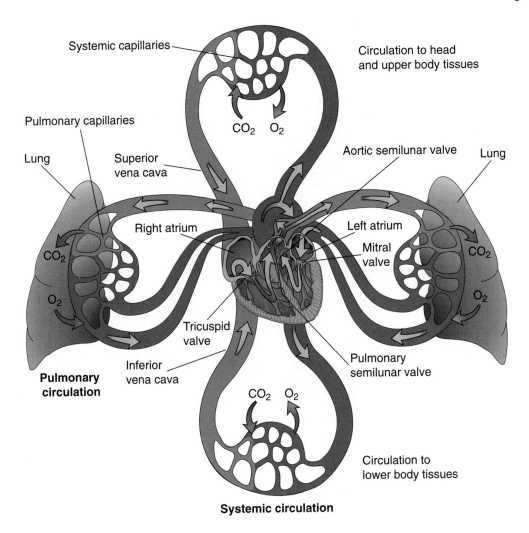

Systemic capillaries

Circulation to head
and upper body tissues

CO_2 O_2

Pulmonary capillaries

Lung

Superior
vena cava

Aortic semilunar valve

Lung

Right atrium

Left atrium

Mitral
valve

CO_2

CO_2

O_2

O_2

Tricuspid
valve

Inferior
vena cava

Pulmonary
semilunar valve

**Pulmonary
circulation**

CO_2 O_2

Circulation to
lower body tissues

Systemic circulation

the tricuspid valve to the right ventricle through the pulmonary semilunar valve and into the pulmonary artery. Unoxygenated blood flows to the lungs, which oxygenates the blood. Then it flows into the pulmonary veins and into the left atrium through the mitral valve to the left ventricle, through the aortic semilunar valve and into the aorta from which oxygenated blood is pumped to the entire body.

The system that causes the pumping action works like an electrical circuit. This conduction system consists of an area called the **sinoatrial (SA) node,** also known as the pacemaker, which determines the rhythm of the heartbeat. (The autonomic nervous system is responsible for the heart rate.) The **atrioventricular (AV) node,** the **AV bundle** (or **bundle of His**), and the **Purkinje fibers** are part of this system and responsible for moving the impulses through the heart. (Follow Figure 11.4, Conduction System of the Heart.) The SA node begins the process (1) and spreads the impulse through the atria, causing the atrial contraction. The AV node (2) moves the impulse to the bundle of His (3) and on to the Purkinje fibers (4), causing the ventricles to contract.

Figure 11.4 - Conduction
System of the Heart

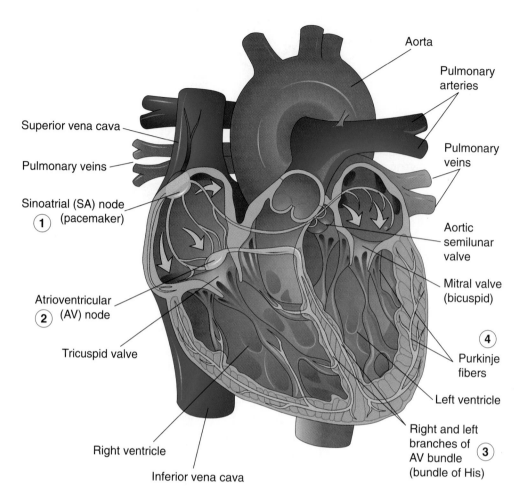

Aorta

Pulmonary
arteries

Superior vena cava

Pulmonary veins

Pulmonary
veins

Sinoatrial (SA) node
① (pacemaker)

Aortic
semilunar
valve

Mitral valve
(bicuspid)

Atrioventricular
② (AV) node

④

Purkinje
fibers

Tricuspid valve

Left ventricle

Right ventricle

Right and left
branches of ③
AV bundle
(bundle of His)

Inferior vena cava

Circulation of Blood: The Blood Vessels

Blood is carried throughout the body by a series of blood vessels. Figure 11.5A shows the major veins and Figure 11.5B shows the major arteries. The **arteries** carry blood away from the heart through the largest artery, the **aorta**, toward vessels that become progressively smaller, **arterioles**, and finally ending in the smallest vessels, **capillaries**, where nutrients and gases are exchanged. Blood then enters the venous system, going into tiny **venules**, which eventually lead into the larger **veins**, the largest being the superior and inferior venae cavae. Veins and arteries are similar in structure. Each is composed of three layers including an outer connective tissue layer, a middle smooth-muscle layer with elastic tissue, and an internal endothelial layer. The internal endothelial layer surrounds the **lumen**, the passage through which the blood flows. Veins have one-way valves that prevent the backflow of blood.

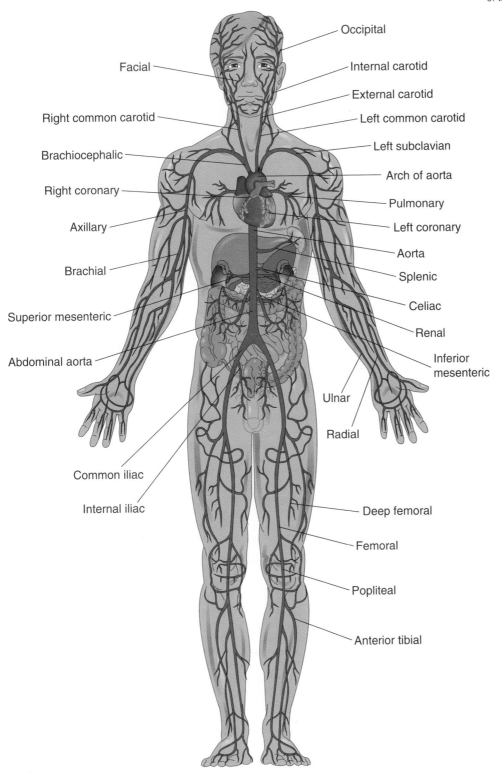

Figure 11.5A - Major Arteries of the Body

Occipital

Facial

Internal carotid

External carotid

Right common carotid

Left common carotid

Brachiocephalic

Left subclavian

Right coronary

Arch of aorta

Axillary

Pulmonary

Left coronary

Brachial

Aorta

Splenic

Superior mesenteric

Celiac

Renal

Abdominal aorta

Inferior mesenteric

Ulnar

Radial

Common iliac

Internal iliac

Deep femoral

Femoral

Popliteal

Anterior tibial

The heart itself has a circulatory system, the **coronary circulation** (root: *coron* for circle or crown from the Latin *coronas* for crown), which brings it nutrients and oxygen. The **right** and **left coronary arteries** deliver the blood into the heart muscle itself. When one or both of these important vessels become clogged, a heart attack results.

Figure 11.5B - Major Veins
of the Body

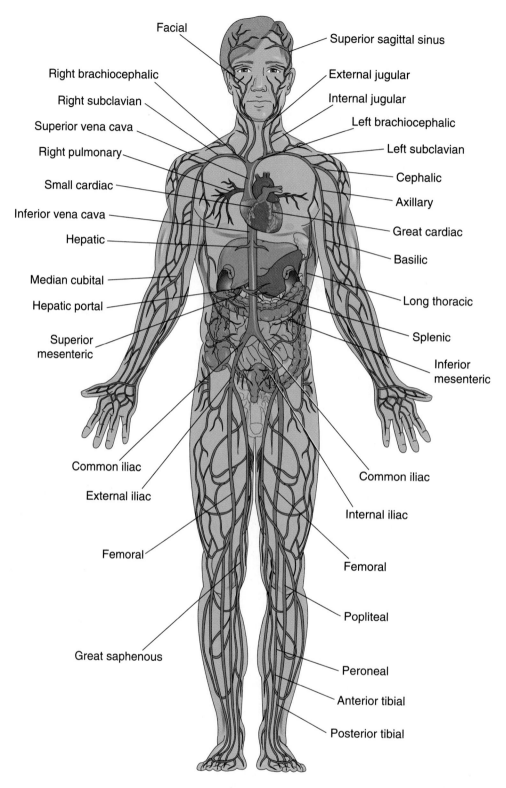

Facial

Superior sagittal sinus

Right brachiocephalic

External jugular

Right subclavian

Internal jugular

Superior vena cava

Left brachiocephalic

Right pulmonary

Left subclavian

Small cardiac

Cephalic

Inferior vena cava

Axillary

Hepatic

Great cardiac

Median cubital

Basilic

Hepatic portal

Long thoracic

Superior
mesenteric

Splenic

Inferior
mesenteric

Common iliac

Common iliac

External iliac

Internal iliac

Femoral

Femoral

Popliteal

Great saphenous

Peroneal

Anterior tibial

Posterior tibial

Each blood vessel type has its own function. In addition to moving blood from
the heart to the capillaries for nutrient and gas exchange, the arteries and arterioles
help to maintain the body's blood pressure. They constrict and dilate to keep the
blood flow within the vessels and throughout the body at an even pressure gradient.
This gradient ensures that the blood flows from the largest vessels to the smallest.

Figure 11.6 - Pulse Points

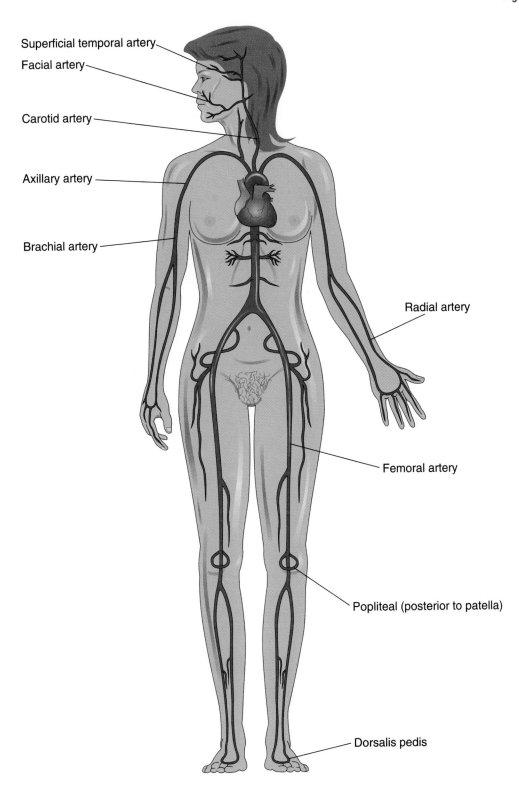

Superficial temporal artery

Facial artery

Carotid artery

Axillary artery

Brachial artery

Radial artery

Femoral artery

Popliteal (posterior to patella)

Dorsalis pedis

The **pulse** felt in different parts of the body is actually an artery expanding and contracting. Figure 11.6 shows the areas of the body where pulses can be felt. The rate, rhythm, and strength of the pulse provide insight into the function of the heart and vessels.

Blood Pressure

High blood pressure, or **hypertension**, means that resistance within the vessels is preventing adequate blood flow. The danger of high blood pressure is the risk that a vessel could rupture and cause a stroke. However, low blood pressure, or **hypotension**, could mean that too little blood is flowing to the organs of the body such as the brain, heart, liver, or kidneys. This lack of oxygenation (resulting from decreased circulation) could cause serious damage to the organs and the body as a whole and perhaps result in death.

What does the actual measurement of blood pressure represent? Blood pressure is written as a fraction; therefore, a person could have a blood pressure of 120/70 (spoken as 120 over 70). The top number is called the **systolic pressure**. It is the maximum arterial pressure during each cardiac cycle. The bottom number is called the **diastolic pressure** and represents the minimum arterial pressure.

Blood flows to all parts of the body via the arteries and veins. The **systemic circulation**, shown in Figure 11.3, is the blood flow from the left ventricle through the body as a whole. The **pulmonary circulation** is the flow of blood from the right ventricle to the lungs via the pulmonary artery (for exchange of gases) and then back to the left atrium through the four **pulmonary veins**.

Table 11.1 lists combining forms associated with the circulatory system; Table 11.2 summarizes the system's common anatomy and physiology terms.

Table 11.1

Combining Forms Relating to the Circulatory System

Combining form	Meaning	Example
angi/o	vessel	angiogram
arteri/o	artery	arterial
arteriol/o	arteriole	arteriole
ather/o	deposit of pasty material	atherosclerosis
atri/o	atrium	atrioventricular
brady-	slow	bradycardia
cardi/o	heart	cardiodynamics
coron/o	crown or circle	coronary bypass
phleb/o	vein	thrombophlebitis
scler/o	hardening	sclerosis
sept/o	partition	septum
sphygm/o	relating to the pulse	sphygmomanometer
sten/o	narrowing, constriction	stenosis
steth/o	chest	stethoscope
thromb/o	blood clot	thrombosis
varic/o	twisted, swollen vein	varicosity
vas/o	vessel	vasoconstriction
vascul/o	vessel	vascularity
ven/o	vein	venule
ventricul/o	ventricle	ventricular

Table 11.2

Anatomy and Physiology Terms Relating to the Cardiovascular System

Term	Meaning	Word Analysis	
aorta ay-**or**-tah	main artery in the body	*aorta*	to lift up
apex **ay**-peks apices (pl) **ap**-ih-seez	pointed portion of the heart at the lower edge directed toward the midline (the base is at the top of the heart)	*apex*	tip
arteriole ahr-**teer**-ee-Ol	small vessels in the body responsible for blood pressure; they lead into the capillaries	*arteri/o* *-ole*	artery small
artery **ahr**-ter-ee	blood vessel that carries blood away from the heart	*arteri/o*	artery
atrioventricular node **ay**-tree-O-ven-**trik**-yoo-ler	area of the heart responsible for the conduction of electrical impulses	*atri/o* *ventricul/o*	atrium ventricle
atrium **ay**-tree-um	upper chamber of the heart	*atri/o* *-ium*	atrium (of the heart) tissue or structure
bicuspid valve bI-**cus**-pid valv	mitral valve (atrioventricular valve) that has two cusps located between the left atrium and ventricle	*bi-* *cuspis*	two point
bundle of His hiss	group of nerve fibers that conduct the electrical impulses through the heart muscle (atrioventricular bundle)	*His*	19th-century German physician
capillary **kap**-ih-lar-ee	smallest unit of the vascular system; location of oxygen and carbon dioxide exchange	*capillarus*	relating to hair (fine)
chordae tendineae **kor**-dee ten-**dih**-nee-ee	stringlike structures that connect the AV valves to the wall of the heart	*chord* *tendineae*	tendinous structure tendons
diastole dI-**as**-tO-lee	relaxation of the heart muscle	*diastole*	dilation
diastolic pressure dI-as-**tol**-ik **preh**-sher	represents the minimum arterial pressure; the bottom number of the recording of the blood pressure	*diastole* *-ic*	dilation pertaining to
epicardium ep-ih-**kar**-dee-um	membrane that forms the inner layer of the pericardium; covers the myocardium	*epi-* *cardi/o* *-ium*	cover heart tissue or structure
lumen **loo**-men	cavity of a blood vessel	*lumen*	light, window
mitral valve **mI**-trel valv	bicuspid valve located between the left atrium and ventricle (named for mitered hat that bishops wear)	*mitra* *-al*	turban pertaining to
pericardium per-ih-**kar**-dee-um	membrane that surrounds the heart	*peri-* *cardi/o* *-ium*	around; surround heart tissue or structure
pulse	dilation of an artery from the contraction of the heart causing blood to be sent into the vessel	*puls*	pulse
Purkinje fibers poor-**kin**-zheh **fI**-bers	specialized cells located in the walls of the ventricles that are part of the heart's conduction system; they relay impulses from the AV node to the ventricles, causing them to contract	*Purkinje*	19th-century Bohemian anatomist

continued on next page

semilunar valves sem-ih-**loo**-ner valvs	valves located between the two ventricular chambers and the large arteries that carry blood away from the heart	semi- lun/a -ar	half; two moon pertaining to
septum	wall separating the right and left chambers of the heart	sept/o -ium	partition tissue or structure
systole **sis**-tO-lee	contraction of the heart muscle	systole	to contract
systolic pressure sis-**tol**-ik	maximum arterial pressure during each cardiac cycle (recorded as the top number in blood pressure)	systole -ic	to contract pertaining to
tricuspid valve trI-**kus**-pid valv	valve located between the right atrium and ventricle	tri- cuspis -oid	three point like or resembling
vein vayn	vessel that carries blood toward the heart	ven/o	vein
vena cava **vee**-nah **kay**-vah	largest vein in the body	ven/o cava	vein plural of cavus (cavity)
ventricles **ven**-trih-kls	actual pumping chambers of the heart	ventricul/o	ventricle
venules **vee**-nyools	small vessels that collect blood from the capillaries and join to form veins	ven/o -ule	vein small

Word Analysis

Identify the anatomical structures on the accompanying diagram by writing the number of the correct term on the structure. On the line beside each term, write the combining form from which the term is formed.

1. aorta _____

2. atrium _____

3. ventricle _____

4. septum _____

5. epicardium _____

6. endocardium _____

7. (pulmonary) veins _____

8. (pulmonary) artery _____

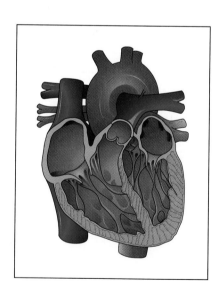

Comprehension Check

Read each sentence and select the best term from the two terms provided. Circle your choice.

1. The medical specialty that diagnoses and treats disorders of the heart is cardiology/hartology.

2. The heart is located in the abdominal/thoracic cavity.

3. Disorders of the blood vessels may be treated by a vascular/vesicular surgeon.

4. The innermost layer of the membrane surrounding the heart is the vascular/visceral pericardium.

5. An inner layer of epithelial tissue in the heart is called the endocardium/epicardium.

6. The two halves of the heart are separated by the speculum/septum.

7. Contractions of the heart are called systole/diastole.

8. The bicuspid/tricuspid valve is located between the right atrium and ventricle.

9. The pulmonary/systemic circulation is the blood flow from the right ventricle to the lungs.

10. The top number in a blood pressure reading is the systolic/diastolic reading.

Matching

Select a term from Column 1 to match the definition in Column 2. Write the number of the term on the line beside its definition.

Column 1		Column 2
1. hypotension	_____	an artery expanding and contracting
2. atria	_____	tiny veins
3. arteries	_____	vessels that carry blood toward the heart
4. veins	_____	part of the heart's conduction system responsible for moving impulses through the heart
5. AV node	_____	low blood pressure
6. arterioles	_____	pumping chamber that sends blood to the body
7. venules	_____	vessels that carry blood to the left atrium
8. left ventricle	_____	vessels that carry blood away from the heart
9. pulse	_____	tiny arteries
10. pulmonary veins	_____	upper chambers of the heart

Select a word part from the list to create the correct term for the definition provided. Note that not all items in the Word Part List will be used.

Word Part List

atrioventricul	thromb	endocard
cardiomy/o	pulmon	cardiopulmon
peri	ven/o	vascul/o
card	chord	
circulat/o	cardi	

1. _____osis means condition of a blood clot.

2. _____itis is an inflammation of the heart muscle.

3. _____ectomy refers to surgical removal of the chordae tendineae.

4. _____pathy means disease of the heart muscle.

5. _____ology refers to study of the heart.

6. _____ar means pertaining to the atrium and the ventricle.

7. _____cardium means surrounding the heart.

8. _____itis is an inflammation of the lining of the heart.

9. _____ary means pertaining to the heart and lungs.

10. _____ry means pertaining to the circulation.

Identify each term as singular or plural by writing a *P* or *S* beside the term; then give the opposite form (i.e., either plural or singular).

1. The <u>apices</u> of all of the hearts in the study were measured. _____ _____

2. All of the <u>valves</u> in his heart were damaged by the toxin. _____ _____

3. These vessels are known as the inferior and superior <u>venae cavae</u>. _____ _____

4. The coronary <u>arteries</u> were clogged with a fatty substance. _____ _____

5. A small <u>capillary</u> was dissected away. _____ _____

6. All of the <u>pulses</u> in the patient's leg were assessed. _____ _____

7. Both <u>ventricles</u> were damaged. _____ _____

8. The atrial and ventricular <u>septa</u> were intact. _____ _____

9. The <u>lumina</u> of the vessels were patent. _____ _____

10. Each <u>vein</u> was carefully removed for transplantation. _____ _____

One concept map below (on the left) illustrates the flow of blood past the major valves of the heart. Complete the map by placing labels in the proper order. The second map below (on the right) describes the muscular heart wall and its covering. Label the sections of the map.

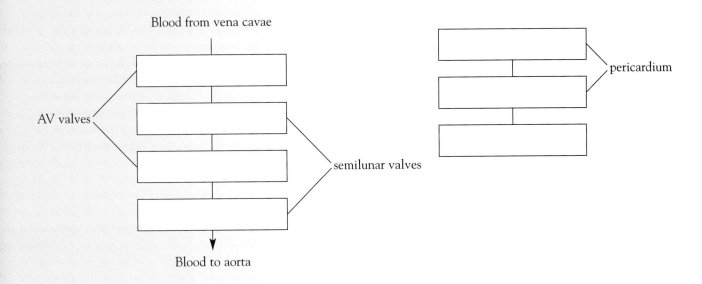

Assessing Patient Health

Wellness and Illness through the Life Span

The first part of the physical examination involves inspection of the patient's skin color, temperature, and texture. Cyanosis, or bluish color, of the skin, mucous membranes, or nail beds may indicate insufficient oxygenated blood flow through the body. Paleness may suggest decreased blood flow; a red face may indicate high blood pressure. All pulses are palpated. A strong, regular pulse should be felt at all pulse points (refer to Figure 11.6). A weak pulse could represent decreased circulation or a blockage leading to the pulse area.

The **stethoscope** is an instrument used to **auscultate**, or listen to, the heart. The normal heart sound is a steady "lub-dub." The "lub," documented as S1, is the first sound heard and represents the closing of the AV valves as the ventricles contract (systole). It is a longer and lower-pitched sound than the "dub," S2, which is the sound of the semilunar valves closing in relaxation (diastole). The examiner listens to the heart on several specific areas of the chest to hear each of the possible sounds of the valves in systole and diastole.

Fetuses and Newborns

The fetal heart begins to beat by about 3 weeks' gestation. Fetal circulation compensates for the nonfunctional lungs by providing oxygen from the placenta. The arterial blood is returned to the right side of the heart. Most of this oxygenated blood goes through an opening in the atrial septum called the **foramen ovale** and flows into the left side of the heart. It is then pumped out through the aorta. The remaining blood is pumped by the right side of the heart through the pulmonary artery to another opening, the **ductus arteriosus**, and then to the aorta. These openings are known as **fetal shunts**.

At birth, the lungs inflate and aeration begins. Circulatory changes take place immediately. The blood is now oxygenated through the lungs, and the foramen ovale closes within about 1 hour of birth because of the lower pressure in the right side of the heart. Within 10 to 15 hours of birth, the ductus arteriosus closes.

The newborn's heart rate may range from 100 to 180 beats per minute and then decrease to about 120 to 140 per minute when awake and about 70 to 90 per minute when asleep. A **murmur**, a type of irregular heart sound, may be heard for several days until the fetal shunts are closed entirely. A persistent murmur may indicate the incomplete closure of a fetal shunt. Skin color is critical in assessing cardiac function, particularly in the newborn. Congenital heart defects may impair cardiac function. For example, the aorta and pulmonary artery may be transposed, or in the opposite locations from where they should be: the aorta is located within the right ventricle, and the pulmonary artery is located within the left ventricle. This defect is called **transposition of the great vessels**. Table 11.3 and Figure 11.7A–E provide descriptions and illustrations of five other defects.

Table 11.3

Congenital Heart Defects

Defect	Description	
atrial septal defect (ASD)	abnormal opening in the atrial septum resulting in excessive pulmonary blood flow **Figure 11.7A** - Atrial Septal Defect	 Atrial septal defect (ASD)
coarctation of the aorta	severe narrowing of the descending portion of the aorta; may have aortic valve defect; the left ventricle overworks **Figure 11.7B** - Coarction of the Aorta	 Coarctation of the aorta
patent ductus arteriosus (PDA)	persistence of the opening of the ductus arteriosus **Figure 11.7C** - Patent Ductus Arteriosus	 Patent ductus arteriosus (PDA)

tetralogy of Fallot	abnormality consisting of four defects: (1) pulmonary artery stenosis, (2) ventricular septal defect, (3) right ventricular hypertrophy, and (4) dextroposition of the aorta **Figure 11.7D** - Tetralogy of Fallot	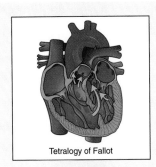 Tetralogy of Fallot
ventricular septal defect (VSD)	abnormal opening in the septum between ventricles **Figure 11.7E** - Ventricular Septal Defect	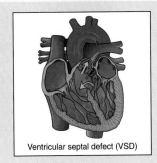 Ventricular septal defect (VSD)

Although valve defects may be present at birth, some occur due to the effects of calcification as the person ages. The murmurs associated with valve defects are listed in Table 11.4. Table 11.5 describes abnormal heart sounds.

Table 11.4

Valve Defects

Type of defect or murmur	Description
aortic regurgitation	blood regurgitates back through the aortic valve into the left ventricle during diastole
aortic stenosis	aortic valve cusps restrict flow of blood during systole owing to calcification
mitral regurgitation	blood regurgitates back through the mitral valve into the left atrium
mitral stenosis	mitral valve does not open properly as a result of calcification
pulmonic regurgitation	blood flows backward through an incompetent pulmonic valve from the pulmonary artery to the right ventricle
pulmonic stenosis	calcification of pulmonic valve restricts forward flow of blood
tricuspid regurgitation	blood regurgitates back through the tricuspid valve into the right atrium
tricuspid stenosis	tricuspid valve does not open properly because of calcification, impeding the flow of blood into the right ventricle during diastole

Table 11.5

Abnormal Heart Sounds

Term	Description
bruit	type of turbulent flow of blood that can be heard in the neck
gallop	very rapid heart beat that sounds like a horse's gallop
murmur	abnormal heart sound that represents turbulent blood flow within the heart
rub	friction heard as a grating sound from inflamed pericardial surface rubbing during heart's contraction
rumble	low-pitched murmur
thrill	type of heart sound that can be felt as a vibration by placing the hand over the heart

Children

The assessment of cardiovascular problems in children includes growth and development, activity level, school performance, skin color, and **clubbing** of fingers and toes (blunt, short, and often cyanotic digits). A child who is not growing appropriately or has decreased energy may have inadequate circulation or poorly oxygenated blood. **Innocent** or **functional** murmurs in childhood are not uncommon. These murmurs have no significance, but the child is usually referred to a pediatric cardiologist for further testing to make that determination.

Pregnant Women

During pregnancy, the blood volume increases by about 40 percent, causing changes within the cardiovascular system. To compensate for the increased blood volume, cardiac output and pulse rate increase and blood pressure changes. Toward the end of pregnancy and in lactating mothers, a murmur termed **mammary soufflé** may be heard because of the increased blood flow through the vessels leading to the mammary artery in the breasts.

Middle-Aged Adults

Middle age brings increased stress emotionally and physiologically. Many persons work extremely hard to provide for themselves and their families, often leaving no time for relaxation, exercise, and good health practices. These factors increase the burden on the cardiovascular system. Poor diet, decreased exercise, and familial factors can lead to **hyperlipemia**, increased blood cholesterol level, early **arteriosclerosis**, hardening of the arteries, and other risks that make a person vulnerable to a heart attack. Even when the body itself gives warning signs and symptoms such as hypertension (high blood pressure) and **angina pectoris** (pain caused by decreased blood flow to the heart muscle), many people pay no attention. A heart attack, or **myocardial infarction**, in this age group can be fatal.

Seniors

As a person matures, the factors of lifestyle, habits, and general health figure significantly in the aging of the cardiovascular system. Smoking, alcohol use, exercise, diet, and stress all play a role, and separating their effects is impossible.

Certain changes occur normally as a person ages. The blood pressure increases by about 25 percent from ages 20 to 80 years because of the normal calcification of the large arteries. The left ventricular wall thickens by about 25 percent to accommodate for the stiffening of the vessels. **Arrhythmias**, irregular heartbeats, may be found in the aging adult. **Ectopic** heartbeats, those outside of the normal conduction pathway from the SA to the AV nodes, also may occur.

Aging causes a gradual thickening of the myocardium, with less mobility in the heart muscle and the entire circulatory system. **Coronary artery disease**, sometimes called hardening of the arteries, increases and accounts for about half of the deaths of older people. These changes make it difficult for the heart and vessels to pump blood and perfuse the body, leading to **congestive heart failure**. This condition is caused by a weak heartbeat, producing increased right atrial pressure and slow right atrial blood outflow. Blood actually backs up in the venous system, affecting the heart, lungs, and kidneys. Many of these problems can be averted by following proper health practices throughout life.

General Illnesses

Bradycardia is a term used to describe a slow heart rate in relation to the individual's age. This condition need not be significant, although it may decrease oxygenated blood to all parts of the body. Some athletes, particularly runners, commonly have slow heart rates. **Tachycardia** describes a rapid heart rate. It is the body's homeostatic mechanism to send (perfuse) enough oxygenated blood through the body.

Cardiomegaly is an enlargement of the heart that can occur for a variety of reasons. Usually the heart becomes enlarged when it must beat with greater force because of a blockage, which makes it difficult to perfuse the body. Table 11.6 lists wellness and illness terms pertaining to the circulatory system, and Table 11.7 summarizes abnormalities in the vasculature.

Table 11.6

Wellness and Illness Terms Relating to the Cardiovascular System

Term	Meaning	Word Analysis	
angina pectoris **an**-jih-nah (an-**jI**-nah) pek-**tor**-is	severe pain in the chest (and often other areas such as arm, jaw, and back) caused by decreased blood flow (insufficient oxygen) to the heart	*angi/o* *-ia*	blood vessel condition of
arrhythmia ah-**rith**-mee-ah	irregular heart rhythm	*a-* *rhythm* *-ia*	abnormal beat condition of
bradycardia bray-dee-**kar**-dee-ah	slow heartbeat	*brady-* *cardi/o* *-ia*	slow heart condition of
cardiomegaly **kahr**-dee-O-**meg**-ah-lee	enlargement of the heart	*cardi/o* *megal/o* *-y*	heart enlarged condition of
clubbing	club-shaped digits resulting from decreased blood flow and oxygenation	*clubbing*	club-shaped
congestive heart failure kon-**jes**-tiv	condition in which the heart and vessels have difficulty pumping blood and perfusing the body	*congestio*	bringing together
cor pulmonale kor pool-mah-**nahl**-ee	enlargement of the right ventricle of the heart resulting from diseases in the lungs and pulmonary arteries	*cor* *pulmon/o*	heart lung
ectopic beats ek-**top**-ik ectopia ek-**tO**-pee-ah	heartbeat outside of the regular rate and rhythm; originates outside of the normal SA node regulation	*ecto-* *-ic*	outer, external pertaining to
endocarditis **en**-dO-kahr-**dI**-tis	inflammation of the endocardium	*endo-* *cardi/o* *-itis*	within, inner heart inflammation
fibrillation fih-bril-**ay**-shun	extremely rapid heartbeats in which the heart muscle fibers are beating at different times and unable to be synchronous	*fibrilla*	small fiber
heart block	partial or complete block of the electrical impulses from the SA node	*N/A*	
infarct **in**-fahrkt	death of a part of the heart because of decreased blood supply	*in-* *fartus*	within to stuff

continued on next page

Term	Meaning	Word Analysis	
ischemia is-**kee**-mee-ah	decreased blood flow	isch/o -emia	deficiency, suppression condition of blood
mammary soufflé **mam**-er-ee **soo**-fl	soft blowing sound heard on auscultation of the pregnant female's heart because of increased vascularity in breasts	mamm/o -ary souffler	breast pertaining to to blow
myocardial infarction mI-O-**kahr**-dee-al in-**fahrk**-shun	decreased blood flow to the heart leading to tissue death of the heart muscle itself	my/o cardi/o -al in- fartus	muscle heart pertaining to into to stuff
myocarditis mI-O-kahr-**dI**-tis	inflammation of the heart muscle	my/o cardi/o -itis	muscle heart inflammation
palpitation pal-pih-**tay**-shun	feeling of the heartbeat within the chest	palpitation	throb
paroxysmal tachycardia par-oks-**iz**-mel tak-ee-**kahr**-dee-ah	sudden onset of rapid heartbeats	paroxysmal tachy- cardi/o -ia	sharp irritation rapid heart condition of
pericarditis per-ih-kahr-**dI**-tis	inflammation of the fluid-filled sac that surrounds the heart	peri- cardi/o -itis	surrounding heart inflammation
tachycardia tak-ee-**kahr**-dee-ah	rapid heartbeat	tachy- cardi/o -ia	rapid heart condition of

Table 11.7

Abnormalities in the Vasculature

Term	Meaning	Word Analysis	
aneurysm **an**-yoo-riz-em	balloonlike swelling or outpouching of an artery	aneurysm	dilation
arteriosclerosis ahr-**teer**-ee-O-skler-**O**-sis	condition in which the walls of the small arteries are hardened	arteri/o scler/o -osis	artery hardening, thickening condition
arteriostenosis ahr-**teer**-ee-O-sten-**O**-sis	narrowing of the arteries	arteri/o sten/o -osis	artery narrowing condition
arteritis ahr-ter-**I**-tis	inflammation of an artery	arteri/o -itis	artery inflammation
atherosclerosis **ath**-er-O-skler-**O**-sis	blockage caused by lipid deposits in the arteries	ather/o scler/o -osis	pasty material hardening condition
embolism **em**-bO-liz-em	obstruction of a vessel	embol- -ism	something within condition of
hyperlipemia **hI**-per-lip-**ee**-mee-ah	increased fatty substances (lipids) in the blood	hyper- lip/o -emia	increased fatty condition of blood
hypertension **hI**-per-**ten**-shun	increased blood pressure	hyper- tensio	increased to stretch

hypotension hI-pO-**ten**-shun	decreased blood pressure	*hypo-* *tensio*	decreased to stretch
phlebitis fleh-**bI**-tis	inflammation of a vein	*phleb/o* *-itis*	vein inflammation
Raynaud's disease (phenomenon, syndrome) ray-**nOz**	cyanosis of the fingers due to arterial contraction; usually caused by cold	*Raynaud*	19th-century French physician
superior vena cava syndrome soo-**peer**-ee-or **vee**-nah **kay**-vah **sin**-drOm	obstruction of the superior vena cava causing swelling of the vessels of the neck, coughing, and difficulty breathing	*superior* *vena* *cava*	above vein plural of cavus (cavity)
thrombophlebitis throm-bO-fleh-**bI**-tis	inflammation in a vein caused by a thrombus formation (blood clot)	*thromb/o* *phleb/o* *-itis*	blood clot vein inflammation
thrombosis throm-**bO**-sis	clot formation in the blood vessels	*thromb/o* *-osis*	blood clot condition
thrombus **throm**-bus	blood clot	*thromb/o*	blood clot
varicose vein **var**-ih-kOs vayn	dilated and twisted vein usually found in the legs	*varic/o* *-ose*	twisted, swollen vein pertaining to
vasoconstriction vas-O-kon-**strik**-shun/ vay-zO-kon-**strik**-shun	narrowing of a vessel	*vas/o* *con-* *strictus*	vein with to draw together
vasodilation vas-O-dI-**lay**-shun/ vay-zO-dI-**lay**-shun	dilation of a vessel	*vas/o* *dilation*	vein to spread out
vasospasm **vas**-O-spaz-em	involuntary contraction in a vein	*vas/o* *spasm*	vein spasm

Word Analysis

On the line in the Word Analysis column, write each term divided into its word parts by hyphens. Identify the parts by type, using a letter for each part (P = prefix, R = root, S = suffix, CV = combining vowel). Then define the term.

Term	Word analysis	Definition
1. stethoscope	_____	_____
2. pericarditis	_____	_____
3. pulmonic	_____	_____
4. stenosis	_____	_____
5. ventricular	_____	_____
6. arteriosclerosis	_____	_____
7. myocardial	_____	_____
8. tachycardia	_____	_____

9. cardiomegaly _____ _____

10. endocarditis _____ _____

Comprehension Check

Circle the correct term from each pair in the following sentences.

1. Mollie was diagnosed with a cerebral aneurysm/arterism.

2. Mr. Donnelley has been experiencing palpations/palpitations for the past week.

3. The cause of death was myocardial infarction/impaction.

4. The ECG revealed several exotic/ectopic beats.

5. The patient's existing respiratory problems were exacerbated by her conclusive/congestive heart failure.

6. Marked clubbing/clutting was noted in the phalanges of both hands.

7. The emergency room physician diagnosed a heart block/bar and requested a cardiology consult.

8. Nitro-Bid was prescribed for the angina/angelina.

9. An ECG was ordered to evaluate the patient's arrhythmias/arrithymia.

10. There was a large area of ischemia/isthemia over the left ventricular/ventricle.

Matching

Match the terms in Column 1 with the definitions in Column 2. Write the number of the term on the line beside its definition.

Column 1		Column 2
1. thrombus	_____	condition of narrowing of an artery
2. cardiomegaly	_____	pertaining to an artery
3. thrombophlebitis	_____	rapid heart rate
4. valvular	_____	pertaining to the heart
5. endocarditis	_____	excess fat in the blood
6. hypotension	_____	blood clot
7. tachycardia	_____	enlargement of the heart
8. hyperlipidemia	_____	low blood pressure
9. arterial stenosis	_____	inflammation of a vein due to a blood clot
10. systole	_____	pertaining to a valve
11. cardiac	_____	contraction of the heart
12. arterial	_____	inflammation of the lining of the heart

Create a term to match the definition given. Suffixes have been provided.

1. specialist in the study of the heart   _____ologist

2. slow heart (beat)   _____cardia

3. pertaining to the heart muscle   _____al

4. condition of narrowing or constriction   _____osis

5. condition of hardening   _____osis

6. record of a blood vessel   _____gram

7. record of the heart   _____gram

8. process of recording the heart   _____graphy

9. around the heart   _____al

10. structure within the heart   _____ium

In the sentences that follow, incorrect prefixes or suffixes are used in the medical terms. Provide the correct prefix or suffix for each term by writing the corrected term on the blank provided.

1. The patient's bacterial endocardioma was treated with antibiotics. _____

2. Blood pressure was 190/110, and the patient was diagnosed with antitension. _____

3. An embolotomy is an obstruction of a vessel. _____

4. Mr. Bowers was brought to the emergency room with a hypercardial infarction. _____

5. Pericardia is a term used to describe a slow heart rate. _____

6. Cardiotrophy is an enlargement of the heart. _____

7. Cardiosclerosis is defined as a condition in which the walls of the small arteries are blocked. _____

8. Mrs. Perkins, who had pain and swelling in her calf, was diagnosed with thrombia. _____

9. The patient's prelipemia was diagnosed with laboratory tests. _____

10. A gastrospasm is an involuntary contraction of a vein. _____

1. List the four major heart valves:

   _____

   _____

   _____

   _____

2. Provide the terms that match the definitions/descriptions:

   _____ Restriction of blood flow due to narrowing

   _____ Backflow of blood due to incomplete closure of valve

3. Using the information from 1 and 2, create a concept map showing eight major types of valvular defects and their descriptions. (Hint: start with the four valve names.)

Diagnosing and Treating Problems

Tests, Procedures, and Pharmaceuticals

Many of the problems that occur with the cardiovascular system are insidious; that is, they often do not display signs and symptoms until the situation is serious. For instance, coronary artery disease is a slow process of plaque buildup in the vessels. Chest pain might provide a warning, but usually the individual does not realize that the heart muscle has been damaged until a heart attack occurs.

Everyone should be periodically screened by a blood test often referred to as a **lipid risk panel**. This test measures the serum **cholesterol**, the **high-density** and **low-density lipoproteins**, and the **triglycerides**. Cholesterol levels represent one of the risks for developing arteriosclerosis. A high blood concentration of cholesterol, low-density lipoproteins, and triglycerides increases the risk for arteriosclerosis.

A common screening method to determine cardiac function is the **electrocardiogram (ECG or EKG)**. This test determines the electrical activity generated through the heart's conduction system. Each time the heart pumps, electrical currents are spread through the tissues on the surface of the body. The ECG is a graphic record that traces these signals (see Figure 11.8). When the heart muscle is damaged or abnormalities occur in the conduction system, the ECG can detect these changes. The **echocardiogram** is an ultrasound of the heart that provides a view of the valves and flow of blood through the heart. This noninvasive procedure, which means that no incision is made, is used to check patients for cardiomyopathy (damage to the muscle tissue of the heart). A nuclear scan, called a MUGA scan, can further depict the workings of the heart.

Normal sinus rhythm (NSR)

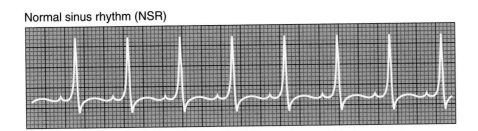

Figure 11.8 - Heart Rhythms in ECG Tests

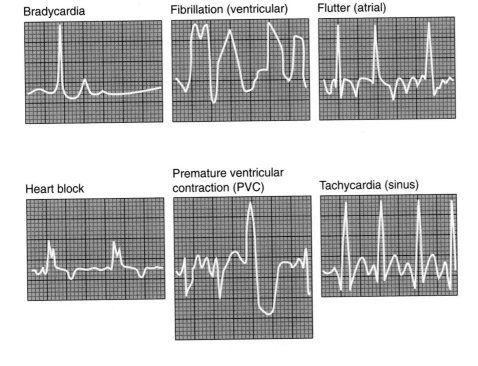

Bradycardia

Fibrillation (ventricular)

Flutter (atrial)

Heart block

Premature ventricular contraction (PVC)

Tachycardia (sinus)

Procedures

Interventional cardiology is a specialty that has evolved within the past 20 years and continues to grow as new procedures are developed. **Cardiac catheterization**, also known as an **angiogram**, threads a flexible tube (catheter) into the heart through one of the large vessels, usually in the groin. A dye is injected into the catheter, and, through fluoroscopy, the heart and vasculature surrounding it can be seen on a monitor, including a blockages, or strictures. Repair can often be achieved during this procedure through a **balloon angioplasty procedure,** or **percutaneous transluminal coronary angioplasty (PTCA)**. In the balloon angioplasty or the PTCA, a catheter with a balloon tip is inserted into the occluded vessel to open it and allow free flow of blood. Other procedures ream the plaque from the vessels. An **endarterectomy** is the removal of the lining of an artery that contains plaque.

Cardiac surgery has evolved from replacement of occluded vessels and valves to transplants involving replacement of the entire heart. Some more common procedures include **angiectomy**, removal of a blood vessel when damaged or occluded, and **coronary artery bypass grafts (CABG)**, replacement of sections of occluded heart vessels with grafts taken from other parts of the body.

Table 11.8

Tests and Procedures Relating to the Cardiovascular System

Term	Meaning	Word Analysis	
angiectomy an-jee-**ek**-tah-mee	removal of a blood vessel	angi/o -ectomy	blood vessel surgical removal
angiogram **an**-jee-O-gram	procedure to determine the flow of blood through the heart and main vessels; a catheter is inserted into a main vessel and threaded into the coronary artery; dye is injected through the catheter and the heart is visualized on a monitor	angi/o -gram	blood vessel recording
angioplasty **an**-jee-O-**plas**-tee	procedure to repair a vessel, usually a main vessel of the heart	angi/o -plasty	vessel shape or repair
balloon angioplasty	procedure in which a balloon-tipped catheter is inserted into the coronary artery and then inflated to push plaque against the vessel walls and free an obstruction	angi/o -plasty	vessel shape or repair
coronary artery bypass graft (CABG) **kor**-ah-nar-ee	procedure to remove sections of occluded vessels of the heart; a large vessel from another part of the body, usually the mammary artery or saphenous vein, is removed and attached to either end of the vessel (anastomosed)	coron/o -ary arteri/o	crown or circle pertaining to artery
echocardiogram ek-O-**kahr**-dee-O-gram	ultrasound that records the function of the valves and flow of blood through the heart	echo cardi/o -gram	reverberating sound heart recording
high-density lipoprotein (HDL) lip-O-**prO**-teen/ II-pO-**prO**-teen	fatty substance (type of lipid) found in the blood that decreases the risk of heart attack	lip/o prote/o	fatty protein
low-density lipoprotein (LDL) lip-O-**prO**-teen/ II-pO-**prO**-teen	fatty substance (type of lipid) found in the blood that increases the risk of heart disease	lip/o prote/o	fatty protein

percutaneous transluminal coronary angioplasty (PTCA) per-kyoo-**tay**-nee-us trans-**loo**-min-al **an**-jee-O-**plas**-tee	procedure in which a balloon- tipped catheter is inserted into the coronary artery and then inflated to push plaque against the vessel walls and free an obstruction	*per-cutis* *-ous* *trans-* *lumen* *-al* *angi/o* *-plasty*	through skin pertaining to across inside of a tubular structure pertaining to blood vessel surgical repair
serum cholesterol **seer**-em kO-**les**-ter-ol	blood test to determine the level of the lipid cholesterol in the blood	*serum* *cholesterol*	whey chemical substance
thallium stress test **thal**-ee-um	the radioactive substance thallium is injected into the patient to enable visualization of the heart's action during activity (walking on a treadmill) and then resting after the exercise	*thallium*	radioactive substance
transesophageal echocardiography trans-eh-sof-ah-**jee**-al **ek**-O-kahr-dee-**og**-raf-ee	test to visualize the back of the heart by passing a tube through the throat and down the esophagus	*trans-* *esophagus* *-eal* *cardi/o* *-graphy*	across, through gullet pertaining to heart process of recording
triglycerides trI-**glis**-er-Ids	fatty substances within the blood	*tri-* *glycer/o* *-ide*	three chemical substance compound

Pharmaceutical Agents

Agents used in cardiology involve those that improve the function of the heart muscle, such as beta-blockers, calcium channel blockers, and antiarrhythmics; some eliminate excess fluid, such as diuretics; or insure the flow of blood through the vessels, such as anticoagulants. Other agents include antihypertensives to decrease blood pressure and hypolipidemics to decrease serum cholesterol levels. Many patients take multiple drugs to achieve therapeutic results or to avoid the undesirable side effects of other drugs. For example, the agent dexrazoxane (Zinecard) is used to try to prevent cardiotoxicity that can be caused by chemotherapeutic agents classified as anthracyclines. Table 11.9 describes the most common drugs used to treat problems with the cardiovascular system.

Table 11.9

Pharmacologic Agents Relating to the Circulatory System

Drug classes	Use	Generic name	Brand names
angiotensin-converting enzyme (ACE) inhibitors	prevent vasoconstriction	captopril enalapril maleate quinapril hydrochloride ramipril	Capoten Vasotec Accupril Altace
antianginals	relieve the pain of acute angina by causing relaxation of vascular smooth muscle and consequent dilatation of peripheral arteries and veins	isosorbide dinitrate nitroglycerin	Isordil Nitrolingual (spray), Nitrostat (sublingual), Minitran (patch)

continued on next page

antiarrhythmic	corrects/improves abnormal rhythms	acebutolol hydrochloride digoxin	Sectral Lanoxin
anticoagulants	keep blood flowing without thromboses; inhibit blood clotting	aspirin enoxaparin (low-molecular-weight heparin) heparin warfarin sodium	Bufferin, Ecotrin Lovenox Hep-Lock Coumadin
beta adrenergic blockers	block certain receptors in the heart to decrease the heart rate and the force of contraction	atenolol propranolol hydrochloride	Tenormin Inderal, InnoPran XL
calcium channel blockers	inhibit calcium flow into muscle cells, leading to muscle relaxation	nifedipine verapamil hydrochloride diltiazem hydrochloride	Adalat CC, Procardia XL Calan, Verelan Cardizem, Dilacor XR
diuretics	decrease fluid retention by promoting increased urinary output (diuresis)	furosemide hydrochlorothiazide	Lasix Aquazide H, Oretic
hypolipidemics	decrease cholesterol level in the blood	fluvastatin sodium lovastatin simvastatin	Lescol Mevacor Zocor
protective agent	prevent cardiotoxicity from doxorubicin	dexrazoxane	Zinecard

Table 11.10

Abbreviations

ACG	angiocardiography
AS	aortic stenosis
ASD	atrial septal defect
ASHD	arteriosclerotic heart disease
BBB	bundle-branch block
CAD	coronary artery disease
CC	cardiac catheterization
CCU	coronary care unit
CF	circumflex (artery)
CHF	congestive heart failure
CPR	cardiopulmonary resuscitation
CV	cardiovascular
DVT	deep vein thrombosis
ECG or EKG	electrocardiogram
ICA	internal carotid artery
IMA	internal mammary artery
IV	intravenous
LAD	left anterior descending coronary artery
LCA	left coronary artery
LCF	left circumflex
LIMA	left internal mammary artery
LMCA	left main coronary artery
LPA	left pulmonary artery

MI	myocardial infarction
MPA	main pulmonary artery
MS	mitral stenosis
MVP	mitral valve prolapse
PA	pulmonary artery
PAT	paroxysmal atrial tachycardia
PDA	posterior descending artery; patent ductus arteriosus
PMI	point of maximal impulse
PVC	premature ventricular contraction
RCA	right coronary artery
RPA	right pulmonary artery
SA	sinoatrial node
VSD	ventricular septal defect

Word Analysis

On the line in the Word Analysis column, write each term divided into its word parts by hyphens. Identify the parts by type, using a letter for each part (P = prefix, R = root, S = suffix, CV = combining vowel). Then define the term.

Term	Word Analysis	Definition
1. angioplasty	_____	_____
2. cardiology	_____	_____
3. arteriogram	_____	_____
4. vascular	_____	_____
5. phlebitis	_____	_____
6. thrombosis	_____	_____
7. venule	_____	_____
8. septal	_____	_____
9. atrial	_____	_____
10. ventricular	_____	_____

Read each sentence and determine whether the terms are spelled correctly. If the spelling is correct, write the word "correct" on the blank. If the spelling is incorrect, select the **correctly spelled** term from the list provided and write your selection on the blank.

CAGB	liqid	PTCA
lipid	cholesterol	CABG
catheterization	echocardiagraphy	triglycerides
vassospasm	beta-blocker	buter-blocker
echocardiography	vasospasm	cardiac
vena cava	vena cova	serum

1. The gunshot injury included damage to the patient's inferior venous cannae. _____

2. Blood supply to the area was decreased due to vastospasm. _____

3. Each of Dr. Benton's patients has a yearly lipstick risk panel. _____

4. The cardial catheterizotomy laboratory is being prepared for the next patient. _____

5. Dr. Thompson's patient is scheduled for a PCAT tomorrow. _____

6. Kerry's specialty is echogardiogramy. _____

7. Mr. Blaise will have the CABAGE procedure this morning. _____

8. The test for serous cholestetoma showed very high lipid levels. _____

9. Serous tricyclics were also elevated. _____

10. Inderal is a widely used belta-blucker. _____

Match the list of procedures and treatments in Column 2 with the diagnosis or reason for the procedure in Column 1. Write the number of the diagnosis or problem in the space beside the name of the related treatment or procedure. Note that some entries in Column 2 are diagnostic procedures.

Column 1

1. visualize the valves and blood flow through the heart

2. visualize heart action during exercise and recovery

3. replace an occluded coronary vessel

4. assess the electrical conduction system of the heart to determine cardiac function

5. repair a vessel

6. remove a damaged blood vessel

Column 2

_____ a. electrocardiogram

_____ b. echocardiogram

_____ c. angioplasty

_____ d. PTCA

_____ e. lipid risk panel

_____ f. diuretics

7. open an occluded coronary vessel   _____   g. CABG

8. visualize the heart and vasculature by fluoroscopy   _____   h. thallium stress test

9. decrease fluid retention by promoting increased urinary output   _____   i. angiography

10. assess the risk of heart disease related to a fatty substance found in the blood   _____   j. angiectomy

Word Building   *Exercise 16*

Find word parts in your text to construct medical terms for the definitions that follow. Note that part of each term has been provided. Write the whole term on the blank provided.

Term	Definition
1. study of the heart	_____ology
2. specialist in the study of the heart	_____ologist
3. record of the electrical activity of the heart	electro_____
4. pertaining to the ventricle	_____ar
5. pertaining to the atrium	_____al
6. pertaining to the aorta	_____ic
7. agent against clotting (coagulation)	anti_____
8. agent against hypertension	anti_____
9. agent against cardiac pain (angina)	_____al
10. surgical removal of a blood vessel	_____ectomy

Spelling Check   *Exercise 17*

Identify each term as singular or plural by writing a *P* or *S* beside the term; then give the opposite form (i.e., either plural or singular).

	P/S	Opposite Form
1. bruit	_____	_____
2. ventricle	_____	_____
3. artery	_____	_____
4. atrium	_____	_____
5. vein	_____	_____
6. vena cava	_____	_____
7. occlusion	_____	_____

8. angioplasty   _____   _____

9. bypass   _____   _____

10. diuretic   _____   _____

Word Maps

Complete the chart of related terms by labeling the blank areas.

Laboratory screening/diagnostic test (lipid risk panel)

1. _____

2. _____

3. _____

4. _____

Noninvasive screening/diagnostic tests

1. _____

2. _____

Invasive diagnostic procedure using transluminal catheter technique

_____

or _____

or _____

Invasive therapeutic procedure using transluminal catheter technique

_____

or _____

or _____ (abbreviation)

Performance Assessment 11

Crossword Puzzle

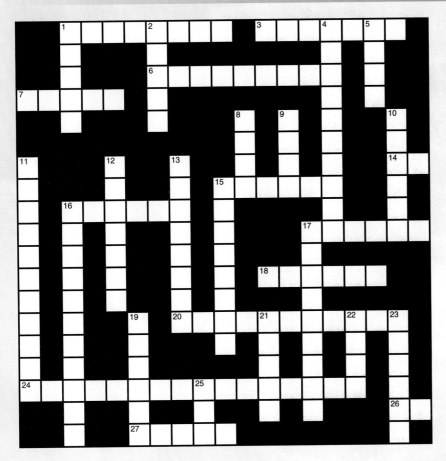

Across

1. dilation of an artery
3. death of a part of the heart
6. inflammation of a vein
7. lip/o
14. sinoatrial node
15. chest pain of cardiac origin
16. abnormal heart sound produced by turbulent blood flow in the heart
17. tiny vein
18. myo
20. instrument for listening
24. hardening of an artery
26. abbreviation for mitral stenosis
27. word part meaning narrowing

Down

1. largest artery in the body
2. tachy
4. listen to sounds produced in the body
5. thrombus
8. phleb/o; vas/o
9. word part meaning surrounding
10. angi/o
11. rapid heart rate
12. pertaining to the heart
13. heart inflammation
15. vessels that carry blood away from the heart
16. inflammation of the heart muscle
17. involuntary contraction of a vein
19. fatty substances
21. cardio
22. word part meaning condition
23. word part meaning surgical removal
25. prefix meaning with

What Do These Abbreviations Mean?

Write the definition of the abbreviation on the line beside the abbreviation.

1. CHF _____

2. CV _____

3. EKG _____

4. VSD _____

5. MS _____

6. IV _____

7. MI _____

8. SA _____

9. CAD _____

10. BBB _____

11. DVT _____

12. ASHD _____

13. PVC _____

14. MVP _____

15. PAT _____

Build the Terms

In this exercise you will construct words from roots, prefixes, and suffixes.

Select word parts from the lists to build a complete medical term for each definition given. Note that not all terms will have a root or combining form, prefix, and suffix. Some word parts may be used more than once.

Combining Forms	Prefixes	Suffixes
cardi/o	hypo-	-itis
arteri/o	tachy-	-logy
atri/o	sub-	-logist
ventricul/o	hypo-	-malacia
electr/o	inter-	-pathy
my/o	dis-	-penia
pulmon/o	a-	-al
angi/o	supra-	-oma
vascul/o	de-	-ic
ven/o	anti-	-ar
aort/o	per-	-gram
arteri/o	bi-	-philic

Note: For this exercise, you will need to use three words for which there are no corresponding combining forms: **volume, systole, and apex.** Use these words, combined with prefixes or suffixes from the list above, to create one of the required terms.

1. study of the heart   _____

2. disease of heart muscle   _____

3. within the ventricle   _____

4. against angina (condition of the blood vessels)   _____

5. record of electrical activity in the heart   _____

6. inflammation of the heart   _____

7. pertaining to the ventricle   _____

8. insufficient volume   _____

9. pertaining to the apex   _____

10. pertaining to the vessels   _____

11. rapid heart (rate)   _____

12. above the ventricle   _____

13. without contraction   _____

14. inflammation of the aorta   _____

Build the Terms

Supply a word part or parts to complete the term, using the context as a guide.

1. _____al means "pertaining to the apex."

2. _____ic means "pertaining to contraction of the heart."

3. _____al means "pertaining to the valve between the left atrium and the left ventricle."

4. _____ium means "structure of the heart muscle."

5. _____ar means "pertaining to the lower chambers of the heart."

6. cardio_____ means "pertaining to the heart and lungs."

7. _____gist means "one who studies the heart."

8. aorto_____ means "record of the aorta."

9. angio_____ means "repair of a vessel."

10. _____al means "pertaining to the wall between the right and left sides of the heart."

What's Your Conclusion?

Read each mini medical record carefully; then select the correct response. Write the letter of your answer in the space provided.

1. 73 y/o Mr. Tennyson comes to the doctor's office, accompanied by his wife. Mrs. Tennyson says that he has complained several times of a "fluttering" feeling in his chest, but has disregarded those until recently, when they've become more frequent. After a physical examination, the doctor tells the patient that he will order blood and urine tests. As a medical office assistant, you try to anticipate the forms the doctor will need. In addition to the blood and urine testing, you anticipate that the physician will want to do

   A. a chest x-ray, an EKG, and an echocardiogram.
   B. an MRI, a KUB, and a CAT scan.

   Your response: _____

2. Harvey M. is a 43 y/o male who, as a farmer, has always led an active life. He has no history of cardiovascular problems and seems to be fit and healthy. The only remarkable aspects of his health history are appendicitis over 20 years ago and several injuries from farming accidents. He denies any recent accidents or injuries to his chest. He was seen in the clinic about two weeks ago for a recheck following an episode of the flu, but was found to have completely recovered. Today he is brought to the Emergency Room after complaining of chest pain. The patient states, "It doesn't hurt if I don't breathe." He has no other symptoms. You are present in the Emergency Room as the doctor examines the patient and note that he winces when the doctor palpates his sternum and rib cage. The doctor orders several tests, including an ECG. That report shows "NSR" and

no abnormalities. The doctor's notes indicate that he has ruled out respiratory disorders and has written "Pain of noncardiac origin" in the chart. You expect that the doctor will:

A. Need to perform additional tests, since the tests that were done didn't locate the source of the problem.
B. Diagnose cholelithiasis, prescribe an NSAID, tell the patient to rest for 48 hours.

Your response: _____

3. The next ER patient is a 65 y/o female who arrives by ambulance from her home. She has a history of diabetes, angina, and hyperlipidemia; she smokes and is overweight. Upon arising this morning, she became dizzy and fainted. She experienced severe substernal chest pain, with pain in her left shoulder, neck, and jaw. Now she is restless, anxious, pale, and diaphoretic. She is mildly hypotensive and her pulse is irregular. The ER physician examines the patient and orders blood and urine tests, CXR, ECG, and echocardiogram. You note that the ECG report mentions "frequent PVCs." You expect that the physician will:

A. Diagnose costochondritis and prescribe an NSAID and rest. She will be returned home.
B. Diagnose acute MI.

Your response: _____

Records Analysis

Read the office chart note that follows. Then answer the following questions.

1. What is the patient's diagnosis?

2. What type of specialist is best suited to manage this patient's condition?

3. What type of the problem did the patient report a week ago?

4. Describe three findings related to the heart from the physical examination of one week ago.

5. What type of tests were performed after the physical exam but before the cardiac catheterization?

6. What were the results of those tests?

7. What is a cardiac catheterization, and why was it performed on this patient?

8. What did the cardiac catheterization reveal?

9. What additional test will this patient have? What may be considered based on the test results?

10. What does "managed medically" mean?

Office Chart Note

PATIENT: S., Richard
DATE: October 19, xxxx

S: Patient states he is 55 y/o and is not aware of any previous heart problems. He is the CFO of a rather large organization and seems to experience considerable stress related to his job. He reports recent episodes of angina, beginning one week ago.

O: This patient is a WDWN male Caucasian who appears his stated age. He has been a patient here for several years and has had no previous history of heart disease. He was last seen approximately two years ago for a complete physical exam. We did a resting ECG at that time that was interpreted as normal. When he reported the angina last week, we did a complete examination and there was no evidence of cardiomegaly, no murmurs, and no extra heart sounds. He did, however, have a mild tachycardia. The remainder of the ROS was unremarkable. An ECG revealed sinus tachycardia and a CXR showed very mild left ventricular hypertrophy. Echocardiography reports indicated that there was no valvular dysfunction, and ejection fraction was calculated at 58%. The patient was referred for a cardiac catheterization procedure to gain additional information. Today's report of the cardiac cath shows a 70 percent stenosis of the left anterior descending coronary artery, immediately after the first septal branch. The remainder of that artery and the other coronary arteries are WNL. Ejection fraction was reported as 58%.

A: Angina due to coronary artery stenosis.

P: We discussed the results of the cardiac cath and plans for the management of this illness. He will be managed medically for the present. We will perform a thallium stress test to determine reaction to exercise and the extent of the anginal symptoms. If there is a marked reversible ischemia, we will consider angioplasty of the left anterior descending coronary artery.

E. Hayes, MD

Using Medical References

The following sentences contain medical terms that were not addressed on the charts in this chapter. Use medical reference books, your medical term analysis skills, and/or a medical dictionary to find the correct definition of each underlined word. Write the definition(s) on the line below the sentence.

1. A phonocardiogram is a noninvasive technique and offers the advantage of minimal or no discomfort for the patient.

2. A holosystolic murmur was detected using the Doppler technique.

3. Left atrial systole will generate a prominent A wave on the apexcardiogram.

4. <u>Echocardiography</u> is valuable in evaluating the <u>cardiac chambers</u>.

_____

5. The patient's <u>pulmonary hypertension</u> responded readily to medical measures.

_____

6. <u>Arterial blood gasses</u> were assessed in the Emergency Room.

_____

7. The patient's low <u>cardiac output</u> has produced increasingly severe symptoms.

_____

8. In diagnosing and treating the patient's condition, we must differentiate <u>essential or primary hypertension</u> and <u>secondary hypertension</u>.

_____

9. The occurrences of the cardiac cycle are sometimes divided into <u>diastolic</u> events and <u>systolic</u> events.

_____

10. <u>Stroke volume</u> can be calculated, using a standard formula.

_____

11. Mrs. Halston's period of unconsciousness was a result of <u>orthostatic hypotension</u>.

_____

12. The patient went into <u>hypovolemic shock</u> as a result of massive blood loss from his injuries in the MVA.

_____

Short Answer

In your own words, in plain language, describe how blood flows through the body.

_____

_____

_____

_____

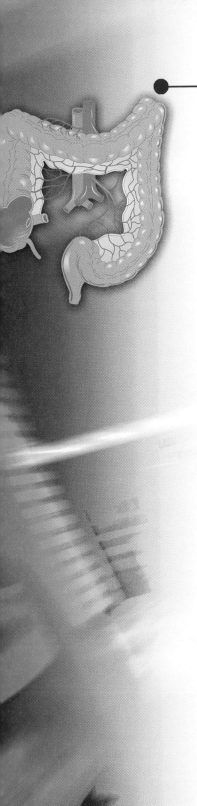

Chapter 12

The Gastrointestinal System

Learning Outcomes

Students will be able to:
- Identify the structures of the gastrointestinal tract.
- Name the elements (steps) of the digestive process.
- Explain the role of digestive enzymes.
- Describe the function of nutrition in maintaining homeostasis.
- Use the terminology of the gastrointestinal system in written and oral communication.
- List gastrointestinal abnormalities and pathologies and their effects.
- Correctly spell and pronounce gastrointestinal tract terminology.
- State the meaning of abbreviations related to the gastrointestinal tract.
- List and define the combining forms most commonly used to create terms related to the gastrointestinal tract.
- Name tests and treatments for major gastrointestinal abnormalities.

Translation, Please? Translation, Please? Translation, Please?

Read the following excerpt from a medical record and try to answer the questions that follow.

The patient was placed on the operating table in the supine position. Pneumoperitoneum was achieved by instillation through a small infraumbilical incision. After identification of the cystic artery and cystic duct, dissection of the hepatoduodenal ligament commenced.

1. Was the patient on his abdomen or back?
2. What is pneumoperitoneum instillation?
3. Where was the incision made?

Answers to "Translations Please?"
1. The patient was on his back. Supine position means on the back.
2. Pneumoperitoneum instillation means adding air to the sac lining the abdominal cavity to create more space during surgery.
3. The incision was infraumbilical, which means below the navel.

Identifying the Specialty

The System and Its Practitioners

To carry out all of its vital functions, the body requires a constant supply of nutrients. The usual way to obtain these nutrients is from the outside by eating food. The function of the **gastrointestinal** (GI) system is to convert food into usable products for the body. The study of the gastrointestinal system is called **gastroenterology**, which includes the processes of digestion, absorption, and elimination.

Among the various specialists who care for diseases of the GI tract are the gastroenterologist; the proctologist, who specializes in the lower GI tract; and surgeons who specialize in surgery of the system's organs.

Figure 12.1 - Organs of the Digestive System

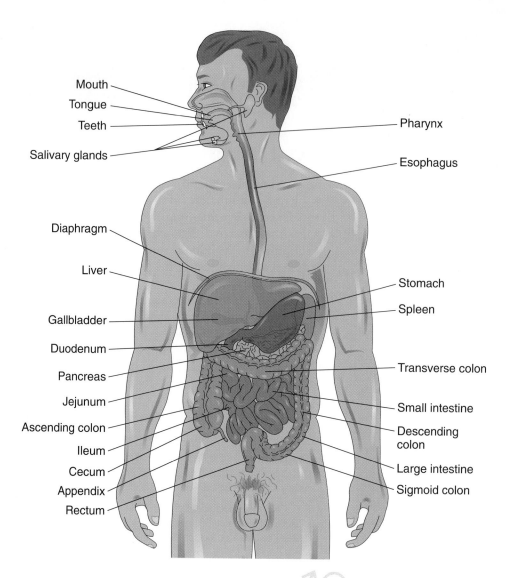

- Mouth
- Tongue
- Teeth
- Salivary glands
- Pharynx
- Esophagus
- Diaphragm
- Liver
- Gallbladder
- Duodenum
- Pancreas
- Jejunum
- Ascending colon
- Ileum
- Cecum
- Appendix
- Rectum
- Stomach
- Spleen
- Transverse colon
- Small intestine
- Descending colon
- Large intestine
- Sigmoid colon

Examining the Patient ♂♀

Anatomy and Physiology of the Gastrointestinal System

Think of the GI tract as a long tube (in adults, approximately 29 feet long) with openings on both ends. The tube must take in and absorb nutrients and eliminate wastes to ensure the survival of the body. Also known as the **alimentary canal**, the GI tract includes the mouth, pharynx, esophagus, stomach, small and large intestines, and accessory organs (the salivary glands, teeth, liver, gallbladder, pancreas, and appendix) (see Figure 12.1).

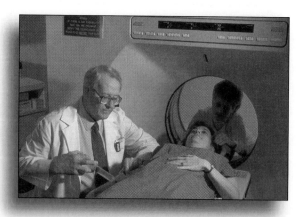

Digestive Process

The process of digestion begins when food enters the mouth. Like all other parts of the GI tract, the mouth has a mucous membrane lining that lubricates the passing food and protects the mouth from the digestive juices within it. The mouth is composed of the roof, which has a hard and soft palate, and a structure at the back called the **uvula**, which—with the soft palate—prevents food from entering the nasal cavity (Figure 12.2A). On the floor of the mouth is the tongue, which is muscle. A thin membrane called the **frenulum** attaches the tongue to the floor of the mouth. The tongue contains the sensory receptors for taste, as described in Chapter 9, "The Special Senses."

Figure 12.2A - Mouth Cavity

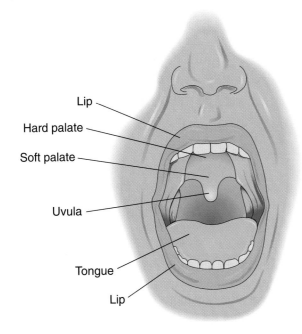

Figure 12.2B - Tongue

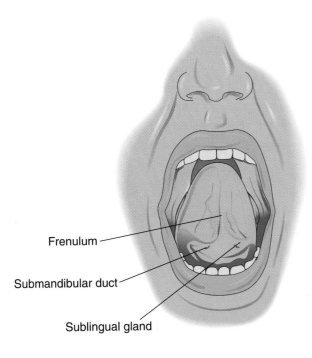

Three pairs of salivary glands (**parotids, submandibulars,** and **sublinguals**) secrete about 1 liter of saliva per day (Figure 12.3). These glands are **accessory structures** of the GI tract and are connected to the GI tract by ducts into which they secrete their saliva. Saliva is composed of mucus, which moistens food in its journey, and **salivary amylase,** a digestive enzyme that begins the chemical digestion of starches and sugars, or **carbohydrates**.

Figure 12.3 - Salivary Glands

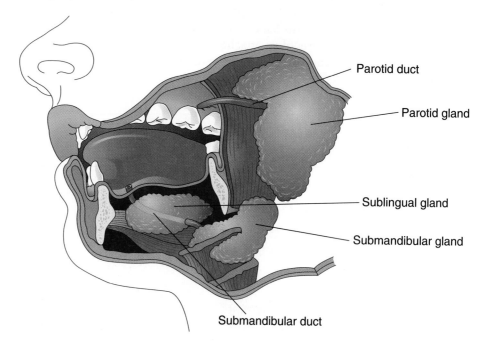

The **teeth** are the organs of **mastication,** or chewing. Teeth break, tear, and crush food and help mix it with mucus and enzymes. Humans are born without teeth, but by about 6 to 8 months of age, the **deciduous** (baby) teeth erupt. Figure 12.4 shows the deciduous and adult teeth and the age of eruption. Humans have 20 deciduous teeth and 32 permanent teeth.

Figure 12.4 - Deciduous (Baby) Teeth and Adult Teeth

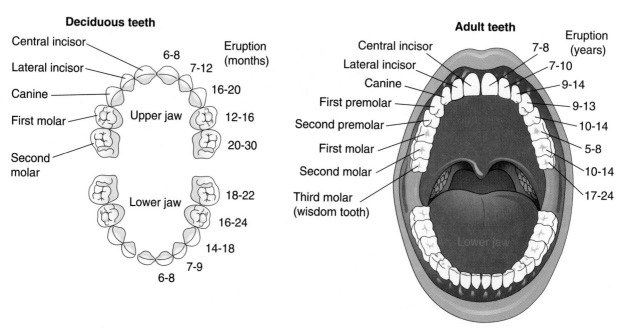

Each tooth consists of the crown, which projects from the gum; the root, which is imbedded in a bony socket, called the **alveolus**; and the neck, which is between the crown and the root. The solid portion of a tooth consists of **dentin** and **enamel**, covering the exposed portion of the crown. A thin layer of connective tissue called cementum surrounds the dentin.

Food passes from the mouth to the **pharynx,** a muscular structure lined with a mucous membrane. Although the pharynx is also part of the respiratory system, food must pass through it to reach the **esophagus**, or the food pipe. The esophagus is about 10 inches long and is the mucous-lined passageway for food as it moves to the next structure, the **stomach** (Figure 12.5). A ring of muscle tissue called the **cardiac sphincter** at the end of the esophagus provides a closure to prevent food from going back up the esophagus as the stomach contracts.

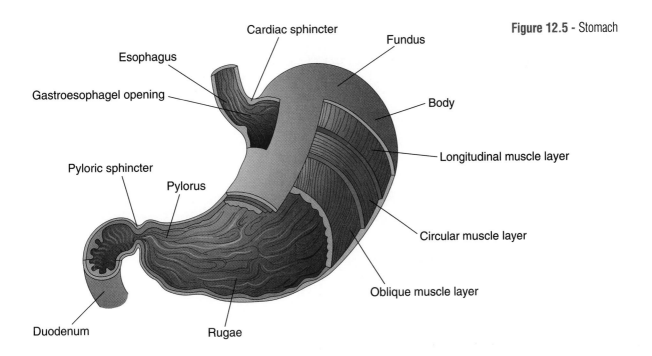

Cardiac sphincter
Esophagus
Gastroesophagel opening
Fundus
Body
Longitudinal muscle layer
Pyloric sphincter
Pylorus
Circular muscle layer
Oblique muscle layer
Duodenum
Rugae

Figure 12.5 - Stomach

The stomach is a pouch that lies within the abdominal cavity under the diaphragm (refer to Figure 12.1). One of the strongest organs of the body, the stomach is composed of three layers of smooth muscle that run in different directions: lengthwise (longitudinal muscle layer), around (circular muscle layer), and obliquely (oblique muscle layer). The stomach is divided into three sections: the **fundus**, which is the upper portion; the **body** in the center; and the **pylorus** at the bottom. A **pyloric sphincter** holds food in the stomach while it is being digested.

The stomach is lined with mucous membranes containing thousands of gastric glands that secrete **gastric juice** and **hydrochloric acid**. When the stomach is empty, the lining is tucked into **rugae**, or folds. When food reaches the stomach, the muscle walls contract to expose the food to the digestive fluids and to continue breaking it down. The final mixture is a semisolid substance called **chyme**. At the end of the digestive process, strong muscle contractions cause **peristalsis**, which propels the chyme farther down into the digestive tract.

The next structure of digestion is the **small intestine**, named for its diameter rather than its 20-foot length. The small intestine is divided into sections—the duodenum, the jejunum, and the ileum (Figure 12.6)—all of which are protected by a mucous lining. Thousands of glands within the intestine secrete digestive juices. This long tube also contains plicae, circular folds covered with fingerlike projections called villi. Smaller structures called microvilli cover each villus to provide a large contact area to promote the absorption of nutrients. Each villus contains a lymph vessel called a lacteal, which absorbs fatty lipid materials from the chyme.

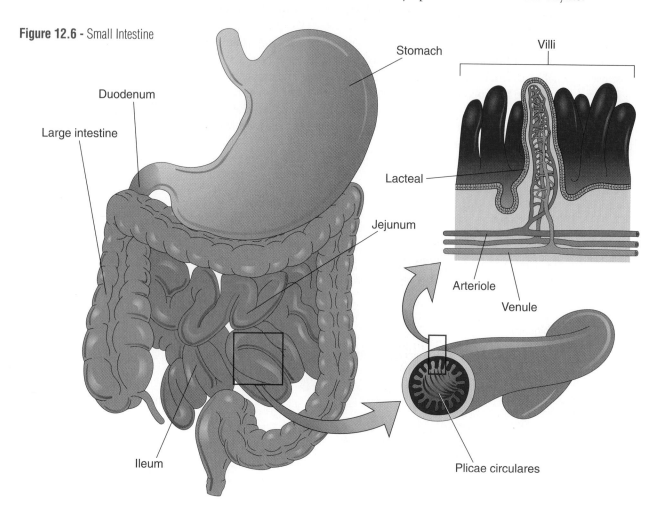

Figure 12.6 - Small Intestine

Chemical digestion takes place in the duodenum. Ducts located in the middle of the duodenum empty digestive juices from the pancreas and bile from the liver. The **pancreas** lies behind the stomach, and, because it secretes pancreatic juice into ducts and hormones into the blood, it is considered both an exocrine and endocrine gland. Pancreatic juice, which is made up of enzymes that can digest the three kinds of food molecules—proteins, fats, and carbohydrates—is extremely important. It also contains an alkaline substance, bicarbonate, which neutralizes hydrochloric acid in the gastric juice.

The **liver** is the largest organ within the abdomen and the largest gland in the body. It is divided into right and left lobes and is considered an exocrine gland because it secretes bile into **hepatic** (from the Greek *hepar* for liver) ducts (Figure 12.7). The process begins with the presence of fat in the chyme that passes into the small intestine. The fat stimulates the secretion of the hormone **cholecystokinin** by the mucosa of the duodenum. This hormone stimulates the **gallbladder** to contract and move **bile** (the substance that breaks down, or **emulsifies**, fats) into the duodenum through the **common bile duct**, which is formed by the joining of the common hepatic duct with the cystic duct (Figure 12.7).

Figure 12.7 - Gallbladder and Bile Ducts

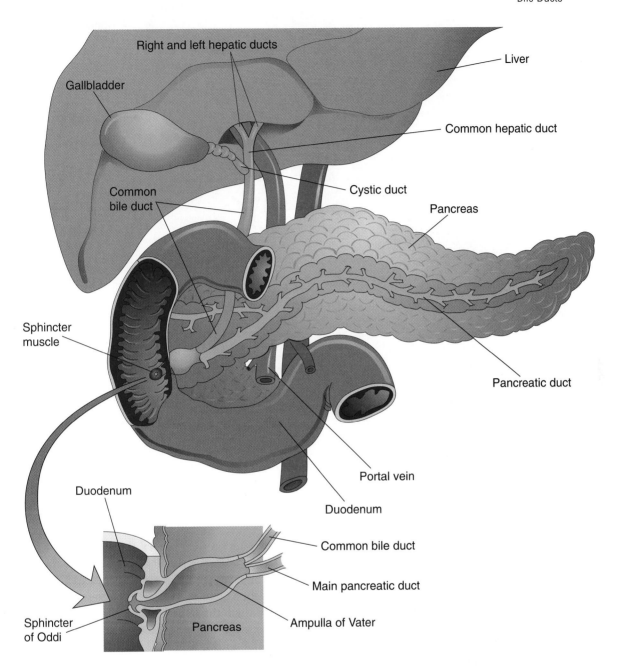

Right and left hepatic ducts

Liver

Gallbladder

Common hepatic duct

Cystic duct

Common bile duct

Pancreas

Sphincter muscle

Pancreatic duct

Portal vein

Duodenum

Duodenum

Common bile duct

Main pancreatic duct

Sphincter of Oddi

Pancreas

Ampulla of Vater

Water and other substances found in the chyme are reabsorbed through the walls of the small intestine, causing the chyme to change to the consistency of **feces**, the formed, sticky substance that is eventually eliminated from the body. The sphincter at the end of the small intestine, called the **ileocecal valve**, holds the undigested material until it passes into the **large intestine**, which is only about 5 feet in total length but wider in diameter than the small intestine.

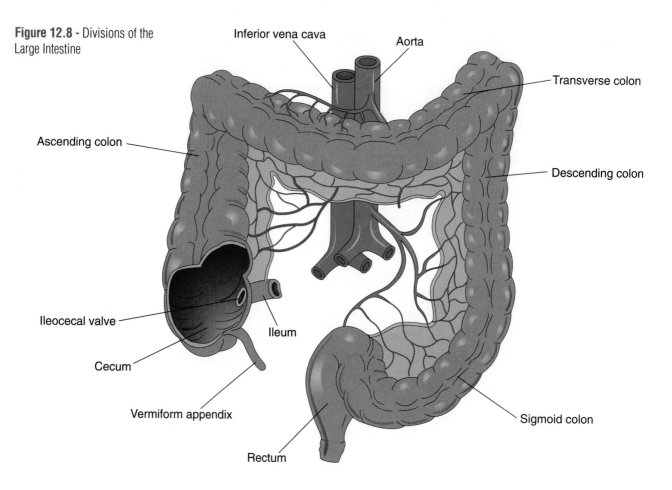

Figure 12.8 - Divisions of the Large Intestine

Inferior vena cava

Aorta

Transverse colon

Ascending colon

Descending colon

Ileocecal valve

Ileum

Cecum

Vermiform appendix

Sigmoid colon

Rectum

Anatomists divide the large intestine into seven divisions, as shown in Figure 12.8:

❶ cecum   ❺ sigmoid colon
❷ ascending colon   ❻ rectum
❸ transverse colon   ❼ anal canal
❹ descending colon

The large intestine contains bacteria that act on the material that has escaped digestion in the small intestine. These bacteria continue the digestive action of the GI tract and also help produce vitamin B complexes and vitamin K, necessary for normal blood clotting. Because the large intestine contains no villi, it has less surface area for absorption, and material is passed through the large intestine slowly, taking from 1 to 5 days. The fecal material travels through the large intestine and is held at the two sphincters at the end of the anal canal until it is passed out of the external opening, the **anus**.

Types of Nutrient Digestion

Digestion occurs in different parts of the GI tract, depending on the type of substance. Mechanical digestion begins with chewing, or mastication, aided by the digestive juices in saliva that begin to break down large molecules. The stomach continues the process with the chemical digestion of **proteins**. The two **enzymes** in the gastric juice, rennin and pepsin, break down proteins into **amino acids**, also called the body's building blocks. Protein digestion is completed in the small intestine.

Carbohydrates are digested in the small intestine where an enzyme, **amylase**, from the pancreas and small intestine begins the process and intestinal enzymes (maltase, sucrase, and lactase) complete the process until carbohydrates are changed to simple sugars, such as **glucose**. **Fats** are undigested until they are emulsified by bile, which breaks them down into fatty acids and glycerol.

The final stage of digestion is the absorption of the molecules—amino acids, glucose, fatty acids, and glycerol. They are transported through the lining of the small intestine and into the blood and lymph to provide the body with the nutrients essential for life.

Additional Gastrointestinal Structures

Not all structures in the abdominal cavity are directly involved with the process of digestion, specifically, the **vermiform appendix**, known simply as the appendix, and the **peritoneum**. The appendix is attached to the cecum and lies close to the wall of the rectum. Although the appendix is composed of lymphatic tissue, it plays only a minor role in the immunologic system.

The **peritoneum** is a serous membrane that lines the abdominal cavity. This membrane includes a **parietal** layer, which covers the cavity walls, and a **visceral** layer, which covers each organ. Peritoneal fluid keeps the two layers from rubbing against each other. The two extensions to the peritoneum are the **mesentery**, which lies between the parietal and visceral layers like a pleated fan covering most of the small intestine, and the greater **omentum**, which hangs down over the intestines like an apron. Table 12.1 lists combining forms pertaining to the GI system, and anatomy and physiology terms relating to the system are presented in Table 12.2.

Table 12.1

Combining Forms Relating to the Gastrointestinal System

Combining form	Meaning	Example
-ase	enzyme	protease
carbo-	carbon atom	carbohydrate
celi/o	abdomen	celiac
cheil/o (chil/o)	lips	cheilitis (chilitis)
chol/o (chol/e)	bile	cholangitis
choledoch/o	common bile duct	choledochitis
col/o	colon	colonoscopy
dent/o	teeth	dentition
duoden/o	duodenum	duodenal
enter/o	intestines	enteritis
gastr/o	stomach	gastroenteritis
gingiv/o	gums	gingivitis
gloss/o	tongue	glossopharyngeal
glyc/o	sugar	glycerol
hepat/o	liver	hepatomegaly
hepatic/o	liver	hepaticodochotomy
herni/o	rupture, hernia	herniorrhaphy
ile/o	ileum	ileostomy
jejun/o	jejunum	jejunectomy
lapar/o	abdomen	laparoscopy
lip/o	fat, lipid	liposuction
lith/o	stone (calcification)	cholelithiasis
odont/o	tooth	orthodontia

continued on next page

pancreat/o	pancreas	pancreatic
pharyng/o	pharynx (throat)	pharyngeal
proct/o	rectum, anus	proctologist
pylor/o	pylorus (gatekeeper)	pyloroplasty
rect/o	rectum	rectal
sial/o	saliva	sialolith
sigmoid/o	sigmoid colon	sigmoidoscopy
splen/o	spleen	splenectomy
stom/a	mouth	stomatitis
typhl/o	cecum	typhlitis
viscer/o	internal organs	viscera

Table 12.2

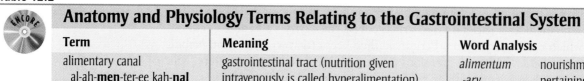

Anatomy and Physiology Terms Relating to the Gastrointestinal System

Term	Meaning	Word Analysis	
alimentary canal al-ah-**men**-ter-ee kah-**nal**	gastrointestinal tract (nutrition given intravenously is called hyperalimentation)	alimentum -ary	nourishment pertaining to
alveolus al-**vee**-ah-lus	a bony socket in which the root of each tooth sits	alveol/o	hollow sac (from alveus, bowl)
amino acid ah-**mee**-nO **as**-id	type of compound that is an essential building block of the human body	amino	chemical substance that refers to an ammonia compound
amylase **am**-ah-lays	type of chemical substance (enzyme) secreted by the pancreas	amyl/o -ase	starch relating to an enzyme
anal canal **ay**-nel kah-**nal**	passageway through which fecal material is passed	anus -al	ring pertaining to
anus **ay**-nus	exit site of the digestive canal from which feces are excreted	anus	ring
bile **bII**	greenish substance secreted by the liver and passed into the duodenum; helps with emulsification of fats	bilus	bile
carbohydrate kahr-bO-**hI**-drayt	type of compound containing carbon atoms that is composed of small molecules such as sugars	carbo- hydr/o -ate	carbon water state of
cardiac sphincter **kahr**-dee-ak **sfink**-ter	muscle ring at the inferior end of the esophagus that prevents food from going back up the esophagus	cardi/o -ac sphincter	heart pertaining to band
cecum **see**-kum	sac that lies below the ileum and is the beginning of the large intestine	cecum	blind
cholecystokinin kO-lee-sis-tO-**kI**-nin	hormone that stimulates contraction of the gallbladder and secretion of pancreatic juice	chol/e cyst/o kin/e	bile bladder, pouch movement, motion
chyme kIm	substance made up of partly digested food passed from the stomach to duodenum	chyme	juice
common bile duct	outlet for bile to be passed into the duodenum; formed by the joining of the common hepatic duct with the cystic duct	bilus	bile

deciduous dee-**sid**-yoo-us	teeth called the baby teeth that fall out; not permanent	*deciduous*	falling off
duodenum doo-O-**dee**-num/ doo-**od**-en-um	first area of the small intestine; cholecystokinin is secreted by the duodenal mucosa	*duodenum*	twelve (duodenum is about 12 finger breadths long)
emulsion ee-**mul**-shun	substance formed by two liquids that do not totally mix (e.g., oil in water)	*emulsify*	to drain out
enzyme **en**-zIm	protein that makes other substances change; enzyme names usually end in *-ase* (e.g., *maltase* changes *maltose*)	*en-* *zyme*	in leaven
esophagus ee-**sof**-ah-gus	structure between the pharynx and stomach	*esophagus*	gullet
fat	greasy substance found in tissues	*fat*	cram
feces **fee**-seez	substance excreted (defecated) from the body; composed of undigested material, waste from food, and other materials	*feces*	dregs
frenulum **fren**-yoo-lum	mucous membrane that anchors the bottom of the tongue to the floor of the mouth	*frenulum*	bridle
fundus **fun**-dus	part farthest away from the opening	*fundus*	bottom
gallbladder **gawl**-blad-er	organ that stores bile	*gall* *bladder*	bile receptacle
gastric juice **gas**-trik joos	secretion from the stomach	*gastr/o* *-ic*	stomach pertaining to
gastroenterology **gas**-trO-en-ter-**ol**-ah-jee	study of the digestive system	*gastr/o* *enter/o* *-logy*	stomach intestine study of
glucose **gloo**-kOs	a type of sugar	*gluc/o* *-ose*	sweet pertaining to
hepatic heh-**pat**-ik	pertaining to the liver	*hepat/o* *-ic*	liver pertaining to
ileum **il**-ee-um	portion of the small intestine from the jejunum to the ileocecal opening	*ileum*	twist
jejunum jeh-**joo**-num	portion of the small intestine between the duodenum and ileum	*jejunum*	empty
lacteal **lak**-tee-el	lymph vessel that absorbs fatty lipid materials from the chyme	*lact/o* *-eal*	milk pertaining to
large intestine in-**tes**-tin	section of the GI tract below the small intestine	*intestine*	intestine
liver **liv**-er	largest gland in the body; secretes bile and filters substances; aids in carbohydrate and protein digestion	*lifer*	liver
mastication mas-tih-**kay**-shun	process of chewing	*masticate*	to chew
mesentery **mez**-en-ter-ee	fan-shaped fold of the peritoneum that covers most of the small intestine	*mesos* *enteron*	middle intestine
microvilli mI-krO-**vil**-I	tiny projections within the small intestine that greatly increase the surface area to better absorb nutrients	*micro-* *villus*	small shaggy hair
omentum O-**men**-tum	fatty layer covering the front of the intestines like an apron	*omentum*	membrane that encloses the bowel

continued on next page

pancreas **pan**-kree-as	gland that extends from the duodenum to the spleen; exocrine portion secretes pancreatic juices directly into the intestine; endocrine portion secretes insulin and glucagon	*pancreas*	all flesh
parietal pah-**rI**-eh-tel	wall of a cavity	*pariet/o* *-al*	wall pertaining to
parotid pah-**rot**-id	salivary gland located near the ear	*parotid*	gland near the ear
peristalsis per-ih-**stal**-sis	action of the intestine characterized by alternating contraction and relaxation to propel food substances forward	*peri-* *stalsis*	around contraction
peritoneum per-ih-tO-**nee**-um	tissue that lines the abdominal cavity	*peritoneum*	to stretch over
plicae **plI**-see	circular folds of the intestines covered with villi	*plica*	fold
protein **prO**-teen	substance from which the body is made	*prote/o*	protein
pyloric sphincter pI-**lor**-ik **sfink**-ter	muscular band that holds food in the stomach while it is being digested	*pylorus* *-ic* *sphincter*	gatekeeper pertaining to band
pylorus pI-**lO**-rus	bottom part of the stomach	*pylorus*	gatekeeper
rectum **rek**-tum	final portion of the GI tract	*rect/o*	rectum
rugae **roo**-gee	the lining of the stomach is tucked into rugae, or folds, that expand when filled to allow for better exposure for absorption	*ruga*	wrinkle
saliva sah-**lI**-vah	secretion from the salivary glands in the mouth that begins the process of digestion	*sialon*	saliva
small intestine in-**tes**-tin	portion of the digestive tract between the stomach and large intestine	*intestin*	intestine
stomach **stum**-ek	sac between the esophagus and the small intestine	*stoma*	mouth
sublingual sub-**ling**-gwal	under the tongue	*sub-* *lingua* *-al*	under tongue pertaining to
submandibular sub-man-**dib**-yoo-ler	below the mandible (jaw)	*sub-* *mandibul/o* *-ar*	under jaw pertaining to
tooth	structure within the mouth that is formed of calcium and breaks down food through mastication	*tooth*	tooth
uvula **yoo**-vyoo-lah	fleshy structure in the back of the throat that prevents food from entering the nasopharynx	*uvula*	cluster of grapes
vermiform appendix **ver**-mih-form ah-**pen**-diks	structure known as the appendix; composed of lymphatic tissue but has only a minor role in the immunologic system; attached to the cecum and lies close to the wall of the rectum	*vermi* *form* *appendix*	worm having the shape or form of bodily outgrowth
villi **vil**-I	hairlike projections within the intestine	*villus*	tiny hairs
visceral **vis**-er-al	refers to the internal organs	*viscer/o* *-al*	internal organs pertaining to

Separate the terms into their individual word parts, using slashes. Identify each word part by writing a "P" for prefix, "R" for root, "S" for suffix, or "CV" for combining vowel under the word part. Then, supply a definition of the entire term.

	Word Analysis	Definition
1. colitis	_____	_____
2. gastroscopy	_____	_____
3. duodenal	_____	_____
4. enteritis	_____	_____
5. cholecystokinin	_____	_____
6. hepatomegaly	_____	_____
7. laparoscopy	_____	_____
8. pancreatic	_____	_____
9. pyloroplasty	_____	_____
10. proctologist	_____	_____
11. sigmoidoscopy	_____	_____
12. splenectomy	_____	_____

Comprehension Check

Circle the correct word from each pair in the following sentences.

1. The patient's cardiac sphincter/cardiac cycle is incompetent and allows stomach contents to pass into the esophagus.

2. The fundic/fundus is the upper portion of the stomach.

3. The stomach produces hydrochloric/hypochloric acid.

4. The terminal portion of the small intestine is the ileum/jejunum.

5. Laparoscopy/Peristalsis propels the chyme farther down the digestive tract.

6. The hepatic/hepatitic ducts were completely obstructed.

7. The parietal/partial peritoneum was torn and had to be sutured.

8. Masticayse/Amylase is an important enzyme.

9. Proteins are composed of amino acids/hydrochloric acids.

10. Dr. Besidan's specialty is gastroenterology/hypogastrology.

11. Chyme/Uvula is a semisolid substance composed of gastric juices and partially digested food.

12. Food passes down the thymus/esophagus and into the stomach.

Matching

Match the term or abbreviation in Column 1 with the correct definition in Column 2. Write the number of the term on the blank provided.

Column 1

1. frenulum

2. carbohydrates

3. pyloric sphincter

4. sublingual

5. mastication

6. cardiac sphincter

7. peristalsis

8. jejunum

9. pharynx

10. duodenum

11. ileum

12. bile

Column 2

a. chewing

b. muscle lined with mucous membrane

c. ring of muscle between the stomach and esophagus that holds food in the stomach while it is digested

d. muscle contractions that propel chyme farther down the digestive tract

e. thin membrane that attaches the tongue to the floor of the mouth

f. portion of the small intestine nearest the stomach

g. portion of the small intestine that joins with the large intestine

h. ring of muscle between the stomach and small intestine that holds food in the stomach while it is digested

i. chemical compounds of starches and sugars

j. substance secreted by the liver and stored in the gallbladder

k. midportion of the small intestine

l. under the tongue

Word Building

In the sentences that follow, the correct combining form is used, but the prefix or suffix does not match the definition. Rewrite the word, supplying the correct word part.

1. colostomy: inflammation of the colon

2. duodenectomy: pertaining to the duodenum

3. gastritis: removal of the stomach

4. pregastric: below the stomach

5. pancreatectomy: pertaining to the pancreas

6. splenitis: removal of the spleen

7. hepatoscopy: pertaining to the liver

8. antipharyngeal: pertaining to the tongue and pharynx

9. proctectomy: study of the rectum

_____

10. sigmoidotomy: examination of the sigmoid
    colon through an instrument

_____

Spelling Check

Write the correct spelling of each misspelled word in each sentence.

_____

1. The study of the gasterintestinal system is called gastroenrterology.

_____

2. The GI tract is also known as the elementary canal.

_____

3. There are three pairs of salaviary glands.

_____

4. The desiduous teeth are also called baby teeth.

_____

5. The lining of an empty stomack is folded into rugby.

_____

6. Each vilus contains a lymph vessel called a lactael.

_____

7. The pancrious lies behind the stomach.

_____

8. Cholesystokinnin is a hormone secreted by the mucousa of the duoduenum.

_____

9. The veriform apendix is sometimes just called the apendix.

_____

10. The viscerial periteonum covers the organs of the abdominal cavity.

_____

The diagram below traces the route nutrients follow through the digestive tract. Fill in the missing information.

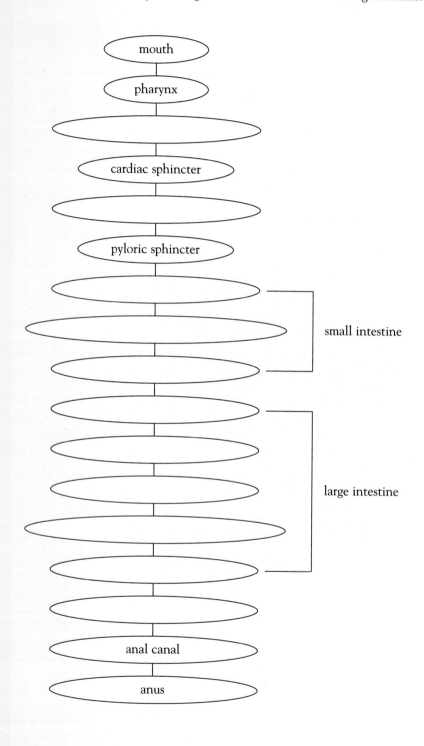

mouth

pharynx

cardiac sphincter

pyloric sphincter

small intestine

large intestine

anal canal

anus

Wellness and Illness through the Life Span

In an assessment, the examiner first observes the patient's general appearance, since nutritional status can be indicated by general size, height, and weight. As is always the case, a complete history is taken to evaluate general health. When the focus is the gastrointestinal system, questions concern nutrition (what is eaten, when, and over how long a period?), digestion (is there is any pain during or after eating, abdominal swelling, bloating, burping, or gassiness?), and elimination (what are the color, texture, and pattern of bowel movements?).

The physical examination begins with the mouth and teeth—proper oral hygiene is important to good digestion. The examination continues with the abdomen to determine size, shape, and characteristics. The examiner then uses the stethoscope to listen to the abdomen for bowel sounds, followed by percussion, which indicates the sizes and shapes of the organs. Lastly, the abdomen is palpated using light touch and then deep touch under the rib area and over the entire abdomen to the pelvis.

The abdomen is divided into four quadrants—right and left upper and lower quadrants—and sometimes into regions—the epigastric, the area between the lower margins of the ribs; the umbilical, the area surrounding the umbilicus (belly button); and the hypogastric or suprapubic, the area above the pubic bone. Figure 12.9 depicts these areas and lists the organs located within each one.

Figure 12.9 - Divisions of the Abdomen

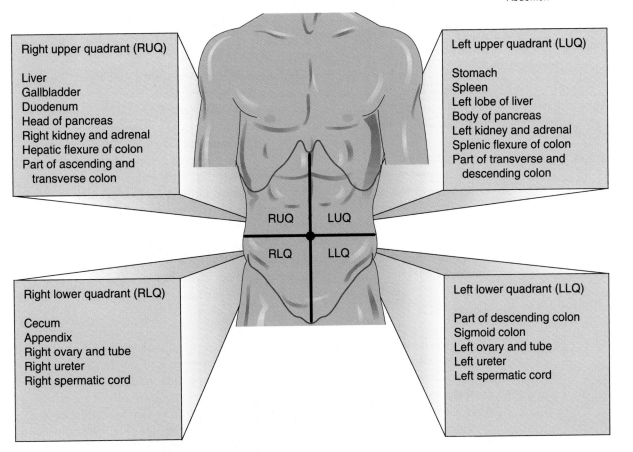

Right upper quadrant (RUQ)

Liver
Gallbladder
Duodenum
Head of pancreas
Right kidney and adrenal
Hepatic flexure of colon
Part of ascending and
    transverse colon

Left upper quadrant (LUQ)

Stomach
Spleen
Left lobe of liver
Body of pancreas
Left kidney and adrenal
Splenic flexure of colon
Part of transverse and
    descending colon

RUQ LUQ
RLQ LLQ

Right lower quadrant (RLQ)

Cecum
Appendix
Right ovary and tube
Right ureter
Right spermatic cord

Left lower quadrant (LLQ)

Part of descending colon
Sigmoid colon
Left ovary and tube
Left ureter
Left spermatic cord

Infants

The premature infant is at great risk for a disorder called **neonatal necrotizing enterocolitis (NEC)**, which is characterized by death of the tissues of the ileum and colon. Possible causes include bacteria and decreased blood supply to the intestines.

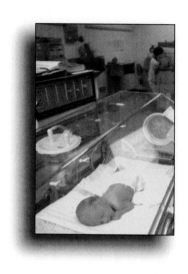

The newborn has a prominent belly button because of the attachment of the umbilical cord *in utero*. The muscles of the abdomen are not developed, making the abdominal wall fairly thin. Infants' abdominal organs are easy to palpate, especially the liver, which is large in the newborn. The abdomen is protuberant, and it may be possible to see an **umbilical** or **inguinal hernia**, if present, especially when the infant cries. A hernia occurs when a portion of the intestine is pushed out through a weakened area of the tissue that would normally contain it. Thus an umbilical hernia can be seen at the belly button and an inguinal hernia in the inguinal area, or groin.

During the first examination of the newborn, the physician checks for an anal opening so that elimination may occur. **Imperforate anus** describes a condition in which an infant has no anal opening. Congenital disorders such as **aglossia** (absence of the tongue); **ankyloglossia**, tongue-tie; and **cleft palate**, an incomplete closure of the middle of the palate, are noted and corrected as soon as possible so that the infant can receive good oral nutrition. The first stool of the newborn, called **meconium**, is greenish-black and sticky and occurs within 24 hours of birth. When the infant eats after birth, the stools change color and texture and become fecal smelling.

A **tracheoesophageal fistula (T-E fistula)** is a congenital disorder in which an abnormal opening between the trachea and the esophagus causes food to enter the trachea, resulting in choking and pneumonia. **Pyloric stenosis**, which first appears in the 6-week-old male child (most commonly), is a condition characterized by a narrowing of the pyloric sphincter, causing projectile vomiting.

Children

The genetic disorder **cystic fibrosis** is diagnosed in infancy or early childhood. It is an inherited disease that causes airway obstruction and pancreatic insufficiency. Patients must take pancreatic enzymes so that food can be absorbed properly. The stool is sticky and foul smelling because of the missing pancreatic enzymes. Respiratory problems associated with the disease are discussed in Chapter 10, "The Respiratory System."

An **intussusception** can occur at any time but most commonly presents in childhood and most often in the male. Intussusception is the enfolding (telescoping) of one part of the intestine into another, causing a blockage. **Crohn's disease** is characterized by diarrhea, cramps, abdominal pain, weight loss, and sometimes fever. It is a chronic disorder of the terminal ileum that involves ulcers, fibrosis of the bowel, and fistulas. **Ulcerative colitis** is a chronic condition that causes anemia, pain, rectal bleeding, and electrolyte imbalance. Symptoms include ulceration of the colon and rectum, with inflammatory changes in the bowel.

Adults

One of the most common GI disorders affecting adults is the **ulcer**, or hole in the mucosa, of the GI tract. Gastric ulcers occur in the stomach area and duodenal ulcers are found in the duodenum, where there is a high concentration of hydrochloric acid from the stomach. Researchers have discovered that a bacterium called *Helicobacter pylori* is largely responsible for ulcers. This organism burrows through the mucous lining of the GI tract, preventing mucus production in that area. The lack of mucus allows the hydrochloric acid to erode the area, forming the ulcer. While stress is a factor in the formation of ulcers, treatment is now directed toward antibiotics that inhibit the bacteria.

Hemorrhoids frequently occur in pregnant women but are a common problem among adults of both sexes. This disorder, often called piles, is characterized by the painful outpouching of veins in the anal area.

Seniors

Diverticula are pouches that develop in the GI tract, causing bleeding and inflammation. Diverticulosis is found in the intestine of middle-aged persons; diverticulitis is an inflammation of a diverticulum, usually within the colon. **Polyps**, masses of tissue or projections from the surface of the intestine that vary in shape, are also found in the GI tract. Another disorder found in older persons is the **hiatal hernia**, sometimes called hiatus hernia. A hernia of the stomach, it pushes out near the esophagus and diaphragm, causing indigestion, pain, and discomfort, especially when the person lies down.

General Illnesses

Hepatitis is an inflammation of the liver caused by viral pathogens found in some foods, such as shellfish, or in blood transmitted through transfusions. A common ailment among adults (although it can occur in any age-group), **heartburn** is caused by the irritation of the esophagus from an acidic stomach. Food reenters the esophagus by a process called **reflux,** causing discomfort, burping, a bad taste in the mouth, pain in the chest, and even **emesis** (vomiting). It can signify ulcer formation or eating too rapidly, or other problems.

Lactose intolerance occurs when the sugar lactose cannot be digested properly in the GI tract. This intolerance can occur at any age and is characterized by gassiness and often diarrhea after the ingestion of dairy products. Individuals can avoid the problems by taking a product called Lactaid, which artificially breaks down the lactose in foods.

Constipation can occur at any age. This problem develops when food passes too slowly through the GI tract so that the water within it is absorbed in the small and large intestines, and the fecal material becomes hard and difficult to pass through the anal canal. **Diarrhea** is the opposite problem. When food passes through the system too quickly, not enough water is absorbed, which results in loose, watery stools. **Ileus** is a mechanical failure of the gut in which there is no peristalsis to move stools through the bowel.

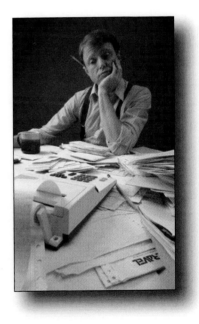

Problems with the gallbladder occur most frequently in the adult, but they may also be found in children with certain hematologic disorders such as sickle cell disease. The most common disorder is **cholecystitis**, an inflammation of the gallbladder when fatty foods are ingested and the secretion from the gallbladder (bile) cannot digest them. **Cholelithiasis**, or gallstone formation, can occur in the gallbladder or the bile ducts.

Oncologic diseases of the GI tract are generally carcinomas. These include head and neck cancers, colorectal cancers, pancreatic carcinoma, stomach cancer, hepatocellular carcinoma. Hepatoblastoma and GI lymphomas are found more commonly in the young. The two main factors affecting the occurrence of **colorectal cancer** are age and diet. Risk increases with age and decreases in those who eat a high-fiber vegetarian diet. Predisposing conditions that increase risk include benign polyps, chronic ulcerative colitis, Crohn's disease, and a family history of colon cancer. Surgery is performed on localized tumors, with radiation and chemotherapy as adjunct treatments.

Figure 12.10 displays the common diseases of the digestive tract and their locations. Table 12.3 defines wellness and illness terms related to the GI system.

Figure 12.10 - Digestive Tract Diseases and Their Locations

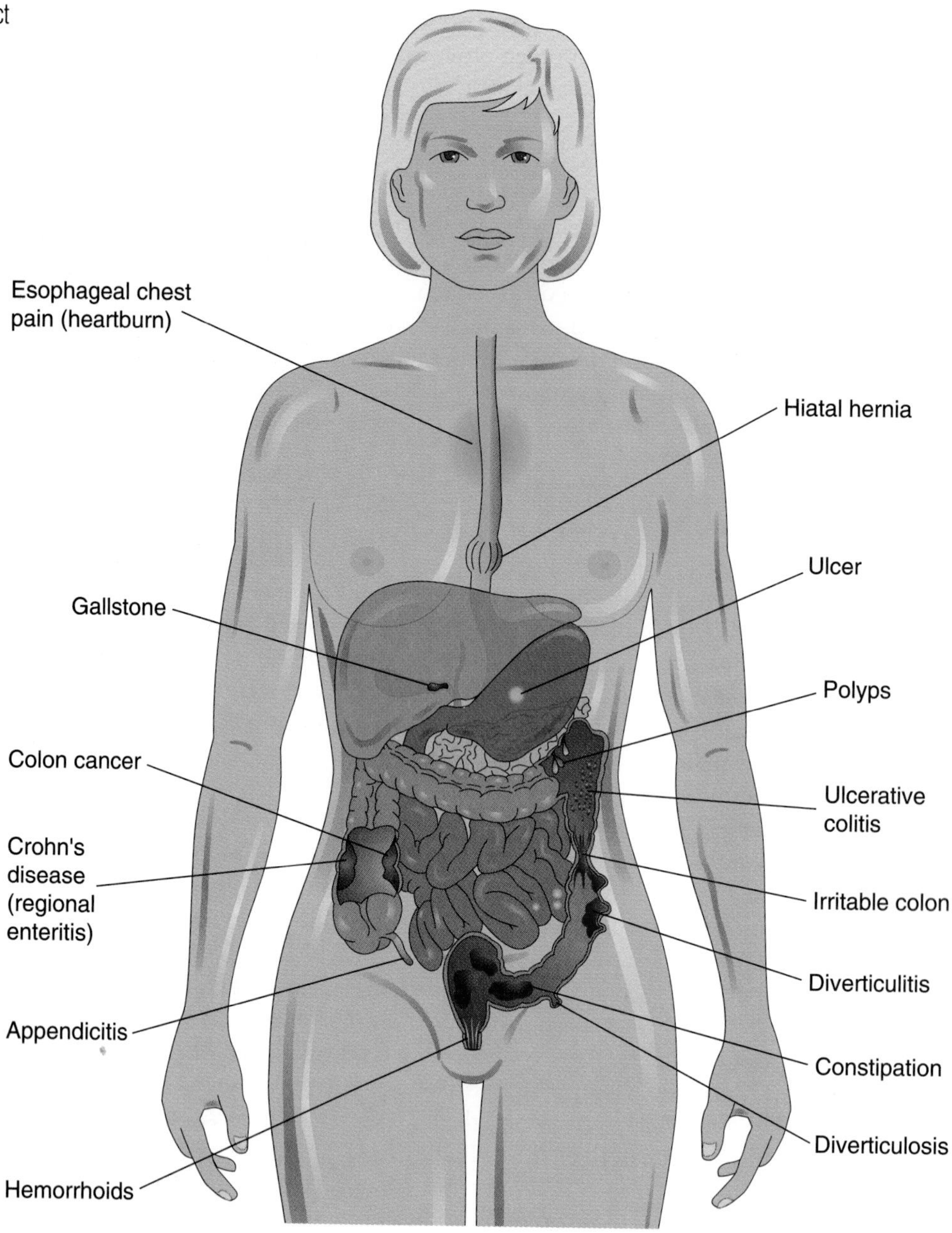

Esophageal chest pain (heartburn)

Gallstone

Colon cancer

Crohn's disease (regional enteritis)

Appendicitis

Hemorrhoids

Hiatal hernia

Ulcer

Polyps

Ulcerative colitis

Irritable colon

Diverticulitis

Constipation

Diverticulosis

Table 12.3

Wellness and Illness Terms Relating to the Gastrointestinal System

Term	Meaning	Word Analysis	
aglossia ah-**glos**-ee-ah	congenital anomaly in which an infant has no tongue	a- gloss/o -ia	without tongue; language condition of
ankyloglossia **an**-kil-O-**glos**-ee-ah	tongue-tied; the tongue is not freely movable	ankl/o gloss/o -ia	bent, fixed tongue; language condition of
appendicitis ah-pen-dih-**sI**-tis	inflammation of the appendix (actual name is vermiform appendix)	appendix -itis	appendage inflammation
cholecystitis kO-leh-sis-**tI**-tis	inflammation of the gallbladder when fatty foods are ingested and the secretion from the gallbladder (bile) is unable to digest them	chol/e cyst/o -itis	bile bladder, pouch inflammation

cholelithiasis kO-leh-lith-**I**-ah-sis	gallstone formation in the gallbladder or bile ducts	chol/e lith/o -iasis	bile stone disease
cleft palate kleft **pal**-et	congenital abnormality consisting of an opening in the palate	cleft palat	opening; fissure palate
constipation kon-stih-**pay**-shun	condition in which food passes too slowly through the GI tract, and water is absorbed from the small and large intestines, causing fecal material to become hard and difficult to pass through the anal canal	con- stipo	with to press together
Crohn's disease krOnz	chronic disorder usually involving the terminal ileum; there are ulcers, fistulas, and fibrotic areas of bowel	Crohn	20th-century American gastroenterologist
cystic fibrosis **sis**-tik fI-**brO**-sis	hereditary disorder characterized by respiratory difficulties and frequent, mushy, foul-smelling stools because of missing pancreatic enzymes	cystic fibr/o -osis	refers to cysts; bladder, pouch fiber (fibrous) condition
diarrhea dI-ah-**ree**-ah	frequent, loose, watery stools from improper absorption of water in the colon	dia- -rrhea	through flow
diverticulum dI-ver-**tik**-yoo-lum diverticulosis dI-ver-tik-yoo-**lO**-sis diverticulitis dI-ver-tik-yoo-**lI**-tis	pouch that develops like a hernia of the mucosa of the GI tract	diverticulum	byroad
emesis **em**-eh-sis	vomit; vomiting	emesis	vomit
heartburn	condition characterized by regurgitation of stomach contents into the esophagus	heartburn	describes the symptom associated with the disorder
hemorrhoid **hem**-or-oyd	characterized by the painful outpouching of veins in the anal area (commonly called piles)	hem/o rhoia	blood flow
hepatitis (viral) hep-ah-**tI**-tis	inflammation of the liver caused by viral pathogens found in food or blood	hepat/o -itis	liver inflammation
hiatal (hiatus) hernia hI-**ay**-tel (hI-**ay**-tus) **her**-nee-ah	hernia of the stomach that pushes out near the esophagus and diaphragm	hiatus hernia	opening rupture
ileus **il**-ee-us	absence of peristalsis, causing obstruction within the intestine	ileus	to roll up tightly
imperforate anus im-**per**-fer-ayt **ay**-nus	congenital anomaly in which there is no anal opening	im- perforo anus	negative to bore through anal orifice
inguinal hernia **in**-gwin-el **her**-nee-ah	portion of the intestine pushed out through a weakened area of the tissue that would normally contain it; inguinal hernia is seen in the inguinal area, or groin	inguinal hernia	relating to the groin rupture
intussusception **in**-tus-sus-**sep**-shun	enfolding of one part of the intestine into another, causing a blockage	intus suscipio	within to take up
jaundice **jawn**-dis	yellowish color of the skin and mucous membranes because of increased bile pigment in the blood	jaune	yellow

continued on next page

lactose intolerance **lak**-tOs in-**tol**-er-ens	lactose, a sugar, cannot be digested properly by the GI tract; characterized by gassiness and often diarrhea after ingestion of dairy products	lactose intolerance	a sugar
meconium meh-**kO**-nee-um	first elimination of the newborn; consists of mucus, bile, and tissue from the intestines	meconium	poppy
neonatal necrotizing enterocolitis nee-O-**nay**-tel **nek**-rO-**tIz**-ing **en**-ter-O-kO-**II**-tis	death of the tissues of the ileum and colon of premature infants, perhaps due to bacteria and decreased blood supply to the intestines	ne/o natal necr/o enter/o col/o -itis	new relating to birth death intestine colon inflammation
polyp **pol**-ip	mass of tissue or projection from the surface of the intestine	polyp	many feet
pyloric stenosis pI-**lor**-ik steh-**nO**-sis	first appears in the 6-week-old male child (most commonly) and is characterized by a narrowing of the pyloric sphincter, causing projectile vomiting	pylor/o -ic sten/o -osis	pylorus pertaining to constriction condition
reflux **ree**-fluks	backward flow of stomach contents (as in heartburn)	re- fluxus	back flow
suprapubic soo-prah-**pyoo**-bik	area of the abdomen above the pubic bones	supra- pub/o -ic	above pubis, pubic pertaining to
tracheoesophageal fistula **tray**-kee-O-ee-sah-**fay**-jee-el **fis**-tyoo-lah	abnormal opening between the trachea and the esophagus that causes food to enter the trachea and cause choking and pneumonia	trache/o esophagus -eal fistula	trachea gullet pertaining to a tube
ulcer **ul**-ser	hole in the mucosa	ulcus	ulcer
ulcerative colitis **ul**-ser-ah-tiv kO-**II**-tis	chronic disease characterized by ulceration of the colon and rectum and an inflammatory process usually in the colon	ulcus -ative col/o -itis	ulcer pertaining to colon inflammation
umbilicus um-**bil**-ih-kus (also um-bil-**I**-kus)	the navel (belly button)	umbilicus	navel
umbilical hernia um-**bil**-ih-kl **her**-nee-ah	portion of the intestine is pushed out through a weakened area of the tissue that would normally contain it; an umbilical hernia can be seen at the belly button	umbilicus hernia	navel rupture

Supply a definition for the combining form in each term. Then supply a definition for the entire term.

	Combining form	Definition	Term definition
1. gastritis			
2. colonoscopy			
3. aglossia			
4. stenosis			
5. pancreatectomy			
6. cholelithiasis			
7. hyperlipidemia			
8. hepatitis			
9. gingival			
10. stomatitis			

Comprehension Check

Exercise 8

Circle the correct term from each pair in the following sentences.

1. The umbilical/umbilicus cord was clamped and cut.

2. The hypergastric/hypogastric area is below the stomach.

3. Intussusception/Ulceration is the enfolding of one part of the intestine into another.

4. Cystic fibrosis/Crohn's fibrosis is a genetic disease.

5. Both T-E fistula/ET fishtula and hypochloric stenosis/pyloric stenosis are congenital disorders.

6. Incarceration/Ulceration of the gastric mucosa/epigastric mucous was widespread.

7. Cholecystitis/Cholelithiasis describes the formation of gallstones.

8. The patient had postanesthesia/postkinesia hyperemesis/hypesis that was difficult to control with antiemetics.

9. The patient underwent an emergency appendicitis/appendectomy.

10. The infant required hernioplasty/hernioptomy during the neonatologist/neonatal period.

Match each definition in Column 2 with a term from Column 1. Write the number of the term on the line beside its definition.

Column 1		**Column 2**
1. umbilicus	_____	painful outpouching of veins in the anal area
2. ulcer	_____	abnormal opening between the trachea and esophagus
3. polyp	_____	yellowish color of skin due to increased bile pigments in the blood
4. suprapubic	_____	vomiting
5. appendicitis	_____	navel
6. emesis	_____	backward flow of stomach contents
7. T-E fistula	_____	hole in the mucosa
8. reflux	_____	mass of tissue that projects from the surface of the intestine
9. jaundice	_____	"above the pubis," area of abdomen above the pubic bones
10. hemorrhoid	_____	inflammation of the appendix

Word Building

Use prefixes, root words, combining forms, and suffixes to create medical terms for the following definitions. Write the term on the blank provided.

1. pertaining to above the pubis   _____

2. under the stomach   _____

3. above the stomach   _____

4. inflammation of the liver   _____

5. inflammation of the colon   _____

6. flow through   _____

7. inflammation of the gallbladder   _____

8. inflammation of the appendix   _____

9. without tongue   _____

10. pertaining to the trachea and esophagus   _____

Circle the correct plural or singular form from each pair in the following sentences.

1. The examination located several diverticula/diverticulum in the sigmoid colon.

2. A total of four polyp/polyps were removed during surgery.

3. The operation was listed as a polypectomy/polypectomies.

4. The abdomen was marked and divided into four quadrant/quadrants.

5. Each specimen was placed in a jar, and the liver/livers were taken to the laboratory.

6. There were four gastroenterologist/gastroenterologists present.

7. Several proteins/protein have been identified as allergens.

8. The child had two hernioplasties/hernioplasty.

9. The hepatic duct/ducts were removed.

10. The villi/villus in the intestines demonstrated morphological abnormalities.

Word Maps   *Exercise 12*

Group the following illness terms under the GI tract area where they occur.

constipation	heartburn	inguinal hernia
diverticulitis	hemorrhoids	intussusception
gastric ulcer	hiatal hernia	umbilical hernia

Stomach	**Intestines**	**Rectum/Anus**
_____	_____	_____
_____	_____	_____
_____	_____	_____
_____		

Diagnosing and Treating Problems

Tests, Procedures, and Pharmaceuticals

Several laboratory blood tests can assess the functioning of organs within the GI tract (see Table 12.4). For example, the following liver function tests can help diagnose liver disease:

- alanine aminotransferase (ALT)
- alkaline phosphatase
- aspartate aminotransferase (AST)
- bilirubin
- lactate dehydrogenase (LDH)
- serum glutamic-pyruvic transaminase (SGPT)

Amylase and **lipase** can be measured in the serum to ascertain pancreatic enzymes. Also, as discussed in Chapter 7, "The Endocrine System," serum glucose tests can evaluate the functioning of the pancreatic islets. Specific blood tests can detect the presence of the antigens that cause viral hepatitis.

Procedures

X-ray procedures are particularly important for diagnosing diseases and conditions in the GI tract. A "**GI series**" refers to a set of various x-rays, including the barium swallow, which visualizes the upper GI system, and the barium enema, which visualizes the lower GI system. **Cholangiography** is a radiologic study to view the gallbladder and its ducts. The procedure in which gallstones are crushed and removed is called **lithotripsy**.

Many of the GI diagnostic procedures center on the use of the **endoscope** and other instruments. The endoscope is a flexible tube with fiberoptics that allows the physician to look inside the esophagus, stomach, and other areas. Some of the common studies (note the suffix *-scopy*) include **gastroscopy** (stomach), **colonoscopy** (colon), **sigmoidoscopy** (sigmoid colon), and **proctoscopy** (rectum and anal area).

Surgical procedures of the GI tract, signaled by the suffix *-ectomy*, include the **gastrectomy**, removal of the stomach or part of the stomach; **appendectomy**, removal of the appendix; **cholecystectomy**, removal of the gallbladder; and **colostomy** and **ileostomy**, in which an opening is made on the abdominal wall and the end of the colon or ileum is attached to the artificial opening. The colostomy and ileostomy are necessary when portions of the large or small intestine are removed because of cancer or other destructive diseases.

Table 12.4

Tests and Procedures Relating to the Gastrointestinal System

Term	Meaning	Word Analysis	
amylase **am**-ah-lays	blood test to measure the amount of amylase, an enzyme secreted by the pancreas	amyl/o -ase	starch relating to an enzyme
appendectomy ap-en-**dek**-tah-mee	removal of the appendix	appendix -ectomy	bodily outgrowth surgical removal
cholangiography kO-lan-jee-**og**-rah-fee	x-ray of the gallbladder and its ducts	chol/o angi/o -graphy	bile vessel process of recording

cholecystectomy kO-leh-sis-**tek**-tah-mee	removal of the gallbladder	*chol/e* *cyst/o* *-ectomy*	bile bladder surgical removal
colonoscopy kO-lon-**os**-kah-pee	endoscopic procedure to visualize the colon	*col/o* *-scopy*	colon examination
colostomy kO-**los**-tah-mee	surgical procedure to remove part of the colon and make an artificial opening on the abdomen for the excretion of feces	*col/o* *-stomy*	colon surgical creation of an artificial opening
endoscopy en-**dos**-kO-pee	examination of interior structures of the body with an endoscope	*end/o* *-scopy*	within examination
gastrectomy gas-**trek**-tah-mee	removal of the stomach or part of the stomach	*gastr/o* *-ectomy*	stomach surgical removal
gastroscopy gas-**tros**-kah-pee	visualization of the stomach with an endoscope	*gastr/o* *-scopy*	stomach examination
GI series	x-ray procedures such as the barium swallow and barium enema in which a contrast medium (barium) is given either orally or rectally; an x-ray is taken to visualize the flow of the barium through the GI tract		
ileostomy il-ee-**os**-tah-mee	surgical procedure to remove a portion of the ileum and attach the remaining end to an opening made on the abdomen	*ile/o* *-stomy*	relating to the ileum surgical creation of an artificial opening
lipase **lip**-ays	test to measure the amount of lipase, a pancreatic enzyme	*lip/o* *-ase*	fat relating to an enzyme
liver function tests	tests to determine the functioning of the liver	*N/A*	
proctoscopy prok-**tos**-kah-pee	visualization of the rectum and anal canal	*proct/o* *-scopy*	rectum, anus examination
sigmoidoscopy sig-moy-**dos**-kah-pee	visualization of the sigmoidal region of the colon	*sigmoid/o* *-scopy*	sigmoid (portion of the colon) examination

Pharmaceutical Agents

Table 12.5 describes the common pharmacologic agents utilized in treating GI tract illnesses.

Table 12.5

Pharmacologic Agents Relating to the Gastrointestinal System

Drug Classes	Use	Generic Names	Brand Names
antacids and antiflatulents	decrease acidity and gas	aluminum hydroxide and magnesium hydroxide	Maalox
		aluminum hydroxide, magnesium hydroxide, and simethicone	Mylanta
		simethicone	Mylicon
		aluminum hydroxide	Amphojel
		sodium citrate and citric acid	Bicitra

continued on next page

antidiarrheals	stop diarrhea	loperamide octreotide acetate diphenoxylate and atropine	Imodium A-D Sandostatin Lomotil
antiemetics	stop or prevent nausea or vomiting	meclizine hydroxyzine prochlorperazine granisetron promethazine metoclopramide chlorpromazine scopolamine ondansetron	Antivert, Bonine Atarax Compazine Kytril Phenergan Reglan Thorazine Hyoscine, Transderm Scōp Zofran
antifungals	fight fungi (plantlike organisms)	nystatin	Mycostatin
anti-infective	fight *Clostridium* *difficile*	vancomycin metronidazole	Vancocin Flagyl
anti-inflammatory agents	treat GI inflammatory disorders	mesalamine sulfasalazine	Asacol Azulfidine

antispasmodics and
anticholinergics
	decrease GI spasms	dicyclomine
		hyoscyamine, atropine,
		    scopolamine, and
		    phenobarbital
			Bentyl
			Donnatal

appetite suppressants	decrease appetite	phentermine dextroamphetamine	Adipex-P Dexedrine
digestive enzymes	replace pancreatic enzymes	pancrelipase (amylase, lipase, and protease) lactase	Pancrease, Ultrase, Viokase Lactaid
duodenal ulcer adherent	coats the stomach lining	sucralfate	Carafate
gallstone dissolution agents	dissolve gallstones	ursodiol metoclopramide	Actigall Reglan
histamine (H_2) receptor antagonists	treat ulcers	famotidine cimetidine ranitidine	Pepcid Tagamet Zantac
laxatives	stimulate the GI tract to produce stool	psyllium docusate senna sodium phosphate enema bisacodyl	Metamucil Colace Senokot Fleet Enema Dulcolax
nutritional supplements	supplement diet	none	Ensure, Osmolite
proton pump inhibitors	inhibit gastric acid secretion	omeprazole esomeprazole lansoprazole	Prilosec Nexium Prevacid
vaccines	prevent hepatitis B prevent hepatitis A	hepatitis B vaccine hepatitis A vaccine	BayHep B Havrix
vitamin supplements	supplement dietary intake	multivitamins	Vicon Forte, Poly-Vi-Flor, Tri-Vi-Flor

Table 12.6

Abbreviations

a.c.	before meals
BaE or BE	barium enema
BM	bowel movement
CF	cystic fibrosis
GB	gallbladder
GERD	gastroesophageal reflux disease
GI	gastrointestinal
HAL	hyperalimentation
HCl	hydrochloric acid
IVC	intravenous cholangiography
LFT	liver function test
LLQ	left lower quadrant
LRQ	lower right quadrant
LUQ	left upper quadrant
NEC	neonatal necrotizing enterocolitis
n.p.o.	nothing by mouth
p.c.	after meals
p.p.	postprandial (after eating)
PPI	proton pump inhibitors
RLQ	right lower quadrant
RUQ	right upper quadrant
TPN	total parenteral nutrition (hyperalimentation)
UGI	upper gastrointestinal
ULQ	upper left quadrant
URQ	upper right quadrant

Word Analysis

Exercise 13

Identify the combining form or forms in each term and write the definition of the combining form in the first blank. Then write the definition of the entire term in the second blank.

Term	Combining Form Definition	Term Definition
1. cholecystectomy	_____	_____
2. gastrectomy	_____	_____
3. dental	_____	_____
4. sigmoidoscopy	_____	_____
5. proctitis	_____	_____
6. ileostomy	_____	_____
7. colitis	_____	_____
8. pharyngitis	_____	_____

9. enteral _____ _____

10. lithiasis _____ _____

Comprehension Check

Read each sentence and circle the correct term from the two terms given.

1. Amylase and lipase can be measured to ascertain the functioning of the pancreas/esophagus.

2. Serum glucose/gluteus tests are performed to determine the function of the pancreatic islets.

3. The patient had a duodenum/cholangiogram before surgery to remove her gallbladder.

4. Dr. Malone ordered a GI series/GERD series for the patient he saw this morning.

5. Dr. Baker will assist Dr. Malone with the emesis/endoscopy.

6. Impression: jejunum/GERD.

7. There was marked URQ/CHF tenderness on palpation.

8. This patient has been receiving hyperalimentation/appendicitis for the past 3 months.

9. Please call the home health agency to arrange for TPN/CF at home for Mr. Burrows.

10. The laboratory will do a pancreatic/postprandial blood glucose measurement.

Matching

Match the abbreviations in column 1 with their spelled-out versions in column 2. Write the number of the abbreviation on the blank provided.

Column 1		Column 2
1. a.c.	_____	a. gastrointestinal
2. n.p.o.	_____	b. upper left quadrant
3. LRQ	_____	c. liver function test
4. GI	_____	d. postprandial
5. IVC	_____	e. upper gastrointestinal
6. CF	_____	f. nothing by mouth
7. p.p.	_____	g. intravenous cholangiography
8. UGI	_____	h. before meals
9. ULQ	_____	i. lower right quadrant
10. LFT	_____	j. cystic fibrosis

Supply the word parts to complete each term, according to the definition provided.

1. _____ectomy means surgical removal of the gallbladder.

2. _____itis is an inflammation of the gallbladder.

3. _____graphy is the process of recording the gallbladder and its ducts (vessels).

4. _____scopy refers to examination of the colon using an instrument.

5. _____stomy is the surgical creation of an artificial opening from the colon to the outside of the body.

6. _____ectomy means removal of the stomach.

7. _____scopy is an examination of the stomach using an instrument.

8. _____scopy is an examination of the rectum using an instrument.

9. _____stomy refers to the surgical creation of an artificial opening from the ileum to the outside of the body.

10. An _____scope is an instrument with a flexible tube used to view the interior of the body.

11. _____tomy refers to an incision into the stomach.

12. _____ectomy means removal of the appendix.

Spell out the following abbreviations on the blanks provided.

1. p.c.   _____

2. HCl   _____

3. NEC   _____

4. N&V   _____

5. BE   _____

6. GB   _____

7. RLQ   _____

8. UGI   _____

9. LLQ   _____

10. HAL   _____

Endoscopic procedures to examine different areas of the gastrointestinal tract have different names, all indicating that an instrument is used to visualize the area. Provide the correct term for the scope examination of each area indicated. In the second column of lines, write the name of a disease associated with the area.

	Procedure	Disease
mouth/oral cavity	_____	_____
esophagus	_____	_____
stomach	_____	_____
small intestine	_____	_____
large intestine (colon)	_____	_____
sigmoid colon	_____	_____
rectum	_____	_____

Performance Assessment 12

Crossword Puzzle

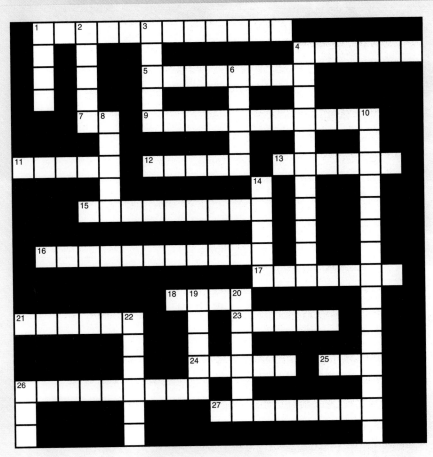

Across
1. inflammation of the appendix
4. word part meaning stomach
5. absence of the tongue
7. abbreviation for after meals
9. below the stomach
11. umbilicus
12. hole in the mucosa
13. jaune
15. flexible, lighted instrument used to view the inside of structures in the body
16. chewing
17. enzyme secreted by the pancreas
18. secreted by the liver and stored in the gallbladder
21. vomiting
23. relating to birth
24. fleshy structure at the back of the throat, prevents food from entering nasopharynx
25. lip/o
26. inflammation of the liver
27. first elimination of the newborn

Down
1. proct/o
2. having any feet
3. necr/o
4. removal of the stomach
6. lactose
8. col/o
10. removal of the gallbladder
14. type of laxative
19. absence of peristalsis, causing obstruction in the intestine
20. example of a nutritional supplement
22. secretion of the salivary glands
26. abbreviation for hyperalimentation

Analyze the Terms

Read each sentence carefully. Then break each underlined word into its individual parts and write a definition for the whole term. Use hyphens to divide the words. Write the divided term and its definition on the line.

1. Mark's class is studying the <u>gastrointestinal</u> system. _____

   _____

2. They dissected the <u>sublingual</u> salivary gland. _____

   _____

3. The <u>pyloric</u> sphincter holds food in the stomach. _____

   _____

4. The patient was diagnosed with a <u>duodenal</u> ulcer. _____

   _____

5. Mr. Kelly has <u>peritonitis.</u> _____

   _____

6. The scheduled surgical procedure is a <u>jejunectomy.</u> _____

   _____

7. The resident assisted with the <u>pyloroplasty.</u> _____

   _____

8. This patient's bleeding was caused by an <u>esophageal</u> _____
   ulceration.

   _____

9. The <u>anoscope</u> was disinfected after use. _____

   _____

10. The <u>visceral</u> structures were all intact. _____

   _____

What Do These Abbreviations Mean?

Provide a definition for each abbreviation. Write the definition on the line beside the abbreviation.

1. a.c.   _____

2. LRQ   _____

3. n.p.o.   _____

4. p.c.   _____

5. GI   _____

6. CF   _____

7. p.p.   _____

8. TPN   _____

9. LFT   _____

10. IVC   _____

11. HAL   _____

12. GB   _____

Build the Terms

Select word parts from the lists to build a complete medical term for each definition given. Note that not all terms will have a root or combining form, prefix, and suffix. Some word parts may be used more than once.

Combining Forms	Prefixes	Suffixes
gastr/o	hyper-	-ectomy
hepat/o	e-	-otomy
jejun/o	sub-	-logist
lapar/o	hypo-	-pathy
lith/o	pre-	-megaly
lip/o	dys-	-ulous
chole/o	an-	-ectomy
dent/o	pre-	-emia
enter/o	de-	-ic
carb/o	anti-	-plasty
herni/o	per-	-iasis
pancreat/o	bi-	-lysis

1. surgical removal of the middle portion of the small intestine   _____

2. excess fat in the blood   _____

3. breakdown of fat   _____

4. disease of the liver   _____

5. specialist in the study of the digestive system   _____

6. pertaining to carbon   _____

7. condition of gallstones   _____

8. surgical removal of the pancreas   _____

9. surgical repair of a hernia   _____

10. incision into the abdomen   _____

11. without teeth   _____

12. enlargement of the liver   _____

Using Medical References

The following sentences contain medical terms that may not have been addressed on the charts in this chapter. Use medical reference books, your medical term analysis skills, and/or a medical dictionary to find the correct definition of each underlined word. Write the definition on the line below the sentence.

1. This patient has been <u>anorexic</u> for the past two weeks.

   _____

2. There is <u>dysphagia</u>, secondary to the CVA of one month ago.

   _____

3. There is a hairline fracture on the <u>buccal</u> surface of the molar.

   _____

4. The patient exhibited massive <u>ascites</u> and abdominal distention.

   _____

5. The patient presented in the Emergency Room with <u>hematemesis</u>.

   _____

6. There is a marked <u>icterus</u> and hepatomegaly.

   _____

7. The patient c/o frequent and excessive <u>eructation</u>.

   _____

8. The patient c/o <u>flatus</u> and <u>encopresis</u>.

   _____

9. The patient reported that his mouth was painful, and severe <u>glossitis</u> was noted upon examination.

   _____

10. The laboratory report revealed <u>steatorrhea</u>.

   _____

11. The physician will perform <u>esophagoscopy</u> in an attempt to locate the source of the patient's chest pain.

   _____

12. <u>Cheiloplasty</u> was performed ten days after the accident.

   _____

Read each mini medical record or scenario carefully; then estimate the doctor's response. Write the letter of your answer in the space provided.

1. This 57 y/o female reports epigastric pain for the past two weeks and occasional N&V. She has been taking Naprosyn for previously diagnosed arthritis and erythromycin for otitis media. Examination of the abdomen revealed no organomegaly, no ascites, and no tenderness. Which of the following diagnoses will be included in the doctor's analysis?

   A. Gastritis, arthritis, otitis media.
   B. Arthritis, otitis, pericarditis.

   Your response: _____

2. Patient is a 73 y/o male c/o "burning pain" in his chest after eating and at night. After a complete examination, the doctor finds no other problem that could account for the symptoms, so you expect that he will:

   A. Schedule the patient for an esophagoscopy and list an initial impression of GERD.
   B. Order an EKG to R/O MI.

   Your response: _____

3. As the medical transcriptionist, you are transcribing the physician's progress notes. In an early portion of her notes, the doctor dictates that the patient is "edentulous" and later states that the patient has several broken teeth. You would:

   A. Send the transcribed notes to the physician for her signature, as usual.
   B. Call the doctor, tell her that you believe you may have misunderstood the dictation, and ask for clarification.

   Your response: _____

Analyzing Medical Records

Read the physician's progress note on the next page; then answer the following questions.

1. What was the nature of the patient's complaint?

2. Where was the patient seen?

3. Describe four findings from the physical examination.

4. What is the analysis? Is this an infectious disease?

5. Was any medication prescribed?

6. Are any tests to be performed?

7. What type of procedure will the patient have?

8. Why is it necessary to hospitalize this patient?

Physician's Progress Note

PATIENT: Carlos V
DATE: April 2, xxxx

S: Pt. states that he is a 42 y/o carpenter. He reports that yesterday afternoon, while at work, he lifted a 75-lb bag of nails and felt a sharp pain in his abdomen, near the navel. The pain eventually lessened, after he rested, but never completely went away, and he returned to work. The pain became worse throughout the day and continued during the night. The patient states that his father recently died of stomach cancer and he is concerned that he might have the same illness.

O: VS WNL. Patient appears to be in distress with moderate to severe abdominal pain. Abdomen is soft, with generalized tenderness upon palpation. Tenderness is most pronounced in the umbilical region and muscle spasms are noted in that area. There is bulging around the umbilicus, with a palpable mass.

A: Incarcerated umbilical hernia.

P: Admit to Lakeshore Memorial Hospital stat. for herniocrophy. Pt. to remain n.p.o. Request surgical consult from Dr. Ryder.

S. J. Klingman, MD

Short Answer

Describe the function of nutrition in maintaining homeostasis

_____

_____

_____

_____

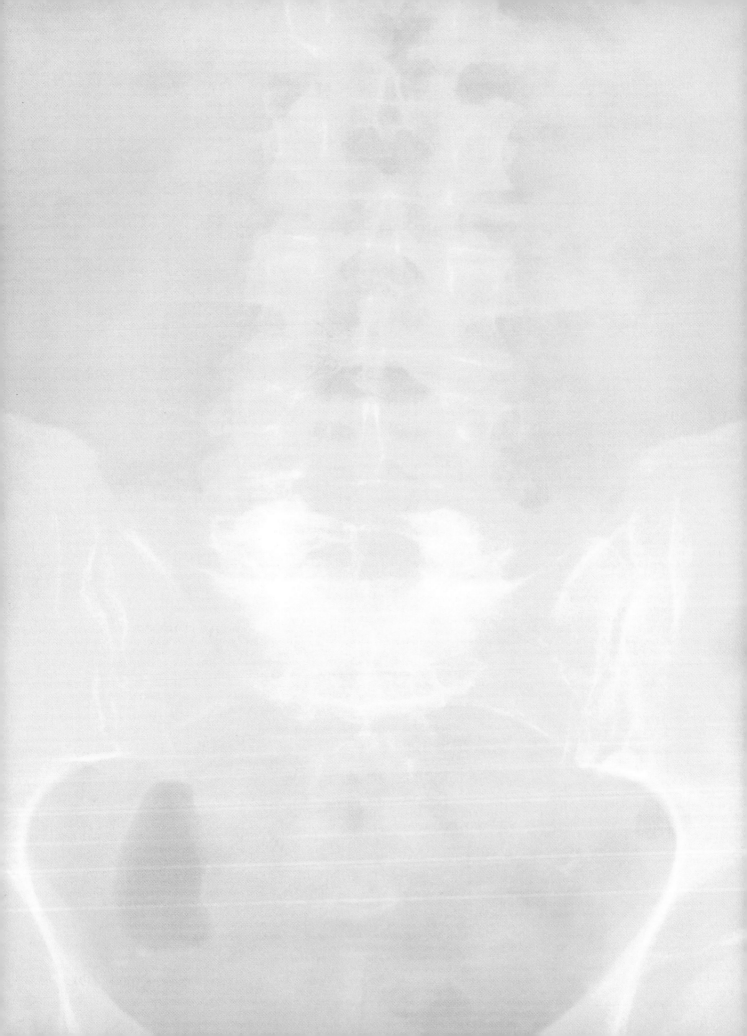

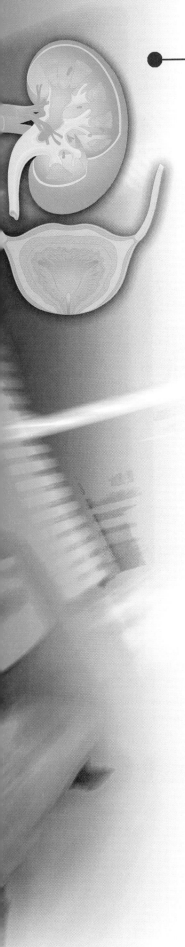

Chapter 13

The Urinary System

Learning Outcomes

Students will be able to:
- Locate and label the structures of the urinary tract on an illustration.
- Describe the process of urine formation.
- Explain the role of the kidneys in maintaining fluid and electrolyte balance.
- State the role of the urinary tract in homeostasis.
- Use the terminology of the urinary system in written and oral communication correctly.
- Correctly spell and pronounce urinary system terminology.
- State the meaning of abbreviations related to the urinary system.
- List and define the combining forms most commonly used to create terms related to the urinary system.
- Name tests and treatments for major urinary system abnormalities.

Translation, Please?Translation, Please?Translation, Please?

Read this excerpt from a physician's progress report, and try to answer the questions that follow.

This 56-year-old male is seen in follow-up for a recent pyelonephritis and microscopic hematuria. He has been referred to urology because of this occasional mild dysuria. He denies any flank or abdominal pain, nausea, or vomiting. There is mild CVA tenderness on examination.

1. Does pyelonephritis refer to pus in the urine or an inflammation of the internal structures of the kidney?
2. Microscopic hematuria refers to tiny amounts of what?
3. Does dysuria mean the inability to urinate or painful urination?
4. Does CVA refer to a cerebrovascular problem or the costovertebral angle?

Answers to "Translation, Please?"
1. Pyelonephritis is inflammation of the internal structures of the kidney—did you notice the "itis"?
2. Microscopic hematuria refers to tiny amounts of blood—recall the meaning of "hema."
3. Dysuria means painful urination. Remember that "dys" refers to pain.
4. CVA refers to the costovertebral angle.

Identifying the Specialty

The System and Its Practitioners

The urinary system filters substances from the blood and eliminates waste. The organs of this system are among the most active structures in the body, filtering about 20 percent of the total blood pumped by the heart each minute. **Urology** is the study of the urinary tract in both sexes and the genital tract in the male, while **nephrology** is the science of the structure and function of the kidney. Because the systems are interdependent, the specialties are often considered together in medical studies. Specialists who deal with the urinary system are **urologists** and **nephrologists**.

Anatomy and Physiology of the Urinary Tract

The main organs of the urinary tract, shown in Figure 13.1, are the **kidneys**, the **ureters**, the **bladder**, and the **urethra**, which ends in the external urinary **meatus**. The kidneys are located in the area just above the waist in the **retroperitoneal** area, that is, behind the peritoneum. The right kidney sits a little lower than the left. The kidneys are completely covered by a thick layer of fat that protects it from injury.

Figure 13.1 - Urinary System

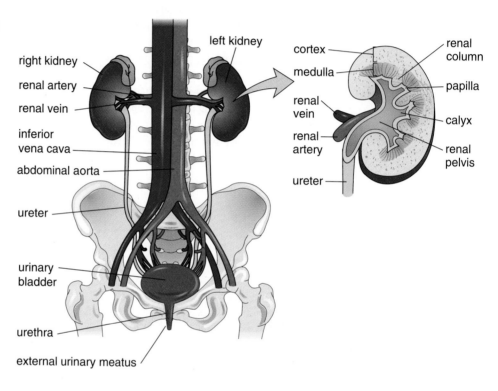

The parts of the kidney are the outer **cortex**, the inner **medulla**, the **pelvis** (which is attached to the ureter that drains urine into the bladder), and a portion of the pelvis called the **calyx** (Figure 13.2). The internal structure is designed to filter substances through millions of microscopic units called **nephrons**.

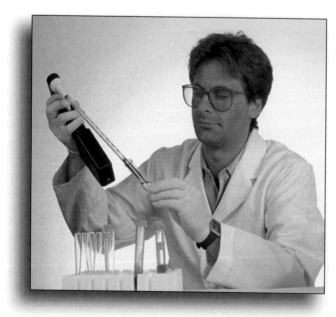

Figure 13.2 - Kidney
Structure

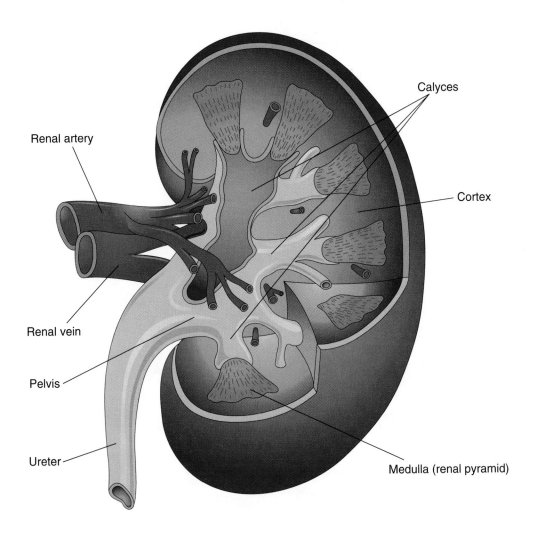

Renal artery

Calyces

Cortex

Renal vein

Pelvis

Medulla (renal pyramid)

Ureter

Each nephron consists of the **renal corpuscle** and the **renal tubule**. Figure 13.3 shows a nephron's structure. The renal corpuscle is subdivided into **Bowman's capsule**, a sac at the top of the nephron, and the twisted structure called the **glomerulus** that is found within Bowman's capsule, that actually serves as the capillary system of the kidney. If the glomeruli were stretched in a single line, they would extend approximately 50 km (31 miles). The renal tubule has four divisions: the **proximal convoluted tubule**, the **loop of Henle** extending from the proximal tubule, the **distal convoluted tubule**, and the **collecting tubule**.

Figure 13.3 - Nephron

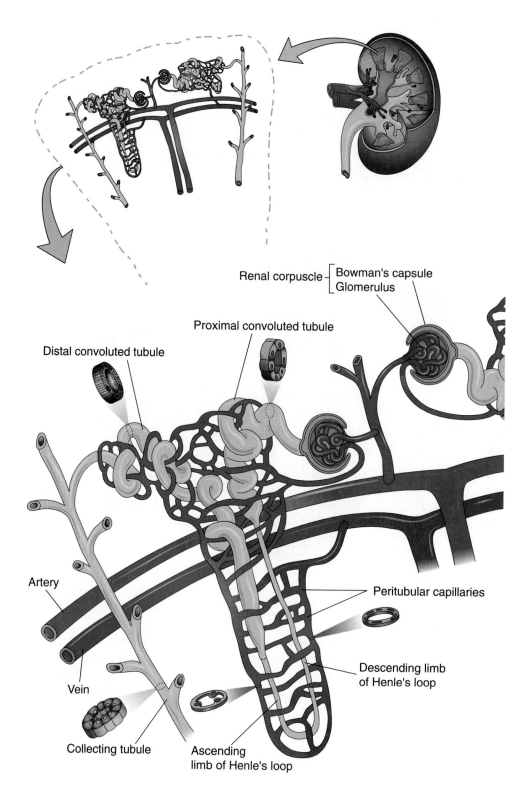

Renal corpuscle — Bowman's capsule
— Glomerulus

Proximal convoluted tubule

Distal convoluted tubule

Artery

Peritubular capillaries

Vein

Descending limb
of Henle's loop

Collecting tubule

Ascending
limb of Henle's loop

Urine Formation

The main function of the kidneys is to produce **urine** (Figure 13.4), but they must also take care of other important tasks such as filtering fluid, electrolytes, and metabolic waste materials from the blood. The kidneys help maintain blood pressure and the delicate balance of fluids and **electrolytes**, the chemical substances in the blood.

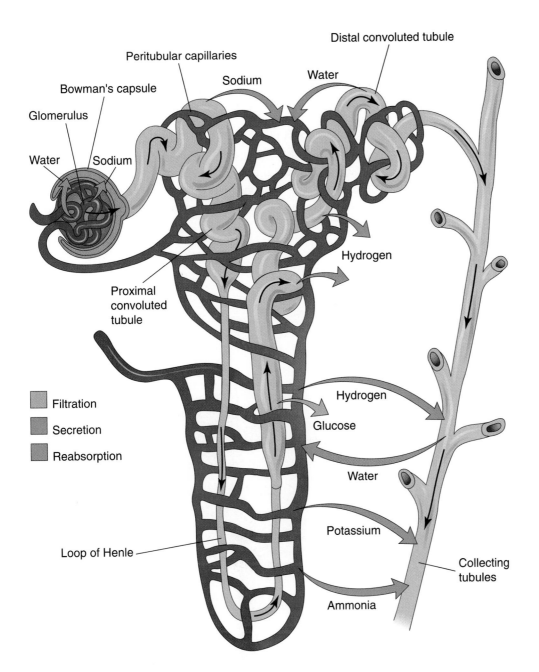

Figure 13.4 - Urine Formation

Peritubular capillaries

Distal convoluted tubule

Bowman's capsule

Sodium

Water

Glomerulus

Water   Sodium

Proximal convoluted tubule

Hydrogen

Filtration

Secretion

Reabsorption

Hydrogen

Glucose

Water

Loop of Henle

Potassium

Collecting tubules

Ammonia

Urine formation begins with the **filtration** of blood in the **glomeruli**. When the glomerular blood pressure becomes high enough, water and dissolved materials are driven out into Bowman's capsule. This is a feedback loop because when the pressure falls below a certain level, filtration and urine production cease. Approximately 125 mL of fluid are filtered through the glomeruli each minute.

The next phase is **reabsorption**, when substances are moved out of the renal tubules into the surrounding **peritubular** capillaries by diffusion, osmosis, and active transport. Reabsorption begins in the proximal convoluted tubules, proceeds through the loop of Henle to the distal convoluted tubules, and ends in the collecting tubules. Approximately 180 liters of water are reabsorbed from the proximal tubules each day.

The final step is **secretion**, during which substances move from the surrounding capillaries into the urine within the distal and collecting tubules. Reabsorption and secretion are almost opposite: reabsorption moves substances out of the urine into the blood; secretion moves substances out of the blood into the urine. These substances include hydrogen and potassium ions, creatinine, ammonia, and some drugs.

The Urinary Bladder

From the collecting tubules, urine drains into the renal pelvis, down the **ureter**, and into the **urinary bladder**. The ureters are narrow (about ¼ inch wide and 12 inches long) and made of thick muscle that contracts to move the urine down. Mucous membranes line the inside.

The urinary bladder (Figure 13.5) lies behind the symphysis pubis within the skeletal pelvis. The elastic fibers and involuntary muscles that make up the urinary bladder allow it to hold large amounts of urine. When empty, the bladder is wrinkled and folded into **rugae**, except for one area on the posterior surface. This area, called the **trigone**, is always smooth. The urinary bladder expands to provide room for the urine and contracts to excrete it.

Figure 13.5 - Bladder Structure

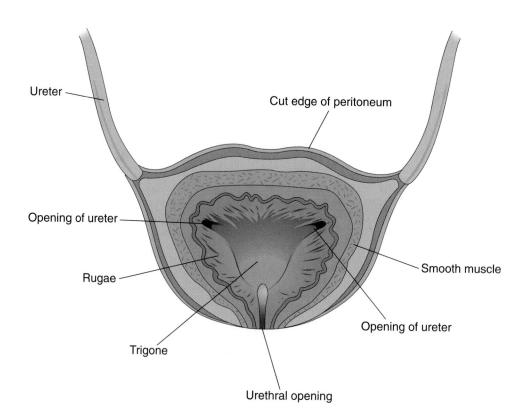

The bladder is connected to the **urethra** and contains the same mucous membrane lining as the ureters. The urethra is only about 1.5 inches long in women and about 8 inches long in men. The **urinary meatus** at the end of the urethra is the external opening for the voiding of urine. Two sphincters (muscle rings) lead from the bladder. The **internal urethral sphincter** is located at the exit of the bladder, and the **external urethral sphincter** encircles the urethra below the neck of the bladder. These sphincters seal off the bladder so urine can accumulate. The internal sphincter is under involuntary nerve control, and the external sphincter is under voluntary control.

The bladder can hold approximately 300 to 400 mL of urine (slightly less than 2 cups). When the volume of urine reaches about 350 mL, sensory nerve receptors in the bladder send a message to initiate the process of urination, although the adult becomes aware of the accumulation of urine at about 150 mL. The emptying reflex causes contraction of the bladder wall and relaxation of the internal sphincter, which allows urine to enter the urethra. Urination occurs when the external sphincter is relaxed.

Medical professionals use several terms for urine excretion: **micturition**, **urination**, and **voiding**. The combining forms for these and other essential urinary system terms are listed in Table 13.1. Table 13.2 lists important anatomical and physiological terms derived from the roots or taken directly from their original form in other languages.

Table 13.1

Combining Forms Relating to the Urinary System

Combining form	Meaning	Example
cyst/o	bladder	cystoscope
electr/o	electric	electrolyte
hydr/o	water	hydration
lith/o, -lith	stone, calcification	nephrolith
meat/o	passageway	meatus
nephr/o	kidney	nephrology
pyel/o	renal pelvis	pyelonephritis
ren/i (o)	pertaining to the kidney	renal
tub/o	tube (little tube)	tubule
ur/e (a), (o)	relating to urea or urine	urea
ureter/o	ureter	ureter
urethr/o	urethra	urethral
urin/o	urine	urinary
ur/o	relating to urine	urogenital

Table 13.2

Anatomy and Physiology Terms Relating to the Urinary System

Term	Meaning	Word Analysis	
bladder **blad**-er	musculomembranous organ that serves as a container for fluid and is distended when filled	blaedre	vessel
Bowman's capsule **bO**-menz **kap**-sel	structure of the renal corpuscle that is the top of a nephron; surrounds the glomerulus	Bowman capsule	English ophthalmologist, anatomist, and physiologist box
calyx/calix cal-icks	one of the branches of the kidney pelvis	calyx	cup of the flower
cortex **kor**-teks	outer portion of an organ such as the kidney	cortex	bark (of a tree)
distal convoluted tubule **dis**-tel **kon**-vO-loot-ed **too**-byool	part of the nephron farthest from Bowman's capsule	distal con/ volutus tub/o	away from with; together to roll tube (denotes a little tube)
electrolyte ee-**lek**-trO-lIt	substance that can conduct electricity within a fluid	electr/o -lysis	electric to dissolve; break up
external urethral sphincter eks-**ter**-nel yoo-**ree**-threl **sfink**-ter	band of muscle fibers that encircles the urethra below the neck of the bladder; under voluntary control	externus urethr/o sphincter	outside urethra band

continued on next page

Term	Definition	Root	Meaning
filtration fil-**tray**-shun	process of passing a substance through a filter to separate the particulate matter	*filtro*	strain through
glomeruli glO-**mer**-yoo-lI	capillary loops within Bowman's capsule	*glomero*	to wind into a ball of yarn
internal urethral sphincter in-**ter**-nel yoo-**ree**-threl **sfink**-ter	band of muscle fibers at the base of the bladder; under involuntary control	*internus* *urethr/o* *sphincter*	away from the surface urethra band
kidneys **kid**-neez	paired organs that produce urine	*nephr/o*	kidney
loop of Henle **hen**-lee	extension of the proximal tubule of the nephron that contains a hairpin loop between two straight limbs	*loupe* Henle	loop German anatomist
medulla med-**ul**-ah	soft, marrowlike structure in the center of the kidney	*medull/o*	medulla (marrow; middle)
micturition mik-tyoo-**rish**-un	elimination of urine from the bladder	*micturio*	desire to make water
nephron **nef**-ron	tubular structure that produces the urine in the kidney	*nephr/o*	kidney
pelvis (in kidney)	area at the upper end of the ureter	*pelvis*	basin
peritubular capillaries pear-eh-**too**-byeh-lar	tiny blood vessels that provide the blood supply for much of the nephron	*peri-* *tubular* *capillaris*	around tube hair
proximal convoluted tubule **proks**-ih-mel **kon**-vO-loot-ed **too**-byool	first segment of the renal tubule (nearest to Bowman's capsule)	*proxim/o*	proximal; nearest
reabsorption ree-ab-**sorp**-shun	process of retaining fluid and electrolytes in the kidney	*re/* *absorptio*	again swallow
renal corpuscle **ree**-nel **kor**-pus-l	area of the nephron located in the cortex; area that contains the glomerular capillaries and Bowman's capsule	*ren/o* *corpus*	kidney body
renal tubule **ree**-nel **too**-byool	part of the nephron composed of the proximal and distal convoluted tubules, the loop of Henle, and the collecting tubule	*ren/o* *tub/o*	kidney tube (denotes a little tube)
retroperitoneal **ret**-rO-per-ih-tO-**nee**-el	relating to area behind (posterior to) the peritoneum	*retro-* *periteino*	behind, backward stretch over
secretion seh-**skree**-shun	movement of substances from surrounding capillaries into the urine within the distal and collecting tubules	*cretus*	separate
tubule **too**-byool	small tube	*tub/o*	tube (denotes a little tube)
ureter yoo-**ree**-ter	tube that sends urine from the renal pelvis to the bladder	*ureter/o*	ureter
urethra yoo-**ree**-thrah	tube to void urine that leads from the bladder to the outside	*urethr/o*	urethra
urinary meatus **yoo**-rin-ar-ee mee-**ay**-tus	opening (orifice) for the voiding (passage) of urine	*urin/o* *meat/o*	urine meatus
urine **yoo**-rin urinate **yoo**-rin-ayt	fluid that is voided from the body; filtered from the blood in the kidney	*urin/o*	urine
void	to eliminate urine	*vocare*	empty

For each term in the left column, write the combining form in the next column, the combining form's definition in the third column and the original term's definition in the right column.

Term	Combining form	Definition	Term definition
1. cystectomy	_____	_____	_____
2. renal	_____	_____	_____
3. ureterectomy	_____	_____	_____
4. urethritis	_____	_____	_____
5. nephrectomy	_____	_____	_____
6. urologist	_____	_____	_____
7. urinary	_____	_____	_____
8. medullary	_____	_____	_____
9. tubular	_____	_____	_____
10. nephritis	_____	_____	_____

Comprehension Check

Exercise 2

Circle the correct term in each sentence.

1. The ureter/urethra carries urine from the bladder to the outside of the body.

2. The glomerulus/glucose is an important part of the nephron.

3. The nephritis/nephron is the functional unit of the kidney.

4. The proximal and distal tubules/tubercles are structures in the renal system.

5. Nephritis/Nephronosis is a disease that can cause scarring in the kidneys.

6. The cortex/medulla is the outer portion of the kidney.

7. Urine drains from the collecting tubules first into the renal pelvis/urinary bladder.

8. Pyelonephritis/Pyonitis is a term that indicates an inflammation with pus in the kidneys.

9. Urea/Urine is the watery fluid produced by the kidneys that contains water and waste products.

10. Urea/Urine is a waste product formed in the liver.

Matching

Select a term from Column 1 to match each definition in Column 2. Write the number of your selection on the line beside the definition.

Column 1

1. urology
2. nephrologist
3. urinary meatus
4. retroperitoneal
5. cortex
6. micturation
7. electrolytes
8. calyx
9. filtration
10. glomeruli

Column 2

_____ a. outermost portion of the kidney

_____ b. chemical substances in the blood

_____ c. "behind the peritoneum"

_____ d. study of the urinary system

_____ e. voiding of urine

_____ f. specialist in the study of the kidneys

_____ g. external opening at the end of the urethra

_____ h. capillary loops within Bowman's Capsule

_____ i. branch of the renal pelvis

_____ j. passing a substance through a filter to separate out particulate matter

Word Building

Use prefixes and suffixes from the lists and the provided combining forms to create a term to match each definition.

Prefixes

hydro-	hyper-
hemat-	post-
dys-	bi-
an-	anti-
poly-	en-
trans-	a-
pre-	intra-

Suffixes

-pathy	-ectomy
-osis	-plasty
-itis	-graphy
-stomy	-ia
-tomy	-al
-logy	-gram
-analysis	-uria

New Terms

1. pyel/o inflammation of the renal pelvis _____

2. nephr/o surgical removal of the kidney _____

3. ren/o pertaining to the kidneys _____

4. ur/o pertaining to urine and the genitals _____

5. cyst/o inflammation of the bladder _____

6. urin/o pertaining to urine _____

7. urethr/o inflammation of the urethra _____

8. tub/o pertaining to a tube _____

9. meat/o pertaining to a passageway   _____

10. lith/o condition of stones   _____

Spelling Check *Exercise 5*

Identify the misspelled terms in the sentences below. Write the correct spelling and the definition of the term on the line following each sentence.

1. Cell morpology throughout the medula was abnormal.   _____

    _____

2. The renul pelivs was dilated.   _____

    _____

3. Cysotoscopy was preformed three days ago.   _____

    _____

4. This patient had an intrevenous pyleogram last week.   _____

    _____

5. Bouman's capasule was easily identified in the microscopic sample.   _____

    _____

6. The reneal tulbuler defect is congenital.   _____

    _____

7. The surgeon sutured a 1 cm tear in the urethreal metaus.   _____

    _____

8. Creatinnine clearance was not reported.   _____

    _____

9. The concentration increased in the loop of Henele.   _____

    _____

10. The peritubuelar capilaries were stenotic.   _____

    _____

This diagram illustrates the production and flow of urine through the urinary system. Add the missing terms.

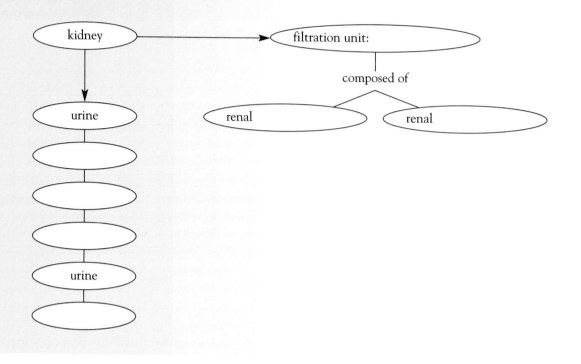

Assessing Patient Health

Wellness and Illness through the Life Span

During the physical examination of a patient with urinary tract problems, the physician palpates the kidney area (**costovertebral angle**) and bladder, evaluates the urine through tests, and questions the patient about any difficulty with urination. Can the patient pass urine? Is there any pain (**dysuria**) involved? Is there any difficulty in starting the urine stream (**hesitancy**)? Is there an inability to hold the urine (**incontinence**)? **Frequency** and **urgency** are terms for the feeling that urine must be passed but actually very little urine is produced; **nocturia** means the need to urinate during the night.

The examiner asks about the amount of urine being produced. **Anuria** means that no urine is produced, and this is considered a medical emergency because the inability to eliminate wastes through urination will cause poisons to build up in the body to fatal levels. Decreased urine production, called **oliguria**, is serious and must be investigated further. **Polyuria** is frequent urination and can indicate diabetes mellitus (see Chapter 7, "The Endocrine System") or other disorders. The examiner also asks about the characteristics of the urine: color, odor, the appearance of unusual substances or particles within the urine such as blood, a condition called **hematuria**. Table 13.3 lists these conditions along with other major illness terms relating to urine production.

Table 13.3

Terms Relating to Urine Production

Term	Meaning	Word Analysis	
anuria an-**yoo**-ree-ah	inability to produce urine	a- -uria	without urine
dysuria dis-**yoo**-ree-ah	pain or difficulty with urination	dys- -uria	painful; difficult urine
frequency (of urination) **free**-kwen-see (yoo-rin-**ay**-shun)	urination that occurs often with little actual production of urine	frequent	often
hematuria hee-mah-**too**-ree-ah/ hem-ah-**too**-ree-ah	blood in the urine	hem/o -uria	blood urine
hesitancy **hez**-ih-ten-see	inability to start the urine stream, or the involuntary interruption of the stream	haesitare	to stick fast
incontinence (of urine) in-**kon**-tih-nens	inability to hold urine	in- contineo	not; in; within hold together
nocturia nok-**too**-ree-ah	urination at night	noct/i -uria	night urine
oliguria ol-ih-**gyoo**-ree-ah	production of very little urine	olig/o -uria	little urine
polyuria pol-ee-**yoo**-ree-ah	production of an increased amount of urine	poly- -uria	frequent urine
urgency **er**-jen-see	feeling of having to pass urine immediately, but with little actual urine production	ergon	work

Infants and Children

One anomaly that may be present in the kidneys of the newborn is **horseshoe kidney**, which is caused by improper prenatal formation of the kidneys. A band of tissue, extending across the spine, attaches the kidneys to each other, making them into one horseshoe-shaped kidney.

Children over the age of three years are at risk for developing acute poststreptococcal **glomerulonephritis**. This occurs after the child has had a throat or skin infection with a group A beta-hemolytic streptococci organism (a type of bacteria). The symptoms include an acute onset of hematuria, edema, hypertension, and oliguria, or even complete kidney failure (anuria). This illness is not as common as it once was because of the early identification and treatment of streptococcal infections in children.

The result of glomerulonephritis can be **nephrotic syndrome**, or **nephrosis**. This disorder is characterized by **proteinuria**, protein in the urine, which results from an increase in permeability of the glomerular capillary wall. The protein lost is usually albumin, causing a specific protein-related condition called **albuminuria**. The resulting loss of albumin from the blood (**hypoalbuminemia**) leads to edema, or swelling. A corresponding reduction in the volume of fluid in the vessels stimulates ADH (antidiuretic hormone) to reabsorb water. This causes reabsorption of sodium and water into the spaces between the cells, causing further edema. There are many causes of nephrotic syndrome, which can become a chronic disorder leading to total kidney failure. Figure 13.6 outlines the path of nephrosis.

Figure 13.6 - Word Map of
Nephrotic Syndrome
(Nephrosis)

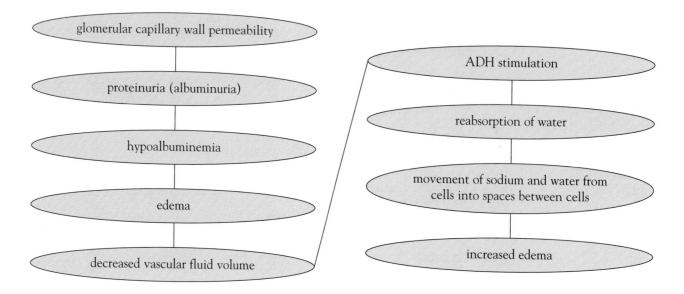

Urinary tract infections (UTI) in childhood are more common in girls than in boys because the female urethra is shorter, and outside organisms can more easily enter the urinary tract by migrating up through the urinary meatus. A UTI can potentially cause an infection anywhere within the system, and the urine's warmth and moisture makes the bladder a particularly vulnerable organ. When a girl has more than one urinary tract infection, testing is recommended to determine if there are any abnormalities or deformities within the urinary system. Urinary tract infections are characterized by dysuria, fever, frequency, urgency, and occasionally **pyuria**. **Pyelonephritis** is an inflammation of the internal structures of the kidney, usually resulting from a bacterial urinary tract infection.

Enuresis, or bedwetting, is not uncommon in school-aged children. If a child who has never been a bed wetter begins enuresis, several issues should be considered. First, laboratory examination of the urine and a physical examination should rule out the possibility of a UTI. If there is no infection or other abnormality, then it may be necessary to look for a psychosocial cause, such as "schoolitis," problems with peers, or family problems, to name a few.

Wilms Tumor is a malignancy of the kidney usually diagnosed in infancy. It is most commonly found in one kidney, but may be found bilaterally. Treatment consists of surgical removal of the tumor and the affected kidney, chemotherapy, and depending upon the extent of disease at diagnosis, radiation therapy.

Adolescents

Systemic lupus erythematosus (SLE), often referred to as **lupus**, is most commonly diagnosed in teenage girls. The first manifestations of the disorder may be **nephritis**, characterized by hematuria and proteinuria with normal renal function in less severe cases. In severe cases, there may be decreased renal function or nephrotic syndrome. Lupus is an autoimmune disorder (see Chapter 6, "The Immune System") that causes the deposit of immune complexes in various organs including the heart, lungs, central nervous system, and kidneys.

Adults

A **calculus**, or stone in the kidney, is called a **nephrolith**. The condition of **nephrolithiasis** (kidney stones) is an extremely painful illness that afflicts adults more often than children. This condition is characterized by **renal colic**, or pain in the abdomen, and severe pain in the flank (kidney area of the back). The stone may pass to the ureters and down the tract, but may cause an obstruction along the way.

Seniors

Problems in the senior age group are often the result of decreased competence of the muscles within the urinary tract. **Incontinence**, the inability to hold urine, can be caused by the loss of muscle control of the urinary sphincters. A condition called **cystocele** is a hernia of the bladder that pushes down into the vagina. **Vesicoureteral reflux** occurs when there is incompetence of one of the urinary sphincters, allowing urine to flow backward—up from the bladder to the ureters. Renal cell carcinoma, a malignancy that affects the kidney, is usually found in adults. These conditions and other major wellness and illness terms relating to the urinary system are listed in Table 13.4.

Table 13.4

Wellness and Illness Terms Relating to the Urinary System

Term	Meaning	Word Analysis	
albuminuria al-byoo-min-**yoo**-ree-ah	presence of the protein albumin in the urine; albumin is found in the serum portion of blood	albumin -uria	the white of an egg urine
costovertebral angle kos-tO-**ver**-tah-brel **ang**-l	area on the back over the 12th rib; pain in the area when thumped with the fist during physical examination may indicate kidney disease	cost/o vertebr/o angulus	the ribs vertebra angle
cystitis sis-**tI**-tis	inflammation causing dysuria and pain in the bladder; usually caused by bacterial infection	cyst/o -itis	bladder inflammation
cystocele **sis**-tO-seel	condition involving a hernia of the bladder that pushes it into the vagina	cyst/o -cele	bladder space or cavity
enuresis en-yoo-**ree**-sis	bed-wetting	en/ ur/e -sis	in urine condition
glomerulonephritis glom-**er**-yoo-lO-neh-**frI**-tis	disease of cells in the kidneys (glomeruli) characterized by inflammatory changes resulting from an infection	glomerulus nephr/i -itis	a ball of yarn kidney inflammation
glycosuria glI-kO-**syoo**-ree-ah	presence of glucose (sugar) in the urine	glyc/o -uria	sugar characteristic of urine
horseshoe kidney	band of tissue extending across the spine that attaches the kidneys to each other and makes them one horseshoe-shaped kidney	horseshoe	shape similar to a horse's shoe
hydronephrosis hI-drO-neh-**frO**-sis	condition characterized by dilation of the pelvis and calices of the kidneys; usually results from an obstruction that prevents the flow of urine	hydr/o nephr/o -osis	water kidney condition
hypercalciuria **hI**-per-kal-sih-**yoo**-ree-ah	increased calcium in the urine; may indicate loss of calcium due to osteoporosis (bone loss)	hyper/ calx -uria	increased lime (calcium) urine

continued on next page

lupus	see *systemic lupus erythematosus*		
nephritis nef-**rI**-tis	inflammation of the kidneys	*nephr/o* *-itis*	kidney inflammation
nephrolith **nef**-rO-lith	kidney stone usually made from calcium	*nephr/o* *-lith*	kidney stone (calculus)
nephrolithiasis nef-rO-lith-**I**-as-is	condition of having kidney stones	*nephr/o* *-lith* *-iasis*	kidney stone (calculus) condition
nephrosis nef-**rO**-sis nephrotic syndrome nef-**rot**-ik	condition of the kidney characterized by protein in the urine	*nephr/o* *-sis*	kidney condition
pyelonephritis pI-el-O-nef-**rI**-tis	inflammation of the internal structures of the kidney usually from bacterial infection	*pyel/o* *nephr/o* *-itis*	relating to the renal pelvis kidney inflammation
pyuria pI-**yoo**-ree-ah	pus in the urine	*py/o* *-uria*	pus urine
renal colic **ree**-nel **kol**-ik	pain in the abdomen and back as a result of a kidney stone	*ren/i* *col/o*	kidney pertaining to the colon
systemic lupus erythematosus sis-**tem**-ik **loo**-pes er-ih-**them**-ah-tO-sus	autoimmune disorder that causes inflammatory connective tissue disease in many areas of the body, including the kidneys, skin and joints	*lupus* *-erythem/a* *-osus (-osis)*	wolf redness condition
uremia yoo-**ree**-mee-ah	excessive accumulation of urea (a waste product) within the blood	*ur/e* *-emia*	urine blood
ureteritis yoo-ree-ter-**I**-tis	inflammation of the ureter(s)	*ureter/o* *-itis*	ureter inflammation
urethritis yoo-reh-**thrI**-tis	inflammation of the urethra	*urethr/o* *-itis*	urethra inflammation
urinary retention **yoo**-rin-ar-ee ree-**ten**-shun	inability to void	*ur/i* *retentio*	urine holding back
urinary tract infection	infection anywhere within the urinary tract	*ur/i* *-ary*	urine relating to
vesicoureteral reflux **ves**-ih-kO-yoo-**ree**-ter-el **ree**-fluks	incompetence of the valve at the ureterovesical junction (between the ureter and bladder) allowing the flow of urine backward from the bladder into the ureter	*vesic/o* *ureter/o* *re-* *fluxus*	relating to a bladder ureter again, back flow

First, write a definition of the combining form on the line provided. Then use the combining form to create a term that matches the definition given, and write the term on the second line.

1. Combining form: ur/o

   Definition: pus in the urine

   Definition: _____

   Term: _____

2. Combining Form: lith/o

   Definition: condition of kidney stones

   Definition: _____

   Term: _____

3. Combining Form: nephr/o

   Definition: study of the kidneys

   Definition: _____

   Term: _____

4. Combining Form: cyst/o

   Definition: inflammation of the bladder

   Definition: _____

   Term: _____

5. Combining Form: urethr/o

   Definition: inflammation of the urethra

   Definition: _____

   Term: _____

6. Combining Form: tub/o

   Definition: pertaining to a tube

   Definition: _____

   Term: _____

7. Combining Form: proxim/o

   Definition: pertaining to nearest

   Definition: _____

   Term: _____

8. Combining Form: ureter/o

   Definition: removal of the ureter

   Definition: _____

   Term: _____

9. Combining Form: medull/o

   Definition: pertaining to the marrowlike structure in the center of the kidney

   Definition: _____

   Term: _____

10. Combining Form: meat/o

    Definition: pertaining to the passage

    Definition: _____

    Term: _____

Study each sentence and note whether the singular or plural form of the term should be used. Write S if the form should be singular, or P if it should be plural; then write the corrected form of the term, if necessary.

	S or P	Corrected Form
1. There are many <u>nephron</u> in a kidney.	_____	_____
2. The <u>glomeruli</u> are malformed.	_____	_____
3. The <u>tubule</u> collect the urine.	_____	_____
4. Both <u>ureter</u> are stenosed.	_____	_____
5. There are three <u>urologist</u> in Dr. Blakeley's office.	_____	_____
6. Three <u>calculus</u> were identified in the distal portion of the left ureter.	_____	_____
7. Albumin is a <u>proteins</u> that appears in the urine in certain abnormalities.	_____	_____
8. Loss of muscle control in one of the urinary <u>sphincters</u> can result in incontinence.	_____	_____
9. The <u>nephrolith</u> was destroyed by lithotripsy.	_____	_____
10. The <u>urethras</u> was severely inflamed.	_____	_____

Select a term from Column 1 to match each definition in Column 2. Write the number of your selection in the blank beside the definition.

Column 1		Column 2
1. cortex	_____	tubelike structure that carries urine from the kidneys to the bladder
2. medulla	_____	excreting urine
3. nephron	_____	body's container for urine, distends when filled
4. glomerulus	_____	"behind the peritoneum"
5. ureter	_____	outermost portion of the kidney
6. urethra	_____	area at the upper end of the ureter
7. renal pelvis	_____	tube that carries urine from the bladder to the outside of the body
8. retroperitoneal	_____	marrowlike inner portion of the kidney
9. bladder	_____	capillary loops within Bowman's capsule
10. voiding	_____	microscopic units within the kidney that filter substances

Word Building

Use prefixes, root words, combining vowels, and suffixes to create medical terms for the definitions given. Write the term in the space beside the definition.

1. inflammation of the ureters   _____

2. pus in the urine   _____

3. inflammation of the urethra   _____

4. inflammation of the internal structures of the kidney, usually from bacterial infection   _____

5. inflammation of the kidneys   _____

6. increased calcium in the urine; may indicate osteoporosis   _____

7. kidney disease characterized by inflammatory changes in the glomeruli   _____

8. inflammation of the bladder   _____

9. pertaining to urine   _____

10. pertaining to the kidneys   _____

Spelling Check

Underline each misspelled term in the following sentences, and then write the term's correct spelling and its definition on the line provided.

1. When laboratory tests revealed piurea, the physician ordered additional diagnostic tests.

2. Nephritis is often characterized by hemeturia and proetinuria.

3. Ssytemic lupus eryethematosis is most commonly diagnosed in teenage girls.

4. Eneuresis is not uncommon in the school-aged child.

5. The cappillary wall of the glomeurulus became increasingly permeable.

6. Neprotic syndrome can be the result of gloermulonephritis.

_____

_____

7. Pyelonephritis usually results from a bacterail uraniry tract infection.

_____

_____

8. The reasorbption of water is an important function of the kidneys.

_____

_____

9. Mr. Patterson's kidney disease has resulted in fluid retention and massive ederma.

_____

_____

10. Mrs. Keele's urinary incontenience is due to a UTI.

_____

_____

Word Maps

This diagram shows how pyelonephritis begins. Supply the missing terms.

bacteria from outside the body

urethra

bacteria

bacteria

Renal disease: | |
| --- |

Diagnosing and Treating Problems

Tests, Procedures, and Pharmaceuticals

The most common screening test for urinary tract problems is **urinalysis**, the study of a freshly voided sample of urine under the microscope. However, if a urinary tract infection is suspected, a **clean-catch** or **catheterized** specimen is obtained. The urinalysis can detect blood, glucose, and/or **creatinine** (a substance that is elevated with kidney dysfunction). The blood test called **blood urea nitrogen (BUN)** can determine the level of urea in the blood, which indicates normal or abnormal kidney function. The **creatinine clearance** measures how well blood is being filtered through the kidneys. The **glomerular filtration rate** is a nuclear scan that also determines how well blood is being filtered through the kidneys.

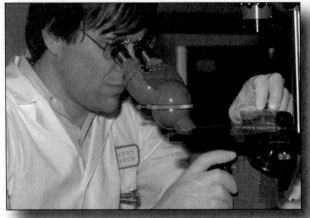

Several x-ray and scanning techniques are used to view the structures within the urinary tract. A simple screening x-ray is known as a **KUB (kidneys, ureters, bladder) x-ray**. An MRI of the kidney area, including abdomen and pelvis, can identify any structural abnormalities or tumor growth. A **renal scan** is an x-ray using a radioactive substance to view the kidneys. The **cystogram** is an x-ray of the bladder; a **cystoscopy** is the procedure where the cystoscope, a type of endoscope, is inserted through the external urinary meatus to view the urethra and bladder. An **intravenous pyelogram (IVP)** is an x-ray taken to view the kidneys and other structures after a dye is injected.

Dialysis is a procedure used to compensate for kidney failure. As noted previously, absence of urine is a medical emergency, and dialysis must be performed. Dialysis involves accessing the blood to clear it of waste products through artificial means. In other words, a machine is used as an artificial kidney. The machine contains a membrane and a fluid bath. A special tube is attached to an artificial vein in the patient, and blood is filtered through the machine, which separates large particles, such as blood cells, from small ones, such as urea and other waste products. The waste products remain in the dialyzing solution, and electrolytes and other essential products are returned intravenously to the patient. A patient with kidney failure may need two to three **hemodialysis** procedures per week.

Another type of dialysis is called **peritoneal dialysis (PD)**. During PD a fluid is introduced directly into the peritoneal cavity through a special opening created in the abdominal wall. The membranes of the peritoneal cavity are used as a filter for the blood and the transfer of waste products and electrolytes. The fluid remains in the peritoneal cavity for several hours before it is drained back into the container.

Surgical Procedures

A **nephrectomy** is the total removal of a kidney; a **cystectomy** is the removal of all or part of the bladder. If a cystocele is present, a **cystopexy** may be performed that attaches the bladder to a supporting structure to prevent it from herniating. A **nephrostomy** may be performed to create an opening from the kidney to the outside of the body so that urine can drain.

Extracorporeal shock wave lithotripsy is a procedure that sends shock waves from ultrasonic energy externally through the kidney and/or ureter to break up kidney stones. In some instances it may eliminate the need for surgery since the crushed stones may be passed through the urethra more easily. Numerous other procedures exist to treat conditions of the urinary system. Their names are created from the combining forms presented earlier in this chapter and the common procedural suffixes such as *-plasty, -ostomy, -ectomy, -pexy,* and *-otomy,* as shown in Table 13.5.

Table 13.5

Tests and Procedures Relating to the Urinary System

Test or procedure	Description	Word analysis	
blood urea nitrogen blud yoo-**ree**-ah **nI**-trO-jen	blood test to measure the urea; an indication of kidney function	*ure/a*	relating to urea, urine
catheterization (urinary) kath-eh-ter-ih-**zay**-shun	procedure using a sterile tube (catheter) inserted through the urinary meatus into the bladder to obtain a sterile urine specimen or to drain urine	*katheter*	send down
clean catch	procedure that uses a voided urine specimen for microscopic analysis after the person has cleaned the urinary meatus with an antiseptic solution	*N/A*	
creatinine clearance kree-**at**-in-een	test that measures how blood is being filtered through the kidney	*creatinine*	substance in the urine
cystectomy sis-**tek**-tah-mee	surgical removal of the bladder	*cyst/o* *-ectomy*	bladder surgical removal
cystogram **sis**-tO-gram	x-ray examination of the bladder using a cystoscope (type of endoscope) threaded up through the urethra to visualize the bladder	*cyst/o* *-gram*	bladder recording
cystopexy **sis**-tO-peks-ee	surgical repair of the bladder by anchoring it to a supporting structure	*cyst/o* *-pexy*	bladder repair; fixation
extracorporeal shock wave lithotripsy **eks**-trah-kor-**pO**-ree-al **lith**-O-trip-see	breaking up of a renal or ureteral stone using ultrasound energy	*extra-* *corpus* *lith/o* *tripsis*	beyond, outside of the body calculus (stone) rubbing
glomerular filtration rate glo-**mer**-yoo-ler	determination of volume of water being filtered from plasma through the kidneys	*glomerulus* *filtro*	to wind into a ball of yarn to strain
hemodialysis **hee**-mO-dI-**al**-ah-sis	procedure to remove waste products from the blood with a machine that uses a filter to separate large molecules from smaller ones	*hem/o* *dia-* *-lysis*	blood through separation
intravenous pyelogram in-trah-**vee**-nus **pI**-el-O-gram	x-ray using contrast medium injected into the vein to view the kidneys and surrounding structures	*intra/* *ven/o* *pyel/o* *-gram*	inside, within pertaining to veins pertaining to the renal pelvis recording
nephrectomy neh-**frek**-tah-mee	removal of the kidney	*nephr/o* *-ectomy*	kidney removal
nephrostomy neh-**fros**-tah-mee	surgical procedure to create an opening from the kidney to the outside to drain urine	*nephr/o* *os-* *-tomy*	kidney opening; mouth incision
peritoneal dialysis per-ih-tO-**nee**-al dI-**al**-ah-sis	procedure using the peritoneal membranes as a filter for the transfer of wastes out of the body and electrolytes into the body	*peritoneum* *dia-* *-lysis*	stretch over through dissolving or breaking apart

renal scan	x-ray using an isotope to view the kidneys	*ren/o* *scan*	kidney imaging technique
urinalysis yoo-rin-**al**-ih-sis	laboratory study of the urine	*urin/o* *an/a* *-lysis*	urine up; apart dissolve; separate; to break apart

Pharmaceutical Agents

The following table describes some of the common pharmacologic agents used to treat problems of the urinary tract.

Table 13.6

Pharmacologic Agents

Class	Use	Generic	Brand
analgesics	relieves urinary pain or burning	phenazopyridine	Pyridium
antibiotics	treats infection	trimethoprim- sulfamethoxazole gentamicin nitrofurantoin nalidixic acid trimethoprim	Bactrim, Septra Garamycin Macrobid, Macrodantin NegGram Primsol, Proloprim
antidiuretic hormone, antihemophilic agent	treats diabetes insipidus and bed-wetting; controls bleeding in certain types of hemophilia	vasopressin desmopressin	Pitressin DDAVP, Stimate
antidote for hypercalcemia	Paget's disease, post- menopausal osteoporosis	calcitonin	Miacalcin
antigout agent, uric acid lowering agent	prevents attacks of gouty arthritis and uric acid kidney stones	allopurinol	Zyloprim
benign prostatic hyperplasia therapy	treats BPH	terazosin doxazosin finasteride	Hytrin Cardura Proscar
cholinergic agent	treats nonobstructive urinary retention	bethanechol	Urecholine
diuretics	promotes urination	furosemide spironolactone chlorothiazide	Lasix Aldactone Diuril
hematinics	promotes red blood cell production	erythropoietin	Epogen, Procrit
potassium replacement	potassium deficiency	potassium chloride	K-Dur, Kay Ciel
urinary alkalinizers	increase urine pH	potassium citrate, sodium citrate, and citric acid solutions	Cytra-3, Polycitra
urinary antispasmodics	inhibit urinary tract spasms	oxybutynin	Ditropan

Table 13.7

Abbreviations

AGN	acute glomerulonephritis
ATN	acute tubular necrosis
BUN	blood urea nitrogen
CVA	costovertebral angle
cysto	cystoscopy
ESWL	extracorporeal shock wave lithotripsy
GFR	glomerular filtration rate
GU	genitourinary
I&O	intake and output
IVP	intravenous pyelogram
KUB	kidneys, ureters, bladder (x-ray)
PD	peritoneal dialysis
RP	retrograde pyelogram
SLE	systemic lupus erythematosus
UA; U/A	urinalysis
UTI	urinary tract infection

Word Building

Exercise 13

Define each combining form listed below; then build a term from it.

	Definition	Term
1. nephr/o		
2. ur/o		
3. ren/o		
4. glomerul/o		
5. py/o		
6. cyst/o		
7. urethr/o		
8. ureter/o		
9. lith/o		

Draw a box around the combining form in each term. Provide a definition for the combining form, then define the whole term.

Term	Definition of Combining Form	Definition of Term
1. nephrologist	_____	_____
2. urinal	_____	_____
3. renal	_____	_____
4. glomerular	_____	_____
5. cystitis	_____	_____
6. urethrectomy	_____	_____
7. cystscopy	_____	_____
8. anuria	_____	_____
9. oliguria	_____	_____
10. nephrotic	_____	_____

Write the medical term for the underlined phrase in each sentence.

1. Dr. Harrison performed a <u>kidney removal</u> this morning. _____

2. Harriet underwent a <u>procedure to remove part of her bladder</u> after she was diagnosed with a tumor in her bladder. _____

3. <u>Removing wastes from the blood using fluids instilled into and then removed from the patient's abdomen</u> is a procedure that can be performed in the patient's home. _____

4. <u>Filtering blood by routing it through a special machine</u> will be required if the kidneys fail. _____

5. The <u>special endoscope for viewing the interior of the bladder</u> was inserted through the external urinary meatus. _____

6. This patient is scheduled for a <u>procedure in which an agent is infused into the blood for the purpose of measuring how fast blood flows through the kidneys</u> test. _____

7. The surgical team will perform a <u>procedure in which the bladder is attached to an adjacent structure</u> in OR3 at 1700. _____

8. Mrs. Henry's physician has ordered a <u>flexible sterile tube to be inserted into her bladder</u> for a urine specimen. _____

9. The patient will have a <u>laboratory test to measure the amount of creatinine being passed through the kidneys</u>. _____

10. This 69 y/o female takes a <u>drug to promote the formation of urine</u> _____
    prescribed by her family physician.

What Do These Abbreviations Mean?   Exercise 16

Provide a definition for each abbreviation.

1. KUB _____

2. MRI _____

3. BUN _____

4. GFR _____

5. IVP _____

6. ESWL _____

7. UA _____

8. UTI _____

9. BPH _____

10. PD _____

Word Building   Exercise 17

Supply the word parts to complete each term.

1. _____ plasty = surgical repair of the ureter

2. cyst _____ = surgical removal of the bladder

3. nephr _____ = surgical removal of the kidney

4. cysto _____ = herniation of the bladder into the vagina

5. litho _____ = crushing of stones

6. uretero _____ = surgical creation of an opening between the ureter and the outside of the body

7. cysto _____ = incision into the bladder

8. cysto _____ = examination of the bladder through an instrument

9. urina _____ = breaking apart of the urine

10. nephr _____ = surgical creation of an opening from the kidney to the outside of the body

11. _____ otomy = surgical incision into the ureter

12. _____ lysis = separation of blood products through filtration (blood through separation)

Indicate whether each term is singular or plural by writing an S or a P after the term. Then supply the opposite form (singular vs. plural) of the term.

S or P   Opposite

1. cystectomies   _____   _____

2. glomeruli   _____   _____

3. catheterizations _____   _____

4. urinalysis   _____   _____

5. analgesic   _____   _____

6. diuretic   _____   _____

7. lithotripsy   _____   _____

8. calculus   _____   _____

9. kidney   _____   _____

10. membranes   _____   _____

Word Maps

Complete the diagram by supplying the missing terms.

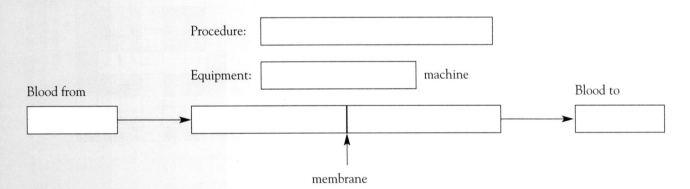

Procedure: [   ]

Equipment: [   ] machine

Blood from   Blood to

[   ] →   [|] →   [   ]

↑

membrane

Performance
Assessment 13

Crossword Puzzle

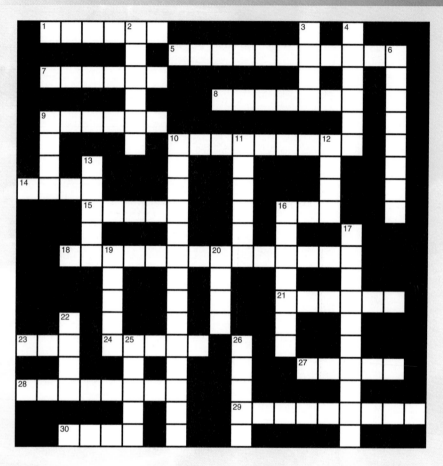

Across

1. opening
5. substance that conducts electricity in a fluid
7. nephr/o, ren/o
8. the body's container for urine
9. outer portion of an organ
10. blood in the urine
14. corpus
15. glyc/o
16. prefix meaning painful
18. structure that surrounds the glomerulus
21. -pexy
23. pyo
24. prefix meaning behind
27. hem/o
28. inflammation of the bladder
29. inflammation of the kidney
30. root for urine

Down

2. tube-like structure that carries urine from the kidney to the bladder
3. to excrete urine
4. pus in the urine
6. bed-wetting
9. pertaining to the colon
10. dilation of the pelvis and calces due to obstruction of urine flow
11. inability to produce urine
12. suffix meaning inflammation
13. root for bladder
16. painful urination
17. pain in the abdomen and back as a result of kidney stone
19. hydro/o
20. word part meaning cavity
22. word part meaning condition
25. prefix meaning outside
26. -lith

Word Analysis

Draw a box around the suffix in each term. Write the definition of the suffix on the line beside the term, then use the next lines to write a definition of the whole term.

1. pyelonephritis

   Suffix Definition _____

   Term Definition _____

   _____

2. renal

   Suffix Definition _____

   Term Definition _____

   _____

3. cystopexy

   Suffix Definition _____

   Term Definition _____

   _____

4. cystorrhaphy

   Suffix Definition _____

   Term Definition _____

   _____

5. necrosis

   Suffix Definition _____

   Term Definition _____

   _____

6. nephrectomy

   Suffix Definition _____

   Term Definition _____

   _____

7. prostatic

   Suffix Definition _____

   Term Definition _____

   _____

8. peritoneal

Suffix Definition _____

Term Definition _____

_____

9. pyelogram

Suffix Definition _____

Term Definition _____

_____

10. urologist

Suffix Definition _____

Term Definition _____

_____

What Do These Abbreviations Mean?

Provide a definition for each abbreviation given. Write the definition on the line beside the abbreviation.

1. ATN _____

2. BUN _____

3. CVA _____

4. cysto _____

5. GFR _____

6. GU _____

7. I&O _____

8. IVP _____

9. KUB _____

10. UA _____

11. UTI _____

12. SLE _____

Build the Terms

Select word parts from the lists to build a complete medical term for each definition given. Note that not all terms will have a root or combining form, prefix, and suffix. Some word parts may be used more than once.

Combining Forms	Prefixes	Suffixes
ur/o	hyper-	-ectomy
glyc/o	e-	-tomy
calic/o	sub-	-logist
urin/o	hypo-	-pathy
nephr/o	pre-	-megaly
ren/o	dys-	-esis
ureter/o	an-	-sclerosis
lith/o	pre-	-uria
glomerulo/o	de-	-trophy
cyst/o	anti-	-plasty
urethr/o	per-	-ectasis
pyel/o	bi-	-lysis

1. surgical incision into a calyx   _____

2. sugar (glucose) in the urine   _____

3. breakdown or separation of urine   _____

4. disease of the kidneys   _____

5. specialist in the study of the urinary system   _____

6. hardening of the glomerulus   _____

7. hardening of the ureter   _____

8. surgical incision into a ureter to remove a kidney stone   _____

9. surgical repair of the bladder   _____

10. dilation of the calyces   _____

11. without urine   _____

12. enlargement of the kidneys   _____

Using Medical References

The following medical terms may not have been addressed in this chapter. Use medical reference books, your medical term analysis skills, and/or a medical dictionary to find the correct definition of each word. Write the definition on the line provided below each term.

1. cortical nephrons

   _____

2. juxtamedullary nephrons

   _____

3. glomerular filtrate

   _____

4. solute

   _____

5. endogenous creatinine

   _____

6. tubular lumen

   _____

7. diffusion

   _____

8. diuresis

   _____

9. pneumaturia

   _____

10. orthostatic proteinuria

   _____

11. perinephritic hematoma

   _____

12. excretory urogram

   _____

What's Your Conclusion?

As you read each mini medical record or scenario, assume that you are a medical transcriptionist. Select the correct response for the situation. Write the letter of your answer in the space provided.

1. In a physician's progress notes, there is an entry about an "arteriovenous shunt in the left forearm." You expect that the doctor will include which of the following in his analysis:

   A. That the patient is receiving hemodialysis.
   B. That the patient is addicted to drugs, as evidenced by needle marks in his left forearm.

   Your response: _____

2. The next pediatric patient is a 5 y/o male who, the doctor's notes indicate, is being seen for a recheck with a note about poststreptococcal glomerulonephritis. You anticipate that the doctor's orders and plan will include which of the following:

   A. UA, BUN, creatinine clearance.
   B. Sputum specimen for C&S.

   Your response: _____

Records Analysis

Read the progress note on the next page; then answer the following questions.

1. What were the patient's primary complaints?

2. What is the purpose of the patient's visit?

3. What three tests has the patient had recently?

4. Describe four objective findings.

5. What is the analysis?

6. Are any tests to be performed? If so, what are they?

7. What type of procedure will the patient have?

8. Why is the patient being referred to an oncologist?

Physician's Progress Note

PATIENT: Delores M.
DATE: August 10, xxxx

S: Pt. is here today for the report of her lab tests and CT scan. She reports that her symptoms of fatigue and weakness are unchanged since last visit. She continues to have no voiding symptoms and no hematuria. She states that she did have the abdominal CT scan, as we discussed. She has appointments for the remainder of her tests on Friday. She has also seen Dr. Latimer for a PAP smear and a mammogram.

O: T 98.6, P 72, R 16, BP 138/90.

Previously taken family and medical histories are noncontributory. Pt. is gravida II, para II. Only remarkable findings on physical examination are mild costovertebral angle tenderness and slight pallor of the skin and mucous membranes. Reports of PAP smear and mammogram are normal. Abdominal CT showed a tumor on the anterior aspect of the left kidney and uterine fibroids. Hgb is 10.5; Hct, 30%.

A: Left nephroma.

P: Schedule bone scan; refer to Dr. Taylor for left nephrectomy; follow up with oncologist.

S. L. Ying, MD

Short Answer

In your own words, describe the process of urine formation.

_____

_____

_____

_____

_____

_____

_____

_____

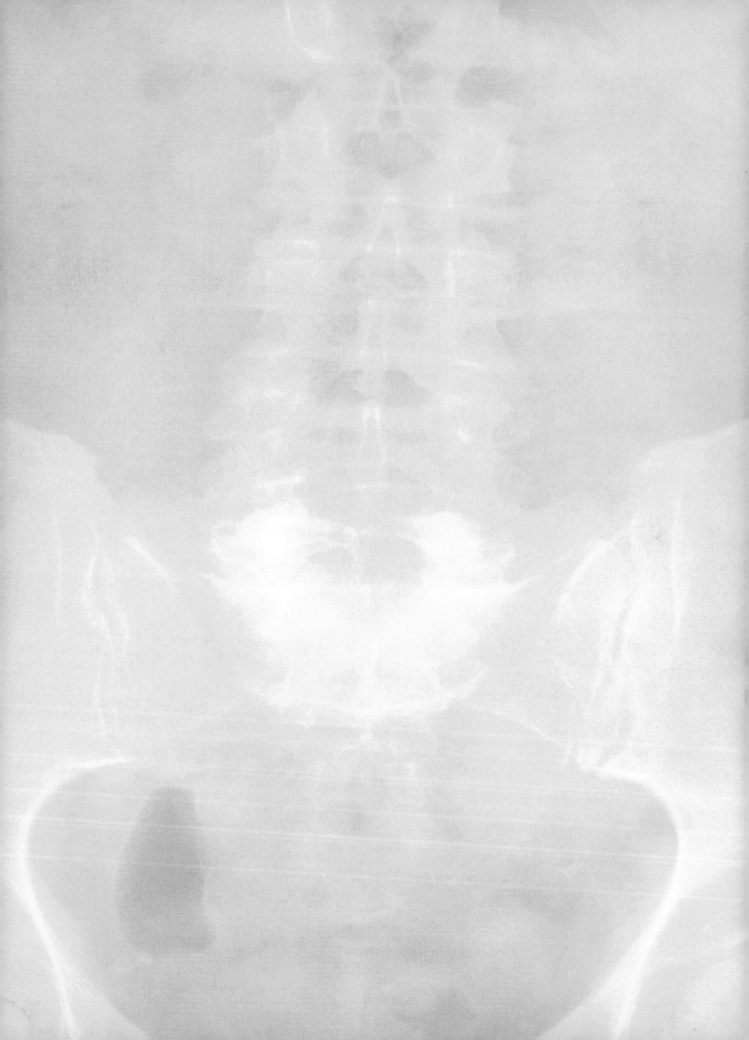

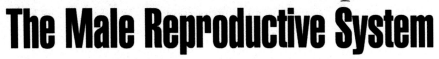

Chapter 14

The Male Reproductive System

Learning Outcomes

- Identify the structures of the male reproductive system.
- List the steps in the process of sperm production.
- Describe the function of the male reproductive organs in the process of fertilization.
- Correctly use the terminology of the male reproductive system in written and oral communication.
- Correctly spell and pronounce male reproductive system terminology.
- State the meaning of abbreviations related to the male reproductive system.
- List and define the combining forms most commonly used to create terms related to the male reproductive system.
- Name tests and treatments for major male reproductive system abnormalities.

Translation, Please? Translation, Please? Translation, Please?

Read this excerpt from a medical record and try to answer the questions that follow.

Patient is to have testicular ultrasound, testicular scan, and left scrotal exploration with possible orchiectomy or bilateral orchidopexy. The complications were discussed, including bleeding, infection, and possibility of the need for future testicular prosthesis.

1. Is testicular ultrasound an invasive procedure?
2. Orchiectomy and orchidopexy have the same root. What is it and what does it mean?
3. What is a bilateral orchidopexy?
4. A testicular prosthesis is an artificial penis. True or false?

Answers to "Translation, Please?"
1. No. This test is performed on the outside of the testicle.
2. Orchi/o or orchid/o means testis (testicle).
3. Orchidopexy is fixation by suturing the testicle into the scrotal sac. Bilateral means that the procedure is performed on both sides, that is, on both testicles.
4. False. A testicular prosthesis is a device that substitutes for a removed testicle.

Identifying the Specialty

The System and Its Practitioners

Most animals and some plants require contributions from both sexes to reproduce and proliferate the species. In humans, the organs that produce the male and female sex cells are called the **gonads**. The male and female sex cells, or **gametes**, are the ova in the female, and the **sperm** in the male. When the ovum (singular of ova) and sperm meet and join, the product is a **zygote**, the cell that starts a new life.

This chapter discusses the male reproductive system, which includes the external components (testes, penis, and scrotum), the internal structures (seminal vesicles, prostate gland, bulbourethral gland, and ductus deferens), and some of the structures of the urinary tract. Figure 14.1 shows the components of the male reproductive system.

The **urologist** is the physician who specializes in treating diseases of the male reproductive system, as well as in the study of the urinary system. Male sexual dysfunction may be treated by the urologist, but male infertility may be managed by an **infertility specialist**.

Figure 14.1 - Male Reproductive System

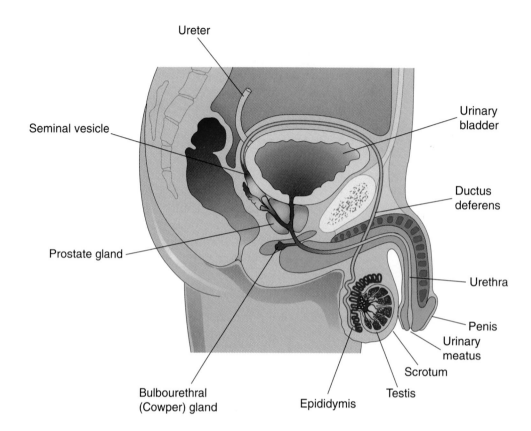

Ureter

Seminal vesicle

Urinary bladder

Ductus deferens

Prostate gland

Urethra

Penis

Urinary meatus

Scrotum

Bulbourethral (Cowper) gland

Epididymis

Testis

Examining the Patient ♂♀

Anatomy and Physiology of the Male Reproductive System

The external organs of the reproductive system are called **genitalia**. The **testes (testicles)** are contained within the **scrotum**, a pouch-like sac suspended outside the body. Each testis is an egg-shaped gland about 1½ by 1 inches in the adult. The testicle is composed of about a thousand long, coiled structures, called **seminiferous tubules**, with special cells that secrete **testosterone**, the male sex hormone, into the area around the tubules.

Figure 14.2 - Structure of the Penis

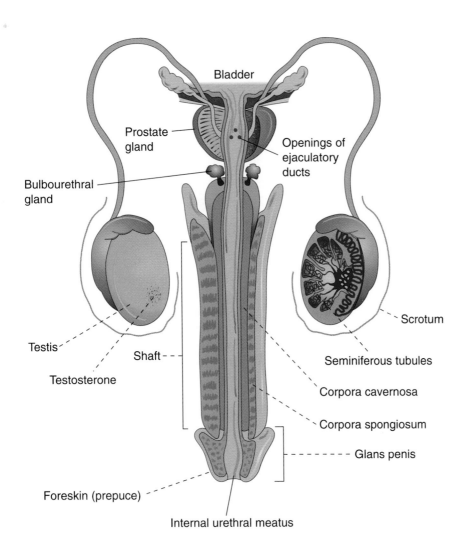

The Penis

The **penis** is the organ that enters the female's vagina during intercourse and deposits sperm. Medical descriptions of the penis assume an orientation in the erect state: the ventral side is away from the body and the dorsal side faces inward. The penis consists of a cylinder-shaped **shaft** with a tip called the **glans penis**. Covering the glans is retractable, loose-fitting tissue known as the **foreskin**, or **prepuce**. The shaft is formed by the **corpus spongiosum** that surrounds the urethra in the back, and the **corpora cavernosa**, two separate structures in front. These tissues are spongy and fill with blood when aroused, causing the penis to become erect.

Figure 14.3 - Sperm Structure

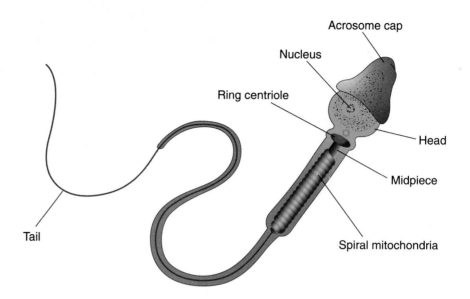

Acrosome cap

Nucleus

Ring centriole

Head

Midpiece

Tail

Spiral mitochondria

Sperm develop within the walls of the seminiferous tubules and are eventually released into the lumen of the tubules on their trip to the outside of the body. Although one of the smallest cells in the body, sperm is highly developed. Figure 14.3 shows the structure of the sperm. A covering on the head of the sperm contains special enzymes to break down the outside of the female's ovum. Genetic material is found in the head of each sperm. Within the **midpiece** of the sperm are the **mitochondria**, the structures that produce energy to nourish the sperm. The **tail** propels the sperm during its journey.

The Pathway of Sperm

Sperm pass through many ducts as they move toward the outside. Their first encounter is the **epididymis**, a long and twisted duct that stores the sperm for ten to twenty days as they develop and mature. The epididymis lies along the top of and behind the testes.

The next structure through which the sperm pass is the **ductus deferens**, or **vas deferens**. This tube leads sperm from the epididymis, away from the scrotum, and into the abdominal cavity. The ductus passes through the inguinal canal as part of the **spermatic cord**, over the top and down the posterior surface of the bladder, to eventually join the duct of the **seminal vesicles**. The seminal vesicles are glands that create about 60 percent of the volume of **semen**, the fluid that contains sperm and other substances. Thick and yellowish, semen contains a type of sugar that provides a source of energy for the sperm. The seminal vesicles join to form the **ejaculatory duct**.

The ejaculatory duct passes through the walnut-shaped **prostate gland**, which is below the bladder. The prostate secretes a milky fluid that aids in the mobility of the sperm and constitutes about 30 percent of the semen. The journey of the sperm continues to the **bulbourethral**, or **Cowper's**, **glands**, pea-sized structures located under the prostate gland. The Cowper's glands empty their secretions into the urethra to lubricate it with a mucus-like secretion, adding about 5 percent of the fluid volume. The final fluid is **ejaculated** outside the body.

Ejaculation is the rapid expulsion of the semen from the penis. About one teaspoon is ejaculated at one time, and this small amount of fluid contains about 100 million sperm. Figure 14.4 diagrams the journey of sperm through the ducts and glands of the male reproductive system. The combining forms for the names of the structures can be found in Table 14.1, and additional terms created from the combining forms are listed in Table 14.2.

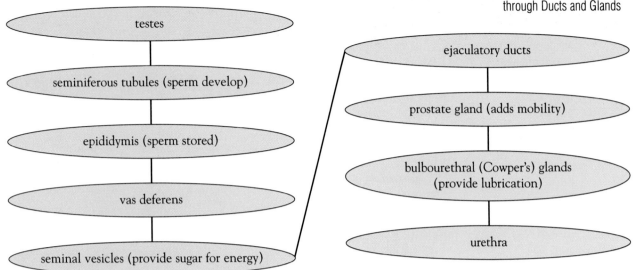

Figure 14.4 - Travel of Sperm through Ducts and Glands

testes

seminiferous tubules (sperm develop)

epididymis (sperm stored)

vas deferens

seminal vesicles (provide sugar for energy)

ejaculatory ducts

prostate gland (adds mobility)

bulbourethral (Cowper's) glands (provide lubrication)

urethra

Table 14.1

Combining Forms Relating to the Male Reproductive System

Combining form	Meaning	Example
andr/o	male, masculine	androgenous
balan/o	glans penis	balanoplasty
gamet/o	gamete	gametocyte
gonad/o	gonad; seed	gonadal
orchi/o	testis (testicle)	orchiocele
orchid/o	testis (testicle)	orchidometer
prostat/o	prostate	prostaglandins
spermat/o	semen, spermatozoa	spermatogenesis
sperm/o	semen, spermatozoa	spermatic
zyg/o	a yoke; joining	zygote

Table 14.2

Anatomy and Physiology Terms Relating to the Male Reproductive System

Term	Meaning	Word Analysis	
bulbourethral glands **bul**-bO-yoo-**ree**-threl Cowper's glands **kow**-perz	pea-sized glands located under the prostate gland; they empty their mucus-like secretions into the urethra to lubricate it	*bulb/o* *urethr/o*	bulb urethra
corpus cavernosum **kor**-pus kav-er-**nO**-sum	one of the two parallel areas of erectile tissue forming the dorsal side of the penis	*corpus* *cavernosum*	body cavern
corpus spongiosum **kor**-pus spun-jee-**O**-sum	middle column of spongy erectile tissue on the ventral side of the penis	*corpus* *spongiosum*	body sponge
ejaculate (n) ee-**jak**-yoo-let	the semen that is expelled	*ejaculatio*	shooting out
ejaculate (v) ee-**jak**-yoo-layt	to suddenly expel	*ejaculatio*	shooting out
ejaculation ee-jak-yoo-**lay**-shun	process of rapid expulsion of semen from the penis	*ejaculatio*	shooting out

continued on next page

ejaculatory ducts ee-**jak**-yoo-lah-tor-ee dukts	tunnels through the prostate gland; formed by the joining of the seminal vesicles	*ejaculatio* *-ory* *duct*	shoot out relating to passage
epididymis ep-ih-**did**-ah-mis	structure attached to the testis that transports, stores, and matures sperm	*epi/* *didymos*	on, above twin
foreskin **fOr**-skin prepuce **pree**-pyoos	loosely folded tissue that covers the glans penis (tip of the penis)	*fore-* *skin* *prepuce*	before; in front Anglo Saxon term foreskin
gamete **gam**-eet	male and female sex cells	*gamet/o*	to marry
genitalia jen-ih-**tay**-lee-ah genitals (pl) **jen**-ih-telz	male and female sex organs	*genitalia*	reproduction
glans penis glanz **pee**-nis	end of the penis	*glans* *penis*	an acorn-shaped structure tail
gonad **gO**-nad	organ that produces male and female sex cells	*gonad/o*	seed
penis **pee**-nis penile (adj) **pee**-nIl	male reproductive organ	*penis*	tail
prostate **pros**-tayt	walnut-shaped gland located below the bladder; secretes a milky fluid that aids in the mobility of the sperm	*prostat/o*	protector
scrotum **skrO**-tem	sac that contains the testes; located below the penis	*scrotum*	sac containing the testes
semen **see**-men	fluid containing the sperm	*semen*	seed
seminal vesicles **sem**-ih-nel **ves**-ih-kls	sacs (glands) that secrete a fluid containing sperm and other substances, including a type of sugar that provides energy for the sperm; the two seminal vesicles join to form the ejaculatory duct	*semen* *-al* *vesic/o*	seed relating to small sac
sperm spermatozoa **sper**-mah-tO-zO-ah	male sex cell that fertilizes the ovum to produce a new life	*sperm/o*	seed
testis (sing) **tes**-tis	male reproductive glands located within the scrotum; male gonads; testicles	*testis*	one of the two reproductive glands within the scrotum
testicle **tes**-tih-kl testicular (adj) tes-**tik**-yoo-ler	male reproductive gland (testis)	*testis*	one of the two reproductive glands within the scrotum
vas deferens vas **def**-er-enz ductus deferens **duk**-tes **def**-er-enz	duct of the reproductive tract; the tube that leads sperm from the epididymis, away from the scrotum and into the abdominal cavity	*vas* *defero*	a vessel to carry down
zygote **zI**-gOt	cell that is the product of the joining of the female ovum and the male sperm	*zyg/o*	joining; yoked

Separate the terms into their word parts, using hyphens. Identify the parts by type, using a letter for each part (P = prefix, R = root, S = suffix, CV = combining vowel), and give a definition for each term.

	Word Analysis	Definition
1. orchiocele	_____	_____
2. spermatic	_____	_____
3. androgenous	_____	_____
4. balanoplasty	_____	_____
5. gonadal	_____	_____
6. prostatectomy	_____	_____
7. gametocyte	_____	_____
8. testicular	_____	_____
9. spermatogenesis	_____	_____
10. zygote	_____	_____

Spelling Check

Exercise 2

Each of the following sentences contains a misspelled term. Circle the misspelled term and then write it correctly on the line provided.

1. The patient's enlarged prostrate gland is preventing urine from passing through the urethra.   _____

2. The female ovum and the male sperm join to form the psygoat.   _____

3. Male and female sex cells are called gamites.   _____

4. A eurologist treats disorders of the male reproductive system.   _____

5. The scroteum is a pouch-like sac suspended from the body.   _____

6. A hematoma was evident on the glens penal.   _____

7. The spomotic cord contains several separate structures.   _____

8. Ejaculation is the process of rapid expulsion of semen.   _____

9. Mitochrondial are essential for energy production in the sperm cell.   _____

10. The epidindymus is attached to the testis.   _____

Match the terms or abbreviations in Column 1 with the definitions in Column 2. Write the number of the term on the line beside the correct definition.

Column 1

1. mitochondria

2. prepuce

3. testosterone

4. genitalia

5. semen

6. spermatic cord

7. ejaculation

8. corpus spongiosum

9. bulbourethral glands

10. foreskin

11. ovum

12. ductus deferens

Column 2

a. loose-fitting tissue covering the glans penis

b. external organs of the male reproductive system

c. process of rapid expulsion of semen

d. tube that leads sperm from the epididymis into the abdominal cavity; same as vas deferens

e. middle column of spongy erectile tissue on the ventral side of the penis

f. located under the prostate gland, they empty secretions into the urethra to lubricate it; same as Cowper's glands

g. male sex hormone

h. same as prepuce

i. cord formed by ductus deferens and associated structures, extends through the inguinal canal and into the scrotum

j. structures that produce energy for the sperm, located in the midpiece

k. fluid containing sperm

l. female germ cell; egg

Supply the missing word part or parts to complete each term.

1. _____oid = like or resembling sperm

2. oligo_____ia = condition of scanty or deficient sperm

3. _____pexy = surgical fixation of a testicle

4. _____ectomy = removal of the epididymis

5. an_____ia = condition of absent testes

6. crypt_____ism = undescended testicle

7. _____itis = inflammation of the prostate gland

8. _____ectomy = removal of all or part of the vas deferens

9. _____ectomy = removal of the prostate gland

10. _____ = tumor of the testicle

Circle the correct term from the pair in each sentence.

1. The male and female sex cells are called gametes/gonads.

2. The product of the joining of ovum and sperm is a prepuce/zygote.

3. At the tip of the penis is the corpus cavernosa/glans penis.

4. Sperm are released into the lumen/mitochondria of the tubules.

5. The first duct that sperm pass through is the epididymis/vas deferens.

6. Glands that create about 60 percent of the volume of semen are bulbourethral glands/seminal vesicles.

7. Pea-size structures under the prostate gland are Cowper's glands/vas deferens.

8. The rapid expulsion of semen from the body is called ejaculation/epididymus.

9. The physician who specializes in treating diseases of the male reproductive system is the testologist/urologist.

10. Human reproductive organs are called ductus/gonads.

Word Maps

Exercise 6

The diagram below depicts the journey of sperm from its origin in the testicle through the urethra. Complete the diagram by supplying the missing terms.

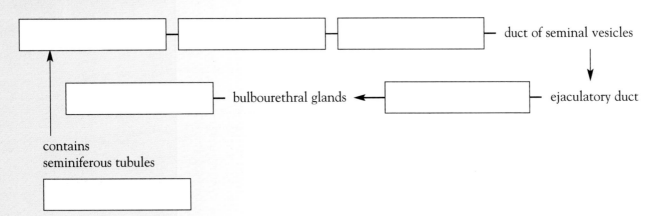

Assessing Patient Health

Wellness and Illness through the Life Span

The testes develop in the abdominal cavity of the fetus. They descend along the inguinal canal in the groin into the scrotum before birth. The size of each testis is about ½ to ¾ inches long by about ⅓ inch wide at birth and increases only slightly during childhood. With the onset of puberty, which can occur as early as age 9 or 10, the testes begin to grow. Shortly thereafter, pubic hair appears and the penile size increases. These changes in development are compared on a rating scale called **Tanner staging**, which healthcare professionals use to establish sexual maturity in children and adolescents (see Figure 14.5).

Figure 14.5 - Tanner Staging: Male

Genital Stage	Pubic hair	Scrotum/Penis	Age at onset (mean + SD)
1	no coarse hair`	prepubetal	
2	longer, silky hair appears at base of penis	scrotum and testes enlarge; skin of scrotum reddens and rugations appear	11.4 ± 1.1 yr
3	hair coarse, kinky, spreads over pubic bone	penis lengthens; testes enlarge further	12.9 ± 1 yr
4	hair of adult quality but not spread to junction of medial thigh with perineum	penis growth continues in length and width; glans develops adult form	13.8 ± 1 yr
5	hair spreads to medial thigh	development completed; adult appearance	14.9 ± 1.1 yr

Male sexual development is completed in three to five years, and the system does not change significantly throughout the years of young and middle adulthood. Sperm production decreases around age 40, but some sperm are produced even at age 90. When men reach their sixth decade, testosterone begins to decline gradually, causing physical changes such as decreased muscle tone and decreased energy levels. As the aging process continues the amount of pubic hair decreases, and penile size and scrotal tone decline.

During a physical examination, the physician palpates the testes to check for lumps or tenderness, inspects the urinary meatus (opening), and palpates the inguinal canal and prostate gland (in adults) to identify enlargement or other changes that may indicate disease.

Infancy

The newborn male may be circumcised several days after birth. **Circumcision** removes the prepuce from the penis. The uncircumcised child must have the foreskin gently retracted for careful examination of the meatus. Abnormalities include malposition of the urethral opening: **epispadias** (opening is on the dorsum of the penis) and **hypospadias** (opening is on the ventral side of the penis). Other congenital anomalies of the male reproductive system include the following categories:

- Abnormalities of the testes, such as **anorchism** (absence of testicles), **cryptorchism** (failure of one or both of the testicles to descend), and **polyorchism** (having more than two testicles);
- Abnormalities in the formation of the genitalia, such as **ambiguous genitalia** (the sex organs of the newborn cannot be identified clearly) and **hermaphroditism** (the infant has male and female sexual tissues).

Table 14.3 describes congenital anomalies of the male reproductive organs. Figure 14.6 illustrates some of these congenital malformations, as well as certain abnormalities that develop as a result of a disease process.

Table 14.3

Congenital Anomalies of the Male Reproductive System

Term	Meaning	Word Analysis	
ambiguous genitalia am-**big**-yoo-us jen-ih-**tay**-lee-ah	sex organs in a newborn that are not clearly male or female	ambi- (ambigo) gen/i	around; both sides (wander) being born; producing
anorchism an-**or**-kiz-em	absence of the testes	an- orch/i	without testes
cryptorchism krip-**tor**-kiz-em	failure of one or both testicles to descend into the scrotal sac	crypt/o orch/i	hidden, concealed testes
epispadias ep-ih-**spad**-ee-as	abnormality in which the urethral opening is on the dorsum of the penis	epi- spadon	on, above a tear, rip
hermaphroditism her-**maf**-rod-ih-tiz-em hermaphrodism her-**maf**-rod-iz-em hermaphrodite her-**maf**-rO-dIt	having both ovarian and testicular tissue; pseudohermaphroditism is the term used when the person *displays* either male or female sexual characteristics, i.e., male pseudohermaphrodite	Hermes Aphrodite pseud/o	Greek god (Mercury), a male Greek goddess (Venus), a female false; denoting a resemblence

continued on next page

hypospadias hI-pO-**spay**-dee-as	abnormality in which the urethral opening is on the ventral side of the penis	*hypo-* *spadon*	below; less a tear, rip
polyorchism pol-ee-**or**-kiz-em polyorchidism pol-ee-**or**-kid-iz-em	having more than two testicles	*poly-* *orch/i* *(orchid/o)*	many testes

Figure 14.6 - Abnormalities of the Male Reproductive Organs

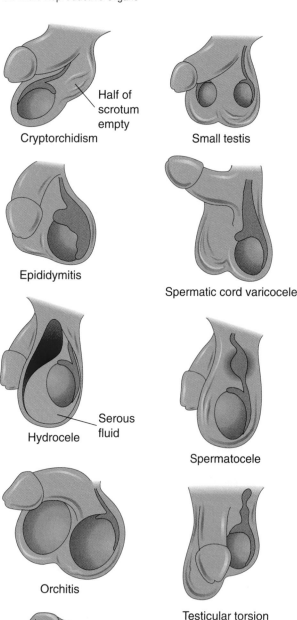

Cryptorchidism — Half of scrotum empty

Small testis

Epididymitis

Spermatic cord varicocele

Hydrocele — Serous fluid

Spermatocele

Orchitis

Testicular torsion

Scrotal edema

Childhood and Adolescence

A condition of early childhood is **varicocele** of the spermatic cord, that is, varicose veins in the spermatic cord, which can cause the affected testicle to be smaller because of decreased circulation to the area. A **hydrocele** is an accumulation of fluid in the testicle of young boys.

A serious condition that occurs later in childhood and in adolescence is **testicular torsion**. This usually occurs on the left side and is caused by an incomplete or faulty attachment of the testis on the wall of the scrotum, allowing it to rotate, usually medially. Emergency surgery is necessary to prevent gangrene. Also occurring in this age group is **priapism**, or prolonged erection, which is often associated with sickle cell anemia (see Chapter 5, "Hematology"). A blockage to the blood flow from the penis causes it to become engorged with blood that cannot exit.

Adults and Seniors

Benign prostatic hyperplasia (BPH) occurs in men as they age. In this condition, the prostate gland becomes increasingly enlarged, squeezing the urethra that passes through it. The swollen prostate can cause painful, frequent, and/or difficult urination. Prostate cancer is a malignant transformation within the prostate gland that is usually diagnosed in the older male. It can be treated with radiation therapy to shrink the tissue, or in some cases with a surgical procedure to remove the prostate.

General Illnesses

A common problem for men is **impotence**, the inability to have an erection. Also known as erectile dysfunction, this condition can occur at any age, although it is more common in older men. The causes may be physical or psychological. Chronic substance abuse along with diseases of the lungs, liver, heart, kidneys, nerves, and vascular system can lead to impotence; certain medications, including antidepressants, antihistamines, and drugs for high blood pressure can also contribute to impotence. Psychological causes include stress, anxiety, and depression.

Another important problem of adult males is **sterility**, which is the term for a category of conditions related to diminished or absent sperm production. **Aspermatogenesis** is the inability to produce sperm; **aspermia** is the inability to produce semen; **oligospermia** is decreased sperm production. Note, however, that a man who is sterile is not necessarily impotent, and vice versa.

Common infections of the male reproductive organs include **balanitis**, inflammation of the glans penis, **orchitis**, inflammation of the testes, **epididymitis**, inflammation of the epididymis, and **prostatitis**, inflammation of the prostate gland. **Phimosis** is a narrowing of the opening of the prepuce preventing its being drawn back over the glans, which may be congenital or caused by scarring from frequent infections.

Testicular carcinoma is found most commonly in the young adult population. It can affect one or both testicles and can be local or disseminated at diagnosis. It is treated by orchiectomy and chemotherapy.

Table 14.4 lists the wellness and illness terms that appear frequently in medical records and in other written and oral communication concerning the male reproductive system.

Table 14.4

Wellness and Illness Terms Relating to the Male Reproductive System

Term	Meaning	Word Analysis	
aspermatogenesis ay-sper-mah-tO-**jen**-ah-sis	failure of sperm production	a- sperm/o -genic, genesis	without seed formation, production
aspermia ah-**sper**-mee-ah	ejaculation without seminal fluid or without spermatozoa	a- sperm/o	without seed
balanitis bal-ah-**nI**-tis	inflammation of the glans penis	balan/o -itis	pertaining to the glans penis inflammation
benign prostatic hyperplasia bee-**nIn** pros-**tat**-ik hI-**per**-play see ah	enlarged prostate tissue causing pressure on the urethra	benign prostat/o hyper- -plasia	kind protect increased formation
circumcision ser-kum-**sih**-zhun	procedure to remove the foreskin of the penis	circum- incisio	around to make a cut
epididymitis ep-ih-did-ih-**mI**-tis	inflammation of the epididymis	epi- didymos -itis	on, above twin inflammation
hydrocele **hI**-drO-seel	collection of fluid within the testis	hydr/o -cele	pertaining to water tumor, hernia
impotence **im**-pah-tens	inability to achieve and/or maintain an erection of the penis	im- potentia	no; negative power
oligospermia ol-ih-gO-**sper**-mee-ah	decreased sperm in the ejaculate	olig/o sperm/o	too little seed
orchitis or-**kI**-tis	inflammation of the testis	orchi/o -itis	pertaining to the testes inflammation
phimosis fI-**mO**-sis phimoses (pl) fI-**mO**-seez	narrowness of the opening of the prepuce preventing its being drawn back over the glans	phimos	muzzle

continued on next page

priapism **prI**-ah-piz-em	prolonged erection	*Priapos*	Greek god of procreation
prostatitis pros-tah-**tI**-tis	inflammation of the prostate gland	*prostat/o* *-itis*	protects inflammation
sterility stah-**ril**-ih-tee	incapable of fertilization	*sterilis*	barren
testicular torsion tes-**tik**-yoo-ler **tor**-shun	rotation of the testis within the scrotum	*testicle* *torsio*	Latin term twisting, rotation
varicocele **var**-ih-kO-seel	varicose veins in the spermatic cord	*varic/o* *-cele*	dilated vein, varicosity pouch, hernia

Word Analysis

Separate each word into its individual parts, using hyphens. Identify the parts by type, using a letter for each part (P = prefix, R = root, S = suffix, CV = combining vowel), then define the term.

	Word Analysis	Definition
1. cryptorchism	_____	_____
2. polyorchism	_____	_____
3. anorchism	_____	_____
4. hydrocele	_____	_____
5. aspermia	_____	_____
6. spermatogenesis	_____	_____
7. balanitis	_____	_____
8. orchitis	_____	_____
9. testicular	_____	_____
10. epididymitis	_____	_____

Select the correct medical term from the list to substitute for the underlined definition in each sentence. Write the correct term on the blank provided at the end of each sentence.

phimosis	benign prostatic hyperplasia	circumcision
orchialgia	testicular torsion	pseudohermaphrodite
priapism	balanitis	aspermia
cryptorchism	epispadias	ambiguous genitalia
impotence		

1. The infant was born with <u>sex organs that are not clearly male or female</u>. _____

2. The child will require surgery for <u>failure of one or both of the testicles to descend into the scrotum</u>. _____

3. Surgery has already been scheduled for <u>condition where the urethral opening is on the dorsum of the penis</u>. _____

4. The patient is a male <u>having both ovarian and testicular tissue, but displaying characteristics of only one gender</u>. _____

5. The <u>procedure to remove the prepuce from the penis</u> was performed several days after birth. _____

6. There is a congenital <u>narrowing of the opening of the prepuce</u> that will require immediate surgical intervention. _____

7. The patient was referred to the clinic because of recent onset of <u>inability to have an erection</u>. _____

8. Mr. Roberts will be evaluated for <u>pain in the testes</u>.

9. This patient was diagnosed with <u>enlarged prostate tissue causing pressure on the urethra</u> and was referred to a urologist for further treatment. _____

10. The child will have emergency surgery for <u>incomplete or faulty attachment of the testis on the wall of the scrotum, allowing it to rotate</u>. _____

Matching

Match the terms or abbreviations in Column 1 with the definitions in Column 2. Write the number of the term on the line beside the correct definition.

Column 1		Column 2
1. oligospermia	_____	having more than two testicles
2. balantis	_____	inflammation of the testicle or testicles
3. antibiotics	_____	inflammation of the prostate
4. hypospadias	_____	opening of the urethra
5. orchitis	_____	small or scanty amount of sperm
6. urinary meatus	_____	enlargement or excessive formation/development
7. polyorchism	_____	agent that kills or inhibits growth of bacteria
8. aspermatogenic	_____	inflammation of the glans penis
9. prostatitis	_____	lacking formation of sperm
10. hyperplasia	_____	urinary meatus is displaced to the ventral side of the penis

Word Building

Construct terms to match the definitions provided, using only the following suffixes:

-itis   -ectomy   -plasty

1. inflammation of the testes   _____

2. inflammation of the glans penis   _____

3. inflammation of the prostate   _____

4. inflammation of the epididymis   _____

5. inflammation of the urethra   _____

6. surgical repair of the testis   _____

7. surgical repair of the glans penis   _____

8. surgical repair of the vas deferens   _____

9. surgical removal of the prostate   _____

10. surgical removal of the vas deferens   _____

Rewrite the misspelled terms, using the correct spelling, and then define the term. If the term is spelled correctly, write OK on the line beside the term and supply the definition.

1. hydrocelle   _____

_____

2. phymosis   _____

_____

3. begnign prostetic hyperplasia   _____

_____

4. balanitis   _____

_____

5. oligiospermia   _____

_____

6. circiumcision   _____

_____

7. prostrate   _____

_____

8. steritlity   _____

_____

9. variocele   _____

_____

10. testicular tortion   _____

_____

Complete the concept maps below by supplying the missing terms.

lack of production of sperm:

[ ]

deficient amount of sperm:

[ ]

absence of sperm:

[ ]

term for male and female sex cells:

[ ]

male sex cell:

[ ]

female sex cell:

[ ]

term for joined sex cells (fertilized egg):

[ ]

becomes [ ]

Diagnosing and Treating Problems

Tests, Procedures, and Pharmaceuticals

When physical examination of the prostate reveals an abnormality, it is important to test for **prostate-specific antigen (PSA)**. This blood test can help diagnose cancer of the prostate. **Prostatic ultrasonography** is performed when there is an abnormality in the prostate gland.

A blood test also can determine the amount of male hormones being secreted, for example, testosterone. **Semen analysis** calculates the amount of sperm that is ejaculated and evaluates sperm viability. Ultrasonography and CT scanning can identify structural abnormalities within the system.

Procedures

One of the most common surgical procedures involving the male reproductive system is circumcision, the removal of all or part of the prepuce of the glans penis (see Table 14.4). **Epididymotomy** is an incision into the epididymis, usually performed to drain fluid resulting from epididymitis. An **epididymovasostomy** is the joining of the epididymis to the vas deferens. An undescended testicle is repaired with a procedure called **orchidorrhaphy**, during which the testicle is fixed within the scrotum. **Orchiectomy** is the surgical removal of one or both testicles.

Procedures involving the prostate gland include **prostatectomy**, or removal of part or all of the gland. A **transurethral resection of the prostate (TURP)** resections the prostate gland through the urethra.

A **vasectomy**, usually performed as a method of birth control, removes a section of the vas deferens to prevent sperm from exiting the body. A **vesiculectomy** is the excision of all or part of the seminal vesicle. These terms and their word parts are listed in Table 14.5.

Table 14.5

Tests and Procedures Relating to the Male Reproductive System

Term	Meaning	Word Analysis	
epididymotomy ep-ih-did-ih-**mot**-ah-mee	incision into the epididymis to drain pus or other fluid	epi/ didymos -tomy	on, above twin incision, cutting
epididymovasectomy ep-ih-did-ih-mO-vah-**sek**-tah-mee	surgical removal of the epididymis and vas deferens	epi/ didymos vas/ -ectomy	on, above twin vessel removal
orchidorrhaphy or-kid-**or**-af-ee	surgical procedure to bring down the undescended testicle and suture it into the scrotum	orchid/o -rrhaphy	testicle suturing
orchiectomy or-kee-**ek**-tah-mee	removal of the testis (testes)	orch/i -ectomy	testicle removal
prostate-specific antigen **pros**-tayt	blood test to determine the presence of malignancy of the prostate gland	prostat/o anti/ -gen	protect against producing
transurethral resection of the prostate trans-yoo-**ree**-thral	surgical procedure to remove all or part of the prostate gland; performed through the urethral opening	trans/ urethr/o re-seco prostat/o	through urethra cut off protect
vasectomy vah-**sek**-tah-mee	surgical removal of a portion of the vas deferens	vas/ -ectomy	vessel removal
vesiculectomy veh-sik-yoo-**lek**-tah-mee	surgical removal of the seminal vesicle	vesic/o -ectomy	small sac removal

Pharmaceutical Agents

Drugs used to treat problems of the male reproductive tract include hormone replacement agents, erectile dysfunction therapy, and treatment for benign prostatic hyperplasia. Antibiotics are used when there is an infection in any of the organs or tissues of this system.

Table 14.6

Pharmacologic Agents

Class	Use	Generic names	Brand names
benign prostatic hyperplasia therapy	treatment of BPH	doxazosin mesylate finasteride terazosin hydrochloride	Cardura Proscar Hytrin
erectile dysfunction therapy	assisting men with producing and/or maintaining an erection	alprostadil (prostaglandin E$_1$) sildenafil vardenafil	Caverject Injection Muse Pellet Viagra Levitra
testosterone replacement hormone	replacement of the male hormone, testosterone	methyltestosterone testosterone transdermal patch testosterone transdermal gel	Android, Testred Androderm, Testoderm AndroGel

Table 14.7

Abbreviations

BPH	benign prostatic hyperplasia
DRE	digital rectal examination
PSA	prostate-specific antigen
STD	sexually transmitted disease
TUR	transurethral resection
TURP	transurethral resection of the prostate or transurethral prostatectomy
VDRL	Venereal Disease Research Laboratory (test for syphilis, an STD)

Word Analysis

Separate each word into its individual parts, using hyphens. Identify the parts by type, using a letter for each part (P = prefix, R = root, S = suffix, CV = combining vowel), then define the term.

	Analysis	**Definition**
1. balanitis		
2. spermatogenic		
3. orchitis		
4. vasectomy		
5. zygote		
6. androgen		
7. gametogenic		
8. gonadal		
9. orchioectomy		
10. prostatitis		

Comprehension Check

Read each sentence and select the most appropriate term from the two choices given. Underline your choice. You may need to use a medical dictionary for this exercise.

1. Mr. Masterson's testosterone/zygote level will be evaluated.

2. A semen analysis/glans penis will also be performed.

3. We will also schedule a prostate-specific antigen test/circumcision to evaluate for prostate cancer.

4. Prostatic ultrasonography/prostate gland will be performed in the morning.

5. An epididymotomy/urinary meatus will be necessary to remove the accumulated fluid.

6. The damage will be repaired by an epididymovasotomy/hypospadias.

7. He is being prepped for surgery, for a transurethral resection of the prostate/oligospermia.

8. The child will undergo an orchidorrhaphy/aspermia for cryptorchism/scrotum.

9. The patient will be treated with testosterone replacement hormone/gametocyte to correct the condition.

10. The patient will have a vasectomy/urologist, as a birth control measure.

Matching

Match the abbreviations in Column 1 with the meanings in Column 2. Write the letter of the abbreviation on the line beside the meaning. You may need to use a medical dictionary.

Column 1		Column 2
1. TURP	_____	digital rectal exam
2. BPH	_____	transurethral resection
3. PSA	_____	Venereal Disease Research Laboratory (test for syphilis)
4. STD	_____	human immunodeficiency virus
5. VDRL	_____	prostate specific antigen
6. TUR	_____	sexually transmitted disease
7. DRE	_____	benign prostatic hyperplasia
8. HIV	_____	transurethral resection of the prostate

Word Building

Supply the word parts to complete each term.

1. _____ectomy = surgical removal of the testes

2. _____ectomy = surgical removal of the prostate gland

3. _____ectomy = surgical removal of all or part of the seminal vesicle

4. _____urethral = through the urethra

5. _____ic = pertaining to the prostate

6. orchido_____ = suturing of the testicle

7. _____otomy = incision into the glans penis

8. _____pexy = surgical fixation of the testicle

9. _____ = excess development or enlargement

10. _____ otomy = joining of the epididymis to the vas deferens

Check for misspelled terms and names in the list below. Make corrections by rewriting the word with the correct spelling, then define it.

1. transurthreal resetcion of the prostrate _____

2. vassectomy _____

3. orchioectomy _____

4. semin alalysis _____

5. terasozin _____

6. finalasteride _____

7. Tesred _____

8. allprostadium _____

9. Prostacar _____

10. doxizosin mesylate _____

Word Maps

Exercise 18

On the illustration below, identify the marked structures and write their names on the first line beside each item, then on the next lines write names of procedures performed on the structure.

structure: _____

procedures: _____

_____

_____ (abbreviation)

structure: _____

procedures: _____

_____

_____ (abbreviation)

structure: _____

procedures: _____

_____

_____ (abbreviation)

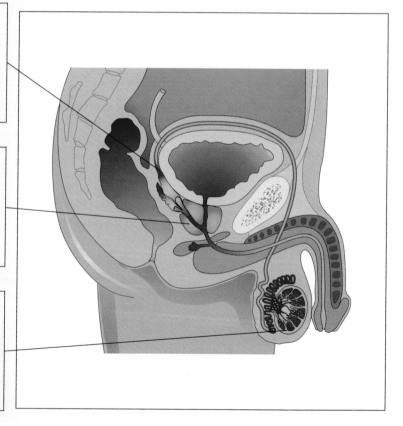

Performance Assessment 14

Crossword Puzzle

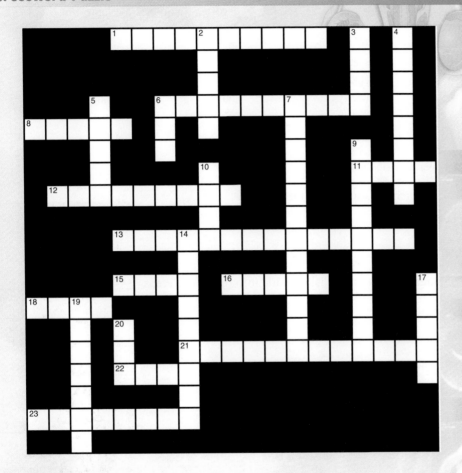

Across

1. tip of the penis
6. varicose veins in the spermatic cord
8. fluid containing secretions of male urogenital tract, including sperm
11. prefix meaning many
12. removal of vas deferens to prevent sperm from reaching the outside of the body
13. suturing of the testicle or testicles
15. semen
16. combining form meaning pertaining to the testes
18. corpus
21. procedure to remove the prepuce from the penis
22. word part meaning pouch, hernia
23. walnut-shaped gland that lies below the bladder

Down

2. male sex cell
3. andr/o
4. egg-shaped gland of male reproduction, source of sperm
5. tail
6. Latin for a vessel
7. undescended testicle or testicles
9. opening of the urinary meatus is on the dorsum of the penis
10. root meaning both
14. accumulation of fluid in the testicle or testicles
17. Latin for acorn
19. root meaning twin
20. scrotum

Build the Terms

Select word parts from the lists to build a complete medical term for each definition given. Note that not all terms will have a root or combining form, prefix, and suffix. Some word parts may be used more than once.

Combining Forms	Prefixes	Suffixes
balan/o	hyper-	-ia
orchi/o	epi-	-graphy
orchid/o	sub-	-ostomy
zyg/o	hypo-	-oma
gamet/o	oligo-	-ectomy
andr/o	dis-	-itis
sperm/o	an-	-al
spermat/o	pre-	-ar
epididym/o	de-	-ic
vas/o	anti-	-phobia
vesic/o	per-	-cyte
gonad/o	bi-	-lysis

1. germ or sex cell _____

2. deficient or scanty amount of sperm _____

3. breakdown of sperm _____

4. process of recording (x-ray) the vas deferens _____

5. creation of an artificial opening into the vas deferens _____

6. fear of males _____

7. tumor of the testicle (sperm) _____

8. pertaining to the gonads _____

9. surgical removal of the epididymis _____

10. inflammation of the epididymis and testicle _____

Word Analysis

Separate each word into its individual parts, using slashes. Identify the parts by type, using a letter for each part (P = prefix, R = root, S = suffix, CV = combining vowel), then define the term.

	Analysis	Definition
1. urologist	_____	_____
		_____
		_____

2. balanoplasty _____ _____
_____
_____

3. urethritis _____ _____
_____
_____

4. gonadal _____ _____
_____
_____

5. spermatic _____ _____
_____
_____

6. prostatectomy _____ _____
_____
_____

7. prostatitis _____ _____
_____
_____

8. hyperplasia _____ _____
_____
_____

9. anorchism _____ _____
_____
_____

10. orchitis _____ _____
_____
_____

What Do These Abbreviations Mean?

Write out the meaning of each abbreviation on the line provided.

1. UA _____

2. UTI _____

3. BPH _____

4. TURP _____

5. PSA _____

6. DRE _____

7. STD _____

8. HIV _____

What's Your Conclusion?

In this exercise you will practice selecting the correct explanation or logical next step. Read each mini medical record or scenario carefully; then select the correct response. Write the letter of your answer in the space provided. (There may be more than one correct response.)

1. A 39 y/o male comes to the physician's office requesting a vasectomy. He and his wife have three children and another pregnancy would risk his wife's health. She was diagnosed with lupus approximately six months ago. The procedure, risks, and benefits were discussed with the patient and he was provided an informational booklet. What form does the patient need to sign prior to the procedure?

    A. Release of information for his insurance to pay for the vasectomy.
    B. Surgical consent form for the procedure.

    Your response: _____

2. A 73 y/o male is seen for a yearly physical examination. The patient reports that he has dysuria and frequency, and the physician performs a DRE. Which of the following might be included in the assessment?

    A. R/O STD.
    B. R/O VDRL.
    C. R/O BPH.
    D. R/O UTI.

    Your response: _____

3. A 34 y/o male is seen in the office, and he reports left testicular pain and mild swelling following flulike symptoms. Upon examination, the left epididymis is tender. You anticipate that the doctor's analysis may include which of the following:

    A. left epididymitis
    B. cystitis

    Your response: _____

Analyzing Medical Records

Read the progress note on the next page and then answer the following questions.

1. Who dictated this document?

2. What are the age and the gender of the patient?

3. Where was the patient seen?

4. Describe the findings from the physical examination.

5. What is the analysis? Is this an infectious disease?

6. Was any medication prescribed? If so, what is the medication and the sig.?

7. What tests are to be performed?

8. When will the patient be seen again?

PATIENT: Martin M.
DATE: August 12, xxxx

S: 34 y/o male states that he has pain in right scrotum, radiating into his back. This has been getting worse. Pt. is a wrangler at a local resort and he states the pain began some time after he was thrown from a horse two days ago. He also had injuries to his left knee and shoulder from the same incident. He believes the knee and shoulder injuries are not serious, but is concerned about the scrotal pain. He denies fever, nausea, vomiting, blood in the urine, and changes in pattern of urination. ROS is otherwise normal.

O: T 98.6° F, P 76, R 16, BP 128/72.
Observable ecchymoses on lateral aspect of left shoulder, with some tenderness. No palpable masses or fractures. Joint is intact, with full ROM, although pt. reports pain with movement. Minimal swelling. Left knee is also tender, with ecchymoses over patellar area. Mild to moderate swelling; full ROM, pain with movement. No crepitus in either joint. Inferior ecchymoses of scrotum; testes and epididymides are normal bilaterally. Small area of induration on right lateral aspect of scrotum, with mild tenderness. Exquisitely tender nodule, approx 0.5 cm on right lateral inferior aspect of scrotum. No other induration or tenderness in upper scrotal area. No palpable masses or tenderness in abdomen or suprapubic area.

A: Bruising of left side, following fall. Probable soft tissue injuries in areas of knee and shoulder. Probable hematoma of scrotum.

P: 1) Testicular ultrasound.
    2) Darvocet-N 100 mg q.4h. p.r.n. pain.
    3) Ibuprofen p.r.n.
    4) Obtain x-rays of left shoulder and knee to R/O bone or joint injuries.
    5) Instruct pt. to RTO or go to ER if scrotal pain or swelling increases or, if fever, nausea, vomiting, blood in urine, or frequent urination occur.
    6) Pt. to RTO in one week.

_____
                              T. Knight, MD

Using Medical References

The following sentences contain medical terms that may not have been addressed on the charts in this chapter. Use medical reference books, your medical term analysis skills, and/or a medical dictionary to find the correct definition of each underlined word. Write the definition on the line below the sentence.

1. Balanitis and balanoposthitis can be complications of gonorrhea.

2. Genital candidiasis has been increasing in frequency.

3. Primary erectile dysfunction is rare and indicates severe pathology.

4. Treatment with human chorionic gonadotropin is being considered.

5. Impression is condylomata acuminata.

6. Trichomoniasis can be treated successfully with metronidazole.

7. The patient exhibits a mucoid subpreputial discharge.

8. <u>Congenital syphilis</u> is entirely preventable with good prenatal care.

9. Over 250 million persons are infected with <u>gonorrhea</u> each year.

10. <u>Pediculosis pubis</u> requires aggressive treatment to avoid spreading.

Short Answer

In your own words and in plain language, describe the process of sperm production.

_____

_____

_____

_____

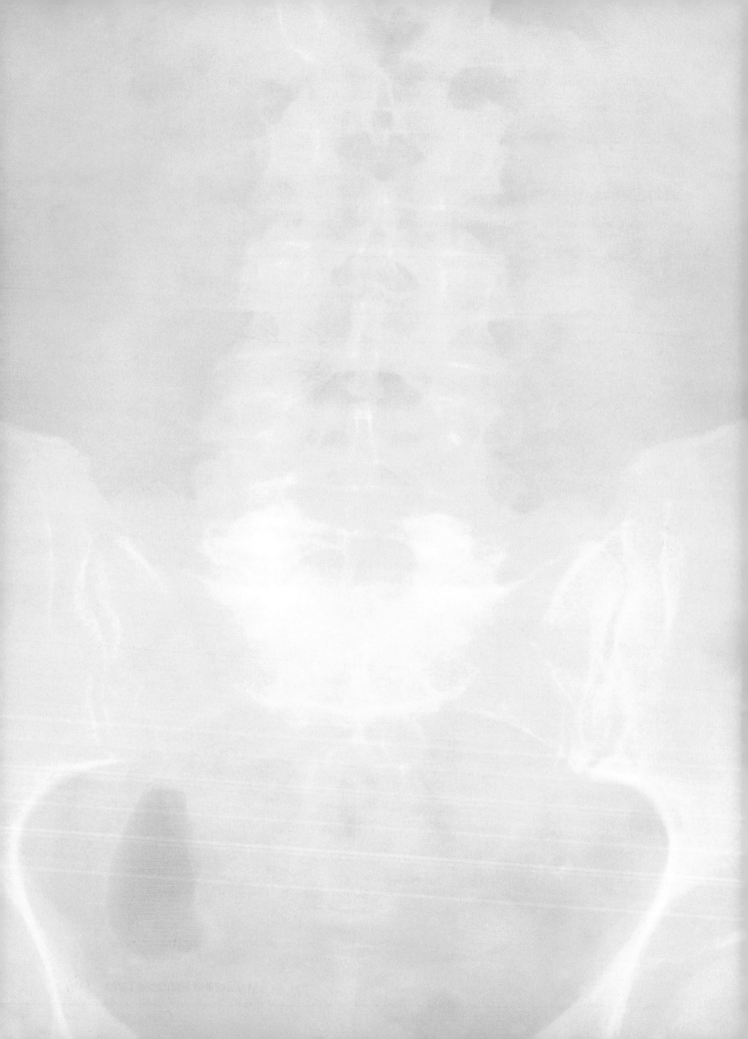

The Female Reproductive System

Learning Outcomes

Students will be able to:
- Identify and label the structures of the female reproductive system.
- List the steps of the reproductive cycle.
- Describe the function of the female reproductive organs in the process of fertilization.
- Use the terminology of the female reproductive system in oral and written communication correctly.
- Correctly spell and pronounce female reproductive system terminology.
- State the meaning of abbreviations related to the female reproductive system.
- List and define the combining forms most commonly used to create terms related to the female reproductive system.
- Name tests and treatments for major female reproductive system abnormalities.

Translation, Please? Translation, Please? Translation, Please?

Read these excerpts from medical records and try to answer the questions that follow them.

> This is a 25-year-old female, gravida 1, para 0, at 39 weeks.
> Endometriosis was causing dyspareunia and metrorrhagia.
> After having four children by natural childbirth, the woman had a uterine prolapse.

1. Gravida 1, para 0 means that this female was in grave condition around her delivery. True or false?
2. Endometriosis is an infectious condition. True or false?
3. Does metrorrhagia refer to vaginal bleeding or a urinary tract infection?
4. Does dyspareunia refer to painful urination or painful intercourse?
5. Does prolapse mean the uterus developed a tear?

Answers to "Translation Please?"
1. False. Gravida 1, para 0 means that the mother had one pregnancy and no births (at the time).
2. False. Endometriosis is a nonmalignant condition in which aberrant uterine tissue grows outside the uterine wall.
3. Metrorrhagia refers to vaginal bleeding.
4. Dyspareunia refer to painful intercourse.
5. No, prolapse means the uterus fell from the pelvic cavity.

Identifying the Specialty

The System and Its Practitioners

Producing offspring requires a joining of the male's sperm and the female's egg, called the ovum. Together, the sperm and the egg produce a zygote, as described in Chapter 14. When things go correctly, this process ends with the female giving birth.

The medical care of the female reproductive system includes several disciplines: **gynecology**, which includes the study of the organs, hormones, and diseases of the female reproductive system; **obstetrics**, the specialty concerned with pregnancy and the delivery of a baby; **neonatology**, the study and treatment of the newborn infant, although today it usually refers to the premature infant; and **pediatrics**, the study and treatment of newborns (neonates), infants, and children.

Examining the Patient ♂♀

Anatomy and Physiology of the Female Reproductive System

The structures of the female reproductive system include the **vagina** (plus the outwardly visible genitalia), **ovaries**, **fallopian tubes**, **uterus**, and **cervix** (Figure 15.1). The **breasts** also are considered part of the system, although they play no direct role in reproduction.

Figure 15.1 - The Female Reproductive Organs

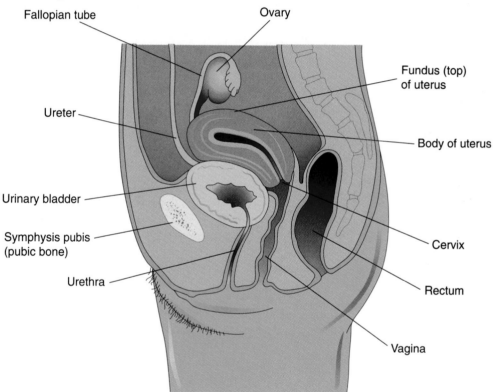

Fallopian tube

Ovary

Ureter

Fundus (top) of uterus

Body of uterus

Urinary bladder

Symphysis pubis (pubic bone)

Urethra

Cervix

Rectum

Vagina

Figure 15.2 - The External Genitalia

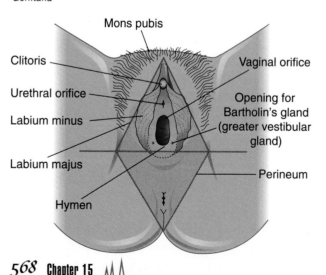

Mons pubis

Clitoris

Urethral orifice

Labium minus

Labium majus

Hymen

Vaginal orifice

Opening for Bartholin's gland (greater vestibular gland)

Perineum

External Genitalia and Vagina

The external genitalia (genitals) are a group of structures known as the **vulva** (Figure 15.2). They consist of the **mons pubis**, a pad of fatty tissue that lies over the **symphysis pubis** (the bone on the lower portion of the pelvis); the **labia majora** (translated as large lips), long, fatty folds containing glands; the **labia minora** (small lips), which join anteriorly; the **vestibule**, an area between the labia minora; the **clitoris**, erectile tissue that is just behind the anterior juncture of the labia minora; and the **Bartholin's glands**, located on either side of the vagina, whose function is to secrete a lubricating substance that prepares the vagina for intercourse.

The urethra, or urinary meatus, is located posterior to the clitoris and anterior to the **vagina**, the opening that leads to the uterus. The area between the vaginal opening and the anus is called the **perineum**. The opening to the vagina is sometimes covered by a membrane called the **hymen.** The vagina is located between the bladder and rectum, and extends inward about 4 inches.

Female Gonads

The actual organs of reproduction, or gonads, of the female (Figure 15.3) are the **ovaries**, a pair of almond-shaped structures located within the pelvic cavity on either side of the **uterus**, which is the organ that holds the fetus during pregnancy. The female's reproductive cells are the **ova**, or eggs, which are produced in the ovaries. The production of ova is called **oogenesis**. Besides producing ova, the ovaries begin secreting the hormones estrogen and progesterone at puberty.

The two **fallopian tubes** are the ducts for the ovaries, although they are not directly attached (see Figure 15.3). The outer end of each of the fallopian tubes is fan-shaped with fingerlike projections called **fimbriae** that open into the abdominal cavity. The 4-inch fallopian tubes lead into the uterus, a small structure about the size of a pear that is composed mostly of muscle called the **myometrium**. The upper portion of the uterus is called the **body (corpus)**, and the lower portion is the **cervix**. At the top is the **fundus**. The inside of the uterus is composed of a mucous membrane lining called the **endometrium**.

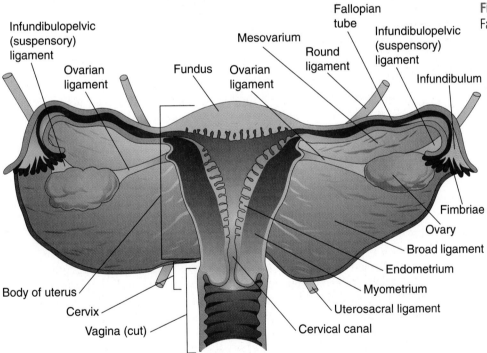

Figure 15.3 - The Ovaries, Fallopian Tubes, and Uterus

Breasts

The female breasts are two glandular structures that produce milk for a newborn in response to hormonal secretion and the stimulation of the infant's sucking. The process is called lactation (from the Latin *lacto*, milk). In addition to glandular tissue, the breasts contain **lactiferous sinuses** that hold the milk, **lactiferous ducts**, which carry the milk to openings in the **nipples**, and fibrous and fatty (adipose) tissue (Figure 15.4).

Figure 15.4 - Breast Structure

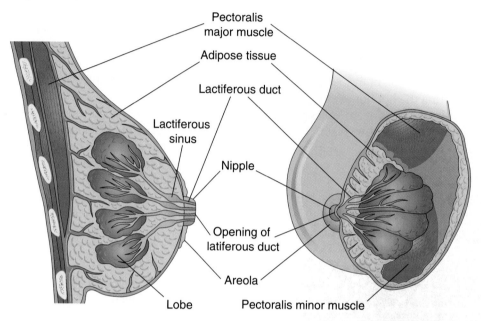

Pectoralis major muscle

Adipose tissue

Lactiferous duct

Lactiferous sinus

Nipple

Opening of latiferous duct

Areola

Lobe

Pectoralis minor muscle

The Reproductive Cycle

Females are born with about one million **ovarian follicles** (large masses of cells that contain an immature female sex cell called an **oocyte**) which secretes the hormone estrogen when it matures. As a girl grows to puberty, only about 400,000 follicles remain (called **primary follicles**). From this group only about 350 to 500 primary follicles develop fully to become mature follicles, or **Graafian follicles**.

The reproductive cycle begins with the ovum's development from primary follicle to **ovulation**. First, the female hormones (follicle-stimulating hormone and luteinizing hormone) are released from the pituitary gland, causing the follicles to mature. A follicle breaks open and releases the ovum, thus beginning the process of ovulation. (The ovum is the largest cell in the body and can be seen with the naked eye.)

Once an ovarian follicle has released its ovum to begin ovulation, it shrinks to become the yellow-colored **corpus luteum**, the structure that secretes progesterone for about eleven days. Progesterone is responsible for the proliferation and vascularization of the lining of the uterus, preparing it for possible pregnancy. If pregnancy does not occur, the corpus luteum shrinks and becomes the whitish structure called the **corpus albicans**. If pregnancy occurs, the corpus luteum continues to grow and secrete various hormones needed for the pregnancy.

The ovum is released from the left or right ovary (alternating monthly) into the abdominal cavity and transported via the fimbriae into the fallopian tube. It continues down the tube, eventually resting in the uterus. The uterus thickens and develops a rich blood supply in preparation for pregnancy. If fertilization does not ensue, in about eleven to thirteen days after ovulation, the uterine lining is sloughed and passes through the vagina, beginning **menstruation**. Also known as a period, this cycle of blood flow occurs approximately every twenty-one to twenty-eight days and

Figure 15.5 - The Stages of Ovulation

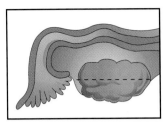

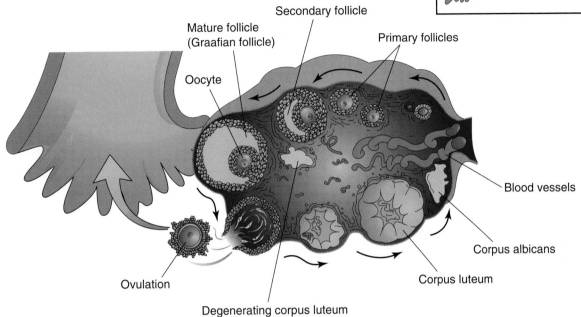

Secondary follicle

Mature follicle
(Graafian follicle)

Primary follicles

Oocyte

Blood vessels

Corpus albicans

Corpus luteum

Ovulation

Degenerating corpus luteum

Table 15.1

Combining Forms Relating to the Female Reproductive Cycle

Combining form	Meaning	Example
amni/o	the amnion (sac around fetus)	amniocentesis
arch/e	first	menarche
blast/o	germ or bud	blastocyst
cervic/o	neck	cervix
embry/o	embryo	embryologist
gyn/o	female	gynatresia
gynec/o	female	gynecologist
hyster/o	uterus	hysterectomy
labi/o	lips	labia
lact/o	milk	lactiferous
mamm/o	breast	mammogram
men/o	menses, menstruation	menstrual
metr/a, o	uterus	metratonia
oophor/o	ovary	oophorectomy
o/o	egg	oocyte
ov/o	egg	ovulate
salping/o	tube	salpingostomy
thel/o	nipple	thelarche
uter/o	uterus	uterine
vagin/o	vagina (sheath)	vaginal
vulv/o	vulva (covering)	vulvectomy

lasts from four to six days. Menstruation begins near the time of **puberty**, the onset of which varies from about age 10 to age 16, and continues monthly from the first period, called **menarche**, until the time when estrogen and progesterone secretion diminishes, called **menopause**, beginning at about age 50.

Phases of the Menstrual Cycle

The 28-day menstrual cycle is divided into four phases, as shown in the following diagram:

Figure 15.6 - Phases of the Menstrual Cycle

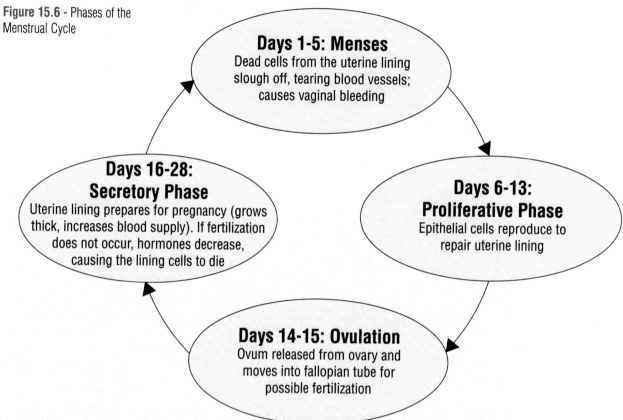

Days 1-5: Menses
Dead cells from the uterine lining slough off, tearing blood vessels; causes vaginal bleeding

Days 6-13: Proliferative Phase
Epithelial cells reproduce to repair uterine lining

Days 14-15: Ovulation
Ovum released from ovary and moves into fallopian tube for possible fertilization

Days 16-28: Secretory Phase
Uterine lining prepares for pregnancy (grows thick, increases blood supply). If fertilization does not occur, hormones decrease, causing the lining cells to die

Table 15.2

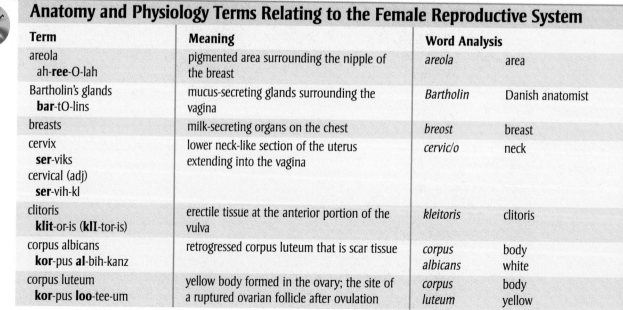

Anatomy and Physiology Terms Relating to the Female Reproductive System

Term	Meaning	Word Analysis	
areola ah-**ree**-O-lah	pigmented area surrounding the nipple of the breast	*areola*	area
Bartholin's glands **bar**-tO-lins	mucus-secreting glands surrounding the vagina	*Bartholin*	Danish anatomist
breasts	milk-secreting organs on the chest	*breost*	breast
cervix **ser**-viks cervical (adj) **ser**-vih-kl	lower neck-like section of the uterus extending into the vagina	*cervic/o*	neck
clitoris **klit**-or-is (**klI**-tor-is)	erectile tissue at the anterior portion of the vulva	*kleitoris*	clitoris
corpus albicans **kor**-pus **al**-bih-kanz	retrogressed corpus luteum that is scar tissue	*corpus* *albicans*	body white
corpus luteum **kor**-pus **loo**-tee-um	yellow body formed in the ovary; the site of a ruptured ovarian follicle after ovulation	*corpus* *luteum*	body yellow

endometrium en-dO-**mee**-tree-em	mucous membrane layer of the uterine wall	*endo-* *metra*	within uterus
fallopian tube fah-**lO**-pee-en toob	tube through which the ovum passes, leading to the uterus	*fallopian*	Greek anatomist, Fallopius
fimbria **fim**-bree-ah	fringe at the end of the fallopian tube	*fimbria*	fringe
follicle **fol**-ih-kl	a spherical portion of cells that form a cavity	*follicle*	a small sac
fundus **fun**-dus	part farthest away from the opening	*fundus*	bottom
Graafian follicle **graf**-ee-en **fol**-ih-kl	follicle in which the oocyte grows to full size	*Graaf*	Dutch physiologist and histologist, R. de Graaf
gynecology gI-neh-**kol**-ah-jee	the study and treatment of the female	*gynec/o* *-logy*	female study of
hymen **hI**-men	membranous skin fold that may cover the external opening of the vagina	*hymen*	membrane
labia majora **lay**-bee-ah mah-**jor**-ah	outer folds of skin surrounding the vagina	*labi/o* *majora*	lips large
labia minora **lay**-bee-ah mih-**nor**-ah	inner folds of skin surrounding the vagina	*labi/o* *minora*	lips small
lactiferous ducts lak-**tif**-er-us dukts	tubular structures in the breast that carry milk to the nipples	*lact/o* *fero* *-ous*	milk to bear pertaining to
menarche men-ark-ee	onset of menses (the first menstrual period)	*men/o* *-arche*	menstruation beginning
menses **men**-seez	female reproductive cycle in which the lining of the uterus is sloughed, causing bleeding; occurs approximately every 28 days	*men/o*	menstruation
menstrual cycle **men**-stroo-el **sI**-kl menstruation men-stroo-**ay**-shun	female reproductive cycle (also known as the period)	*men/o*	menstruation
mons pubis monz **pyoo**-bis	fatty elevation of tissue over the symphysis pubis	*mons* *pubis*	mountain a pubic hair
myometrium mI-O-**mee**-tree-em	muscular wall of the uterus	*my/o* *metr/o*	muscle uterus
neonate **nee**-O-nayt	the period for the first month immediately after birth; the neonatologist usually specializes in the premature infant	*neo-* *natus*	new born
obstetrics ob-**stet**-riks	study and treatment of pregnancy and birth	*obstetrix*	midwife
oocyte **O**-O-sIt	immature egg cell	*o/o* *cyt/o*	egg, ovary cell
oogenesis O-O-**jen**-eh-sis	production of the female gametes (ova)	*o/o* *-genesis*	egg, ovary to produce
ovum **O**-vem	egg; the female's reproductive cell	*ov/o*	egg
ovulation ov-yoo-**lay**-shun	menstrual cycle step in which the ovum is released from the ovarian follicle	*ov/o* *-ation*	egg process

continued on next page

perineum per-ih-**nee**-em	area between the vagina and the anus	*perineum*	area between the vagina and anus
salpinx (sing) **sal**-pinks	fallopian tube	*salping/o*	tube
symphysis pubis **sim**-fih-sis **pyoo**-bis	joint between the pubic bones	*symphysis pubes*	growing together the hair that grows on the genitals
uterus **yoo**-ter-us	muscular organ in the pelvic cavity that contains the growing fetus	*uter/o*	uterus
vagina vah-**jI**-nah	opening to the uterus	*vagin/o*	vagina
vestibule **ves**-tih-byool	area between the clitoris and the opening of the vagina	*vestibulum*	entrance
vulva **vul**-vah	female external genitalia	*vulv/o*	vulva

Word Analysis

On the line beside each term, write the combining form that refers to the structure.

1. uterus _____

2. fallopian tube _____

3. vagina _____

4. cervix _____

5. ovary _____

6. fundus _____

7. urethra _____

8. pubic bone _____

9. rectum _____

10. ureter _____

Identify the anatomical structures on the diagram below by writing the number of the term directly on the structure.

1. body of uterus

2. fallopian tube

3. vagina

4. cervix

5. ovary

6. fundus of uterus

7. urethra

8. pubic bone

9. rectum

10. ureter

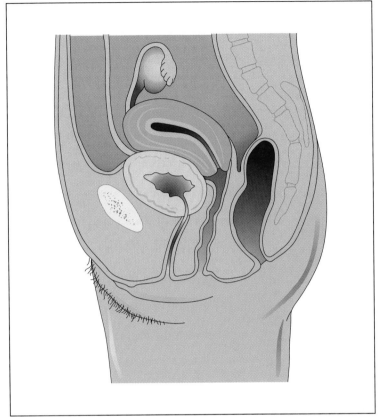

Circle the correct term(s) to complete each sentence. Be sure to read the entire sentence and use the context of the sentence to make your selection.

1. Within the vestibule/vagina is the clitoris/climateric.

2. The mons pubis/pelvum lies just over the zygote/symphysis pubis.

3. The skin covering the labia majora/labia minora is pigmented and has hair on the outer surface.

4. The fundus/urinary meatus is located posterior to the clitoris.

5. The vagina/ovulation appeared normal; there were no injuries or signs of diseases.

6. The estrogens/ovaries were positively identified prior to removal.

7. The neonatologies/fallopian tubes are not directly attached to the ovaries.

8. The fimbriae/endometriae open into the abdominal cavity.

9. The uterus/uteri was judged to be underdeveloped.

10. The gynecology/myometrium was intact, and the endometrium/puberty was undisturbed.

Matching

Match the definition to the correct term. Write the correct term on the line next to the definition.

1. _____ pigmented area surrounding the nipple of the breast
    corpus luteum

2. _____ mucus-secreting glands surrounding the vagina
    fimbriae

3. _____ yellow body formed in the ovary following the rupture of an ovarian follicle
    Graafian

4. _____ lower neck-like portion of the uterus
    areola

5. _____ tube that the ova passes through to the uterus
    hymen

6. _____ fringe-like structures at the end of the fallopian tubes
    Bartholin's

7. _____ follicle where the oocyte grows to full size
    perineum

8. _____ upper portion of the uterus, farthest from the opening
    cervix

9. _____ membranous skin fold that may cover the vagina
    mons pubis

10. _____ female cycle where the lining of the uterus is sloughed
    fundus

11. _____ fatty elevation of tissue over the symphysis pubis
    fallopian

12. _____ area between the vagina and the anus
    menses

Word Building

Write the missing word parts in the blanks to create the correct term for the definition given.

1. _____ian = pertaining to the ovaries

2. _____al = pertaining to the cervix

3. _____itis = inflammation of the endometrium

4. _____rrhea = faulty, difficult or painful menstruation

5. a_____ = absence of menstruation

6. _____ology = study of the female reproductive system

7. ____cyte = egg cell

8. _____otomy = incision into the fallopian tube

9. _____ual = pertaining to menstruation

10. _____ist = specialist in the female reproductive system

Circle the correct word from the choices given.

1. The follicles/follicle had ruptured and the egg/eggs were/was released.

2. All of the fimbria/fimbriae were/was malformed.

3. All the uterine funduses/fundi examined were/was similar in size.

4. The cervices/cervix of all the women were/was also of similar size.

5. The areola/areolae was/were excised bilaterally.

6. The Bartholin's gland/Bartholin's glands was/were absent.

7. In addition to the congenital malformation of the two uteri/uterus, there were/was also two cervix/cervices.

8. There is/are five gynecologist/gynecologists in this clinic.

9. The vulva/vulvae of both infants were/was atrophied.

10. Twelve ovums/ova were/was harvested and processed for freezing.

Word Maps   *Exercise 7*

The diagram below illustrates the development of an ovum and its ovarian follicle. Complete the diagram by supplying the missing terms.

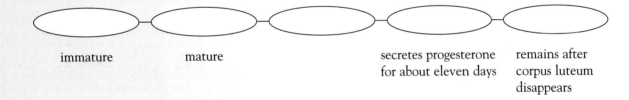

immature   mature   secretes progesterone for about eleven days   remains after corpus luteum disappears

Examination of adult female reproductive organs includes the breasts and the external and internal genitalia. During a breast examination, the physician usually teaches the woman how to perform breast self-exam (BSE) on a monthly basis to check for lumps or other changes that require further investigation. Next, the woman is draped with a sheet and placed in lithotomy position. The genitalia are inspected and then an instrument called a **speculum** is inserted into the vaginal opening to allow visualization and palpation.

The examiner performs a bimanual ("two hands") examination of the vagina and cervix, inserting one or two fingers of a gloved and lubricated hand into the vagina and placing the other hand on the patient's abdomen. The examination allows the physician to assess the size, shape, and position of the uterus, and may aid in the discovery of any masses, abnormalities, or tenderness.

Figure 15.7 - Breast Self Examination

Breast Self Exam

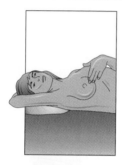

LYING DOWN
Place a pillow under your shoulder. Put your right hand under head. Check your entire breast area with the finger pads of your left hand. Use small circles and follow an up and down pattern. Use light, medium, and firm pressure over each area of your breast. Gently squeeze the nipple for any discharge. Repeat these steps on your left breast.

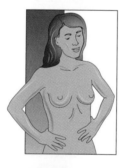
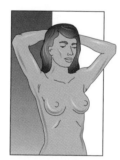

BEFORE A MIRROR
Check for any changes in the shape or look of your breasts. Note skin dimpling or nipple discharge. Inspect your breast in four steps; arms at side, arms overhead, hands on hips, and bending forward.

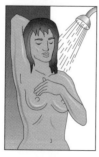
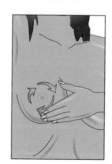

IN THE SHOWER
Raise your right arm, With soapy hands and fingers flat, check your right breast. Use the method described in the "Lying Down" step. Repeat on your left breast.

Infancy, Childhood

Congenital anomalies that may be present in the newborn female include absence of the vagina (vaginal **agenesis**); uterine anomalies; and cervical **atresia**, absence of the cervix. Unless there is an anomaly of the external genitalia, problems with the internal structures are not noted until adolescence, when the girl does not develop appropriately or achieve menarche.

Preadolescence and Adolescence

The time of puberty is marked by increased physical growth and sexual maturity. The girl develops secondary sex characteristics, beginning with breast development called **thelarche**. A physical examination at this time includes an evaluation of sexual development according to Tanner staging (as is the male). Figures 15.8 and 15.9 show the Tanner stages for the female. Problems associated with lack or delay of maturation must be investigated and can indicate hormonal abnormalities or congenital malformation as described above.

Figure 15.8 - Tanner Staging: Breast Development

Prepubertal
small nipple present

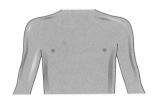

Breast bud stage
small amount (bud) of
breast tissue and
nipple develops
11.2 years ± 1.1 year

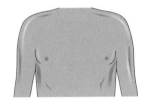

Elevation of breast contour
breast tissue growth continues;
areolae enlarge
12.2 years ± 1.1 year

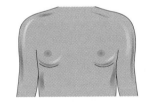

Development of secondary mound
areolae and papilla form
a secondary mound
13.1 years ± 1.2 years

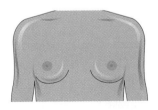

Adult form
development is complete;
areola is flush with breast
15.3 years ± 1.7 years

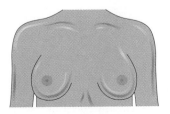

Figure 15.9 - Tanner Staging: Pubic Hair Development

Prepubertal
no corse hair in pubic area

Development of silky hair
long, silky hair appears along labia
11.7 years ± 1.2 years

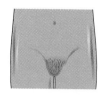

Spread of hair over mons pubis
coarse, kinky hair spreads over pubic bone
12.4 years ± 1.1 year

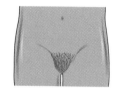

Devolopment of adult hair
hair of adult quality but has not spread to junction of medial thigh with perineum
13 years ± 1 year

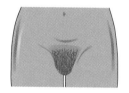

Spread of hair to thigh
hair development complete; hair also exists on medial thigh
14.4 years ± 1.1 year

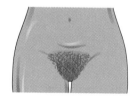

Puberty is the time of the first period (**menarche**). Several problems can occur with the menstrual period, as described in Table 15.3. Most of the terms are formed by adding a prefix or suffix to the root terms *men/o, -rrhagia,* and *-rrhea.*

Table 15.3

Abnormalities with Menstruation

Term	Meaning	Word Analysis	
amenorrhea ah-men-O-**ree**-ah	absence of menses	*a/* *men/o* *-rrhea*	without menses (menstruation) flow
dysmenorrhea dis-men-O-**ree**-ah	painful or difficult menstruation (period)	*dys/* *men/o* *-rrhea*	painful, difficult menses flow
hypermenorrhea hI-per-men-O-**ree**-ah	long or excessive bleeding during period	*hyper/* *men/o* *-rrhea*	increased menses flow

hypomenorrhea hI-pO-men-O-**ree**-ah	short or decreased bleeding during period	*hypo/* *men/o* *-rrhea*	decreased menses flow
menometrorrhagia **men**-O-**met**-rO-**ray(rah)**- jee-ah	irregular or excessive bleeding during and between periods	*men/o* *metr/o* *-rrhagia*	menses uterus discharge
menorrhagia men-O-**ray**-jee-ah	increased or excessive menstrual flow	*men/o* *-rrhagia*	menses discharge
menorrhalgia men-O-**ral**-jee-ah	painful menstruation	*men/o* *-rrhea* *algi/o*	menses flow pain
metrorrhagia met-rO-**ray(rah)**-jee-ah	irregular bleeding between periods	*metr/o* *-rrhagia*	uterus flow
oligomenorrhea ol-ih-gO-men-O-**ree**-ah	scanty menstrual flow	*olig/o* *men/o* *-rrhea*	little menses flow

The Adult

The adult female should have an annual examination by a gynecologist. In addition to palpating and visualizing the reproductive organs, the physician performs an endocervical swab called the **Pap (Papanicolaou) smear** to screen for cervical cancer. A **mammogram**, the radiographic examination of the breasts to screen for cancer, is part of the routine examination.

The cervix of the female varies with the woman's age and the number of pregnancies she has had. The term for pregnancy is "gravida," which refers to the number of times a woman has been pregnant. "Para" (from the Latin word, *pario*, to bring forth) is the term that refers to the number of births a woman has had. When caregivers refer to the number of pregnancies and births a woman has had, they use the following terminology:

- Gravida I, para 0 means the woman has been pregnant once, but has had no births (although she may be pregnant at the time of the exam);
- Gravida II, para II means the woman has been pregnant twice and given birth twice;
- Nulliparous means having had no births; multiparous is a term for having had many births;
- *Primi*, the Latin prefix, may be used to describe a woman who has had one birth, as in primipara.

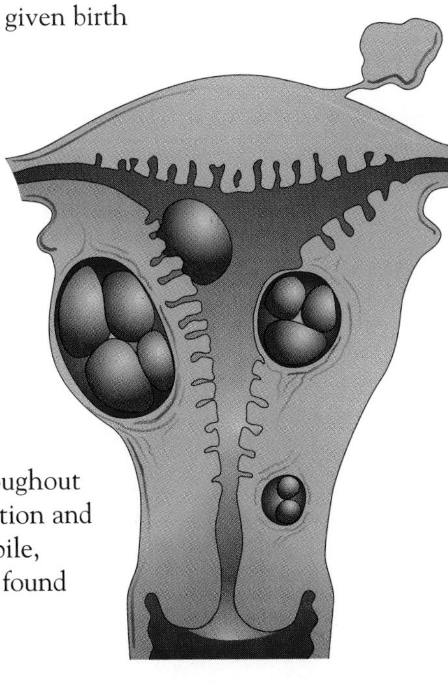

Chapter 16 will discuss pregnancy, childbirth, and parturition in more detail.

Endometriosis is a nonmalignant condition in which aberrant uterine tissue grows outside the uterine wall. Symptoms include extreme menstrual pain, abnormal bleeding, infertility, and painful intercourse, called **dyspareunia**. Another common disorder is **pelvic inflammatory disease (PID)**, an inflammatory condition, usually infectious, of the pelvic cavity that may be localized or spread throughout the reproductive organs. This can lead to acute **salpingitis**, inflammation and infection of the fallopian tubes. **Fibroids** (Figure 15.10) are firm, mobile, painless nodules in the uterine wall. They are usually benign and are found most commonly in the 30- to 45-year old.

Figure 15.10 - Fibroids

Human papillomavirus (HPV) is a sexually transmitted disease (STD) that is characterized by small growths on the genitalia. Certain types of HPV are associated with increased risk of cervical cancer; therefore, frequent Pap smears are indicated. Other common STDs include gonorrhea, syphilis, herpes, and chlamydial infections.

The Aging Female

Many changes occur as a result of decreasing hormone levels in the aging female. This is known as **menopause** or **climacteric**. It is characterized by irregular periods, which eventually cease altogether. The ovaries stop producing progesterone and estrogen. Table 15.4 summarizes the changes associated with the menopause (also called the "change of life").

Changes in the pelvic musculature can cause **cystocele**, in which the bladder protrudes into the vagina; **uterine prolapse**, in which the uterus protrudes into the vagina, and **rectocele**, in which the rectum prolapses into the vagina. These terms are included in the wellness and illness terms listed in Table 15.5.

PID can be diagnosed at any age as a result of an infection, usually from an STD that has been untreated.

Table 15.4

The Physiologic Changes of Menopause

uterus	shrinks in size because of decreased myometrium
	prone to prolapse or protrusion (falls from the pelvic cavity because of relaxing of sacral ligaments and weakened musculature)
ovaries	atrophy (shrink) although ovulation may occur sporadically
vagina	becomes shorter and narrower
	decreases in elasticity because of increased connective tissue
	thinning of the walls
	drier
	fragile because of epithelial atrophy
external genitalia	decreased fat on mons pubis
	decreased pubic hair
	decrease in size of labia and clitoris

Table 15.5

Wellness and Illness Terms Relating to the Female Reproductive System

Term	Meaning	Word Analysis	
agenesis (vaginal) ay-**jen**-eh-sis	absence of the vagina; failure of formation of the vagina	a/ genesis	without production
atresia (cervical) ah-**tree**-zhah	absence of the cervical opening	a/ tresis	without a hole
climacteric klI-**mak**-ter-ik/klI-mak-**ter**-ik	term for menopause	klimakter	the rung of a ladder
cystocele **sis**-tO-seel	condition involving a hernia of the bladder that pushes it into the vagina	cyst/o -cele	relating to the bladder a hernia; swelling
dyspareunia dis-pah-**roo**-nee-ah	pain during sexual intercourse	dys/ pareunos	pain, difficult lying beside
endometriosis en-dO-mee-tree-**O**-sis	benign condition in which there is aberrant uterine tissue growing outside the uterine wall	end/o metr/o -osis	within uterus condition

endometrium en-dO-**mee**-tree-um	mucous membrane layer of the uterine wall	end/o metr/o ium	within uterus tissue or structure
fibroids **fI**-broyds myomas my-**oh**-maz	firm, mobile, nonmalignant nodules in the uterine wall	fibr/o eidos myo- -oma	pertaining to fibroid tissue resembling muscle tumor
human papillomavirus pap-ih-**lO**-mah-vI-res	a sexually transmitted disease that is associated with small growths on the genitalia	humanus papula -oma virus	human, man pimple tumor poison
menarche men-**ar**-kee	onset of menses (the first menstrual period)	men/o -arche	pertaining to the menses first
menopause **men**-O-pawz	period of time when a woman's hormones are decreasing, causing many changes	men/o pausis	pertaining to the menses cessation
prolapse (uterine) prO-**laps**	the sinking of an organ into another orifice	prolapsus	a falling
puberty **pyoo**-ber-tee	onset of changes in the body that herald the physiologic maturity of the person	pubertas	grown up
rectocele **rek**-tO-seel	prolapse of the rectum through the vagina	rect/o -cele	pertaining to the rectum hernia; swelling
salpingitis sal-pin-**jI**-tis	inflammation of the fallopian tube(s)	salping/o -itis	a tube inflammation
sexually transmitted disease (STD)	viral or bacterial infections that are transmitted between sexual partners	sexus transmitted disease	qualities, structures that distinguish male and female passed on to illness
speculum (sing) **spek**-yoo-lem	instrument that is inserted into an orifice to provide visualization	specio	look at
thelarche thee-**lar**-kee	beginning of breast development	thel/o -arche	nipple first

Word Analysis

In the following terms, identify the root by drawing a box around it. Write the definition for each root, and then the definition for the entire term.

Term	Root Word Definition	Term Definition
1. cervical	_____	_____
2. thelarche	_____	_____
3. hypermenorrhea	_____	_____
4. metrorrhagia	_____	_____
5. oligomenorrhea	_____	_____

6. endometriosis _____ _____

7. salpingitis _____ _____

8. cystocele _____ _____

9. fibroid _____ _____

10. menarche _____ _____

Comprehension Check

Circle the correct term in each sentence.

1. The patient's cervical amenorrhea/atresia was noted at the time of the examination.

2. The speculum/rectocele was inserted into the vaginal opening.

3. A bilateral/bimanual examination of the vagina and cervix was performed.

4. The time of menopause/puberty is marked by increased physical growth.

5. The patient reports dysmenorrhea/dysmetrosis for the past three months.

6. This patient is being referred for a salpingum/mammogram.

7. The patient is gravida/gravila I, patra/para 0.

8. This patient describes a severe dysalpingo/dyspareunia for the past four weeks.

9. She will have a Papanicolaou/papillomavirus smear for cervical cancer.

10. The patient will require surgery for her uterine/thelarche prolapse.

Matching

Select the term from Column 1 to match the definition in Column 2. Write the number of your selection on the line beside the definition.

Column 1		**Column 2**
1. vaginal agenesis	_____	firm, mobile, nonmalignant nodules in the uterine wall
2. cystocele	_____	onset of body changes that herald physiologic maturity of the person
3. endometriosis	_____	milk-secreting organs on the chest
4. fibroids	_____	protrusion of the bladder through the vagina
5. menarche	_____	inflammation of the fallopian tubes
6. puberty	_____	lower neck-like section of the uterus extending into the vagina
7. salpingitis	_____	instrument used to visualize the vagina and cervix
8. cervix	_____	onset of menses (the first menstrual period)

9. mammary glands   _____   absence of the vagina

10. speculum   _____   condition of the lining of the uterus

Word Building

Use prefixes, roots, combining vowels, and suffixes to create the medical term for each definition. Write the term in the space beside the definition.

1. painful or difficult menstruation   dys_____

2. irregular or excessive bleeding during and between periods   _____metro_____

3. short or decreased bleeding during period   hypo_____

4. increased or excessive bleeding during period   _____rrhea

5. irregular bleeding between periods   metro_____

6. radiologic examination of the breasts   _____gram

7. process of ovulating   _____ion

8. period of time when a woman's hormones are decreasing, causing many physical changes   _____pause

9. prolapse of the rectum through the vagina   _____cele

10. beginning of breast development   _____arche

Spelling Check

From the choices given, circle the correct plural or singular form for each word.

1. The external genital/genitalia are/is normal.

2. Several fibroid/fibroids were/was palpable in the uterine wall.

3. Frequent Pap smears/smear are/is indicated.

4. The fallopian tubes/tube were/was affected bilaterally.

5. Both gynecologist/gynecologists agreed that the surgery was necessary.

6. The reproductive organs/organ were/was examined and found to be normal.

7. She has had four mammograms/mammogram this year.

8. There is one specula/speculum in the examining room.

9. Sexually transmitted diseases/disease are/is on the increase.

10. The abdomen was opened and the salpinx/salpinges were/was identified.

The chart below lists body changes associated with the beginning of menstruation and the cessation of menstruation. Complete the chart by writing the changes beside the organ name.

Changes with Menarche

breasts _____

uterus _____

vagina _____

external genitalia _____

Changes with Menopause

ovaries _____

uterus _____

vagina _____

external genitalia _____

Diagnosing and Treating Problems

Tests, Procedures, and Pharmaceuticals

Laboratory tests of the female reproductive system include blood tests for measuring hormone levels. These tests can determine proper functioning at all stages of life, including childhood, adolescence, pregnancy, and menopause.

Procedures

Procedures involve all the organs of the system, including the external genitalia and the internal structures. The most common procedure is **dilatation and curettage (D&C)**, performed to obtain endometrial or endocervical tissue for cytologic examination. The D&C is also performed to control abnormal uterine bleeding. In the procedure, the cervix is dilated and a curette is used to obtain uterine scrapings, which are then studied under the microscope to determine if diseased cells are present. **Colposcopy** is ordered when there is an abnormal Pap smear. Tissue is removed and a biopsy is performed.

Sterilization to prevent pregnancy is performed by cutting or cauterizing the fallopian tubes, known as **bilateral tubal ligation**. A **hysterectomy** is a surgical procedure to remove the uterus. If the fallopian tubes and ovaries are removed, the procedure is known as a total hysterectomy with **bilateral salpingo-oophorectomy**.

Table 15.6 summarizes the major tests and procedures relating to the female reproductive system.

Table 15.6

Tests and Procedures Relating to the Female Reproductive System

Term	Meaning	Word Analysis	
bilateral salpingo-oophorectomy bI-**lat**-er-el **sal**-pin-gO-**O**-O-for-**ek**-tah-mee	procedure to remove the ovaries and fallopian tubes	*bilateral* *salping/o* *oophor/o* *-ectomy*	both sides tube ovary removal of a structure
bilateral tubal ligation bI-**lat**-er-el **too**-bl ll-**gay**-shun	procedure to cut and/or cauterize the fallopian tubes	*bilateral* *ligatura*	both sides tie or band

colposcopy kol-**pos**-kah-pee	examination of the cervix using an endoscope	*colp/o* *-scopy*	vagina examination
dilation and curettage (D&C) dI-**lay**-shun and **kyoo**-reh-tahj	procedure to dilate and scrape the cervical area	*dilato* *curettage*	spread out scrape
human chorionic gonadotropin (HCG) **hyoo**-men kor-ee-**on**-ik gon-ad-O-**trO**-pin	blood test to determine pregnancy, a hormone produced by the placenta	*chorion* *gone* *trope*	membrane enclosing the fetus seed a turning
hysterectomy his-ter-**ek**-tah-mee	surgical removal of the uterus	*hyster/o* *-ectomy*	uterus surgical removal
mammogram **mam**-ah-gram	radiographic study of the breast	*mamm/o* *-gram*	breast recording
Pap smear	the cytologic study of a scraping of the cervix	*Pap*	George Papanicolaou, an anatomist and cytologist

Pharmaceutical Agents

The list of pharmaceuticals used to treat conditions relating to the female reproductive system includes agents and devices used for contraception, i.e., the prevention of pregnancy, agents to increase fertility, to relieve menopausal symptoms, and to manage endometriosis; and agents to induce labor. Lastly, there are drugs used for routine management after delivery of the placenta or to control increased vaginal bleeding. See Table 15.7 for the generic and brand names.

Table 15.7

Pharmacologic Agents

Class	Use	Generic names	Brand names
contraceptives (devices)	prevent pregnancy	diaphragm	All-Flex Arcing Spring Diaphragm; Ortho Diaphragm Kit-Coil Spring; Para Gard T 380 A
contraceptives (emergency)	prevent pregnancy	levonorgestrel	Plan B
contraceptives (implant)	prevent pregnancy	levonorgestrel implant (progestin)	Mirena
contraceptives (injectable)	prevent pregnancy	medroxyprogesterone	Depo-Provera
contraceptives (oral)	prevent pregnancy	ethinyl estradiol and drospirenone ethinyl estradiol and levonorgestrel ethinyl estradiol and norethindrone ethinyl estradiol and norgestimate ethinyl estradiol and norgestrel mestranol/norethindrone norgestrel	Yasmin PREVEN, Nordette Norinyl 1+35, Ovcon Ortho-Cyclen, Sprintec Lo/Ovral, Ovral Norinyl 1+50, Ortho-Novum 1/50 Ovrette

continued on next page

contraceptives (patch)	prevent pregnancy	ethinyl estradiol and norelgestromin	Ortho Evra
contraceptives (ring)	prevent pregnancy	ethinyl estradiol and etonogestrel	NuvaRing
endometriosis management, etc	treat endometriosis	norethindrone acetate danazol	Aygestin, Camila Micronor, Norlutate Danocrine
fertility agents	improve, encourage fertility	clomiphene menotropins (injection)	Clomid Pergonal
gonadatropin-releasing hormone (synthetic)	breast cancer treatment	goserelin acetate injection	Zoladex
induce labor	commence/intensify uterine contractions	oxytocin	Pitocin
menopausal symptoms	decrease symptoms of menopause, vaginal dryness	estrogen (conjugated/equine) estradiol transdermal (patch) system estradiol vaginal cream	Premarin Estraderm Estrace
post-pregnancy hemorrhage		methylergonovine	Methergine
vaginal topical preparations	treat fungal infections	butoconazole vaginal cream clotrimazole vaginal tablets miconazole (vaginal suppositories)	Gynazole-1 Gyne-Lotrimin Monistat
	treat bacterial infections	sulfabenzamide, sulfacetamide, and sulfathiazole cream	V.V.S.
	broad spectrum antibiotics	povidone-iodine medicated douche clindamycin phosphate vaginal cream	Betadine Cleocin

Table 15.8

Abbreviations

AB, ab	abortion
BTL	bilateral tubal ligation
BSO	bilateral salpingo-oophorectomy
D&C	dilation and curettage
DUB	dysfunctional uterine bleeding
GC	gonorrhea
GYN	gynecology
HPV	human papilloma virus
HRT	hormone replacement therapy (usually refers to replacement at menopause)
HSG	hysterosalpingography
IUD	intrauterine device
LMP	last menstrual period
OB	obstetrics
PID	pelvic inflammatory disease
PMP	previous menstrual period
STD	sexually transmitted disease
TAH	total abdominal hysterectomy
TAH/BSO	total abdominal hysterectomy with bilateral salpingo-oophorectomy
VH	vaginal hysterectomy

Separate each term into its individual parts, using hyphens. Identify the parts by type using a letter for each part (P = prefix, R = root, S = suffix, CV = combining vowel), and then provide a definition for the entire term.

1. amenorrhea _____ _____

   _____

2. metrorrhagia _____ _____

   _____

3. salpingectomy _____ _____

   _____

4. lactogenesis _____ _____

   _____

5. cervical _____ _____

   _____

6. gynecology _____ _____

   _____

7. hysterectomy _____ _____

   _____

8. oophorectomy _____ _____

   _____

9. colposcopy _____ _____

   _____

10. mastitis _____ _____

   _____

Read each sentence and select the best of the two terms given.

1. The patient experiences severe mastodynia/cervical.

2. Mrs. Keene will have a puberty/hysteroscopy on Tuesday.

3. A complex interaction of hormones causes salpingectomy/lactogenesis.

4. The patient will have surgery for a vesicovaginal fistula/thelarche.

5. A parovarian cyst/HPV was identified and will be removed.

6. The Pap smear identified cervical dysplasia/speculum.

7. The patient was diagnosed with vagina/endometritis soon after puberty.

8. Dilation and curettage/salpingitis were performed to obtain tissue samples.

9. Labia minora/Colposcopy will be necessary following the abnormal Pap smear.

10. The surgeons performed a bilateral salpingo-oophorectomy/Bartholin's glands.

What Do These Abbreviations Mean?

Exercise 16

Write the meaning for each definition in the space provided. (Try to do it from memory!)

1. D&C _____

2. OB _____

3. TAH _____

4. GC _____

5. DUB _____

6. BTL _____

7. HSG _____

8. LMP _____

9. PMP _____

10. VH _____

Construct terms to match the definitions provided, using only the following suffixes:

-cele   -ectomy-   rrhaphy

1. herniation of the bladder into the vagina   _____

2. herniation of the rectum into the vagina   _____

3. herniation of the urethra into the vagina   _____

4. surgical removal of the uterus   _____

5. surgical removal of the ovaries   _____

6. surgical removal of the fallopian tubes and ovaries   _____

7. surgical removal of the breast   _____

8. suture of the vagina   _____

9. suture of the vulva   _____

10. suture of the fallopian tube   _____

Spelling Check

Exercise 18

Indicate whether each term is plural or singular; then provide the opposite term. (For each plural term, provide the singular form; for each singular term, give the plural.)

	P/S	Opposite term
1. episiotomy	_____	_____
2. oophorectomy	_____	_____
3. mammography	_____	_____
4. contraceptives	_____	_____
5. uterus	_____	_____
6. ovary	_____	_____
7. areola	_____	_____
8. fundus	_____	_____
9. cervix	_____	_____
10. follicles	_____	_____

On the illustration of the female body below, identify the structures listed. Then on the lines next to the structure name, write a related surgical term and a corresponding test or screening term.

breasts   _____   _____

uterus   _____   _____

ovaries   _____   _____

fallopian tubes   _____   _____

vagina   _____   _____

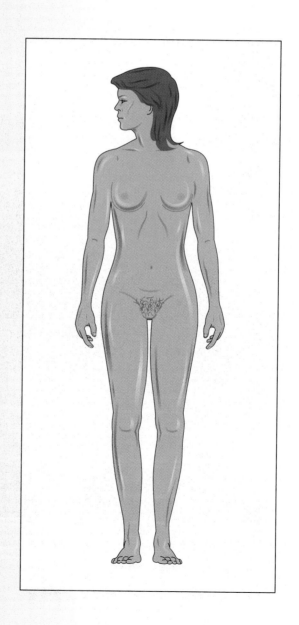

Crossword Puzzle

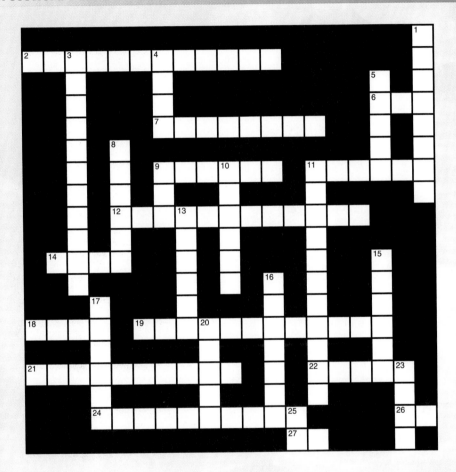

Across

2. difficult or painful menstruation
6. eggs
7. inflammation of the breast
9. combining form for cessation
11. pigmented area surrounding the nipple of the breast
12. removal of the ovary or ovaries
14. lateral
18. combining form for female
19. surgical removal of the uterus
21. surgical removal of the breast or breasts
22. suffix meaning flow
24. absence of menstruation
26. abbreviation for gonorrhea
27. prefix for both

Down

1. _____ follicles
3. inflammation of the fallopian tubes
4. largest cell in the body
5. combining form for vagina
8. fertilized ovum
9. endocervical swab; _____ smear
10. curettage
11. pertaining to inability to ovulate
13. type of STD
15. female sex cell
16. incapable of fertilization
17. prefix for against
20. -oma
23. combining form for pain
25. abbreviation for abortion

Build the Terms

Select word parts from the lists to build a complete medical term for each definition given. Note that not all terms will have a root or combining form, prefix, and suffix. Some word parts may be used more than once.

Combining Forms	Prefixes	Suffixes
lact/o	an-	-ia
gynec/o	epi-	-graphy
vagin/o	sub-	-ostomy
vulv/o	hypo-	-oma
hyster/o	tetra-	-ectomy
mast/o	a-	-itis
oophor/o	an-	-al
ov/o	pre-	-genesis
salping/o	de-	-logy
cervic/o	anti-	-phobia
men/o	per-	-cyte
ovari/o	bi-	-lysis
o/o	pan-	-rrhagia
metr/o	endo-	-otomy

1. egg (female germ or sex cell)   _____

2. fear of woman   _____

3. breakdown of a fallopian tube   _____

4. beginning of milk production   _____

5. incision into a breast   _____

6. process of recording (x-ray) the breast   _____

7. study of female reproductive system   _____

8. pertaining to the ovaries   _____

9. surgical removal of an ovary and fallopian tubes   _____

10. inflammation of the endometrium   _____

Separate each term into its individual parts, using hyphens. Label each part (P = prefix, R = root, S = suffix, CV = combining vowel), and then provide a definition for the entire term.

1. gametocyte _____

_____

2. neonatology _____

_____

3. oogenesis _____

_____

4. follicular _____

_____

5. ovarian _____

_____

6. vulvectomy _____

_____

7. aminocentesis _____

_____

8. embryologist _____

_____

9. salpingostomy _____

_____

10. menstrual _____

_____

What Do These Abbreviations Mean?

Write the meaning of the abbreviation on the line provided.

1. ABX _____

2. D&C _____

3. GC _____

4. PMP _____

5. VH _____

6. GYN _____

7. HRT _____

8. TAH _____

9. HPV _____

10. PID _____

What's Your Conclusion?

In this exercise you will practice selecting the correct explanation or logical next step. Read each mini medical record or scenario carefully, and then select the correct response. Write the letter of your answer in the space provided.

1. You are a medical secretary and the physician you work for has asked you to open a thick envelope, which has just been delivered from the lab. The doctor wants you to review the reports and gather telephone numbers of patients he will need to call about their test results. The first paper is the report of a Pap smear, with a notation of cervical dysplasia.

   A. Cervical dysplasia is perfectly normal, so there will be no need for the doctor to call the patient.
   B. Locate the patient's chart, note the phone number on the outside, and place it with the lab report on the doctor's desk so that he can call the patient as soon as possible.

   Your response: _____

2. Mrs. Chan comes to the clinic with symptoms of menorrhalgia, dyspareunia, and menometrorrhagia. These symptoms are consistent with:

   A. PID
   B. Endometriosis
   C. Folliculitis
   D. Severe thelarche

   Your response: _____

3. It is lunchtime and you are the only staff member in the doctor's office when the telephone rings. The caller is a 58-year-old woman who has previously been a patient of your employer. She has not had a Pap smear in eight years and is

calling to confirm that she does not need to schedule an appointment for one, since she is of postmenopausal age and had a hysterectomy several years ago.

A. You tell her that her age and hysterectomy do not necessarily mean that she does not need a Pap smear. You suggest that she schedule an appointment so she can discuss her concerns with the doctor.

B. You tell her that she is correct and she does not need to be concerned about a Pap smear, and then thank her for calling.

Your response: _____

Analyzing Medical Records

Read the progress note on the next page; then answer the following questions.

1. Where was this patient seen? Why did she see the doctor?

2. Describe the findings from the physical examination today.

3. What is the analysis?

4. Was any medication prescribed? What type of test will the patient have?

5. Why is it important that the patient have the test soon?

Physician's Progress Note

PATIENT: Janna M
DATE: October 5, xxxx

S: 23 y/o female states that she has been performing monthly breast self-exams, as she was previously instructed in this office. Yesterday, as she was examining her left breast, she noticed a lump in the lower, lateral aspect of the left breast. She states that the area of the lump is slightly uncomfortable in a vague sort of way. She reports that she is not sexually active and she is not using any type of contraception.

O: T 98.7, P 76, R 15, BP 124/76.
This patient was seen in the office approximately six months ago for her yearly physical exam. No abnormalities were found, and her health was judged to be very good at that time. In particular, there were no palpable masses in her breasts and no external abnormalities of the breasts or nipples. We discussed breast self-examination and several other health-promoting measures appropriate for a young woman. We did a baseline mammogram at that time, and the mammography report showed normal breasts. Today's examination reveals a firm, non-movable 2.5 cm nodule in the five o'clock position, in the left lateral aspect of the left breast. There is a slight peau d'orange appearance of the skin over the nodule, but no edema, no lesions, and no erythema. Axillary lymph nodes are not palpably enlarged. Right breast appears normal. ROS: findings unremarkable.

A: 1) Left breast mass.
2) R/O carcinoma of the breast

P: Mammogram today, with evaluation to be delivered to my office ASAP. Pt. to RTO tomorrow. Will make further plans based on mammography findings.

T. Harriman, MD

Using Medical References

The following sentences contain medical terms that may not have been addressed on the charts in this chapter. Use medical reference books, your medical term analysis skills, and/or a medical dictionary to find the correct definition of the underlined word(s). Write the definition on the line below the sentence.

1. Abnormal uterine bleeding includes polymenorrhea and metrorrhagia.

_____

2. The bleeding is due to endometrial hyperplasia.

_____

3. The patient will require surgery for ovarian carcinoma.

_____

4. Acute salpingitis causes severe lower abdominal pain.

_____

5. Pain of <u>extragenital</u> origin may be related to problems in the urinary tract or gastrointestinal system.

_____

6. <u>Pruritus</u>, burning, <u>edema</u>, and pain may be indications of <u>vulvitis</u>.

_____

7. Chronic <u>cervicitis</u>, <u>uterine eversion</u>, tumors, and <u>fistulas</u> can lead to <u>leukorrhea</u>.

_____

8. In the case of suspected <u>gonorrhea</u>, specimens for <u>bacteriologic</u> and <u>microscopic</u> study should be obtained.

_____

9. <u>Salpingitis</u> may lead to <u>tubal abscess</u>, which can rupture into the <u>peritoneal</u> cavity.

_____

10. She was to undergo dilation of the cervical <u>os</u> secondary to dysmenorrhea.

_____

Short Answer

In your own words, explain what happens in the female reproductive system after an ovum is released.

_____

_____

_____

_____

_____

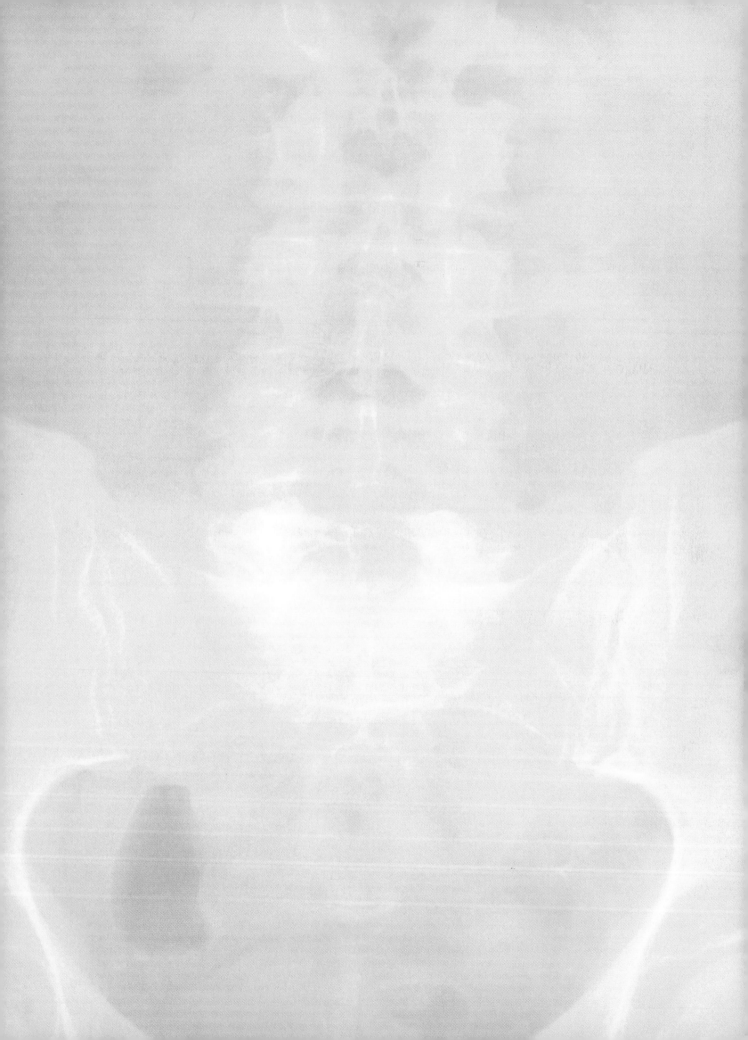

Chapter 16

Pregnancy, Birth, and Postpartum

Learning Outcomes

Students will be able to:

- Identify the normal stages of pregnancy.
- List the types of breech presentations.
- Define the stages of labor.
- Describe the changes in the female body immediately after childbirth.
- Correctly use the terms of pregnancy, birth, and postpartum in written and oral communication.
- Correctly spell and pronounce pregnancy, birth, and postpartum terminology.
- State the meaning of abbreviations related to pregnancy, birth, and postpartum.
- List and define the combining forms most commonly used to create terms related to pregnancy, birth, and postpartum.
- Name tests and treatments for major pregnancy, birth, and postpartum abnormalities.

The process of conception, described in Chapter 15, occurs when the male's sperm meets and fertilizes the female's egg. The resulting tiny zygote, barely as big as the period at the end of this sentence, grows about 200 billion times its size to become the newborn child. The entire process from conception to childbirth averages about 9 months, or about 280 days from the first day of the last menstrual period. However, the **gestational age**, a period based on the moment of conception, is the calculation most often used to determine the expected arrival date (expected date of delivery or confinement—EDD or EDC). This calculation assumes conception occurs near ovulation, or midway through the menstrual cycle, which is about 14 days from the first day of the last menstrual cycle. Thus, the pregnancy lasts 266 days, or 38 weeks. Note that this calculation is only an estimate, since pregnancies can vary by two weeks or more on either side of the average duration.

PREGNANCY

During sexual intercourse, semen is ejaculated into the vagina. Millions of sperm within the seminal fluid swim through the vagina, cervix, and uterus, and into one of the fallopian tubes, where a small fraction of them reach the ovum. This process takes from three to fifteen hours. (Sperm are capable of fertilizing from about thirty hours to three days after ejaculation, and the ovum can be fertilized for about twenty-four hours after ovulation.)

The fertilized ovum, or **zygote**, begins the process of cell division, **mitosis.** After about three days, it becomes a solid mass of cells called a **morula.** By the time the morula, which continues to divide, reaches the uterus, it contains the developing embryo and becomes a hollow ball of cells called a **blastocyst**, which implants itself in the wall of the uterus. The process from fertilization to implantation takes about six days. The blastocyst develops into a structure with two cavities, the **yolk sac** and **amniotic cavity.** In humans, the yolk sac produces blood cells, and the amniotic cavity becomes the fluid-filled cavity in which the fetus floats while it develops.

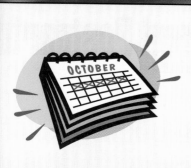

Quick Method for Calculating EDD: Nägele's Rule

- Determine the first day of the last menstrual period (example: January 10)
- Add 7 days (January 17)
- Count back 3 months (October 17)
- Add 1 year; the resulting date is the EDD (October 17 of the next year)

Ninety percent of expectant mothers deliver within 2 weeks of their date, but no more than 10 percent deliver on their date.

After implantation of the blastocyst on the endometrium, the **placenta** develops (about the 5th week after fertilization) and is complete by the 13th week after fertilization. The placenta is the organ for the exchange of nutrients and waste products, passing oxygen and hormones between the mother and the baby. A thin layer of placental tissue separates fetal blood from maternal blood and prevents toxins from entering the fetus. Some substances able to penetrate this barrier are certain viruses and legal and illegal drugs, including alcohol, caffeine, cocaine, nicotine, and many, many more.

Embryonic Phase

Pregnancy is divided into three 3-month periods called **trimesters**. The first trimester, known as the **embryonic phase**, begins with fertilization and concludes at the end of the eighth week of gestation. During this time, three layers of specialized cells called **primary germ layers** develop, each of which eventually produces a definitive structure of the human body. The layers are called **endoderm**, or inside layer; **ectoderm**, or outside layer; and **mesoderm**, or middle layer. Table 16.1 shows the structures that are formed by each of these layers. Any abnormality in the formation of a layer can cause an abnormality in the structures it forms.

Table 16.1

The Embryonic Layers and their Developing Structures

Embryonic Layer	Structure	Word Analysis	
Endoderm	lining of GI tract from pharynx to rectum; epithelium of trachea, bronchi, lungs, liver, pancreas, urinary bladder	endo- derm	within skin
Ectoderm	mucous membrane, tooth enamel, hair, nails, mammary glands, nervous system; neural tube formation	ecto- derm	outside skin
Mesoderm	heart, blood vessels, spleen, blood and lymph cells, bones, muscles; umbilical vessels pass through the connecting structure to the placenta	meso- derm	middle skin

Fetal Phase

In the **fetal phase**, which extends from week 9 to week 39, the term *embryo* is replaced by the word *fetus*. By four months of gestation, every organ system is complete and from that time until term (about 280 days), the fetus grows. The uterus expands about 50 to 100 times its original size, occupying most of the mother's abdominal cavity (Figure 16.1). Table 16.2 traces the general development of the fetus (Figure 16.2) from the embryonic phase to birth. Table 16.3 summarizes the changes that occur in the woman's body during pregnancy.

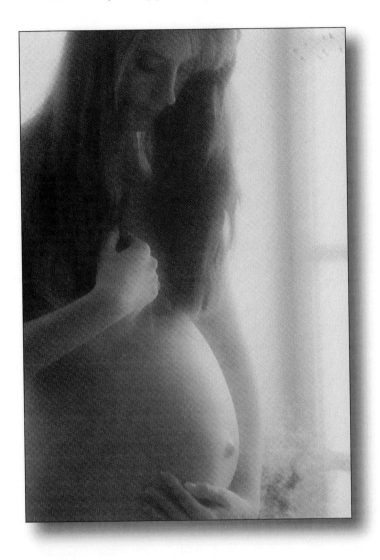

Figure 16.1 - Expanded Uterus of Pregnancy

How is the gender of the child determined?

♀ ♂ ♀ ♂ ♀ ♂ ♀ ♂ ♀ ♂ ♀ ♂

Females have two X sex chromosomes, and males have one X and one Y sex chromosome. At the time of fertilization, each parent donates one sex chromosome. If the X chromosome from the male is carried on the sperm that fertilizes the ovum, the child will have two Xs and be a female. If the Y chromosome from the male fertilizes the egg, the child will be a male with the X and Y sex chromosomes. (The female can only donate an X chromosome.)

Figure 16.2 - Fetus in Utero

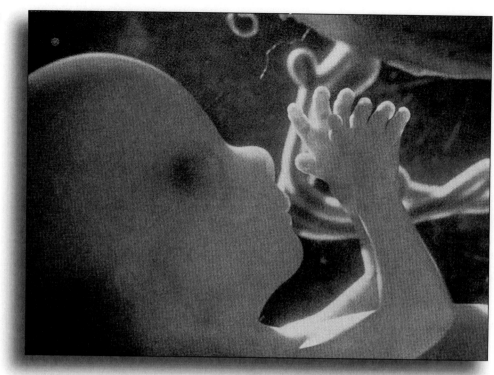

Table 16.2

Fetal Development

Gestational period	Weight and length	Developing characteristics
Embryonic phase		
weeks 1–3	1/16 inch	embryo curls to C-shape; forebrain develops; heart prominence; arm and leg buds; primitive ears and eyes; yolk sac becomes primitive gut; early development of lungs and kidneys
weeks 4–7	1/3 inch	continued brain development; retina, heart chambers, fingers, toes, eyes; palate and upper lip form; GI tract develops, but is still part of the umbilical cord; urogenital tract
Fetal stage (end of 8th week to birth)		
weeks 8–10	1⅛ inches 1/15 ounce	growth and maturation of structures that have already begun to form; skeleton begins to calcify
weeks 11–12	4½ inches ⅔ ounce	facial features, eyelids, intestine separates from umbilical cord; palate fusion; genital structures visible; nail beds and tooth buds form
weeks 13–16	7½ inches 3⅓ ounces	limbs and trunk grow; fetus becomes active; placenta is prominent
weeks 17–20	8¾ inches 10 ounces	eyebrows, lanugo, vernix caseosa; scalp hair; hears sounds
week 24	12 inches 1¼ pounds	external ear; wrinkled, translucent skin with apparent capillaries; lanugo; alveoli form
week 28	14 inches 2¼ pounds	appearance of subcutaneous fat; nail growth begins; testes descend; eyes open; increased hair on scalp
week 32	16 inches 3¾ pounds	nail growth to tips of fingers and toes; female genitalia develop further; breast areolae become visible; creases on soles begin to form
week 36	18 inches 4½ pounds	skin thickens; lanugo disappears; breast tissue develops; male genitalia continue development; sole creases complete
term (end of week 38)	20 inches 6½ pounds	facial lanugo disappears; vernix caseosa decreases; areolae more distinct; ears well formed; genitalia complete formation

Table 16.3

The Changing Female Body during Pregnancy

Change	Description	Word analysis	
General			
menstrual cycle suspended		*mensis*	month
"morning sickness"	nausea and vomiting; if pathological (extreme or protracted) it is diagnosed as hyperemesis	*naus* *vomitus* *hyper* *emesis*	ship (seasickness) to vomit excessive to vomit
fatigue		*fatigo*	to tire
frequency of urination		*frequens*	repeated, often, constant
Genitalia			
Goodell's sign	cervix softens	*Goodell*	For William Goodell, American gynecologist
Chadwick's sign	vaginal mucosa and cervix appear cyanotic	*Chadwick*	For James Read Chadwick, American gynecologist
Hegar's sign	Uterine isthmus softens	*Hegar*	For Alfred Hegar, German gynecologist
Breasts			
pigmentation	increased pigmentation of areolae and nipples	*pigment* *ation*	coloring making of
striae gravidarum	stripes or lines (stretch marks)	*striae* *gravidarum*	stripe pregnant
engorgement	active breast tissue fills with fluid and expands, including ducts and fatty tissue	*gurges*	a whirlpool
colostrum secretion	a thin first milk that can be expressed after 4th month; milk (lactation, or milk production) begins after parturition	*colostrum*	also called foremilk
Abdomen			
linea nigra	hyperpigmentation on midline of the abdomen	*linea* *nigra*	line dark; black
striae gravidarum	commonly called "stretch marks"	*striae* *gravida*	stripe pregnancy
Face			
chloasma	hyperpigmentation on face; the mask of pregnancy	*khloasma*	greenness
Musculoskeletal			
lordosis	anteroposterior curvature of the spine; protuberant abdomen causes changes in posture	*lordos* *-osis*	bent backward condition
kyphosis	extensive flexion of the spine; protuberant abdomen causes changes in posture	*kyphos* *-osis*	bent condition

continued on next page

anterior cervical flexion	change in center of gravity causes head to protrude to maintain balance	*anterior*	front
		cervi	neck
		cal	adjective indicator
		flex	bend
		-ion	noun indicator
waddling gait	wide-based gait due to change in center of gravity and increased relaxin secretion which affects joints	*wade*	walking with short steps
		gata	path

QUICKENING The first time the mother feels the fetus move within her is called **quickening**, and it usually occurs about week 16 of gestation if she is multiparous and week 18 if she is nulliparous. The **amnionic fluid** ("bag of waters") around the baby increases at about the midpoint of the pregnancy. **Braxton Hicks** contractions occur throughout the pregnancy, but are usually not painful. They can be felt on the outside of the abdomen by about the 28th week of gestation.

LIGHTENING The fetus develops *in utero* and is known as the **passenger** as the time of birth nears. About two weeks before giving birth, the mother will feel **lightening**, the baby dropping down into position for birth. The following terms are used to describe the relationship of the passenger to the mother's pelvis, called the **passageway**:

- **Lie:** Relationship of the long axis of the fetus to the long axis of the mother—if the fetal spine is perpendicular to the maternal spine, it is a transverse lie; if the fetus' and mother's spines are parallel, the lie is longitudinal.

- **Attitude:** Amount of flexion of the fetal head, body, and extremities (should be complete flexion).

- **Presentation:** Part of the fetus that comes through the passageway first; cephalic presentation is headfirst and represents about 96% of births; breech is a feet- or buttocks-first presentation, and occurs in about 4% of births; shoulder or transverse presentations account for a few number of births.

- **Station:** Measurement relating the fetal presenting part to the ischial spines of the mother's pelvis. When the largest diameter of the presenting part (usually the head) is level with the ischial spines, the baby is **engaged**, and the station is 0 (which is at the center of the pelvic outlet); above the spines is -1 cm, -2, -3, -4, and -5 (which represents the pubic-bone level). The measurements of +1 cm, +2, +3, +4, and +5 represent stations below the center.

Labor

The process of birth is also called **parturition** and begins with uterine muscle contractions. The fetus is in the "head-down" (**vertex**) position and rests against the cervix. Contractions cause the amniotic sac to rupture (also referred to as a woman's "water breaking"), beginning the process of **labor**, which includes the following stages:

- **Stage 1** Onset of uterine contractions until cervix is completely dilated (opened)
- **Stage 2** Maximum cervical dilation until exit of baby through vagina
- **Stage 3** Expulsion of placenta through vagina
- **Stage 4** Period of 1 to 4 hours after delivery of placenta

Word Analysis

Separate each term into its individual word parts, indicating the type of word part using the letters P (prefix), S (suffix), R (root word), and CV (combining vowel). Then write the definition of the term.

	Word Parts	**Definition**
1. embryonic		
2. endoderm		
3. ectoderm		
4. mesoderm		
5. oocyte		
6. genital		
7. abdominal		
8. lordosis		
9. parturition		
10. pigmentation		
11. trimester		
12. mitosis		

Comprehension Check

Select the correct term from the two choices provided in each sentence.

1. The process of conception/ovum is a miraculous event.

2. The ETC/EDC is the anticipated date of the baby's birth.

3. The date of the last gestational/menstrual cycle is used in calculating a woman's due date.

4. The placenta/endoderm is responsible for the exchange of nutrients and waste between the fetus and the mother.

5. Pregnancy is divided into three menarches/trimesters.

6. Females have two X/Y chromosomes.

7. In the embryonic phase/fetal phase, the organ systems are complete.

8. The process of cell division is called zygote/mitosis.

9. The morula/yolk sac becomes a ball of cells called a mesocyst/blastocyst.

10. Gestational age is based on the moment of conception/first day of the last menstrual period.

Matching

Select the phase or stage in Column 1 that matches the developmental characteristic(s) in Column 2. Write the number of your answer on the line beside the characteristic.

Column 1

1. Week 24
2. Week 32
3. Embryonic Phase
4. Fetal Stage
5. Week 36
6. term
7. Week 28
8. about 266 days
9. 3 to 15 hours
10. 24 hours after ovulation

Column 2

_____ time for sperm to reach ovum

_____ end of 8th week to birth

_____ period an ovum can be fertilized

_____ facial lanugo disappears

_____ through Week 7

_____ nail growth to tips of fingers and toes

_____ length of pregnancy based on moment of conception

_____ 18 inches long

_____ 14 inches long

_____ alveoli form

Name That Term

Write the stage of labor that matches each description.

Description   **Stage**

1. Onset of uterine contractions until cervix is completely dilated.   _____

2. Period of 1-4 hours after delivery of placenta.   _____

3. Maximum cervical dilation until exit of baby.   _____

4. Expulsion of placenta through vagina.   _____

Word Puzzle

Use these misspelled clues to write the correctly spelled term in the puzzle.

Across
- 3. zygoat
- 5. pheetis
- 7. moroula
- 11. partition
- 12. ektadrem
- 13. mukousa
- 15. oravum
- 16. kifosis
- 18. aroelea
- 19. kromisoam

Down
- 1. colustrim
- 2. blasticytes
- 4. clhaosma
- 5. fertalizashun
- 6. endodrem
- 7. misaderme
- 8. syinotic
- 9. quickning
- 10. mistosis
- 14. imebryo
- 17. youk

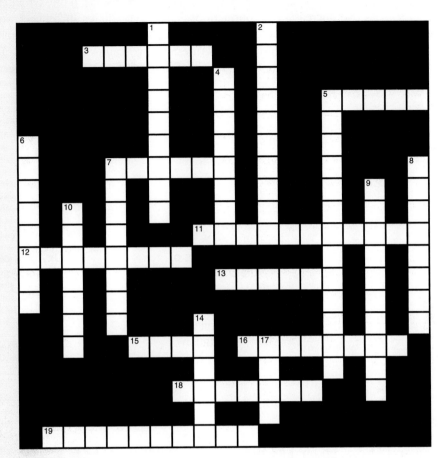

Word Maps

Place the following words into one of three categories: conception, fetal life, or pregnancy

striae gravidarum embryo fertilize chloasma kyphosis ovum morula mesoderm seminal fluid

Conception	Development	Pregnancy
_____	_____	_____
_____	_____	_____
_____	_____	_____

The **myometrium**, part of the uterine wall, becomes more sensitive to oxytocin in late pregnancy. Once labor begins, the secretion of oxytocin increases, which in turn increases the contractions. The cervix dilates and effaces, and the vagina distends with the aid of another hormone, **relaxin**. This positive feedback loop (refer to Chapter 7, "The Endocrine System") causes the sequence of events that result in the baby's birth, and stops at delivery. Figure 16.3 illustrates the oxytocin positive feedback loop.

Figure 16.3 - Oxytocin Positive Feedback Loop

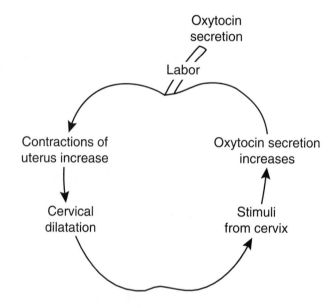

Labor and Delivery Problems

Occasionally, problems occur with labor and/or delivery. These difficulties include absence of contractions, or decreased labor, and difficult labor, called **dystocia**. Abnormalities with the placenta can occur, such as **placenta previa**, an abnormal placement of the placenta that causes hemorrhage, or **abruptio placenta**, a premature separation of the placenta from the uterine wall. These are emergency situations for the mother and the infant. Difficult labor, placental problems, and breech presentations usually require a **cesarean** birth (a surgical intervention) to deliver the neonate.

Care of the Newborn after Birth

At birth, the newborn must have immediate care. The first task is to establish and maintain the infant's respiration. The airway (mouth and nose) must be cleared, and the infant must breathe on its own. Next, the newborn must be dried off and kept warm by placing it on the mother's abdomen or chest, and covering it. A cap may be placed on the baby's head to prevent heat loss. The neonate is screened at one minute and five minutes with an **Apgar score**, a numerical value system that indicates the infant's condition. Of course, any abnormalities with cardiac and/or respiratory status are addressed immediately. Table 16.4 displays the Apgar scoring system. A score of 8–10 points is normal.

Table 16.4

Apgar Score

Points	0	1	2
heart rate	absent	under 100	over 100
respiratory effort	absent	slow, irregular	good (screams)
muscle tone	limp	good in limbs	active movement
response stimulation	none	makes grimaces	coughing or sneezing
skin color	pale	rosy trunk, blue extremities	rosy

THE POSTPARTUM PERIOD

The time after delivery is called the **postpartum** (*post* = after; *partum* = delivery) period, and it includes the fourth stage of labor or the one to four hours after the delivery of the placenta. During postpartum, the woman is referred to as the **parturient**. At this time, the **episiotomy** incision or any tearing of the perineum is repaired. The mother is cleaned and covered to minimize cold and shaking from chills. Many changes in the parturient take place in the immediate postpartum period. The physician assesses the position of the **fundus**, or base of the uterus by palpating the abdomen and also notes the vaginal discharge, called **lochia**.

Table 16.5

The Terms of Pregnancy, Labor, Delivery, and Postpartum

Term	Meaning	Word Analysis	
abruptio placentae ah-**brup**-she-o play-**sen**-tea	abnormal premature placental separation from the uterine wall	abruptio plakoenta	breaking off flat cake
amniotic fluid **am**-knee-ah-tic	the fluid that surrounds the baby *in utero*	amnio -tic	bowl shaped
Apgar score	the method of screening the neonate	Apgar	Virginia Apgar, anesthesiologist
blastocyst **blast**-oh-sist	a stage in the formation of the embryo	blastos kustis	bud or germ bladder
Braxton Hicks (contractions)	contractions that occur during pregnancy, but do not lead to birth	Braxton Hicks	John Braxton Hicks, English gynecologist
cesarean section	surgical delivery of the fetus	lex cesarea	(allowed under) Roman law
embryo **m**-brie-oh	the early stage of the human organism	embruon	to be full to bursting
episiotomy E-pea-zee-ot-a-**mee**	a surgical intervention to prevent tearing of the vulva, usually during childbirth	episeion tome	pubic region incision
fetus (sing)	the unborn child between the 8th week of gestation until birth	fetus	offspring
gestation jes-**tay**-shun	pregnancy	gestation	carrying
gravida **grav**-eh-dah	refers to the number of pregnancies	gravida	pregnancy
labor	the process of giving birth	labor	work
lochia low-**key**-ah	vaginal discharge after delivery of the fetus	lokhos	childbirth

continued on next page

meiosis my-**oh**-sis	cell division process resulting in cells that contain half the number of chromosomes as the parent cell	meiosis	lessening
morula more-**ooh**-ah	a stage in the divisions of the zygote before implantation	morum	mulberry
nulligravida **nuh**-le-grav-id ah	a female who has never conceived a child	nulla gravida	never pregnancy
nullipara nuh-**lip**-a-rah	a female who has not given birth to a child	nulla parare	never to give birth
oxytocin **ox**-e-toe-sin	a hormone that causes uterine contractions and promotes milk release	oxy toc in	acid birth chemical
para **pair**-ah	the term that refers to the number of births	parare	to give birth
parturition par-too-**rish**-on	the process of giving birth	parturitio	childbirth
placenta play-**sent**-ah	the organ that provides transfer of substances between the fetus and mother	plakoenta	flat
placenta previa play-**sent**-ah **pre**-vee-ah	placenta is implanted in the lower area of the uterus causing difficulty during the birth	plakoenta previa	flat before
postpartum	the period after the delivery of the placenta	post- partus	after birth
relaxin ree-**lax**-inn	a hormone secreted by the corpus luteum; causes softening and lengthening of the symphysis pubis and cervix during pregnancy	re lax in	again; back loosen chemical
trimesters	the three periods of three months during pregnancy	tri mester	three month; moon
vertex presentation **ver**-tex	occipital cephalic presentation of the fetus	vert	turn
yolk	one of the nutrients for the embryo that arise from the ovum	yolk	yellow

TESTS AND PROCEDURES

A simple blood pressure test is important in determining whether the expectant woman has hypertension (high blood pressure). About 5 percent of pregnant women develop such high blood pressure that it becomes hazardous to them and their unborn child. This is called preeclampsia (or toxemia). The high blood pressure leads to protein becoming present in their urine that is detected by urinanalysis. If the high blood pressure becomes severe, the mother and unborn child are at high risk for stroke, coma, liver damage, and convulsions (eclampsia). The only real treatment is delivery of the baby.

Ultrasound imaging technology has many applications during pregnancy. Some of the common indications include verifying fetal age (fetal growth during the first trimester is highly predictable), determining whether twins, triplets (or more) are present, checking for ectopic pregnancy, screening for abnormalities, and more. No study has shown that having ultrasound performed poses a risk to mother or fetus.

A pregnant woman will have blood drawn to determine electrolyte and hematocrit levels, and will be screened for gestational diabetes. In addition to all of the other dangers of diabetes, uncontrolled gestational diabetes has been associated with macrosomia (fetal birthweight of 10 lbs. or more). A maternal blood sample can be used to screen for birth defects using the alfa fetoprotein level, which can reveal a neural tube defect (spina bifida), chromosomal abnormalities (including Down syndrome), and more. In addition, the level of HCG (human chorionic gonadatropin) and another substance, estriol, can be determined from the same sample, and the three measurements are used to more precisely calculate the risk of fetal abnormalities.

Amniocentesis

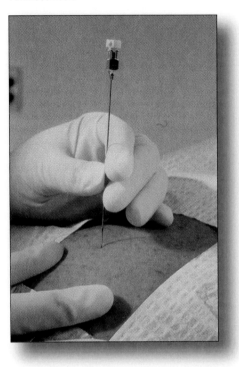

Amniocentesis (aspiration of the fluid from the amniotic sac) is the most common test for ruling out birth defects. This procedure may be performed at 15 to 18 weeks and is between 99 and 100 percent accurate in determining fetal genetic abnormalities. However, the risk of miscarriage is 2.6 percent when performed in the first trimester, and 0.8 percent when performed in the second trimester.

One test that is 99 percent accurate in ruling out chromosomal abnormalities is chorionic villus sampling. This test can be done at week ten, earlier than amniocentesis. The test uses one of the tiny villi that attach the placenta to the uterine wall, and although there is a risk of miscarriage or fetal limb defects from performing this test, the risk is lower than that associated with early amniocentesis testing.

Fetal monitoring has become common during labor and delivery. Sensors measure the heart rate of the fetus. The heart rate is printed on paper tracings, and these strips become part of the medical record. The information is important when the delivery team is determining whether there is any fetal distress, or if an unplanned cesarean section (surgical delivery of the fetus) is indicated.

INFANT MORTALITY

Infant mortality (defined as death within one year of birth) remains a problem all over the world. The 2005 infant mortality statistic for the United States is estimated to be 6.5 deaths per 1000 live births. By one agency's ranking, this puts the U.S. at 184 out of 226 countries or locations, meaning 42 had lower mortality. The infant mortality rate had climbed (for the first time since the 1950s) from 6.8 in 2001 to 7.0 in 2002, possibly because of the increased incidence of females delaying childbearing into their late 30s and 40s. Some causes of infant mortality include birth defects, preterm delivery, and low birth weight. A large proportion of mothers still do not have access to prenatal care, which accounts for much of the mortality rate. The U.S. Department of Health and Human Services has set particular objectives in the Healthy People 2010 initiative to promote national maternal and child health and decrease infant mortality disparities between ethnic and socioeconomic groups. Healthcare personnel as well as consumers will work toward those goals.

Table 16.6

Abbreviations

CPD	cephalopelvic disproportion
CS, C-section, C/S	cesarean section
Cx	cervix
EDC	estimated date of confinement (due date)
EDD	estimated date of delivery
FECG	fetal electrocardiogram
FHR	fetal heart rate
FTND	full-term, normal delivery
FTNSVD	full-term, normal, spontaneous, vaginal delivery
HCG	human chorionic gonadotropin
IUP	intrauterine pregnancy
NB	newborn
UC	uterine contractions
VBAC	vaginal birth after cesarean section

Comprehension Check

Exercise 7

Select from the two terms to find a match for the definition provided, and circle the correct term.

1. hormone secretion increases after labor begins — oxytocin/testosterone

2. difficult labor — relaxin/dystocia

3. premature separation of the placenta from the uterine wall — abruptio placenta/distention

4. abnormal placement of the placenta, causing hemorrhage — zygote/placenta previa

5. screening tool for assessing newborn's condition — Apgar score/Braxton Hicks

6. fluid that surrounds the baby in the uterus — vertex/amniotic

7. early stages of the human organism — lochia/embryo

8. flexed cephalic presentation — flexation/vertex

9. postpartum — period after delivery of the infant/ of the amnion

10. hormone secreted by corpus luteum — luteumin/relaxin

Matching

Select the term from Column 1 that matches the definition in Column 2. Write the number of the answer on the line beside the definition.

Column 1

1. blastocyst
2. gestation
3. ectoderm
4. mitosis
5. postpartum
6. trimester
7. vertex presentation
8. parturition
9. zygote
10. morula

Column 2

_____ solid mass of dividing cells

_____ three periods of three months each, during a pregnancy

_____ completely flexed cephalic presentation of head of fetus

_____ fertilized ovum

_____ pregnancy

_____ period after the delivery of the placenta

_____ hollow ball of cells

_____ process whereby cells divide

_____ forms nervous system and more

_____ process of giving birth

Abbreviations

Read each sentence, then write the appropriate abbreviation in the blank.

1. The fetal heart rate, or _____, was 160.

2. There were no complications, and Linda had a full term, normal, spontaneous, vaginal delivery, or a _____.

3. The newborn, _____, infant weighed 7 lbs., 6 oz.

4. Christie had a vaginal birth after a cesarean section, or a _____.

5. Louisa's urine was positive for human chorionic gonadotrophin, or _____.

6. Terri had a C-section because of cephalopelvic disproportion, or _____.

7. Imaging revealed a _____, or normal intrauterine pregnancy.

8. The _____, or fetal electrocardiogram, revealed no abnormalities.

Divide each word into its parts. Write the meaning of the parts on the line next to the word.

1. relaxin _____

2. nulligravida _____

3. dystocia _____

4. postpartum _____

5. trimester _____

6. placenta _____

7. oxytocin _____

8. nullipara _____

9. gestation _____

10. parturient _____

Performance Assessment 16

Crossword Puzzle

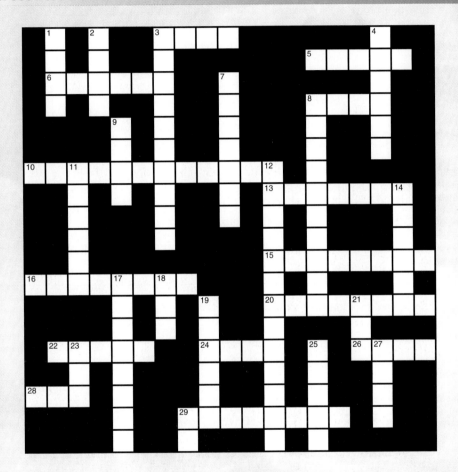

Across

3. prefix meaning after
5. nulla
6. Greek root for bent backward
8. amnio
10. female who has never conceived a child
13. process of cell division
15. hormone that stimulates the flow of milk
16. Greek for a flat cake
20. female hormone
22. Greek for thread
24. walk
26. nutrient for the embryo that arises from the ovum
28. blastos
29. related to the neck

Down

1. myometrium
2. word part meaning turn
3. period following delivery of the placenta
4. yolk color
7. refers to number of pregnancies
8. hollow ball of cells
9. suffix meaning condition
11. vaginal discharge after delivery of a baby
12. puncture of the amniotic sac to remove sample of amniotic fluid
14. stripes
17. lining of the GI tract, epithelium of trachea, bronchi, lungs, liver, pancreas, urinary bladder
18. prefix meaning three
19. fertilized ovum
21. word part meaning acid
23. abbreviation for intrauterine device
25. score indicating infant's condition
27. dilate
29. abbreviation for cervix

What's Your Conclusion?

Both Martha and David had a family history of genetic abnormalities. Now, Martha is pregnant with the couple's first child. They are concerned that their baby may have one or more abnormalities. What procedure do you think their doctor would recommend?

Martha is in labor. Although no genetic abnormalities were identified, the couple and their doctor are still concerned about the baby. Early in labor the heart rate seemed fast. In addition, the physician has identified possible complications with delivery. What procedure do you think Martha will have during her labor?

Using Medical References

The following sentences contain medical terms that may not have been addressed on the tables in this chapter. Use medical reference books, your medical term analysis skills, and/or a medical dictionary to find the correct definition of each underlined word. Write the definition on the line below the sentence.

1. The patient was diagnosed with <u>preeclampsia</u> and admitted to the hospital.

   _____

2. The procedure identified several abnormally large <u>graafian</u> follicles.

   _____

3. The patient required an <u>episiotomy</u> to deliver the infant's head.

   _____

4. There was abnormal development of the <u>chorion</u>.

   _____

5. "<u>Afterbirth</u>" is a term commonly used by those outside the healthcare professions.

   _____

6. A <u>tocolytic</u> agent was administered because the pregnancy was only in the second trimester.

   _____

7. Progesterone is necessary for <u>lactation</u>.

   _____

8. <u>Colostrum</u> is especially nourishing for the newborn.

   _____

9. The patient was given an <u>abortifacient</u>.

_____

10. Examination revealed that <u>involution</u> of the uterus was progressing.

_____

Essence of the Topic

Thinking in physical development terms, describe special types of problems that can occur when the pregnant patient is under 18 years of age, when the patient is 20-35 years old, and when the patient is over 40. You may need to research this topic in other sources.

As you reflect on the types of illnesses and conditions associated with this medical area, what questions related to the origin or cause of the problems occur to you? Write a minimum of three questions. Then select one question and research the latest scientific findings regarding this issue. (See Chapter 1 for a list of medical Web sites that may provide pertinent information.)

Technology and Careers

Research the new jobs evolving in this special topic area and describe how technology plays a role in each job. Include the names of the equipment and technologies used.

Thinking in terms of where you want to be employed (hospital, clinic, private practice, etc.), what new technologies are in use or in development? In your analysis, differentiate office system technologies and clinical technologies. In your view, which technologies will most change how you work?

Short Answer

In your own words, describe the changes in the female body immediately after childbirth.

_____

_____

_____

_____

Appendix A: Exercise Answers

CHAPTER 1

Exercise 1

1. c, 2. f, 3. a, 4. g, 5. b, 6. e, 7. h, 8. i, 9. d, 10. j

Exercise 2

1. gynec = females, 2. leuko = white, cyto = cells, 3. tracheo = trachea, 4. cardio = heart, 5. hemato = blood, 6. gastro = stomach, entero = intestines, 7. cysto = bladder, 8. cardio = heart, 9. angio = vessels, 10. physio = physical, 11. thrombo = clot, cyto = cell, 12. erythro = red, derma = skin, 13. fibrino = fiber, 14. bacterio = bacteria, 15. cephalo = head, pelv = pelvis.

Exercise 3

1. carditis, itis = inflammation; 2. pulmonary, ry = pertaining to; 3. rheumatic, ic = pertaining to; 4. arthrosis, osis = condition; 5. cardiomegaly, megaly = enlargement; 6. renal, al = pertaining to; 7. anemia, ia = condition or process; 8. hypertrophy, trophy = development; 9. dysplasia, ia = condition or process; 10. pustule, ule = small; 11. arteriole, ole = small; 12. macula, ula = small; 13. lithiasis, asis = formation or presence of; 14. vermiform, form = shape or resembling, 15. hemolysis, lysis = breakdown.

Exercise 4

1. metry = process of measuring; 2. meter = measure or measurement; 3. scopy = process of viewing with an instrument; 4. gram = record; 5. graphy = process of recording; 6. iatric = treatment; 7. centesis = puncture to withdraw fluid, 8. desis = stabilization or binding; 9. plasty = repair; 10. rrhaphy = suturing; 11. stomy = creation of an artificial opening; 12. tomy = cut or incision; 13. tripsy = crushing; 14. scope = instrument used for viewing; 15. graph = record or instrument used for making a record.

Exercise 5

1. osteoblasts, 2. erythrocyte, 3. periosteum, 4. anesthetize, 5. hemostasis, 6. cephalgia, 7. arthrodynia, 8. cystocele, 9. hematemesis, 10. osteoid, 11. carcinogenic, 12. hepatoma, 13. photophobia, 14. orthopnea, 15. hemorrhagic.

Exercise 6

1. monochromatic, 2. bilateral, 3. ambidexterous, 4. trigeminy, 5. quadriplegia or tetraplegia, 6. polycythemia, 7. multidisciplinary, 8. megaloblasts, 9. oliguria, 10. microcardia, 11. hemiplegia, 12. apnea, 13. tachycardia, 14. bradycardia, 15. pandemic.

Exercise 7

1. hyper, 2. hypo, 3. sub, 4. super, 5. supra, 6. ultra, 7. ad, 8. ab, 9. circum, 10. de, 11. trans, 12. epi, 13. para, 14. post, 15 re.

Exercise 8

1. m or n, 2. i or o, 3. o or I, 4. g or j, 5. j or g, 6. e, 7. d, 8. a, 9. k, 10. c, 11. h, 12. f, 13. b, 14. l or n or m, 15. n or m or l.

Exercise 9

1. mastectomy, 2. cardiologist, 3. pericardial, 4. sarcoma, 5. dysphagia, 6. cephalic, 7. hepatorrhaphy, 8. prenatal, 9. necrosis, 10. neonatologist

Exercise 10

1. correct, 2. tracheotomy, 3. cardiologist, 4. abdominocentesis, 5. tachycardia, 6. correct, 7. correct, 8. correct, 9. leucocytes, 10. cyanosis.

Exercise 11

1. uro/logist; uro = urine, logist = someone who studies; a specialist in urology
2. thrombo/cyto/sis; thrombo = clot, cyt = cell, osis = condition; an increase in the number of circulating platelets
3. cephal/ic; cephal = head, ic = relating to; toward the head
4. extra/cellul/ar; extra = outside, cellul = cells, ar = pertaining to; outside the cells
5. gastro/rrhaphy, gastro = stomach, rrhaphy = suturing; suture of a perforation of the stomach.
6. osteo/myel/itis; osteo = bone, myel = marrow, itis = inflammation; inflammation of the bone and associated marrow
7. brady/card/ia; brady = slow, card = heart, ia = condition; slowness of the heart
8. oste/oma, oste = bone, oma = tumor or swelling; a tumor of bone cells
9. necro/tic, necro = death, tic = relating to; relating to death or dead tissue
10. hypo/gastr/ic; hypo = below, gastr = stomach, ic = relating to; relating to below the stomach.

Exercise 12

1. f, 2. k, 3. l, 4. a, 5. n, 6. m, 7. e, 8. c, 9. d, 10. o, 11. b, 12. j, 13. i, 14. g, 15. h

CHAPTER 2

Exercise 1

1. j, 2. l, 3. p, 4. i, 5. o, 6. h, 7. a, 8. d, 9. b, 10. f, 11. g, 12. n, 13. m, 14. k, 15. e, 16. c

Exercise 2

1. away from, 2. back, 3. medial; closer to the midline, 4. superficial, closer to the surface, 5. occurring on both sides, 6. farther from the point of attachment, 7. pertaining to the wall, 8. prone, lying horizontally and facing down, 9. lithotomy, lying on back, knees bent, feet

in stirrups, 10. lying on back with knees bent and head lower than trunk, 11. a view or cut lengthwise from anterior to posterior, 12. flexion, bending a join, 13. straightening a joint, 14. moving closer to the body, 15. bent up and away.

Exercise 3
a. 2, b. 4, c. 1, d. 8, e. 10, f. 9, g. 3, h. 11, i 6, j. 12, k. 5, l. 7, m. 14, n. 15, o. 13

Exercise 4
clockwise starting from the top is frontal, mental, pectoral, brachial, antecubital, carpal, digital, genital, femoral, plantar, crural, inguinal, palmar, antebrachial, axillary, acromial, buccal

Exercise 5
top left box: right hypochrondriac region; liver
top central box: epigastric region; liver, gallbladder, stomach
top right box: left hypochrondriac region; stomach, spleen
middle left box: right lumbar region; large intestine
middle central box: umbilical region; small intestine, large intestine
middle right box: left lumbar region; small intestine, large intestine
bottom left box: right inguinal region; large intestine
bottom central box: hypogastric region, large intestine, small intestine, appendix
bottom right box: left inguinal region, large intestine, small intestine

Exercise 6
1. angiography, 2. bronchography, 3. ultrasonography, 4. myelography, 5. radioimmunoassay, 6. radiography, 7. salpingography, 8. sonogram, 9. pyelography, 10. fluoroscopy

Exercise 7
1. urinalysis, 2. radioactive, 3. etiology, 4. inflammation, 5. radiogram, 6. pandemic, 7. roentgen, 8. culture, 9. Morphology, 10. bandage, 11. histology, 12. pathogens, 13. serology, 14. sterile, 15. dressing

CHAPTER 3

Exercise 1
1. skin, 2. skin, 3. skin, 4. skin, 5. sweat glands, 6. horny tissue, 7. fat, 8. pigment, 9. sebum, 10. skin

Exercise 2
1. adipose, 2. confluent, 3. intradermally, 4. apocrine, 5. Dermatology, 6. integument, 7. follicles, 8. Turgor, 9. Sebum, 10. Nevus

Exercise 3
1. i, 2. b, 3. a, 4. g, 5. c, 6. e, 7. d, 8. j, 9. f 10. h

Exercise 4
1. cutane-ous, 2. dermato-logist, 3. epi-derm-is, 4. derm-al, 5. lipo-lysis, 6. melano-cyte, 7. sub-cutane-ous, 8. sebo-rrhea, 9. histo-logy, 10. dermato-logy

Exercise 5
1. nevi, 2. follicles, 3. Melanocytes, 4. papillae, 5. Ephelides, 6. nerves, 7. receptors, 8. vessels, 9. phases, 10. nails

Exercise 6
1. i, 2. f, 3. a, 4. d, 5 . h, 6. g, 7. e, 8. c, 9. j, 10. b

Exercise 7
1. melano = pigment, cyte = cell, a pigment-producing cell, 2. ec = out of, chyme = juice, osis = condition, a condition of blood leaking from a vessel, 3. cyan = blue, osis = condition, blue appearance, 4. chron = time, ic = pertain to, a condition through time, 5. pust = pus, ule = small, small pus-filled lesion, 6. squam = scale, ou = pertaining to, pertaining to scales, 7. xer = dry, osis = condition, dry skin, 8. onycho = nail, lysis = kill, loosening of the nail, 9. carcin = cancer, oma = malignancy, malignant cancer, 10. dermat = skin, itis = inflammation, inflammation of the skin

Exercise 8
1. Physiologic jaundice, 2. erythema toxicum, 3. nevus flammeus, 4. Striae, 5. sebaceous glands, 6. closed comedones, 7. hyperpigmented, 8. decreased, 9. subcutaneous, 10. Alopecia

Exercise 9
1. j, 2. g, 3. h, 4. i, 5. a, 6. c, 7. f, 8. b, 9. e, 10. d

Exercise 10
1. dermatitis, dermat = skin, itis = inflammation, 2. seborrhea, sebo = oil, rrhea = flow, 3. acrocyanosis, acro = tip, cyan = blue, osis = condition, 4. angioma, angi = vessel, oma = tumor, 5. carotenemia, caroten = orange pigment, emia = pertaining to blood, 6. folliculitis, follicul = a small sac, itis = inflammation, 7. ecchymosis, ec = out, chyme = juice, osis = condition of, 8. hidrosis, hidr = sweat glands, osis = condition, 9. keratosis, kerat = horny cells, osis = condition, 10. xerosis, xer = dry, osis = condition

Exercise 11
1. xerosis, 2. purpura, 3. eczema, 4. nigra, 5. impetigo, 6. nodule, 7. pustule, 8. verruca, 9. xanthoma, 10. vitiligo

Exercise 12
1. macule, 2. papule, 3. ulcer, 4. plaque, 5. wheal, 6. urticaria, 7. vesicle, 8. pustule, 9. fissure, 10. lichenification

Exercise 13
1. adip-ose fat tissue, 2. dermat-itis, inflammation of the skin, 3. cyanot-ic, bluish skin, 4. squam-ous, scaly cancer of the skin, 5. nevus, mole, 6. ante-cubit-al, pertaining to the front of the elbow, 7. actin-ic kerat-osis, a premalignant lesion, 8. melan-oma, cancer of the cells that produce melanin, 9. vesi-cle, a small filled sac, 10. par-onych-ia, an infection alongside the nail

Exercise 14
1. Dead tissue—debridement means removal of dead tissue, 2. Crust—eschar is a thick crust from a burn,

3. Separating—slough is the separation of dead tissue from live tissue, 4. No—a first degree burn is damage to top layer of skin, 5. Area—the body is divided into regions of 9% each, 6. Worst burn— third degree burns involve all skin layers, 7. Clean— antimicrobials kill or remove microorganisms, 8. Chemicals—abradants wear away by mechanical action, 9. Skin—topicals are applied to a specific place, 10. Treat infection—an antimitotic impairs cell division

Exercise 15
1. f, 2. a, 3. g, 4. h, 5. i, 6. e, 7. b, 8. j, 9. c, 10. d

Exercise 16
1. dermatology, 2. anesthesia, 3. seborrhea, 4. intradermal, 5. dermabrasion, 6. microbial, 7. retinoid, 8. antifungal, 9. antibacterial, 10. antiseptic

Exercise 17
1. angiomas, 2. keratoses, 3. carcinomas or carcinomata, 4. comedos, comedones, 5. condylomata, 6. chemical peels, 7. follicles, 8. milia, 9. lineae, 10. lentigines

Exercise 18
Newborns: acrocyanosis: blue extremities; mila: tiny epidermal cysts; erythema toxicum: self-limited rash. Pregnant women: chloasma: brown hyperpigmented patch; vascular spiders: tiny red lines; linea nigra: brownish-black line. Seniors: alopecia: loss or lack of hair; melanoma: malignancy of pigment cells; senile purpura: purple discolation.

CHAPTER 4

Exercise 1
A. crani/o, B. mandibul/o, C. stern/o, D. cost/o, E. scapul/o, F. humer/o, G. radi/o, H. uln/o, I. Ili/o, J. femor/o, K. patell/o, L. tibi/o, M. fibul/o, N. tars/o

Exercise 2
1. e, 2. i , 3. g, 4. a, 5. b, 6. j, 7. c, 8. d, 9. f, 10. h

Exercise 3
1. rheumat+logy, 2. ortho+ped+tics, 3. endo+scopy, 4. ossify+ication, 5. epiphys+eal, 6. arthro+tic, 7. burs+itis, 8. orth-osis, 9. osteo+logy, 10. fibr+ous

Exercise 4
1. Ligaments, 2. vertebrae, 3. Osteoblasts, 4. scapulae, 5. phalanges, 6. Trabeculae, 7. Synarthroses, 8. Carpals, 9. rheumatologists, 10. Fasciculus

Exercise 5
1. periosteum, 2. medullary cavity, 3. articular cartilage, 4. articulate, 5. synovial membrane, synovial fluid, 6. lumbosacral area, 7. epiphyseal plate, 8. chiropractor, 9. extension, flexion, 10. insertion

Exercise 6
1. osteoarthritis, 2. fasciculus, 3. homeostasis, 4. tendon, 5. involuntary, 6. ligaments, 7. osteocytes, 8. lactic acid, 9. podiatrist, 10. striations

Exercise 7
Muscle Type, skeletal, cardiac, smooth
Location, attached to skeleton, heart, intestine, GI system blood vessels, uterus
Type of Nerve Control, voluntary, involuntary, involuntary

Exercise 8
Across: 2. osteoclast 5. sternum 7. epiphysis 9. striations 10. femur 12. cranium 14. synovial 16. diarthrosis 18. cartilage 19. sarcomeres 20. fasciculus
Down: 1. periosteum 3. scapula 4. tribecula 6. rheumatology 8. bone 11. myofilaments 13. bursa 15. ilium 17. ossify 18. carpal

Exercise 9
1. fibr+osis, reparative or reactive tissue, 2. arthr+itis, inflammation of a joint, 3. burs+itis, inflammation of a bursa, 4. necr+osis, death of tissue, 5. dis+articul+lation, amputation of limb by cutting ligaments, 6. osteo+por+osis, bone with low calcium content, 7. poly+dactyl+y, extra digits, 8. ankyl+osis, stiffening of a joint from fibrosis, 9. tibia, larger of the two lower leg bones, 10. eip+condyl+itis, inflammation of an epicondyle

Exercise 10
1. Carpal tunnel syndrome, 2. suture lines, 3. syndactyly, 4. Tibial torsion, 5. osteoporosis, 6. Flexion, 7. tenosynovitis, 8. Arthrodynia, 9. ganglion, 10. Avascular

Exercise 11
1. ankylosis, 2. bunion, 3. kyphosis, 4. osteoporosis, 5. calcaneus, 6. metatarsus valgus, 7. arthroscopy, 8. juvenile rheumatoid arthritis, 9. scoliosis, 10. greenstick fracture

Exercise 12
1. osteomyelitis, 2. femoral, 3. skeletal, 4. osteoma, 5. osteodynia, 6. bursitis, 7. avascular, 8. arthritis, 9. osteoplasty, 10. antiinflammatory

Exercise 13
1. biopsies, 2. antigen, 3. diagnoses, 4. metatarsi, 5. fontanels, 6. ganglion, 7. bursa, 8. dislocation, 9. tibiae, 10. genua valgum

Exercise 14
1. deformity of the thoracic spine—children/adolescents, 2. inflammation of rib cartilage—adults, 3. curvature of spine—children/adolescents, 4. inflammation of tibia tubercle—adolescents, 5. chronic, inflammatory disease of spine—adults, 6. severe pain in left foot or toe—adults, seniors, 7. inflammation of joints caused by excessive uric acid—adults/seniors, 8. loss of bone mass in entire skeleton—seniors, 9. congenital deformity of extra fingers/toes—infants, 10. inflammation of tendon sheath or wrist caused by repetitive motion—adults/seniors

Exercise 15

1. logist, 2. scopy, 3. pathy, 4. chondr, 5. ar, 6. sis, 7. itis, 8. al, 9. otic, 10. itis

Exercise 16

1. diagnostic test for muscle contractility, 2. MD trained in orthopedics, 3. thick fibrous membrane covering almost the entire surface of a bone, 4. living bone cells, 5. process of cartilage turning into bone, 6. a fluid filled sac that cushions, 7. bony, 8. anteroposterior curvature of the spine, 9. a break, 10. aspirin

Exercise 17

1. d, 2. h, 3. b, 4. f, 5. g, 6. j, 7. i, 8. c, 9. e, 10. a

Exercise 18

1. osteo+logy, 2. a+vascul+ar, 3, necro+tic, 4. endo+chondr+al, 5. tendon+itis, 6. cartilag+inous, 7. oste+oid, 8. gangl+oid, 9. anti+inflammato+ry, 10. re+sect

Exercise 19

1. s, erythrocytes, 2. s, resections, 3. p, myofilament, 4. p, graft, 5. p, sprain, 6. s, tibiae, 7. p, disease, 8. p, osteocyte, 9. p, ligament, 10. s, bunions

Exercise 20

1) feet: gout: arthrocentesis: allopurinol

2) joints: JRA: ESR: immunosuppressants

3) spine: osteoporosis: photon: absorptiometry: calcium supplements

CHAPTER 5

Exercise 1

1. an (P)/emia (R) = without blood (decreased red blood cells)
2. micro (P)/cyt (R)/ic (S) = condition of small cells
3. hypo (P)/chrom (R)/ic (S) = condition of lacking color (hemoglobin)
4. nucle (R)/ar (S) = pertaining to nucleus
5. splen (R)/ectomy (S) = surgical resection or removal of the spleen
6. hepato (R)/megaly (S) = enlargement of the liver
7. granulo (P)/cyte (R) = granular cell
8. blasto (R)/genesis (S) = origin of immature cell
9. hemato (R)/logist (S) = specialist in the study of blood
10. erythro (P)/cyte (R) = red blood cell

Exercise 2

1. Erythropoiesis, 2. Hypoxia, 3. Macrocytic, 4. Leukocytes, 5. Hematology, 6. Organomegaly, 7. Phagocytosis, 8. reticulocytes, 9. Hemostasis, 10. Hematophylic

Exercise 3

a. 2, b. 10, c. 8, d. 1, e. 9, f. 3, g. 4, h. 6, i. 5, j. 7

Exercise 4

1. blastocyte, 2. leukocyte, 3. phagocytosis, 4. serous, 5. basophilia, 6. hepatomegaly, 7. hematologist, 8. chromatography, 9. macrophage, 10. schistocyte

Exercise 5

1. serum, 2. plasma, 3. albumin/globulins, 4. oxyhemoglobin, 5. macrocytes/microcytes, 6. hypoxia, 7. platelets , 8. hemostasis, 9. leukocytes, 10. vascular constriction

Exercise 6

line 1: whole blood, line 2: plasma/cellular components, line 3: serum/fibrinogen/RBCs/WBCs/thrombocytes

Exercise 7

1. splen/o = spleen,enlargement of the spleen; 2. hem = blood; globin = globe (total), disease of the hemoglobin; 3. hem = blood, the destruction of red blood cells; 4. blast = immature cell or erythr = red, an abnormal decrease of red blood cell precursors; 5. thromb = blood clot; cyt = cell, an abnormal decrease in the number of platelets; 6. pigment = color, less-than-normal coloration of the skin; 7. men = menstruation, increased or excessive menstrual blood flow; 8. thromb = blood clot, blood clot; 9. vascul = blood vessel, within the blood vessel; 10. hem = blood, bleeding.

Exercise 8

1. anemia, 2. epistaxis, 3. menorrhagia, 4. occult, 5. splenomegaly, 6. polycythemia vera, 7. hemolysis, 8. erythroblastosis fetalis, 9. hematologist, 10. autoimmune disease

Exercise 9

a. 7, b. 4, c. 10, d. 2, e. 8, f. 1, g. 3, h. 9, i. 6, j. 5

Exercise 10

1. intravenous, 2. hemorrhagic, 3. thrombosis, 4. anemia, 5. morphology, 6. hypochromic, 7. macrocyte, 8. leukocytopenia, 9. granulocytosis, 10. autoimmune

Exercise 11

1. hemosiderosis – a condition of iron overload from repeated blood transfusions; 2. hemolysis – destruction of red blood cells; 3. infarction – tissue death due to insufficient blood supply; 4. hemoglobinopathy – disorder of hemoglobin (the oxygen-carrying compound in red blood cells); 5. hematologic – pertaining to study of the blood; 6. Extramedullary – outside the bone marrow; 7. Splenomegaly and hepatomegaly – enlargement of the spleen; enlargement of the liver; 8. anemia – lack of RBCs

Exercise 12

enlarged spleen	enlarged liver	pale lips, nail beds, pale inside mouth
splenomegaly	hepatomegaly	pallor
sequestered RBCs, extramedullary hematopoiesis, hemolysis	hemolysis, congestive heart failure. extramedullary hematopoiesis	anemia

Exercise 13

1. red, erythrocyte, Her erythrocyte count was low.

2. spleen, splenectomy, He was to undergo a splenectomy. 3. blood, hemoglobin, He had his hemoglobin level checked before surgery. 4. blood clot, thrombocyte, He was transfused with thrombocytes. 5. cell, cytology, The sample got a cytology workup. 6. immature cell, erythroblastosis, The fetus was diagnosed with erythroblastosis fetalis. 7. serum, serology, The serology report is back from the lab. 8. white, leukocytes, There was an increase in the number of leukocytes. 9. liver, hepatomegaly, The examination revealed a remarkable level of hepatomegaly. 10. shape, morphology, The cells had unremarkable morphology.

Exercise 14
1. plasmapheresis, 2. hematologist, 3. prothrombin time, 4. antibodies, 5. bone marrow, 6. reticulocyte, 7. CBC, 8. anticoagulant, 9. heparin, 10. streptokinase

Exercise 15
a. 5, b. 8, c. 1, d. 10, e. 9, f. 3, g. 4, h. 7, i. 2, j. 6

Exercise 16
1. prothrombin, 2. monocyte, 3. thrombolytic, 4. hematopoiesis, 5. granulocyte, 6. anticoagulant, 7. antithrombotic, 8. erythrocyte

Exercise 17
1. hematocrit, 2. hemoglobin, 3. mean corpuscular hemoglobin, 4. monocyte, 5. polymorphonuclear neutrophils, 6. prothrombin, 7. absolute neutrophil count, 8. mean corpuscular volume, 9. red blood cell, 10. segmented neutrophils

Exercise 18

Drug Class	Use
anticoagulant,	
antithrombotics	prevents clotting
	prevents clotting
thrombolytic	breaks down clots
antifibrinolytic	prevents breakdown of clot
antihemophilic factors	promotes clotting
hemostatic	promotes clotting

Generic	Brand
heparin	Heparin
warfarin sodium	Coumadin
streptokinase,	Streptase
urokinase	Abbokinase
aminocaprioic acid	Amicar
factor replacements named	Humate-P
for factor they replace	Koate,
	Konyne
desmopressin	DDAVP

Exercise 19
1. Hematology, 2. Hemophilia, 3. Thrombic, 4. Hematoma. 5. Monocyte, 6. Hematopoiesis, 7. Microcytic, 8. Splenomegaly, 9. Hypochromic, 10. Hemorrhage.

Exercise 20
Across 2. fluid 4. embolus 9. syndrome 10. pallor 12. anatomy 14. plasma 16. anemia 18. oncology 21. microcyte 22. organ 23. platelets 24. acute;
Down 1. vessels 2. fetus 3. kidney 5. hemolysis 6. purpura 7. megakaryocytes 8. transfusion 11. corpuscle 13. hemoglobin 15. leukocytes 16. agglutinate 17. enzyme 19. syndrome 20. biopsy

CHAPTER 6

Exercise 1
1. thym/o, 2. tonsil/o, 3. inguin; lymph/o, 4. splen/o, 5. lymph/o; ves/o

Exercise 2
1. mediastinum – anterior portion of the chest; 2. pharyngeal tonsils – lymphatic tissue located in the posterior wall of the nasopharynx, sometimes called adenoids; 3. palatine tonsils – lymphatic tissue located on each side of the throat; 4. spleen – organ located in the ULQ of the abdomen, behind the stomach; lymphoid – like or resembling tissue of the lymphoid system; 5. splenectomy – surgical removal of the spleen; 6. lymph node – small areas of lymphatic tissue found throughout the body; 7. macrophages – mature white blood cells of the monocyte type; 8. immunologist – specialist in the immune system; 9. antigen – substance that induces a state of sensitivity or immune response; 10. inflammatory response – nonspecific immunity that occurs when the body is damaged or when foreign organisms enter

Exercise 3
1. phagocytosis, 2. cellulitis, 3. splenectomy, 4. lymphadenopathy, 5. bacteriology, 6. autologous, 7. lymphatic, 8. thymocyte, 9. pathology, 10. histotoxic

Exercise 4
a. 4, b. 5, c. 6, d. 9, e. 1, f. 10, g. 2, h. 7, i. 3, j. 8

Exercise 5
1. histology, 2. morphology, 3. macrophage, 4. antibody, 5. lymphatic, 6. splenic, 7. neutrophil, 8. monocyte, 9. lymphocyte, 10. humoral

Exercise 6
1. Interferons interfere 2. Thymosin 3. Macrophages 4. cisterna chyli 5. chyle 6. thymus 7. palatine 8. Immunoglobulins 9. immunologist 10. immunity

Exercise 7

nonspecific immunity: <u>mechanical barriers</u> and inflammatory response; specific immunity: <u>species</u>, genetic; acquired, <u>active</u>, <u>artificial</u>; immunization stimulates body's antibody production; <u>passive</u>, maternal, <u>antibodies are received in mother's milk</u>; <u>artificial</u>, injected with antibodies

Exercise 8

1. tox = poison, study of poisons; 2. immun = immune (resistant), study of disease resistance; 3. bactr = bacteria (tiny organism), pertaining to bacteria; 4. inflame = cause to burn, decrease inflammation; 5. virus = poison (disease-causing microbe), pertaining to viruses; 6. hem = blood, erythrocyte destruction; 7. rheum = movement of fluid (rheumatism); 8. gen = create, pertaining to genes; 9. immun = immune (resistant), deficient immune response; 10. lymph = lymph (clear fluid), tumor of lymphoid tissue

Exercise 9

1. palpates, 2. immune, 3. enlarged, 4. lymphoid, 5. antibodies, 6. pernicious, 7. HIV, 8. lymphoma, 9. TB, 10 CMV

Exercise 10

a. 3, b. 10, c. 6, d. 8, e. 2, f. 9, g. 7, h. 1, i. 4, j. 5

Exercise 11

1. systemic, 2. leukocytosis, 3. lymphatic, 4. hepatitis, 5. hepatic, 6. adenitis, 7. lymphoid, 8. pharyngitis, 9. lymphectomy, 10. osteopathology

Exercise 12

1. immunologists, 2. Macrophages, 3. Involution, 4. Adenoids, 5. antigen, 6. Adenopathy, 7. leukocyte, 8. Eosinophil, 9. thymocytes, 10. thoracic

Exercise 13

box 1: cell DNA; box 2: viral RNA, box 3: viral RNA; box 4: T cell destruction, box 5: immunodeficiency, box 6: more cell invaded

Exercise 14

1. lymphoma, 2. splenectomy, 3. adenitis, 4. angioplasty, 5. immunologist, 6. monocyte, 7. cytology, 8. phagocytosis, 9. macrocyte, 10. thymic

Exercise 15

1. tonsillectomy; 2. immunologist; 3. lymphocytes; 4. pathophysiology; 5. efferent; 6. spleen; 7. autologous; 8. involution; 9. macrophages; 10. thymus

Exercise 16

a. 4, b. 6, c. 7, d. 1, e. 9, f. 4, g. 2, h. 3, i. 5, j. 8

Exercise 17

1. microbiology, 2. anemia, 3. antihistamine, 4. nodal, 5. antibiotic, 6. thymic, 7. lymphoid, 8. antiviral, 9. bacterial, 10. adenoidectomy

Exercise 18

1. monocytic, 2. tonsils, 3. adenoid, 4. correct, 5. immunity, 6. anemic, 7. retrovirus, 8. immunodeficiencies, 9. infections, 10. radiology

Exercise 19

line 1: antihistamine/antifungal, line 2: inhibits viruses/kills or inhibits fungus, line 3: bacterial infection/viral infection/fungal infection, line 4: acyclovir/diphenhydramine

CHAPTER 7

Exercise 1

1. aden/itis = inflammation of a gland; 2. adren/al = pertaining to the adrenal glands; 3. pancreat/itis = inflammation of the pancreas; 4. andr/oid = like or resembling male; 5. gluco/meter = instrument to measure glucose; 6. melano/carcinoma = cancer of pigment-producing cells; 7. thyroid/ectomy = surgical removal of the thyroid gland; 8. andro/gen/ous = pertaining to male gender *or* both genders; 9. hyper/glyc/emic = condition of excessive sugar in the blood; 10. thym/ic = pertaining to the thymus

Exercise 2

1. placenta, 2. hormones, 3. calcitonin, 4. hypothalamic, 5. testes, 6. ovaries, 7. homeostasis, 8. thymus, 9. islet, 10. cortex

Exercise 3

a. 5, b. 7, c. 10, d. 8, e. 2, f. 11, g. 1, h. 6, i. 3, j. 12, k. 9, l. 4

Exercise 4

1. antidiuretic hormone, 2. hypothalamus, 3. endocrinologist, 4. melanocyte-stimulating hormone, 5. adrenal gland, 6. pancreatic islets, 7. hyperglycemia, 8. hypercalcemia, 9. melanocyte, 10. metabolism

Exercise 5

1. Progesterone; steroid, 2. ovaries; reproductive, 3. mineralcorticoids; metabolism, 4. Melatonin; pineal, 5. islets; Langerhans; pancreas, 6. metabolic; hormones, 7. Insulin, 8. menstrual; estrogen, 9. calcium; calcitonin, 10. adrenal; cortices

Exercise 6

line 1: islets of Langerhans, line 2: beta cells / delta cells, line 3: glucagons / insulin / somatostatin

Exercise 7

3, 1, 5, 7, 2, 4, 6

Exercise 8

5, 7, 2, 6, 3, 1, 4

Exercise 9

1. hyperpituitarism, 2. polydipsia, 3. polyphagia, 4. parasthesia, 5. hyperpigmentation, 6. hypotension, 7. hyperthyroidism, 8. dyspnea, 9. hypogonadism, 10. macrosomia

Exercise 10

1. chromosomal, 2. axillary, 3. hermaphroditism, 4. dysfunction, 5. glycosuria, 6. dehydrated, 7. diuresis, 8. ketoacidosis, 9. tachycardia, 10. edematous

Exercise 11
a. 4, b. 5, c. 6, d 7, e. 1, f. 9, g. 2, h. 10, i. 8, j. 3

Exercise 12
1. atrophy, 2. lipolysis, 3. thyrotoxicosis, 4. somatotrophic, 5. adrenal medulla , 6. hyperplasia, 7. thymocyte, 8. thymoma, 9. adenocarcinoma, 10. colloid

Exercise 13
1. glucagon, 2. secretion, 3. metabolic, 4. antagonism, 5. parathormone, 6. glucocorticoid, 7. pancreas, 8. medullae, 9. ovaries, 10. progesterone, 11. ACTH, 12. IDDM

Exercise 14
box 1: medulla, box 2: corticosteroid hormones, box 3: glucocorticoids, box 4: sex hormones, box 5: epinephrine, box 6: norepinephrine

Exercise 15
1. adrenal glands, 2. gland, 3. thyroid, 4. cortex (outer), 5. ketones, 6. sweetness or sugar; glucose, 7. relationship to the body, 8. gonads or reproductive organs, 9. stretching or tone

Exercise 16
1. disease in populations due to a deficiency of iodine; 2. low or insufficient sodium (salt) in the blood; 3. low or insufficient potassium in the blood; 4. mineral salts in the body; 5. cavity in the skull that holds the pituitary gland; 6. a female hormone produced by the ovaries; 7. thyroid stimulating hormone; 8. "Adam's apple," the cartilage that covers the larynx; 9. hormone that causes contraction of the gallbladder and release of bile; 10. hormone that stimulates secretion of gastric acid and stomach enzymes for digestion

Exercise 17
a. 3, b. 6, c. 9, d. 8, e. 1, f. 7, g. 10, h. 4, i. 5, j. 2

Exercise 18
1. endocrinopathy, 2. melanocyte, 3. lipolysis, 4. pancreatic, 5. hypothyroidism, 6. hypercalcemia, 7. antidiabetic agent, 8. parathyroid, 9. dyspnea, 10. hyperpnea, 11. hyperkalemia, 12. glucosuria

Exercise 19
1. thyrotropin-releasing hormone, 2. radioimmunoassay, 3. triiodothyronine, 4. thyroxine, 5. prolactin-inhibiting hormone, 6. potassium, 7. luteinizing hormone, 8. postprandial, 9. fasting blood sugar, 10. glucose tolerance test

Exercise 20
line 1: hyperglycemia/hypoglycemia; line 2: polyuria, polydipsia, and weight loss/sweating, palpitations, hunger, tachycardia, headache; line 3: insulin/eat food, usually sugar

CHAPTER 8

Exercise 1
alges/i, cephalagia; electr/o, electroencephalogram; kinesi/o, kinetic; myel/o myelitis; neur/o, nervous; cephal, encephalitis; crani/o craniotomy, gli/o, neuroglia; cyt/o, astrocyte; somat/o somatic

Exercise 2
1. neurologist, 2. electroencephalogram, 3. meningitis, 4. ganglioneuroma, 5. astrocytes, 6. autonomic, 7. dendrites, 8. cerebrospinal, 9. axon, 10. innervated

Exercise 3
1. astrocyte, 2. olfactory, 3. cerebrum, 4. neurologist, 5. hemiplegia, 6. temporal, 7. cerebrospinal, 9. autonomic nervous system, 10. meninges

Exercise 4
1. dyskinesic, 2. astrocyte, 3. neurotomy, 4. intracranial, 5. cephalic, 6. meningitis, 7. glioma, 8. somatic, 9. ganglioma, 10. myeloplasty

Exercise 5
1. myelin–fatty sheath that surrounds, protects, and maintains axons of neurons; 2. cerebellar–pertaining to the cerebellum, which helps coordinate voluntary movements and maintains balance and posture; 3. craniotomy–surgical incision into the cranium (skull); 4. axons–part of a neuron that conducts nerve impulses between neurons; 5. encephalopathy–disease of the brain; 6. dendrites–portion of the neuron that receives information from other neurons and sensory cells; 7. neurotransmitter–chemical in the nervous system that carries a signal across the synapse; 8. acetylcholine–a neurotransmitter located at synapses in the spinal cord and in the junction between nerves and muscles; 9. parasympathetic nervous system–division of the autonomic nervous system; slows heartbeat, lowers blood pressure, contracts eye pupils of the eye, and stimulates movements of the digestive tract; 10. medulla oblongata–portion of the brainstem that connects the spinal cord with the brain

Exercise 6
line 1: central nervous system/peripheral nervous system; line 2: somatic nervous system/autonomic nervous system; line 3: sympathetic nervous system/parasympathetic

Exercise 7
1. neur = nerve; 2. cephal = head to foot; 3. mening = outpouching of the membrane covering brain and spine; 4. cerebr = cerebrum of brain, vascul = vessel, blood vessels of the brain; 5. myel = spinal cord, loss of insulating material between nerves; 6. taxis = order, disorderly movement; 7. cephal = head, brain, without a brain; 8. troph = nutrition, changes of size or development, 9. aisthesis = sensation, altered sensation; 10. neur = nerve, relating to nerves

Exercise 8
1. nerves, 2. ventricles, 3. reflexes, 4. cortices, 5. dystrophies, 6. tremor, 7. aurae, 8. attack, 9. synapses, 10. seizures

Exercise 9
a. 9, b. 12, c. 6, d. 16, e. 19, f. 23, g. 2, h. 26, i. 18, j. 5

Exercise 10
1. dermatomes, 2. glossopharyngeal nerve, 3. plantar reflex, 4. infantile automatisms, 5. plantar grasp reflex, 6. spinal, 7. senile tremors, 8. petit mal seizure, 9. spastic paraplegia, 10. athetosis

Exercise 11
1. flaccid quadriplegia; 2. palsy; 3. decorticate; 4. ataxia, aphasia; 5. cerebrovascular accident; 6. epilepsy, postictal; 7. dysphagia, CVA; 8. multiple sclerosis; 9. spina bifida 10. anencephalic

Exercise 12
line 1: preictal/ictal/postictal; line 2: aura

Exercise 13
1. acrophobia, 2. agoraphobia, 3. claustrophobia, 4. hemophobia, 5. allodoxaphobia, 6. xenophobia, 7. thermophobia, 8. entomophobia, 9. astraphobia, 10. radiophobia

Exercise 14
1. ADHD, 2. acrophobia, 3. affective disorders, 4. mania and depression, 5. neurosis, 6. Phobia, 7. bulemia nervosa, 8. psychiatrist, 9. claustrophobia, 10. post-traumatic stress syndrome, 11. schizophrenia, 12. psychosis

Exercise 15
1. crani/o, skull; 2. neur/o, nerves; 3. rhiz/o, root; 4. lob-, lobe; 5. ventricul/o, ventricle; 6. radic-, root; 7. tom/o, section; 8. chord/o, spinal cord

Exercise 16
1. CAT, 2. Romberg, 3. cerebrospinal, 4. EEG, 5. brain scan, 6. chordotomy, 7. ventriculotomy, 8. neuroplasty, 9. anticonvulsants, 10. stimulants

Exercise 17
1. amyotrophic lateral sclerosis, 2. central nervous system, 3. deep tendon reflex, 4. cerebrospinal fluid, 5. multiple sclerosis, 6. peripheral nervous system, 7. magnetic resonance imaging, 8. lumbar puncture, 9. electroencephalogram, 10. transient ischemic attack

Exercise 18
1. cerebrovascular, 2. electroencephalogram, 3. lumbosacral, 4. neuromuscular, 5. neurosensory, 6. ataxia, 7. kinesiology, 8. intracranial, 9. encephalopathy, 10. neuroglioma, 11. cerebellar, 12. sacral

Exercise 19
1. P/seizure, 2. S/palsies, 3. S/dermatomes, 4. P/neuroplasty, 5. S/ventriculotomies, 6. S/barbiturates, 7. P/amphetamine, 8. S/anticonvulsants, 9. P/neurotransmitter, 10. P/neurologist

Exercise 20
hemiplegia: paralyzed arm and leg; paraplegia: paralyzed legs; spastic paraplegia: partially paralyzed legs; hemiparesis: partially paralyzed arm and leg; quadraplegia: paralyzed legs and arms; paraparesis: partially paralyzed legs

Chapter 9

Exercise 1
1. ophthal/o, ophthalmology; 2. palpebr/o (or blephar/o), blepharitis; 3. lacrim/o (or dacry/o), lacrimoma; 4. corne/o (or kerat/o), corneoplasty; 5. conjunctiv/o, conjunctivitis; 6. irid/o, iridectomy; 7. corne/o (or kerat/o), corneal; 8. palpebr/o (or blephar/o), palpebral; 9. phot/o, photophobia; 10. retin/o, retinitis

Exercise 2
1. palpebrae, 2. nasolacrimal, 3. Extraocular, 4. retina, 5. refracted, 6. Vitreous, 7. sclera, 8. optometrist, 9. limbus, 10. iris

Exercise 3
1. extraocular, 2. periorbital, 3. conjunctivitis, 4. intraocular, 5. corneal, 6. retinitis, 7. epicanthic, 8. pupillography, 9. funduscope, 10. Ophthalmalgia

Exercise 4
1. ophthalmoscope, 2. ophthalmology, 3. corneal, 4. orbital, 5. pupillary, 6. iritis, 7. blepharitis, 8. macular, 9. blepharal, 10. phacoectomy

Exercise 5
1. Vision, 2. lenses, 3. ophthalmologist, 4. Laser, 5. optician

Exercise 6
See Figure 9.1

Exercise 7
1. iridectomy, pertaining to the iris; 2. keratotomy, pertaining to the cornea; 3. blepharoptosis, pertaining to the eyelid; 4. ophthalmoscope, pertaining to the eye; 5. keratitis, pertaining to the cornea; 6. Cataracts, pertaining to a waterfall; 7. lacrimotomy, pertaining to tears; 8. phacoerysis, pertaining to the lens; 9. macular, pertaining to the macula; 10. scleritis, pertaining to the sclera

Exercise 8
1. glaucoma, 2. chalazion, 3. ophthalmologists, 4. retinoblastoma, 5. esophoria, 6. presbyopia, 7. sty, 8. esotropia, 9. astigmatism, 10. hyperopia

Exercise 9
a. 9, b. 5, c. 8, d. 3, e. 1, f. 10, g. 7, h. 6, i. 4, j. 2

Exercise 10
1. blepharopexy, 2. blepharoptosis, 3. ophthalmic, 4. iritis, 5. keratomy

Exercise 11
1. keratoplasty–surgical repair of the cornea; 2. ophthalmologist–specialist in diagnosis and treatment of eye disorders; 3. myopia– difficulty seeing distant objects; 4. conjunctivitis–inflammation of the conjunctiva; 5. vitreous–thick, clear, jellylike substance within the eyeball; 6. retinitis–inflammation of the retina, 7. diplopia–double vision; 8. cataract–clouding of the lens of the eye

Exercise 12
light stimulus, cornea, retina, fovea centralis, optic nerve, visual cortex of brain

Exercise 13
1. blepharo, eyelid, repair of the eyelid; 2. palpebr/o, eyelid, pertaining to the eyelid; 3. retin-, retina, inflammation of the retina; 4. ophthalm/o, the eye, a device for viewing the interior of the eye; 5. lacrim-. tears, pertaining to the tears; 6. ophthalm/o, the eye, a physician who specializes in diseases of the eye; 7. ocul-, the eye, within the eye; 8. irid/o, the iris, paralysis of iris muscle; 9. choroid, the middle layer of eyeball tissue, inflammation of the choroid; 10. vitre clear fluid of the eye, removal of the vitreous humor

Exercise 14
1. ophthalmologist, 2. retina, 3. keratoplasty, 4. tonometry, 5. vitreous humor, 6. optic nerve, 7. conjunctivitis, 8. retinal, 9. limbus, 10. fundus

Exercise 15
a. 2, b. 8, c. 6, d. 7, e. 2, f. 1, g. 4, h. 5, i. 3, j. 3

Exercise 16
1. ocul-ar, 2. intra-ocul-ar, 3. conjunctiv-itis, 4. scler-al, 5. peri-orbit-al, 6. retino-pathy, 7. lacrima-tion, 8. kerat-itis, 9. tono-metry, 10. kerato-mileusis

Exercise 17
1. cataracts, 2. palpebrae, 3. sclerae, 4. sties or styes, 5. retinopathies, 6. maculae, 7. irides, 8. limbi, 9. canthi, 10. singular is chalazion

Exercise 18
line 1: double vision; line 2: myopia, hyperopia; line 4: esotropia or esophoria, exotropia or exophoria, amblyopia

Exercise 19
1. tympan (R) /o (CV) /scler (R) /osis (S), hardening of the tympanic membrane; 2. peri (P) /auricul (R) /ar (S), around the external ear; 3. oto (R) /scope (S), device for viewing the inside of the ear; 4. bi (P) /aur (R) /al (S), pertaining to both ears; 5. end (P) / o (CV) / lymphat (R) /ic (S), pertaining to the endolymph; 6. ossi (R) / cle (S), one of the bones of the ear; 7. myring (R) / o (CV) / tomy (S), surgical incision into the tympanic membrane; 8. tub (R) / o (CV) / tympan (R) / ic (S), pertaining to the eustachian tube and tympanic membrane; 9. labyrinth (R) / itis (S), inflammation of the labyrinth; 10. post (P) /auricul (R) / ar (S), behind the ear

Exercise 20
a. 10, b. 5, c. 9, d. 3, e. 8, f. 4, g. 2, h. 7, i. 1, j. 6

Exercise 21
1. otoscope, 2. saccule, 3. tympanic, 4. periauricular, 5. vestibular, 6. perilymph, 7. fenestra ovalis, 8. nasopharynx, 9. otorhinolaryngologist, 10. ceruminolytic

Exercise 22
1. prescription, 2. labyrinth/endolymph, 3. auditory, 4. canals/vestibule, 5. cochlea, 6. myringotomy

Exercise 23
1. auricle or pinna: outer ear; 2. auditory meatus: opening of ear canal; 3. tympanic membrane: eardrum at end of outer ear canal; 4. eustachian tube: tube leading into throat; 5. ossicular chain: malleus, incus, stapes; 6. cochlea: spiral-shaped structure in inner ear

Exercise 24
1. ot/o, ear, inflammation of the middle ear; 2. myring/o, tympanic membrane, incision into the tympanic membrane; 3. osse/o, bones of the middle ear, pertaining to the ossicles; 4. labyrinth, structure of the inner ear, removal of the labyrinth; 5. tympan, the tympanic membrane, a tube that opens the middle ear to the external ear; 6. auricul, the ear, a skin tab anterior to the external ear; 7. canal, external auditory canal, repair of the external auditory canal; 8. cochle, pertaining to the cochlea, a measurement of electrical potentials; 9. fenestra, an opening, making an opening; 10. staped, stirrup-shaped, a breaking apart of the stapes

Exercise 25
1. tympanectomy, 2. AD, 3. Vestibular, 4. Neuroplasty, 5. tinnitis, 6. myringotomy, 7. otoscope, 8. Rinne's, 9. media, 10. cochlear

Exercise 26
1. Meniere's disease, 2. cholesteatoma, 3. tinnitus, 4. audiometry, 5. otoscopy, 6. tympanectomy

Exercise 27
1. oto-logy, 2. an-ot-ia, 3. labyrinth-itis, 4. mastoid-ectomy, 5. oto-rrhagia

Exercise 28
1. auricle, 2. cochlea, 3. endolymph, 4. meatus, 5. ossicle, 6. saccule, 7. tragus, 8. vestibule

Exercise 29
line 1: external auditory meatus, tympanic membrane; line 2: ossicular chain, oval window; line 3: auditory nerve, brain

Exercise 29
1. olfactory bulb, 2. gustatory, 3. dysgeusia, 4. osmesis, 5. anosmia, 6. proprioception, 7. Meissner's corpuscle, 8. olfactory

Chapter 10

Exercise 1
1. pulmon/ary, relating to the respiratory system; 2. aero/phagia, air eating; 3. pneumon/itis, inflammation of the respiratory system; 4. bronch/i/ole, an airway smaller than a bronchus; 5. trache/ostomy, a cut into the trachea; 6. rhino/rrhea, (mucus) flowing from the nose; 7. dys/phonia, difficulty creating sound; 8. pharyng/eal, relating to the throat; 9. thorac/o/tomy, surgical incision into the chest; 10. laryngo/scope, a device of visualizing the larynx; 11. oxygen/a/tion, supplying with oxygen; 12. alveoli/ar, relating to alveoli

Exercise 2
1. epiglottis 2. nasal 3. pleuritis 4. apnea 5. pulmonologist, 6. alveolitis 7. intercostal 8. exhaled 9. apex 10. Surfactant

Exercise 3
1. diffusion 2. carbon dioxide 3. apex 4. trachea 5. nasal septum 6. larynx 7. intercostal 8. nose, mouth 9. pleura 10. thoracic

Exercise 4
1. hypercapnea 2. bronchiolitis 3. nasopharynx 4. bronchial 5. paranasal 6. cartilaginous 7. epiglottal 8. bronchial 9. inhalation 10. hypoxia

Exercise 5
1. cilia, respiratory; 2. pharynx, 3. larynx, cartilage; 4. bronchi, respiratory; 5. apex; 6. exhaled, expiration; 7. intercostals, 8. diaphragm, thoracic; 9. surfactant, alveoli, 10. diffusion

Exercise 6
line 1: trachea; line 2: primary bronchi; line 3: bronchioles; line 4: alveoli

Exercise 7
Upper: nares, oropharynx, trachea, superior concha; Lower: bronchioles, alveoli; Not in the respiratory tract: astrocyte, myelin sheath, neurilemma

Exercise 8
1. steth = chest, device to examine (by listening to) the chest; 2. cyan = blue, condition of blue skin; 3. pne = breath, able to breath best in an upright position; 4. pne = breath, breathing fast; 5. glottis = mouth of windpipe, structure that closes trachea when swallowing; 6. pulmon = lung, relating to the lungs and air exchange; 7 pneum = lungs, air blocking the lungs from inflation; 8. sinus = hollow, inflammation of the sinuses; 9. tubercul = tubercle, disease that forms tubercles; 10. bronchiol = bronchiole, inflammation of the bronchioles

Exercise 9
1. fibrosis, 2. RSV, 3. URI, 4. emphysema, 5. COPD, 6. asthma, 7. IRDS, 8. Aspiration, 9. Atelectasis, 10. Pleurisy

Exercise 10
a. 5, b. 7, c. 10, d. 1, e. 9, f. 2, g. 3, h. 4, i. 6, j. 8

Exercise 11
1. rhinitis, 2. tracheotomy, 3. thoracoplasty, 4. thoracoscopy, 5. laryngeal, 6. pleuritis, 7. apnea, 8. bronchitis, 9. pneumonectomy, 10. bronchocele

Exercise 12
1. P/bronchus, 2. P/alveolus, 3. S/lungs, 4. S/pulmonectomies, 5. S/diaphragms, 6. P/cilium, 7. S/pleurae, 8. S/capillaries, 9. S/sinuses, 10. P/tonsil

Exercise 13
dys/pnea, eu/pnea, tachy/pnea, brady/pnea, ortho/pnea, hyper/pnea, hypo/pnea

Exercise 14
Fetus/infant children: cystic fibrosis, respiratory syncytial virus, croup, acute epiglottitis, IRDS; seniors bronchogenic carcinoma, emphysema, chronic obstructive lung disease, bronchitis

Exercise 15
1. bronch-ioles, small airways; 2. laryngo-scope, a device to examine the larynx; 3. nas-al, pertaining to the nares (nose); 4. pulmon-o-log-ist, a person who studies the pulmonary system; 5. spir-o-metry, measurement of respiratory volumes; 6. rhin-itis, inflammation of the nose; 7. thora-cost-omy, a surgical cutting into the thorax and costal muscles; 8. tracheo-bronch-itis, an inflammation of the trachea and bronchioles; 9. tubercu-lar, relating to tubercles or tuberculosis; 10. pleur-itis, inflammation of the pleural menbranes

Exercise 16
1. COPD, 2. antitussive, 3. antipyretic, 4. Intubation, 5. ventilation, 6. Antibiotic, 7. decongestant, 8. tidal volume, 9. ibuprofen, 10. DNR

Exercise 17
a. 4, b. 10, c. 7, d. 1, e. 9, f. 6, g. 5, h. 3, i. 8, j. 2

Exercise 18
1. fibrosis, 2. laryngotracheobronchitis, 3. dyspnea, 4. respiratory, 5. bronchiectasis, 6. cystic, 7. laryngoscope, 8. lobectomy, 9. laryngotomy, 10. intubation, 11. pharyngeal, 12. thoracentesis

Exercise 19
1. organism, 2, correct, 3. airway, 4. gaseous, 5. viruses, 6. tissue, 7. inhalation, 8. correct, 9. correct, 10. pathogen

Exercise 20
Diagnostic: bronchoscopy, laryngoscopy, endoscopy, spirometry, pulmonary function tests; Therapeutic: lobectomy, intubation, thoracentesis, lobotomy, thoracotomy, tracheostomy, laryngectomy, laryngotomy, rhinoplasty

Chapter 11

Exercise 1
1. aorta = main artery at top, aort/o; 2. atrium = either of two upper chambers, atri/o; 3. ventricle = either of two lower chambers, ventricul/o; 4. septum = divider between halves of heart, sept/o; 5. epicardium = outer membrane covering heart, cardi/o; 6. endocardium = membrane lining cavities of heart, cardi/o; 7. pulmonary veins = red tubular structures, ven/o or phleb/o; 8. pulmonary artery = blue tubular structure, arteri/o

Exercise 2
1. cardiology, 2. thoracic, 3. vascular, 4. visceral, 5. endocardium, 6. septum, 7. systole, 8. tricuspid, 9. pulmonary, 10. systolic

Exercise 3
9, 7, 4, 5, 1, 8, 10, 3, 6, 2

Exercise 4

1. thrombosis, 2. carditis, 3. chordectomy, 4. cardiomyopathy, 5. cardiology, 6. atrioventricular, 7. pericardium, 8. endocarditis, 9. cardiopulmonary, 10. circulatory

Exercise 5

1. P/apex, 2. P/valve, 3. P/vena cava, 4. P/artery, 5. S/capillaries, 6. P/pulse, 7. P/ventricle, 8. P/septum, 9. P/lumen, 10. S/veins

Exercise 6

on left–box 1: tricuspid valve; box 2: pulmonary valve; box 3: mitral or bicuspid valve; box 4: aortic valve; on right—box 1: epicardium; box 2: endocardium; box 3: myocardium

Exercise 7

1. steth (R) /o (CV)/ scope (S) = instrument for listening to the chest; 2. peri (P) / card (R) /itis(S) = inflammation of the covering of the heart; 3. pulmon (R) / ic (S) = relating to the lung; 4. sten (R) /osis (S) = condition of narrowing, 5. ventricul (R) /ar (S) = relating to the ventricle; 6. arteri (R) / o (CV) scler (R)/osis (S) = condition of hardening of the artery; 7. my (R) / o (CV) cardi (R) /al (S) = relating to heart muscle; 8. tachy (P) / cardi (R) / ia (S) = fast heart rate; 9. cardi (R) /o (CV) meg (R) /a (CV) ly (S) = pertaining to a large heart; 10. endo (P) /cardi (R) / itis (S) = inflammation of the lining of the heart

Exercise 8

1. aneurysm, 2. palpitations, 3. infarction, 4. ectopic, 5. congestive, 6. clubbing, 7. heart block, 8. angina, 9. arrhythmias, 10. ischemia; ventricle

Exercise 9

9, 12, 7, 11, 8, 1, 2, 6, 3, 4, 10, 5

Exercise 10

1. cardiologist, 2. bradycardia, 3. myocardial, 4. stenosis, 5. sclerosis, 6. angiogram, 7. cardiogram, 8. cardiography, 9. pericardial, 10. endocardium

Exercise 11

1. endocarditis, 2. hypertension, 3. embolism, 4. myocardial, 5. bradycardia, 6. cardiomegaly, 7. arteriosclerosis, 8. thrombosis, 9. hyperlipidemia, 10. vasospasm

Exercise 12

1. mitral, tricuspid, pulmonic, aortic; 2. stenosis, regurgitation; 3. tricuspid: stenosis—calcification impedes blood flow into right ventricle during diastole; regurgitation—backflow of blood into right atrium; pulmonic valve: regurgitation—backflow of blood from pulmonary artery into right ventricle; stenosis—calcification restricts forward blood flow; mitral/bicuspid valve: regurgitation—backflow of blood into left ventricle; stenosis—calcification prevents proper opening of valve; aortic valve: stenosis—valve cusps restrict blood flow during systole; regurgitation—backflow of blood from aorta into left ventricle during diastole

Exercise 13

1. angi (R)-o (CV)-plasty (S), repair of a vessel; 2. cardi (R)-o (CV)-logy (S), study of the heart; 3. arteri (R)-o (CV)-gram (S), image of an artery; 4. vascul (R)-ar (S), pertaining to vessels; 5. phleb (R)-itis (S), inflammation of a blood vessel; 6. thromb (R)-osis (S), condition of a clot; 7. ven (R)-ule (S), a small vein; 8. sept (R)-al (S), relatinfg to the septum; 9. atri (R)-al (S), relating to an atria; 10. ventricul (R)-ar (S), relating to a ventricle

Exercise 14

1. inferior vena cava; 2. vasospasm; 3. lipid; 4. cardiac catheterization; 5. PTCA: percutaneous transluminal angioplasty; 6. echocardiography; 7. CABG: coronary artery bypass graft; 8. serum cholesterol; 9. serum triglycerides; 10. beta blocker

Exercise 15

a. 4, b. 1, c. 5, d. 7, e. 10, f. 9, g. 3, h. 2, i. 8, j. 6

Exercise 16

1. cardiology, 2. cardiologist, 3. electrocardiogram, 4. ventricular, 5. atrial, 6. aortic, 7. anticoagulant, 8. antihypertensive, 9. antianginal, 10. angiectomy

Exercise 17

1. S/bruits, 2. S/ventricles, 3. S/arteries, 4. S/atria, 5. S/veins, 6. S/venae cavae, 7. S/occlusions, 8. S/angioplasties, 9. S/bypasses, 10. S/diuretics

Exercise 18

1. cholesterol, 2. high-density lipids, 3. low-density lipids, 4. triglycerides
1. electrocardiogram, 2. echocardiogram; angiogram/cardiac catheterization/CCC/ balloon angioplasty/percutaneous transluminal coronary angioplasty/PTCA

Chapter 12

Exercise 1

1. col (R) / itis (S): inflammation of the colon; 2. gastr (R) / o (CV) / scopy (S): examination of the stomach through an instrument; 3. duoden (R) / al (S): pertaining to the duodenum; 4. enter (R) / itis (S): inflammation of the intestines; 5. chole (R) /cysto (R) / kinin (S): hormone secreted by the mucosa in the lining of the duodenum; 6. hepat (R) / o (CV) / megaly (S): enlargement of the liver; 7. lapar (R) / o (CV) / scopy (S): examination of the abdomen through an instrument; 8. pancreat (R) / ic (S): pertaining to the pancreas; 9. pylor (R) / o (CV) / plasty (S): surgical repair of the pylorus; 10. proct (R) / o (CV) / logist (S): one who specializes in the study of the rectum; 11. sigmoid (R) / o (CV) / scopy (S): examination of the sigmoid colon through an instrument; 12. splen (R) / ectomy (S): surgical removal of the spleen

Exercise 2

1. cardiac sphincter, 2. fundus, 3. hydrochloric, 4. ileum, 5. peristalsis, 6. hepatic, 7. parietal, 8. amylase, 9. amino acids, 10. gastroenterology, 11. chyme, 12. esophagus

Exercise 3
a. 5, b. 9, c. 6, d. 7, e. 1, f. 10, g. 11, h. 3, i. 2, j. 12, k. 8, l. 4

Exercise 4
1. colitis, 2. duodenal, 3. gastrectomy, 4. hypogastric, 5. pancreatic, 6. splenectomy, 7. hepatic, 8. glossopharyngeal, 9. proctology, 10. sigmoidoscopy

Exercise 5
1. gastrointestinal, gastroenterology; 2. alimentary; 3. salivary; 4. deciduous; 5. stomach, rugae; 6. lacteal; 7. pancreas; 8. Cholecystokinin, mucosa, duodenum; 9. vermiform appendix, appendix; 10. visceral peritoneum

Exercise 6
missing terms: esophagus, stomach, duodenum, jejunum, ileum, cecum, ascending colon, transverse colon, descending colon, sigmoid colon, rectum

Exercise 7
1. gastr/o = stomach, inflammation of the stomach lining; 2. col/o = colon, visualization of the colon; 3. gloss/o = tongue, absence of the tongue; 4. sten/o = narrowing, condition of narrowing; 5. pancreat/o = pancreas, removal of the pancreas; 6. chol/o = bile, presence of gallstones; 7. lip/o = fat, high level of lipids in the blood; 8. hepat/o = liver, inflammation of the liver; 9. gingiv/o = gums, pertaining to the gums; 10. stom/a = mouth or opening, inflammation of the lining of the mouth

Exercise 8
1. umbilical, 2. hypogastric, 3. intussusception, 4. cystic fibrosis, 5. T-E fistula, pyloric stenosis, 6. ulceration; gastric mucosa, 7. cholelithiasis, 8. postanesthesia, hyperemesis, 9. appendectomy, 10. hernioplasty; neonatal

Exercise 9
10, 7, 9, 6, 1, 8, 2, 3, 4, 5

Exercise 10
1. suprapubic, 2. hypogastric, 3. epigastric, 4. hepatitis, 5. colitis, 6. diarrhea, 7. cholecystitis, 8. appendicitis, 9. aglossia, 10. tracheoesophageal

Exercise 11
1. diverticula, 2. polyps, 3. polypectomy, 4. quadrants, 5. livers, 6. gastroenterologists, 7. proteins, 8. hernioplasties, 9. ducts, 10. villi

Exercise 12
Stomach: gastric ulcer, heartburn, hiatal hernia; Intestines: constipation, diverticulitis, inguinal hernia, intussusception, umbilical hernia; Rectum/Anus: hemorrhoids

Exercise 13
1. cholecyst-, gallbladder, removal of the gallbladder; 2. gastr-, stomach, removal of the stomach; 3. den-, teeth, pertaining to the teeth; 4. sigmoid-, sigmoid colon, visualization of the sigmoid colon; 5. proct-, rectum, inflammation of the rectum; 6. ile-, ileum, opening from the ileum to the outside; 7. col-, colon, inflammation of the colon; 8. pharyng, pharynx, inflammation of the pharynx; 9. enter-, intestine, pertaining to the intestine; 10. lithi- stone, condition of stones

Exercise 14
1. pancreas, 2. glucose, 3. cholangiogram, 4. GI series, 5. endoscopy, 6. GERD, 7. URQ, 8. hyperalimentation, 9. TPN, 10. postprandial

Exercise 15
a. 4, b. 9, c. 10, d. 7, e. 8, f. 2, g. 5, h. 1, i. 3, j. 6

Exercise 16
1. cholecystectomy, 2. cholecystitis, 3. cholangiography, 4. colonoscopy, 5. colostomy, 6. gastrectomy, 7. gastroscopy, 8. proctoscopy, 9. ileostomy, 10. endoscope, 11. gastrotomy, 12. appendectomy

Exercise 17
1. after meals, 2. hydrochloric acid, 3. neonatal necrotizing enterocolitis, 4. nausea and vomiting, 5. barium enema, 6. gallbladder, 7. right lower quadrant, 8. upper gastrointestinal, 9. left lower quadrant, 10. hyperalimentation

Exercise 18
Procedures (top to bottom): none, esophagoscopy, gastroscopy, endoscopy, colonoscopy, sigmoidoscopy, proctoscopy; Diseases (top to bottom): gingivitis, esophagitis, gastritis, ileitis, diverticulitis, polyposis, hemorrhoids

Chapter 13

Exercise 1
1. cysto-, bladder, removal of the bladder; 2. ren-, kidney, pertaining to the kidney; 3. ureter-, ureter, removal of the ureter; 4. urethr-, urethra, inflammation of the urethra; 5. nephr-, kidney, removal of the kidney; 6. uro-, urine, specialist of the urinary system; 7. urin-, urine, pertaining to the urinary system; 8. medull-, middle, pertaining to the medulla; 9. tubul-, tubes, pertiaining to the tubules; 10. nephr, kidney, inflammation of the kidney

Exercise 2
1. urethra, 2. glomerulus, 3. nephron, 4. tubules, 5. nephritis, 6. cortex, 7. renal pelvis, 8. pyelonephritis, 9. urine, 10. urea

Exercise 3
a. 5, b. 7, c. 4, d. 1, e. 6, f. 2, g. 3, h. 10, i. 8, j. 9

Exercise 4
1. pyelitis, 2. nephroectomy, 3. renal, 4. genitourinal, 5. cystitis, 6. urinal, 7. urethritis, 8. tubular, 9. meatal, 10. lithosis

Exercise 5
1. morphology, medulla, 2. renal pelvis, 3. cystoscopy, performed, 4. intravenous pyelogram, 5. Bowman's capsule, 6. renal tubular, 7. urinary meatus, 8. creatinine, 9. Henle, 10. peritubular capillaries

Exercise 6
ureter, urine, bladder, urine, urethra, filtration unit: nephron; composed of renal corpuscle and renal tubule

Exercise 7
1. urine, pyuria; 2. stone, lithiasis; 3. kidney, nephrology; 4. bladder, cystitis; 5. tube that passes urine from the bladder to the outside, urethritis; 6. pertaining to a tube, tubular; 7. nearer to the point of origin or attachment, proximal; 8. tube from kidney to bladder, ureterectomy; 9. inner substance, medullary; 10. opening, meatal

Exercise 8
1. P/nephrons, 2. P, 3. P/tubules, 4. P/ureters, 5. P/urologists, 6. P/calculi, 7. S/protein, 8. P, 9. S, 10. S/urethra

Exercise 9
5, 10, 9, 8, 1, 7, 6, 2, 4, 3

Exercise 10
1. ureteritis, 2. pyuria, 3. urethritis, 4. pyelonephritis, 5. nephritis, 6. hypercalciuria, 7. glomerulonephritis, 8. cystitis, 9. urinary, 10. renal

Exercise 11
1. pyuria, pus in the urine; 2. hematuria, blood in the urine; proteinuria, protein in the urine; 3. systemic lupus erythematosus, an autoimmune disorder; 4. enuresis, bedwetting; 5. capillary, tiny blood vessel; glomerulus, capillary loops in Bowman's capsule; 6. nephrotic, condition of the kidney; glomerulonephritis, inflammation of the glomerulus; 7. bacterial, relating to bacteria; urinary, relating to the urinary system; 8. reabsorption, draw water back from urine; 9. edema, swelling from water retention; 10. incontinence, inability to control bladder

Exercise 12
missing items: urinary bladder, ureter, kidney, renal disease: nephritis

Exercise 13
1. kidney, nephritis; 2. urine, oliguria; 3. kidney, renogram; 4. glomerulus, glomerulonephritis; 5. pus, pyuria; 6. bladder, cystectomy; 7. urethra, urethrotomy, 8. ureter, ureterectomy; 9. stone, lithotripsy

Exercise 14
1. nephr, kidney, a kidney specialist; 2. urin, urine, pertaining to urine; 3. ren, kidney, pertaining to the kidney; 4. glomeru, glomerulus, pertaining to the glomerulus; 5. cyst, bladder, inflammation of the bladder; 6. urethr, urethra, removal of the urethra; 7. cyst, bladder, visualizing the inside of the bladder; 8. uri, urine, no urine output; 9. uri, urine, little urine output; 10. nephr, kidney, a condition of the kidney

Exercise 15
1. nephrectomy, 2. cystectomy, 3. peritoneal dialysis, 4. hemodialysis, 5. cystoscope, 6. glomerular filteration rate, 7. cystopexy, 8. catheter, 9. creatinine clearance test 10. diuretic

Exercise 16
1. kidneys, ureters and bladder, 2. magnetic resonance imaging, 3. blood urea nitrogen, 4. glomerular filtration rate, 5. intravenous pyelogram, 6. extracorporeal shock-wave lithotripsy, 7. urinalysis, 8. urinary tract infection, 9. benign prostatic hyperplasia, 10. peritoneal dialysis

Exercise 17
1. ureteroplasty, 2. cystectomy, 3. nephrectomy, 4. cystocele, 5. lithotripsy, 6. ureterostomy, 7. cystotomy, 8. cystoscopy, 9. urinalysis, 10. nephrostomy, 11. ureterotomy, 12. hemodialysis

Exercise 18
1. P/cystectomy, 2. P/glomerulus, 3. P/catheterization, 4. S/urinalyses, 5. S/analgesics, 6. S/diuretics, 7. S/lithotripsies, 8. S/calculi, 9. S/kidneys, 10. P/membrane

Exercise 19
Procedure: Hemodialysis; Equipment: dialysis machine; blood from patient, fluid bath (membrane) fluid bath, blood to patient

Chapter 14

Exercise 1
1. orchi (R) / o (CV) / cele (S): hernia of a testicle,
2. spermat (R) / ic (S): pertaining to sperm,
3. andro (R) / gen (R) /ous (S): giving birth to males,
4. balan (R) / o (CV) / plasty (S): surgical repair of the glans penis,
5. gonad (R) / al (S): pertaining to the gonads,
6. prostat (R) / ectomy (S): removal of the prostate,
7. gamet (R) / o (CV) / cyte (S): gamete (ovum or sperm),
8. testic (R) / ular (S): relating to the testicle,
9. spermato (R) / gen (R) /esis (S): production of sperm,
10. zygo (R) / te (S): pertaining to a zygote

Exercise 2
1. prostate; 2. zygote; 3. gametes; 4. urologist; 5. scrotum; 6. glans penis; 7. spermatic; 8. ejaculation; 9. mitochondrial; 10. epididymis

Exercise 3
a. 2, b. 4, c. 7, d. 12, e. 8, f. 9, g. 3, h. 10, i. 6, j. 1, k. 5, l. 11

Exercise 4
1. spermoid, 2. oligospermia, 3. orchiopexy, 4. epididymectomy, 5. anorchia, 6. cryptorchidism, 7. prostatitis, 8. vasectomy, 9. prostatectomy, 10. seminoma

Exercise 5
1. gametes, 2. zygote, 3. glans penis, 4. lumen, 5. epididymis, 6. seminal vesicles, 7. Cowper's glands, 8. ejaculation, 9. urologist, 10. gonads

Exercise 6
testes, epididymis, vas deferens, seminal vessicles, prostate gland, urethra

Exercise 7

1. crypt (P) / orch (R) / ism (S), undecended testicles;
2. poly (P) / orch (R) / ism (S), more than two testicles;
3. an (P) / orch (R) / ism (S), absence of testicles;
4. hydro (P) / cele (R), accumulation of fluid in the testicle; 5. a (P) / sperm (R) / ia (S), ejaculation without seminal fluid or without spermatozoa; 6. spermato (R) / gen (R) / esis (S), the process of sperm formation;
7. balan (R) / itis (S), inflammation of the glans penis;
8. orch (R) / itis (S), inflammation of the testis;
9. testicul (R) / ar (S), pertaining to the testicles;
10. epididym (R) / itis (S); inflammation of the epididymis

Exercise 8

1. ambiguous genitalia, 2. cryptorchism, 3. epispadias, 4. pseudohermaphrodite, 5. circumcision, 6. phimosis, 7. impotence, 8. orchialgia, 9. benign prostatic hyperplasia, 10. testicular torsion

Exercise 9

7, 5, 9, 6, 1, 10, 3, 2, 8, 4

Exercise 10

1. orchitis, 2. balanitis, 3. prostatitis, 4. epididymitis, 5. urethritis, 6. orchioplasty, 7. balanoplasty, 8. vasoplasty, 9. prostatectomy, 10. vasectomy

Exercise 11

1. hydrocele: collection of fluid within the testis;
2. phimosis: narrowness of the opening of the prepuce;
3. benign prostatic hyperplasia: enlarged prostate;
4. correct: inflammation of the glans penis; 5. oligospermia: scanty or deficient sperm; 6. circumcision: procedure to remove the foreskin; 7. prostate: gland below the bladder; 8. sterility: incapable of fertilization; 9. varicocele: varicose veins in the spermatic cord; 10. testicular torsion: twisted testis within the scrotum

Exercise 12

(left): aspermatogenesis, oligospermia, aspermia; (right): gametes, sperm, ovum, zygote, embryo

Exercise 13

1. balan (R) / itis (S), inflammation of the glans penis;
2. spermato (R) / genic (S), pertaining to the formation of sperm;
3. orch (R) / itis (S), inflammation of the testicles;
4. vas (R) / ectomy (S), removal of the vas deferens;
5. zygo (R) / te (S), product of sperm and egg joining;
6. andro (R) / gen (S), male hormone;
7. gameto (R) / genic (S), pertaining to the formation of a gamete;
8. gonad (R) / al (S), pertaining to the gonads;
9. orchio (R) / ectomy (S), removal of the testicle;
10. prostat (R) / itis (S), inflammation of the prostate

Exercise 14

1. testosterone, 2. semen analysis, 3. prostate-specific antigen, 4. prostatic ultrasonography, 5. epididymotomy, 6. epididymovasotomy, 7. prostate, 8. orchidorrhaphy, cryptorchism, 9. hormone, 10. vasectomy

Exercise 15

7, 6, 5, 8, 3, 4, 2, 1

Exercise 16

1. orchiectomy, 2. prostatectomy, 3. vesiculectomy, 4. transurethral, 5. prostatic, 6. orchidorrhaphy, 7. balanotomy , 8. orchiopexy, 9. hyperplasia, 10. epididymovasotomy

Exercise 17

1. transurethral resection of the prostate: removal of part or all of prostate gland through the urethra; 2. vasectomy: removal of all or part of vas deferens; 3. orchiectomy: removal of testis; 4. semen analysis: test to assess amount and viability of sperm; 5. terazosin: generic drug to treat benign prostatic hyperplasia (BPH); 6. finasteride: generic drug to treat BPH; 7. Testred: testosterone replacement agent; 8. alprostadil: agent for erectile dysfunction therapy; 9. Proscar: generic drug to treat BPH; 10. doxazosin mesylate: generic drug to treat BPH

Exercise 18

box 1: seminal vesicle, vesiculectomy; box 2: prostate gland, prostatectomy, TURP; box 3: testicle/procedures: orchidorrhaphy, orchiectomy, orchiopexy

Chapter 15

Exercise 1

1. uter/o, 2. salping/o, 3. vagin/o, 4. cervic/o, 5. oophor/o, 6. fundus, 7. urethr/o, 8. symphysis pubis, 9. rect/o, 10. ureter/o

Exercise 2

1. uterus: large, muscular structure; 2. fallopian tube: tube connecting ovary and uterus; 3. vagina: opening to outside (below urethra); 4. cervix: at mouth of uterus; 5. ovary: small, circular structure near top of illustration; 6. fundus: top of uterus; 7. urethra: urinary opening above vagina; 8. pubic bone: oval-shaped bone in front of bladder; 9. rectum: tubular area opening posteriorly; 10. ureter: tube leading to bladder

Exercise 3

1. vestibule, clitoris, 2. mons pubis, symphysis pubis, 3. labia majora, 4. urinary meatus, 5. vagina, 6. ovaries, 7. fallopian tubes, 8. fimbriae, 9. uterus, 10. myometrium, endometrium

Exercise 4

1. areola, 2. Bartholin's, 3. corpus luteum, 4. cervix, 5. fallopian, 6. fimbriae, 7. Graafian, 8. fundus, 9. hymen, 10. menses, 11. mons pubis, 12. perineum

Exercise 5

1. ovarian, 2. cervical, 3. endometritis, 4. dysmenorrhea, 5. amenorrhea, 6. gynecology, 7. oocyte, 8. salpingotomy, 9. menstrual, 10. gynecologist

Exercise 6

1. follicle, egg, was; 2. fimbriae were; 3. fundi, were; 4. cervices, were; 5. areolae were; 6. Bartholin's gland

was, or Bartholin's glands were; 7. uteri, were, cervices; 8. are, gynecologists; 9. vulvae, were; 10. ova were

Exercise 7
primary follicle, Graafian follicle, ovulation, corpus luteum, corpus albicans

Exercise 8
1. cervic/o = cervix, pertaining to the cervix; 2. thel/o = nipple, beginning breast development; 3. men/o = menstruation, long or excessive bleeding during menstruation; 4. metr/o = uterus, irregular bleeding between periods; 5. men/o = menstruation, scant menstrual flow; 6. metr/o = uterus, uterine tissue growing outside of the uterine wall; 7. salping/o = tube, inflammation of the fallopian tube; 8. cyst/o = bladder or pouch, outpouching of the bladder into the vagina; 9. fibr/o = fiber, nodules in the uterine wall; 10. men/o = menstruation, onset of menstruation

Exercise 9
1. atresia, 2. speculum, 3. bimanual, 4. puberty, 5. dysmenorrhea, 6. mammogram, 7. gravida; para, 8. dyspareunia, 9. Papanicolaou, 10. uterine

Exercise 10
4, 6, 9, 2, 7, 8, 10, 5, 1, 3

Exercise 11
1. dysmenorrhea, 2. menometrorrhagia, 3. hypomenorrhea, 4. hypermenorrhea, 5. metrorrhagia, 6. mammogram, 7. ovulation, 8. menopause, 9. rectocele, 10. thelarche

Exercise 12
1. genitalia, are, 2. fibroids, were, 3. smears, are, 4. tubes, were OR tube was, 5. gynecologists, 6. organs, were OR organ was, 7. mammograms, 8. speculum, 9. diseases are, 10. salpinx was OR salpinges were

Exercise 13
Menarche: breasts enlarge, become slightly tender; uterus increases in size; vagina becomes longer, wider, thicker, and more moist; external genitalia increase in size and develop pubic hair. **Menopause:** ovaries atrophy, may ovulate occasionally; uterus shrinks in size, can prolapse; vagina becomes shorter, narrower, drier, less elastic, thinner; external genitalia have decreased fat on mons pubis, decreased pubic hair, decreased size of labia and clitoris.

Exercise 14
1. a (P) / meno (R) / rrhea (S), absence of menses; 2. metro (R) / rrhagia (S), irregular bleeding between periods; 3. salping (R) / ectomy (S); removal of the fallopian tubes; 4. lacto (R) / gen (R) / esis (S); milk production; 5. cervic (R) / al (S), pertaining to the cervix; 6. gynec (R) / o (CV) / logy (S), specialty and study of females; 7. hyster (R) / ectomy (S), removal of the uterus; 8. oophor (R) / ectomy (S), removal of the ovaries; 9. colp (R) / o (CV) / scopy (S); examination of the cervix using an endoscope; 10. mast (R) / itis (S), inflammation of the breasts

Exercise 15
1. mastodynia, 2. hysteroscopy, 3. lactogenesis, 4. vesicovaginal fistula, 5. parovarian cyst, 6. cervical dysplasia, 7. endometritis, 8. curettage, 9. colposcopy, 10. bilateral salpingo-oophorectomy

Exercise 16
1. dilation and curettage, 2. obstetrics, 3. total abdominal hysterectomy, 4. gonorrhea, 5. dysfunctional uterine bleeding, 6. bilateral tubal ligation, 7. hysterosalpingography, 8. last menstrual period, 9. previous menstrual period, 10. vaginal hysterectomy

Exercise 17
1. cystocele, 2. rectocele, 3. urethrocele, 4. hysterectomy, 5. oophorectomy, 6. salpingo-oophorectomy, 7. mastectomy, 8. colporrhaphy, 9. episiorrhaphy, 10. salpingorrhaphy

Exercise 18
1. S/episiotomies, 2. S/oophorectomies, 3. S/mammographies, 4. P/contraceptive, 5. S/uteri, 6. S/ovaries, 7. S/areolae, 8. S/fundi, 9. S/cervices, 10. P/follicle

Exercise 19
breasts: mastectomy, mammogram; uterus: hysterectomy, PAP smear; ovaries: oopherectomy, abdominal ultrasound; fallopian tubes: tubal ligation, salpingotomy; vagina: colposcopy, vaginal swab (for STD)

Chapter 16

Exercise 1
1. embryon (R) / ic (S), relating to an embryo; 2. endo (P) / derm (R), embryonic layer "within skin"; 3. ecto (P) / derm (R), embryonic layer, "outside skin"; 4. meso (P) / derm (R), embryonic layer, "middle skin"; 5. oo (R) / cyte (S), immature egg cell; 6. genit (R) / al (S), relating to the genitalia; 7. abdomin (R) / al (S), relating to the abdomen; 8. lord (R) / osis (S), anteroposterior curvature of the spine; 9. parturi (R) / tion (S), process of birth; 10. pigment (R) / ation (S), coloring; 11. tri (P) / mester (R), three months; 12. mitos (R) / is (S), a process of cell division

Exercise 2
1. conception, 2. EDC, 3. menstrual, 4. placenta, 5. trimesters, 6. X, 7. fetal phase, 8. mitosis, 9. morula, blastocyst, 10. moment of conception

Exercise 3
9, 4, 10, 6, 3, 2, 8, 5, 7, 1

Exercise 4
1. Stage 1, 2. Stage 4, 3. Stage 2, 4. Stage 3

Exercise 5
Across: 3. zygote, 5. fetus, 7. morula, 11. parturition, 12. ectoderm, 13. mucosa, 15. ovum, 16. kyphosis, 18. areolae, 19. chromosome, **Down:** 1. colostrum, 2. blastocyst, 4. chloasma, 5. fertilization, 6. endoderm,

7. mesoderm, 8. cyanotic, 9. quickening, 10. mitosis,
14. embryo, 17. yolk

Exercise 6
Conception ovum, seminal fluid, fertilize, morula;
Development embryo, mesoderm; **Pregnancy** striae
gravidarum, chloasma, kyphosis

Exercise 7
1. oxytocin, 2. dystocia, 3. abruptio placenta, 4. placenta
previa; 5. Apgar score, 6. amniotic; 7. embryo, 8. vertex,
9. period after delivery of the infant, 10. relaxin

Exercise 8
10, 6, 7, 9, 2, 5, 1, 4, 3, 8

Exercise 9
1. FHR, 2. FTNSVD, 3. NB, 4. VBAC, 5. HCG, 6. CPD,
7. IUP, 8. FECG

Exercise 10
1. relax/in, loosen, chemical;
2. nulli/gravida, never, pregnancy;
3. dys/toc/ia, bad, birth, condition of;
4. post/partum, after, childbirth,
5. tri/mester, three, months;
6. placenta, cake or flat;
7. oxy/toc/in, chemical term, birth, chemical
8. nulli/para, never, given birth;
9. gestation, pregnancy;
10. parturi/ent, childbirth giver

Appendix B: Word Parts

a- . . . . without
ab- . . . . away from
abdomin/o . . . . abdomen
-ac . . . . cardiac
acous/o . . . . hearing
ad- . . . . toward, to, near
aden/o . . . . gland
adip/o . . . . fat
adren/o . . . . adrenals
aer/o . . . . air
-al . . . . pertaining to
-algia . . . . pain
alveol/o . . . . hollow sac
ambi- . . . . both
ambly/o . . . . dull
amni/o . . . the amnion (sac around
                              fetus)
an- . . . . without
andr/o . . . . male, masculine
angi/o . . . . vessel
anis/o . . . . unequal
ankyl/o . . crooked, fusion, stiffness
ante- . . . . before
anti- . . . . against, opposed to
aque/o . . . . water
-ar . . . . pertaining to
arch/e . . . . first
arteri/o . . . . artery
arteriol/o . . . . arteriole
arthr/o . . . . joint
articul/o . . . . joint
-ase . . . . enzyme
-asis . . . . formation, presence of
asthen/o . . . . loss of strength
astr/o . . . . star-shaped
-ate . . . . . . make; use; subject to
ather/o . . . deposit of pasty material
atri/o . . . . atrium
audi/o . . . . hearing, sound
aur/o . . . . ear
auricul/o . . . . ear
auto- . . . . self
bacter- . . . . bacteria
bacteri/o . . . . bacteria
balan/o . . . . glans penis
bas- . . . . base
bas/o . . . . Greek for base, basis
bi- . . . . two, both
bio- . . . . life
blast/o . . . . immature cell
-blast . . . . . . young cells or tissue
blephar/o . . . . eyelid
brady- . . . . slow
bronch/o . . . . airway
bronchiol/o . . . . bronchiole
carbo- . . . . carbon atom
carcin- . . . . cancer
carcin/o . . . . cancer
cardi- . . . . heart
cardi/o . . . . heart

-cele . . . . pouch
celi/o . . . . abdomen
-centesis . . . puncture to withdraw
                      fluid or tissue
cephal- . . . . head
cephal/o . . . . head
cerebell/o . . . . cerebellum
cerebr/o . . . . cerebrum
cervic/o . . . . neck
cheil/o (chil/o) . . . . lips
chol/o (chol/e) . . . . bile
choledoch/o . . . . common bile duct
chondr/o . . . . cartilage
chrom/o . . . . Greek for color
circum- . . around, circular motion
-cle . . . . small
col/o . . . . colon
colp/o . . . . vagina
con- . . . . with
conjunctiv/o . . . . conjunctiva
contra- . . . . . against, opposed to
corne/o . . . . cornea
coron/o . . . . crown or circle
corp- . . . . body
cost- . . . . ribs
crani/o . . . . head
cutane/o . . . . skin
cyan/o . . . . blue
cyst/o . . . . sac or cyst containing
      fluid (also urinary bladder)
cyt/o . . . . cell
-cyte . . . . cell
dacry/o . . . . tear
dactyl/o . . . . fingers or toes
de- . . . . not, from, down
dent/o . . . . teeth
derm/o . . . . skin
dermat/o . . . . skin
-desis . . . stabilization or binding
di- . . . . two
dia- . . . . across or through
dipl/o . . . . double
dis- . . . . separate, apart
duoden/o . . . . duodenum
-dynia . . . . pain
dys- . . . . faulty, painful, difficult
-e . . . . noun marker
e- . . . . out, outside, away
-eal . . . . pertaining to
ec- . . . . out, outside, away
echin/o . . . . prickly
ecto- . . . . out, outside, away
-ectomy- . . . . . excision, surgical
                              removal
electr/o . . . . electricity
embry/o . . . . embryo
-emesis . . . . vomiting
-emia . . . . condition of the blood
emmetr/o . . . . correct measure
en- . . . . inside or in

encephal/o . . . related to the brain
endo- . . . . inside or in
enter/o . . . . intestines
epi . . . . upon, above
erythr/o . . . . red
estr/o . . . . female
eu- . . . . normal
-eum . . . . tissue or structure
ex- . . . . out, outside, away
exo- . . . . out, outside, away
extra- . . . . out, outside, away
fibr/o . . . . fiber
fibrin/o . . . . fiber
-form . . . . . shape or resembling
gamet/o . . . . gamete
gangli/o . . . . . swelling, collection
gastr- . . . . stomach
gastr/o . . . . stomach
-genesis . . . . origin
-genic . . . . origin
gingiv/o . . . . gums
glauc/o . . . . blue-gray
gli/o . . . . gluey substance
gloss/o . . . . tongue
gluc/o . . . . glucose (sugar)
glyc/o . . . . sugar
gnath/o . . . . jaw
gonad/o . . . . . seed (reproductive
                              organs)
-gram . . . . record
granul/o . . . . . . granular, granules
-graph . . record or instrument used
              for making a record
-graphy . . . . . process of recording
gyn/o . . . . female
gynec/o . . . . female
hem/o . . . . blood
hemat/o . . . . blood
hemi- . . . . half (usually right/
                          left halves)
hepat/o . . . . liver
hepatic/o . . . . liver
herni/o . . . . rupture, hernia
hidr/o . . . . sweat glands
hydr/o . . . . water
hyper- . . . . above or excessive
hypo- . . . . . less, deficient; below
hyster/o . . . . uterus
-ia . . . . condition or process
-iasis . . . . . formation of, presence
-iatric . . . . treatment
-ic . . . . pertaining to
ichthy/o . . . . fish (scales)
ile/o . . . . ileum
ili/o . . . . ilium; hip
immun/o . . . . immune
immune/o- . . . . immune
in- . . . . inside or in
infra- . . . . less than; under, below
inter- . . . . between

intra- . . . . inside or in
irid/o . . . . iris
-ism . . . . . condition or process
-itis . . . . inflammation
-ium . . . . . tissue or structure
-ize . . . . . make; use; subject to
jejun/o . . . . jejunum
kary/o . . . . nucleus
kerat/o . . . horny tissue (also refers
        to the cornea of the eye)
kinesi/o . . . . movement
labi/o . . . . lips
lacrim/o . . . . tears
lact/o . . . . milk
lapar/o . . . . abdomen
laryng/o . . . . larynx
leuk/o . . . . white
lip/o . . . . fat
lith/o, -lith . . . . . stone, calcification
-logist . . . . . . one who specializes
-logy . . . . study of
lumb/o . . . . lower back
lymph/o . . . . lymph
-lysis . . . breakdown or dissolution
                              process
macro- . . . . large
mal- . . . . bad, abnormal
-malacia . . . . softening
mamm/o . . . . breast
mandibul/o . . . . lower jaw
mast/o- . . . . breast
meat/o . . . . passageway
medull/o . . . . medulla
mega- . . . . large, excessive
-megaly . . . . enlargement
melan/o . . . . black
men/o . . . . . . menses, menstruation
mening/o . . . . . membrane covering
        brain and spinal column
meso . . . . middle
meta- . . . . change; beyond
-meter . . . measure or measurement
metr/a, o . . . . uterus
-metry . . . . . process of measuring
mi/o . . . . less
micro- . . . . very small
mono- . . . . one
morph/o . . . . shape
multi- . . . . many, several
muscul/o . . . . muscle
my/o . . . . muscle
mydr/o . . . . widen
myel/o . . . . bone marrow
myel/o . . . . spinal cord
myring/o . . . . . tympanic membrane
nas/o . . . . nose
necr/o . . . . death
neo- . . . . new
nephr/o . . . . kidney
nerv- . . . . nerve

neur- . . . . .nerve
neur/o- . . . . .nerve
neutr/o . . . . .neutral
nucle/o . . . . .nucleus
o/o . . . . .egg
occipit/o . . . . .back of the head
ocul/o . . . . .eye
odont/o . . . . .tooth
-oid . . . . .like, resembling
-ole . . . . .small
olig- . . . . .few, scant
-oma . . . . . . .tumor or neoplasm
onc/o . . . . .tumor
onych/o . . . . .nail
oophor/o . . . . .ovary
ophthalm/o . . . . .eye
opt/o . . . . .eye/vision
orchi/o . . . . .testis (testicle)
orchid/o . . . . .testis (testicle)
organ/o . . . . .organ
orth/o . . . . .straight
-ose . . . . .pertaining to
-osis . . . . .condition
osse/o . . . . .bony
oste/o . . . . .bone
ot/o . . . . .ear
-ous . . . . .pertaining to
ov/o . . . . .egg
ox/o . . . . .oxygen molecule
pachy- . . . . .thick
palpebr/o . . . . .eyelid
pan- . . . . .all
pancreat/o . . . . .pancreas
para- . . . . .along, beside
pariet/o . . . . .relationship to a wall
path/o- . . . . .disease
pelv/io . . . . .basin; pelvis
pelv/o . . . . .pelvis
-penia . . . . . .abnormal reduction
or lack of
per- . . . . .through
peri- . . . . .around
-pexy . . . . .surgical fixation
phac/o . . . . .lens of the eye
phag/o . . . . .eating
-phage . . . . .eat, swallow
-phagia . . . . . . .process of eating
or related to eating

pharyng/o . . . . .throat
phas/o . . . . .speech
-phile . . . . .affinity for
-philia . . . . .attraction for
phleb/o . . . . .vein
-phobia . . . . .fear
phon/o . . . . .sound
phot/o . . . . .light
phren/o . . . . .diaphragm
pil/o . . . . .hair
-plasia . . . . .formation
plasm/o . . . . .formed; plasma
-plasty . . . . .repair
pleur/o . . . . .rib area
pne/o . . . . .breath
-pnea . . . . .breathing
pneum/o . . . . .lung, air
pod/o . . . . .foot
-poiesis . . . . .formation
poikil/o . . . . .irregular
poly- . . . . .many
post- . . . . .after
pre- . . . . .before
presby/o . . . . .old age
pro- . . . . .before
proct/o . . . . .rectum, anus
prostat/o . . . . .prostate
psych/o . . . . . . .mental, the mind
-ptosis . . . . .drooping
pulmon/o . . . . .lung
pupill/o . . . . .pupil
purpur/o . . . . .purple
pyel/o . . . . .renal pelvis
pylor/o . . . . .gatekeeper
quadra- . . . . .four
rachi/o . . . . .spine
radi/o . . . . .x-rays
re- . . . . .again, back
rect/o . . . . .rectum
ren- . . . . .kidneys
ren/i (o) . .pertaining to the kidney
reticul/o . . . . . . .reticulum (a fine
network of cells)
retin/o . . . . .retina
retro- . . . . . .backward or behind
rhin/o . . . . .nose
-rrhage . . . . .bursting forth or
rapid flow

-rrhaphy . . . . .suturing
-rrhea . . . . .bursting forth or
rapid flow
-rrhexis . . . . . .rupture or breaking
-ry . . . . .pertaining to
sacr/o . . . . .sacrum
salping/o . . . . .tube
sarc/o . . . . .flesh
scapul/o . . . . .scapula
schist/o . . . . .split
scler/o . . . . .hardening
-scope . . . . .instrument used for
viewing
-scopy . . . .process of viewing with
an instrument
scot/o . . . . .dark
seb/o . . . . . . .pertaining to secretion
from the sebaceous glands
semi- . . . . .part of a whole
sept/o . . . . .partition
ser/o . . . . .fluid part of blood
sial/o . . . . .saliva
sider/o . . . . .iron
sigmoid/o . . . . .s shaped
skelet- . . . . . . .skeleton (bones)
somat/o . . . . .body
-spasm abrupt, forceful contraction
sperm/o . . . . . .semen, spermatozoa
spermat/o . . . . .semen, spermatozoa
spher/o . . . . .sphere-shaped
sphygm/o . . . . .relating to the pulse
splen/o . . . . .spleen
spondyl/o . . . . .vertebrae
squam/o . . . . . .pertaining to scales
-stasis . . . . .stop, stand
sten/o . . . .narrowing, constriction
stern/o . . . . .chest
steth/o . . . . .chest
stom/a . . . . .mouth
stomat/o . . . . .mouth
-stomy or -ostomy . . . .creation of
an artificial opening
sub- . . . . .less than; under, below
super- . . . .excessive, more; above
supra- . .excessive, outside; beyond
sym- . . . . .with
syn- . . . . .with
tachy- . . . . .fast

tars/o . . . .tarsal bones in the foot
tempor/o . . . . .time
tend/o; tendin/o . . . . .tendon
tetra- . . . . .four
thel/o . . . . .nipple
thorac/o . . . . .chest
thromb/o . . . . .blood clot
thym/o . . . . .thymus
thyr/o . . . . .thyroid
-tic . . . . .pertaining to
-tomy . . . . .cut or incision
tox/o . . . . .poison
trache/o . . . . .windpipe
trans- . . . . .across or through
tri- . . . . .three
-tripsy . . . . .crushing
-trophy . . . . .development
-tropic (tropin) . . .turning toward,
changing
tub/o . . . . . .tube (little tube)
tympan/o . . . . .drum
typhl/o . . . . .cecum
-ula . . . . .small
-ule . . . . .small
ultra- . . . . .excessive; beyond
uni- . . . . .one, single
ur/e (a), (o) . . . .relating to urea or
urine
ur/o . . . . .relating to urine
ureter/o . . . . .ureter
urethr/o . . . . .urethra
urin/o . . . . .urine
uter/o . . . . .uterus
uve/o . . . . .uvea
vagin/o . . . . .sheath
varic/o . . . . . .twisted, swollen vein
vas/o . . . . .vessel
vascul- . . . . .vessels
vascul/o . . . . .vessel
ven/o . . . . .vein
ventricul/o . . . . .ventricle
vertebr/o . . . . .vertebra
viscer/o . . . . .internal organs
vitre/o . . . . .glassy
vulv/o . . . . .covering
xanth/o . . . . .yellow
-y . . . . . . .condition or process of
zyg/o . . . . .a yoke; joining

Appendix C: Abbreviations

↓	decrease or decreasing
°	degrees Fahrenheit or Celsius
<	less than
>	greater than
♀	female
♂	male
A	assessment or analysis
ā	before
↑	increased or increasing
AB, ab	abortion
ABG	arterial blood gas
ABR	auditory brainstem response
a.c.	before meals
AC	air conduction
ACC	accommodation
ACG	angiocardiography
ACTH	adrenocorticotropic hormone
AD	right ear (*auris dexter*)
ad lib	as desired
ADH	antidiuretic hormone (vasopressin)
ADHD	attention-deficit hyperactivity disorder
AE	above the elbow amputation
AFB	acid-fast bacilli
AFP	alpha fetoprotein
AGN	acute glomerulonephritis
AHF	antihemophilic factor VIII
AHG	antihemophilic globulin factor VIII
AIDS	acquired immunodeficiency syndrome
AK	above the knee amputation
ALL	acute lymphoblastic leukemia
ALS	amyotrophic lateral sclerosis
a.m.	before noon
AML	acute myeloblastic leukemia (also known as acute myelogenous leukemia)
amt.	amount
ANC	absolute neutrophil count
ANS	autonomic nervous system
AOM	acute otitis media
AP	anterior posterior (used with x-ray views)
AP	anteroposterior
APML	acute promyelocytic leukemia
aq	water
ARDS	acute respiratory distress syndrome
AROM	active range of motion
AS	aortic stenosis OR left ear (*auris sinister*)
ASD	atrial septal defect
ASHD	arteriosclerotic heart disease
ATN	acute tubular necrosis
AU	both ears (*auris uterque*)
AZT	azidothymidine
®	bilateral
BaE or BE	barium enema
baso	basophil
BBB	bundle-branch block
BC	bone conduction
BE	below the elbow amputation
b.i.d.	twice a day
BiPAP	bilevel positive airway pressure
BK	below the knee amputation

BM	bowel movement
BMT	bone marrow transplant
BP	blood pressure
BPH	benign prostatic hyperplasia
BRM	biologic response modifier
BRP	bathroom privileges
BSO	bilateral salpingo-oophorectomy
BTL	bilateral tubal ligation
BUN	blood urea nitrogen
bx	biopsy
C	Celsius, centigrade
c̄	with
c/o	complains of (patient's report of a symptom)
C1, C2, etc.	cervical vertebrae (numbered according to area of the spine)
Ca	calcium
CA	chronological age
CAD	coronary artery disease
CAT	computerized axial tomography
CBC	complete blood count
CC	cardiac catheterization OR chief complaint
CCU	coronary care unit
CDH	congenital dislocation of the hip
CEA	carcinoembryonic antigen
CF	circumflex (artery) OR cystic fibrosis
CHF	congestive heart failure
CLL	chronic lymphocytic leukemia
cm	centimeter
CML	chronic myelogenous leukemia
CMV	cytomegalovirus
CNS	central nervous system
CO2	carbon dioxide
COLD	chronic obstructive lung disease
COPD	chronic obstructive pulmonary disease
CP	cerebral palsy OR chest pain
CPAP	continuous positive airway pressure
CPD	cephalopelvic disproportion
CPR	cardiopulmonary resuscitation
CPR	cardiopulmonary resuscitation
CRF	corticotropin-releasing factor
CS, C-section, C/S	cesarean section
CSF	cerebrospinal fluid OR colony stimulating factor
CT	computed tomography
cu mm	cubic millimeter
CV	cardiovascular
CVA	cerebrovascular accident OR costovertebral angle
Cx	cervix
CXR	chest x-ray
cysto	cystoscopy
D	diopter
d.	day
D&C	dilation and curettage
dB	decibel
D/C	discontinue

DCR	dacryocystorhinostomy	GC	gonorrhea
derm.	dermatology	GERD	gastroesophageal reflux disease
DI	diabetes insipidus	GFR	glomerular filtration rate
DIC	disseminated intravascular coagulation	GH	growth hormone
diff	differential	GHRH	growth hormone–releasing hormone
DIP joint	distal interphalangeal joint	GI	gastrointestinal
DJD	degenerative joint disease	gr	grain
DKA	diabetic ketoacidosis	gt (sing) or	drop
DM	diabetes mellitus	gtt (pl)	
DNR	do not resuscitate	GTT	glucose tolerance test
DPT	diphtheria, pertussis, tetanus	GU	genitourinary
	immunization	GVHD	graft-versus-host disease
dr	dram (1/8 ounce)	GYN	gynecology
DRE	digital rectal examination	h.	hour
DTR	deep tendon reflex	H&P	history and physical
DUB	dysfunctional uterine bleeding	HAL	hyperalimentation
DVT	deep vein thrombosis	HBV	hepatitis B virus, hepatitis B vaccine
Dx	diagnosis	HCG	human chorionic gonadotropin
EAC	external ear canal	HCl	hydrochloric acid
ECCE	extracapsular cataract extraction	HCT/Hct	hematocrit
ECG or EKG	electrocardiogram	HD	hip disarticulation
EDC	estimated date of confinement (due date)	HEENT	head, eyes, ears, nose, throat
EDD	estimated date of delivery	HGB/Hgb	hemoglobin
EEG	electroencephalogram OR	HGH	human growth hormone
	electroencephalography	HIV	human immunodeficiency virus
EENT	eyes, ears, nose, and throat	HLA	human-leukocyte antigen
ELISA	enzyme-linked immunosorbent assay	HNP	herniated nucleus pulposus (disk)
Em	emmetropia	HP	hemipelvectomy
EMG	electromyography	HPI	history of present illness
ENT	ears, nose, and throat	HPV	human papilloma virus
EOM	extraocular movements	HRT	hormone replacement therapy (usually
eosin/eos	eosinophil		refers to replacement at menopause)
ERG	electroretinography	h.s.	hour of sleep
ERV	expiratory reserve volume	HSG	hysterosalpingography
ESR	erythrocyte sedimentation rate	HSV	herpes simplex virus
ESWL	extracorporeal shock wave lithotripsy	Ht	height
ETOH	ethyl alcohol (beverage alcohol)	HVA	homovanillic acid
F	Fahrenheit	hx	personal medical history
FBS	fasting blood sugar	i	one
FECG	fetal electrocardiogram	I&D	incision and drainage
FEF	forced expiratory flow	I&O	intake and output
FEF$_{25-75}$	forced midexpiratory flow during the	ICA	internal carotid artery
	middle half of the FVC	ICCE	intracapsular cataract extraction
FEV	forced expiratory volume	ICU	intensive care unit
FEV$_1$	forced expiratory volume in 1 second	IDDM	insulin-dependent diabetes mellitus
FEV$_3$	forced expiratory volume in 3 seconds	Ig	immunoglobulin
FHR	fetal heart rate	ii	two
fl oz	fluid ounce	iii	three
FS	frozen section	IMA	internal mammary artery
FSH	follicle-stimulating hormone	IMP	impression (related to diagnosis)
FTND	full-term, normal delivery	IOL	intraocular lens
FTNSVD	full-term, normal, spontaneous, vaginal	IOP	intraocular pressure
	delivery	IP	inpatient OR interphalangeal joint
FVC	forced vital capacity	IPPB	intermittent positive pressure breathing
FVL	flow volume loop	IQ	intelligence quotient (normal = 90–110)
fx	fracture	IRDS	infant respiratory distress syndrome
g	gram	IRV	inspiratory reserve volume
GAF Scale	Global Assessment of Functioning is a	IS	incentive spirometry OR intracostal space
	subjective assessment tool used to rate	ITP	immune thrombocytopenic purpura
	ability to function on a scale of 1–100,	IUD	intrauterine device
	where 1 = poor mental health and inability	IUP	intrauterine pregnancy
	to function and 100 = good mental health	IV	intravenous
	and ability to function well	IVC	intravenous cholangiography
GB	gallbladder	IVP	intravenous pyelogram

K	potassium
KD	knee disarticulation
kg	kilogram
KOH	potassium hydroxide
KS	Kaposi's sarcoma
KUB	kidneys, ureters, bladder (x-ray)
L or l	liter
Ⓛ	left
L&A	light and accommodation
L1, L2, etc.	lumbar vertebrae
LAD	left anterior descending coronary artery
LASIK	laser-assisted in situ keratomileusis
lb or #	pound
LCA	left coronary artery
LCF	left circumflex
LFT	liver function test
LH	luteinizing hormone
LIMA	left internal mammary artery
LLQ	left lower quadrant
LMCA	left main coronary artery
LMP	last menstrual period
LP	lumbar puncture
LPA	left pulmonary artery
LRQ	lower right quadrant
LUQ	left upper quadrant
lymphs	lymphocytes
MA	mental age
MAI	Mycobacterium avium–intracellulare complex
MCH	mean corpuscular hemoglobin
MCHC	mean corpuscular hemoglobin concentration
MCP joint	metacarpophalangeal joint
MCV	mean corpuscular volume
MDI	metered-dose inhaler
mg	milligram
MI	myocardial infarction
mL	milliliter
mm	millimeter
mono	monocyte
MPA	main pulmonary artery
MRI	magnetic resonance imaging
MS	mitral stenosis OR multiple sclerosis
MSH	melanocyte-stimulating hormone
MVP	mitral valve prolapse
my	myopia
Na	sodium
NB	newborn
NEC	neonatal necrotizing enterocolitis
NKA	no known allergies
NKDA	no known drug allergies
n.p.o.	nothing by mouth
NSCLC	non-small cell lung cancer
O_2	oxygen
OA	osteoarthritis
OB	obstetrics
OCD	obsessive compulsive disorder
OD	right eye (oculus dexter); doctor of optometry
OH	occupational history
½	one half
OP	outpatient
OR	operating room
ortho	orthopedics
OS	left eye (oculus sinister)
OT	oxytocin
OU	both eyes (oculus uterque)
oz	ounce
∅	none
P	pulse
p.r.	by rectum
p.r.n.	as needed
PA	posterior anterior (used with x-ray views) OR pulmonary artery
PAN	periodic alternating nystagmus
PAP	positive airway pressure
PAR	postanesthesia recovery
PAT	paroxysmal atrial tachycardia
p.c.	after meals
PCP	Pneumocystis carinii pneumonia
PD	Parkinson's disease OR peritoneal dialysis
PDA	posterior descending artery; patent ductus arteriosus
PDDNOS	pervasive developmental disorder not otherwise specified
PE	physical examination
PE tubes	pressure-equalizing tubes
PEEP	positive end-expiratory pressure
PEF	peak expiratory flow
per	by or through
PERLA	pupils equal, reactive to light and accommodation
PERRLA	pupils equal, round, reactive to light and accommodation
PERRLA	pupils equal, round, reactive to light and accommodation
PET	positron emission tomography
PFT	pulmonary function test
PH	past history
PI	present illness
PID	pelvic inflammatory disease
PIH	prolactin-inhibiting hormone
PIP joint	proximal interphalangeal joint
plts/PLT	platelets
P.M.	after noon
PMH	past medical history
PMI	point of maximal impulse
PMN	polymorphonuclear neutrophil
PMP	previous menstrual period
PNS	peripheral nervous system
p.o.	by mouth
polys	polymorphonuclear neutrophils
postop	recovery room
p.p.	postprandial
PPI	proton pump inhibitors
PPT	postprandial test
preop	preoperating area
PRH	prolactin-releasing hormone
PRK	photorefractive keratectomy
PRL	prolactin
p.r.n.	as needed
PROM	passive range of motion
PSA	prostate-specific antigen
PSCT	peripheral stem cell transplant
pt	patient
PT	prothrombin time
PTCA	percutaneous transluminal coronary angioplasty

PTH	parathyroid hormone (parathormone)	T1, T2, etc.	thoracic vertebrae
PTT	partial thromboplastin time	T_3	triiodothyronine
PVC	premature ventricular contraction	T_4	thyroxine
Px	alternative abbreviation for physical examination	TAH	total abdominal hysterectomy
		TAH/BSO	total abdominal hysterectomy with bilateral salpingo-oophorectomy
q.	each or every		
q.2h.	every two hours	TB	tuberculosis
q.d.	every day	TB	tuberculosis
q.h.	every hour	TENS	transcutaneous electric nerve stimulation
q.i.d.	four times a day	TFT	thyroid function test
q.o.d.	every other day	THA	total hip arthroplasty
q.s.	quantity sufficient	THR	total hip replacement
R	respirations	TIA	transient ischemic attack
®	right	t.i.d.	three times a day
RA	rheumatoid arthritis	TM	tympanic membrane
RBC	red blood cell	TPN	total parenteral nutrition (hyperalimentation)
RCA	right coronary artery		
RDS	respiratory distress syndrome	Tr	traction
REM	rapid eye movement	TRH	thyrotropin-releasing hormone
RIA	radioimmunoassay	TSH	thyroid-stimulating hormone
RLQ	right lower quadrant	TUR	transurethral resection
R/O	rule out	TURP	transurethral resection of the prostate or transurethral prostatectomy
ROJM	range of joint motion		
ROP	retinopathy of prematurity	TV	tidal volume
ROS	review of systems	Tx	treatment
RP	retrograde pyelogram	UA; U/A	urinalysis
RPA	right pulmonary artery	UC	uterine contractions
RRR	regular rate and rhythm (refers to heart)	UCHD	usual childhood diseases
RTC	return to clinic	UGI	upper gastrointestinal
RTO	return to office	ULQ	upper left quadrant
RUQ	right upper quadrant	ung.	ointment
RV	residual volume	URI	upper respiratory infection
Rx	prescription or recipe	URQ	upper right quadrant
s̄	without	UTI	urinary tract infection
S1, S2, etc.	sacral vertebrae	UV	ultraviolet
SA	sinoatrial node	VA	visual acuity
SAD	seasonal affective disorder	VBAC	vaginal birth after cesarean section
SCC	spinal cord compression	VC	vital capacity
SCLC	small cell lung cancer	VC	vital capacity
SD	shoulder disarticulation	VDRL	Venereal Disease Research Laboratory (test for syphilis, an STD)
sed rate	sedimentation rate		
segs	segmented neutrophils	VF	visual field
SH	social history	VH	vaginal hysterectomy
SIADH	syndrome of inappropriate antidiuretic hormone	VMA	vanillylmandelic acid
		VS	vital signs
sig.	label; instructions	VSD	ventricular septal defect
SLE	systemic lupus erythematosus	w.a.	while awake
SNS	somatic nervous system	WAIS	Wechsler Adult Intelligence Scale
SOB	shortness of breath	WBC	white blood cell
SOB	shortness of breath	WDWN	well-developed, well-nourished
SPECT	single photon emission computed tomography	WISC	Wechsler Intelligence Scale for Children
		wk	week
ss	one-half	WNL	within normal limits
SR	symptoms review	Wt	weight
ST	esotropia	x	times or for
stat.	immediately	XT	exotropia
STD	sexually transmitted disease	yr	year
STD	sexually transmitted disease		
STD	sexually transmitted disease		
subq; SQ	subcutaneous		
SVCS	superior vena cava syndrome		
Sx	symptom		
T	temperature		
T&A	tonsillectomy and adenoidectomy		

Index

Note: Figures are denoted with an f; tables are denoted with a t.

of hematopoietic system, 189
of integumentary system, 92–93
metastatic sequence in, 202t
of musculoskeletal system, 147
prostate, 548
risk assessment for, 202
testicular, 549
treatment goals and options with, 205
tumor staging for, 203
Cancer cells
anatomy of, 201
metabolism of, 202
Canthus, 340, 340
Capillaries, 389, 426, 428
Carbohydrates, 468
digestion of, 464
Carbon dioxide, exchange of oxygen and, 390, 391f
Carcinogenesis, 201
Carcinogens, 201
Cardiac catheterization, 445
Cardiac cycle, 422
Cardiac muscle, 134
Cardiac muscle tissue, 36
Cardiac output, 422
Cardiac sphincter, 465, 465f
Cardiac surgeon, 420
Cardiologist, 420
Cardiology, 420
Cardiomegaly, 439
Cardiovascular surgeons, 420
Cardiovascular system, 419–460
abbreviations for, 448–449t
anatomy and physiology of, 420–430
anatomy and physiology terms relating to, 431–432t
diagnosing and treating problems in, 444–447
general illnesses in, 439
major structures of and medical specialties for, 38f
practitioners and, 419–420
roots for, 3
tests and procedures relating to, 446–447t
wellness and illness terms relating to, 439–440t
wellness and illness through life span and, 435–439
Carpals, 122
Carpal tunnel syndrome, 146
Cartilage, 124
Cataract, 349
Catecholamines, 259, 294
Catheterized urine specimen, 521
Caudal location, 46, 46f
CBC. See Complete blood count
CDC. See Centers for Disease Control and Prevention
Cell body, 294, 296f
Cell-mediated immunity, 220
Cells, 33, 34, 35–36
blood, 171t
bone, 124
cancer, development of, 202
of immune system, 220
Centers for Disease Control and Prevention, 270
Central nervous system, 289, 290
Central sulcus, of brain, 292f
Centrioles, 35
Cephalic location, 46, 46f
Cephalic presentation, 606
Cerebellar function evaluation, 324
Cerebral cortex, 290

functional areas of, 293f
Cerebral palsy, 309
Cerebral thrombosis, 183
Cerebrospinal fluid, 290
Cerebrovascular accident, 309
Cerebrum, 290, 292f
Cerumen, 361
Cervical atresia, 578
Cervical cancer, screening for, 581, 582
Cervical spinal column region, 54, 54f
Cervix, 568, 568f, 569, 569f, 601
CF. See Cystic fibrosis
Chalazion, 350
Chemical names, in prescription drug names, 67
Chemical peel, 104
Chemotherapy, 189, 205
common regimens, 205–206t
Cherry angiomas, 91
Chest sounds, 397t
Chest x-rays, 404
Chewing, 468
Chicken pox, 230
Child health, promoting, 613
Childhood infections, common, 230
Children
abnormalities of male reproductive system in, 547
cardiovascular problems in, 438
ear problems in, 367–368
endocrinological disorders in, 270
female reproductive disorders in, 578
gastrointestinal disorders in, 478
hematologic disorders in, 182–185
immune disorders in, 230
musculoskeletal system of, 143
neurological disorders in, 309
respiratory problems in, 398–399
urinary system disorders in, 513–514
Chiropractic, 119
Chiropractor, 119
Chlamydial infections, 582
Chloasma, 91
Cholangiography, 486
Cholecystectomy, 486
Cholecystitis, 479
Cholecystokinin, 466
Cholelithiasis, 479
Cholesteatomas, 368
Cholesterol levels, 444
Chondrocytes, 124
Chordae tendineae, 421
Chordotomy, 325
Chorea, 313f
Chorionic villus sampling, 613
Choroid, 341
Chromosomal abnormalities, ruling out, 613
Chronic disease, 144
Chronic obstructive lung disease, 399
Chronic obstructive pulmonary disease, 399
Chyle, 219
Chyme, 465, 466, 467
Cilia, 385
Ciliary body, 341
Circular muscle layer, of stomach, 465, 465f
Circulatory system, 426–429
combining forms relating to, 430t
major structures of and medical specialties for, 38f
pharmacologic agents relating to, 447–448t
Circumcision, 547, 554
Circumduction, 50, 50f
Cisterna chyli, 219

Clean-catch urine specimen, 521
Cleft palate, 478
Climacteric, 582
Clitoris, 568, 568f
Closed comedones, 90
Closed reduction, 155
Clotting, 174
evaluating, 195
Clotting cascade, 175f
Clubbing, 438
Clubfoot, 142
CNS. See Central nervous system
Coagulants, 196
Coarctation of the aorta, 436t
Coccyx, 54, 54f
Code of medical ethics, 2
COLD. See Chronic obstructive lung disease
Collagen, 81
Collecting tubule, 503, 504f
Colloid, 257
Colon cancer, Dukes' staging for, 203
Colonoscopy, 486
Colony-stimulating factors, 171
Colorectal cancers, 479
Colors, combining forms for description of, 7t
Colostomy, 486
Colposcopy, 586
Combining forms, 3, 6
colors described with, 7t
common
related to anatomy, 7t
related to diseases and conditions, 6t
relating to circulatory system, 430t
relating to ear, 363t
relating to endocrine system, 260t
relating to eye, 343t
relating to female reproductive cycle, 571t
relating to gastrointestinal system, 469–470t
relating to hematology-oncology, 175–176t
relating to immunity, 223t
relating to integumentary system, 84
relating to male reproductive system, 541t
relating to muscular system, 135–136t
relating to nervous system, 297–298t
relating to respiratory system, 391t
relating to skeletal system, 126t
relating to urinary system, 507t
Comedo, 79
Common bile duct, 466, 466f
Communication, skin and, 83
Complement fixation, 221
Complement proteins, 221
Complete blood count, 170, 194
Compound suffixes, 15
Computed tomography, 57, 59, 59f, 60f, 404
Computerized axial tomography (CAT) scan, 324
Conception, 601
Conchae, 385, 385f
Conditions
common, combining forms related to, 6t
suffixes indicating, 10t
Condyloid diarthroses, 126, 127f
Cones, 341
Congenital anomalies/disorders
in female infants, 578
of male reproductive system, 547–548t
of musculoskeletal system, 142–143
Congestive heart failure, 438
Conjunctiva, 341, 350
Conjunctivitis, 350
treatment of, 357

Emphysema, 399
Emulsification of fats, 466
Enamel, tooth, 465
Endarterectomy, 446
Endocardium, 420, *422f*
Endochondral ossification, 125
Endocrine cancers, 272
Endocrine glands, 254
    functions of, 255–260
Endocrine imbalances, visual signs of, 266
Endocrine system, 253–288
    abbreviations for, 278–279
    anatomy and physiology of, 254
    anatomy and physiology terms relating to, 261–263*t*
    combining forms relating to, 260*t*
    description of and practitioners for, 253
    diagnosing and treatment of, 276–277
    general illnesses of, 272
    major structures of and medical specialties for, *38f*
    pharmaceutical agents for, 277
    surgical procedures relating to, 277*t*
    tests and procedures relating to, 276*t*
    wellness and illness through life span and, 266–272
Endocrinologist, 253
Endocrinology, 253
Endoderm, 602
Endolymph, 362
Endometriosis, 581
    managing, 587
Endometrium, 569, *569f*
Endoplasmic reticulum, 35
Endoscope, 486
Endoscopic surgery, 64
Endoscopy, 404
Endosteum, 123, *123f*
Engagement of baby, 606
ENT specialist, 360
Enuresis, 514
Enzyme-linked immunosorbent assay, 239
Enzymes, 468
Eosinophils, 170, 173
Epicanthic fold, 340, *340f*
Epicardium, 420
Epicondylitis, 146
Epidermis, 80, 81
Epididymis, 540
Epididymitis, 549
Epididymotomy, 554
Epididymovasostomy, 554
Epiglottis, 383, 386, *386f*
Epinephrine, 259
Epiphyseal line, 125
Epiphyseal plate, 125
Epiphysis, 123, *123f*
Episiotomy, 611
Epispadias, 547
Epistaxis, 184
Epithelial tissue, 36, 37
EPO. *See* Erythropoietin
Equilibrium, 361
Erectile dysfunction, 548
    treatment of, 555*t*
ERV. *See* Expiratory reserve volume
Erythema toxicum, 90
Erythroblastosis fetalis, 182
Erythrocytes, 170
Erythrocyte sedimentation rate, 154
Erythrocytes (red blood cells), 171
Erythropoietin, 171, 196
Eschar, 104
Esophagus, 383, 462, *462f*, 465

Esotropia, 348
ESR. *See* Erythrocyte sedimentation rate
Estrogen, 260, 570
    decline in, 582
    in pregnant women, 144
Ethmoid sinus, 385, *385f*
Eustachian tubes, 361, *361f*
    in children, 398
Eversion, 50, *50f*
Ewing's sarcoma, 147
Exchange transfusions, 182
Excoriated rash, 92
Exercise, bodily use of energy during, 135, *135f*
Exhalation, 389
Exocrine glands, 254
Exotropia, 348
Expected date of delivery (or confinement), 601
    Nägele's Rule for calculation of, 602
Expiration, 384
Expiratory reserve volume, 404
Extension, 49, *50f*
External auditory meatus, 361
External ear, *361f*, 361–362
External urethral sphincter, 506
Extracorporeal shock wave lithotripsy, 521
Extramedullary hematopoiesis, 181, 182
Extrapyramidal tract, 309
Eye
    anatomy and physiology of, 340–342
    anatomy and physiology terms relating to, 343–344*t*
    combining forms relating to, 343*t*
    external structure of, *340f*
    general diseases and conditions of, 350
    internal structure of (sagittal and interior views), *342f*
    movement of, with cranial nerves, *348f*
    structure of, from outside in, 340–341
    tests and procedures relating to, 356–357*t*
    vision, and other functions of, 341–342
    wellness and illness terms relating to, 350–351*t*
    wellness and illness through life span, 347–350
Eyelids, 340

F

Fallopian tubes, 568, *568f*, 569, *569f*, 570, 601
Fanconi's anemia, 185
Farmer's lung, 231
Farsightedness, 350
Fasceculi, 134
Fasciculation, *313f*
Fasting blood sugar, 276
Fats, 469
    emulsification of, 466
FBS. *See* Fasting blood sugar
FDA. *See* Food and Drug Administration
Feces, 467
Female gonads, 569
Female reproductive cycle, combining forms relating to, 571*t*
Female reproductive organs, assessment of, 578
Female reproductive system, 567–599
    abbreviations for, 588*t*
    anatomy and physiology of, 568–571
    anatomy and physiology terms relating to, 572–574*t*
    diagnosing and treating problems with, 586–587
    external genitalia, *568f*, 568–569
    organs of, *568f*

pharmacologic agents for, 587–588*t*
    practitioners for, 567–568
    tests and procedures relating to, 586–587*t*
    wellness and illness terms relating to, 582–583*t*
    wellness and illness through life span and, 578–582
Females, pelvises of, 144, *145f*
Femur, 122
Fertility, increasing, 587
Fertilization, 570, 601
Fetal age, verifying, 612
Fetal development, 604*t*
Fetal monitoring, 613
Fetal phase, of pregnancy, 602–603
Fetal shunts, 436
Fetal skeleton, 140
Fetus, 602
    blood cells in, 181
    cardiovascular problems in, 435–436
    endocrinological disorders in, 267–268
    respiratory problems in, 398
    in utero, *604f*, 606
Fibrinogen, 170
Fibroids, uterine, 581, *581f*
Fibromyalgia, 146–147
Fibrosis, 144
Filtration of liquids, urine formation and, 505
Fimbria, 569, *569f*
Fixation, 154
Flaccid quadriplegia, 315, *315f*
Flatfoot, 143
Flexion, 49, *50f*
Fluoroscopy, 57, 58
Follicles, in thyroid gland, 257
Follicle-stimulating hormone, 570
Fontanels, 142
Food and Drug Administration, 103
Foramen ovale, 435
Foreskin (prepuce), 539, *539f*
Form, suffixes indicating, 10*t*
Formation, suffixes indicating, 10*t*
Formed elements, 170
Fovea, 341
Fovea centralis, 341
Fowler's position, 49, *49f*
Fractures
    during adolescence, 144
    surgical treatment of, 154
Fremitus, 397
Frenulum, 463, *463f*
Frequency, 512
Frontal lobe, of brain, 291, 292
Frontal (or coronal) plane, 49, *49f*
Frontal sinus, 385, *385f*
Functional heart murmurs, 438
Fundus, 465, *465f*, 569, *569f*, 611
Fungiform, 374

G

Gallbladder, 462, *462f*, 466, *466f*
    disorders of, 479
Gallium scan, 239
Gallstone, *480f*
    formation of, 479
Gamete, 537, 567
Ganglion, 147
Gas exchange, 390
    through cardiovascular system, 424–425, *425f*
Gastrectomy, 486
Gastric juice, 465
Gastroenterologist, 461
Gastroenterology, 461

Gastrointestinal bleeding, in infants and children, 182
Gastrointestinal (GI) system, 461–499
    abbreviations for, 489t
    anatomy and physiology of, 462–469
    anatomy and physiology terms relating to, 470–472t
    assessment of, 477
    combining forms relating to, 469–470t
    major structures of and medical specialties for, 39f
    pharmacologic agents relating to, 487–488t
    practitioners for, 461
    tests and procedures relating to, 486–487t
    wellness and illness terms relating to, 480–482t
    wellness and illness terms through life span and, 477–479
Gastroscopy, 486
G-CSF. See Granulocyte colony-stimulating factor
Gender, determination of, 603
Generic names, in prescription drug names, 67
Genitalia
    female, 568f, 568–569
    male, 538
Genu valgum, 143
Genu varum, 143
Gestational age, 601
Gestational diabetes, 612
GHRH. See Growth hormone-releasing hormone
Girls, growth chart for, 269f
GI series, 486
Glans penis, 539, 539f
Glaucoma, 349
Glia, 296
Gliding diarthroses, 126, 127f
Globulins, 170
Glomerular filtration rate, 521
Glomeruli (glomerulus), 503, 504f, 505
Glomerulonephritis, 513
Glottis, 386
Glucagon, 260
Glucocorticoids, 259
Glucose, 469
Glucose-6-phosphate dehydrogenase (G-6-PD), 184
Glucose tolerance test, 276
Glucosuria, 270
GnRH. See Gonadotropin-releasing hormone
Goiter, 271
Gold compounds, 156
Golgi apparati, 35
Gonadotropin-releasing hormone, 256
Gonads, 537
    female, 569
Gonorrhea, 582
Gout, 145
Gouty arthritis, 145
Graafian follicles, 570, 571f
Grade, of tumor, 203
Granulocyte colony-stimulating factor, 196
Granulocyte-macrophage colony-stimulating factor (GM-CSF), 196
Granulocytes, 170, 173
Graves' disease, 271
Gravids, 581
Gray matter, 290
Greek-based words, plurals for, 23
Greek roots, 4
Growth factors, 196
Growth hormone-releasing hormone, 256

GTT. See Glucose tolerance test
Gustatory receptors, 374
Gynecologist, 581
Gynecology, 567
Gyri, on brain surface, 290

H

Haemophilus influenzae type b (Hib), 230, 398
Hair, 79, 81–82
    anatomy and physiology terms relating to, 85–86t
    combining forms relating to, 84t
    general conditions of, 95
Hair follicles, 81
    and related structures, 82f
Hair papilla, 82
Hair removal, 82
Hair shaft, 82
Hairy nevi, 92
Hammer toes, 146
Hand-foot syndrome, 183
Hay fever, 231
hCG. See Human chorionic gonadatropin
Head, eyes, ears, nose, and throat (HEENT) examinations, 48
Head, sagittal view of, 386f
Head and neck cancers, 479
Healthy People 2010, 613
Hearing, 339
    process of, 363
    system of and its practitioners, 360
Hearing aids, 360
Heart, 419–420, 420
    abnormal sounds in, 437t
    blood flow through, 423–425
        atrial systole, 423f
        ventricular systole, 424f
    conduction system of, 426f
    congenital defects of, 436, 437–438t
    gas exchange and, 424–425, 425f
    internal view of, 422f
    rhythms of, in ECG tests, 445f
    surrounding structures of, 421f
    valve defects in, 437t
Heart attacks, 427
Heartburn, 479
Heart murmur, 436
Heart sounds, listening to, 435
Heat production, muscle and, 135
Helicobacter pylori, 478
Hemangioma, 92
Hematologic disorders, hereditary, 183t
Hematologist, 169
Hematologist-oncologist, 189
Hematology and oncology, 169–216
    abbreviations in, 197t
    combining forms relating to, 175–176t
    definition of, 169
    diagnosing and treating problems in, 194–196
    pharmacologic agents in, 196t
    wellness and illness through life span and, 181–186
Hematoma, 185
Hematopoiesis, 170–171
    tree, 182f
Hematopoietic stem cell transplantation, 205
Hematopoietic system
    cancers of, 189
    tests of, 194
Hematuria, 512
Hemisphere, of brain, 290
Hemodialysis, 521
Hemoglobin, 171

Hemoglobinopathy, 183
Hemolysis, 181
Hemolytic anemia, 184
Hemolyzed red blood cells, 184
Hemophilia, 184–185
Hemorrhage, 183
Hemorrhoids, 479, 480f
Hemosiderosis, 184
Hepatic ducts, 466, 467f
Hepatitis, 479
Hepatitis B, 230
Hepatocellular carcinoma, 479
Hepatomegaly, 181
Hereditary hematologic disorders, 183t
Hereditary immune system diseases, 230
Hereditary spherocytosis, 184
Hermaphroditism, 268, 547
Herpes, 582
Herpes lesions, 105
Herpetic paronychias, 95
Hesitancy, of urine stream, 512
HGB. See Hemoglobin
Hiatal (or hiatus) hernia, 479, 480f
High blood pressure, 430
High-density lipoproteins, 444
Hinge diarthroses, 126, 127f
Hippocrates, 1, 2
Hippocratic Oath, 2
Hirsutism, 95
Histologists, 36
Histology, 36
HIV. See Human immunodeficiency virus
Hodgkin's lymphoma, 190
Homeostasis, 135, 255
Homovanillic acid, 276
Horizontal plane, 49
Hormonal abnormalities
    manifestations of, 267t
    prefixes in, 266
Hormone replacement agents, male, 555t
Hormones, 171, 253
Horseshoe kidney, 513
HPV. See Human papilloma virus
Human chorionic gonadotropin, 260, 613
Human immunodeficiency virus, 232
    preventing spread of, 233
Human leukocyte antigen (HLA) B-27, 154
Human papilloma virus, 582
Humerus, 122
Humoral immunity, 220
Humpback, in teenagers, 144
HVA. See Homovanillic acid
Hydantoins, 325
Hydrocele, 548
Hydrocephalus, 308
Hydrochloric acid, 465
Hydrocortisone, 277
Hymen, 568f, 569
Hypercalcemia, 154
Hyperemia, 350
Hyperglycemia, 260, 270
Hyperlipemia, 438
Hyperopia, 350
Hypertension, 430
    during pregnancy, 612
Hypertropia, 348
Hypoalbuminemia, 513
Hypoglycemia, 268, 272
Hypoglycemic effect, 260
Hypolipidemics, 447
Hypospadias, 547
Hypotension, 430
Hypothalamus, 255, 256, 294
Hypothyroidism, congenital, 267

skin of, 91
  urinary system disorders in, 515
  visual disorders in, 349–350
Senses, overview of, 339
Sensory neurons, 295
Septum, 420
Sequestered blood cells, 181
Serum, 170
Serum alkaline phosphatase, 154
Serum calcium, 154
Serum glucose tests, 486
Serum glutamic pyruvic transaminase test, 486
Severe combined immunodeficiency, 230
Sex chromosomes, gender determination and, 603
Sex hormones, 259
Sexual development, male, 545, 546f, 547f
Sexual dysfunction
  male, 548
    treatment of, 538
Sexual intercourse, 601
Sexually transmitted disease, 582
SGPT test. See Serum glutamic pyruvic transaminase test
Shaft
  hair, 82
  penile, 539, 539f
Shotty, 229
Shoulder (or transverse) presentations, 606
Sickle cell anemia, 182, 183
  priapism and, 548
Sigmoidoscopy, 486
Silver nitrate, 357
Sims' position, 48, 48f
Single photon emission computed tomography, 324
Sinoatrial (SA) node, 425, 426f
Sinuses, 385, 385f
Sitting position, 48, 48f
Size, suffixes indicating, 10t
Skeletal muscles
  attachments of, 134f
  major, and movements controlled by
    anterior view, 132f
    posterior view, 133f
  structure of, 134f
Skeletal (or striated) muscle tissue, 36
Skeletal system
  anatomy and physiology of, 122–126
  combining forms for, 126t
Skeleton
  anatomy and physiology terms relating to, 128–129t
  bone types of, 122
  fetal, 140
Skin, 79
  of adolescents, 90
  anatomy and physiology terms relating to, 85–86t
  anatomy of, 80f, 80–81
  cardiovascular health and, 435
  combining forms relating to, 84t
  cosmetic treatments for, 104–105t
  functions of, 80
  of infants, 89–90
  layers of, 80–81
  of middle-aged adults, 91
  physiology of, 83–84
  of pregnant women, 91
  procedures and surgeries relating to, 104, 104t
  protection of, 83
  of seniors, 91
  temperature control and, 84

Skin cancer, 92–93
  sun exposure and, 103
Skin glands, 81
Skin lesions
  primary, and associated abnormalities, 93t
  secondary, and associated abnormalities, 94t
Skin problems, diagnosis and treatment of, 103–104
Skull, 290
SLE. See Systemic lupus erythematosus
Small cell lung cancer, 399
Small intestine, 462, 462f, 465, 466f
Smell, 339
  anatomy and physiology of, 374–375
Smooth muscle, 134
Smooth muscle tissue, 36
SNOMED CT (SNOMED Clinical Terms), 71, 72
SNOMED (Systematized Nomenclature of Medicine), 71, 72
SNS. See Somatic nervous system
Social workers, 317
Somatic nervous system, 294
Somatostatin, 256, 260
Sonography, 57, 58, 58f
Soundalikes, 24
Sound waves, movement of, 363f
Sour taste, 374, 374f
Special senses, major structures and medical specialties for, 43f
Specialties, suffixes used in names of, 9t
Species immunity, 222
Specific immunity, 221
  types of, 223t
SPECT. See Single photon emission computed tomography
Speculum, 578
Spelling
  accurate, 25
  of plurals, 23
Sperm, 537, 567, 601
  pathway of, 540
  structure of, 540f
  travel of, through ducts and glands, 540, 541f
Spermatic cord, 540
Sperm production, decline in, 547
Sphenoidal sinus, 385, 385f
Spherocytes, 184
Spider nevi, 92
Spina bifida, 309, 613
Spinal columns, divisions of, 54, 54f
Spinal cord, 294
Spinal nerves, 289, 294, 304, 306f
Spinal tap, 324
Spinal tracts, 294
Spirometer, 404
Spleen, 218, 219
  enlarged, 229
Splenectomy, 185
Splenomegaly, 181
Sports injuries, during adolescence, 144
Sprains, during adolescence, 144
Squamous cell carcinoma, 92
Stages, of tumors, 203
Stapes, 361, 361f
Staphylococcus aureus, 350
Station, 606
STD. See Sexually transmitted disease
Stem cell transplantation, 205
Sterility, male, 549
Sterilization, female, 586
Sternum, 122

Steroid hormones, 254
Steroids, 156
Stethoscope, 435
Stomach, 462, 462f, 465, 465f
Stomach cancer, 479
Strabismus, 348
Stratum corneum, 81, 83
Stratum germinativum, 81
Striae (stretch marks), in pregnant women, 91, 91f
Striated muscle, 36, 134
Striations, 134
Stroke, 309, 430
  causes of, 186
Sty, 350
Subcutaneous layer, 81
Subcutaneous medication administration, 69t, 70f
Sublingual salivary glands, 464, 464f
Subluxation, 146, 147
Submandibular salivary glands, 464, 464f
Suffixes, 8–11, 20
  of adjectives, 24
  combining forms and, 6
  commonly used general, 13t
  compound, 15
  conditions or processes indicated by, 10t
  defined, 3
  diagnostic procedures described by, 11t
  form, size, and formation indicated by, 10t
  meaning "related to" or "pertaining to," 9t
  in medical term, 3
  in names of specialties and practitioners, 9t
  in radiology terms, 60
  therapeutic procedures indicated by, 11t
Sulci, 291
Sun exposure, skin cancer risks and, 103
Superficial location, 47
Superficial reflexes, 307f
Superior location, 46, 46f
Superior venae cavae, 422f, 423
Supination, 50, 50f
Supine position, 47, 47f
Surfactant, 389
Surgery
  endoscopic, 64
  laparoscopic, 64
Surgery terms, general, 64–65t
Surgical procedures
  for cancer, 205
  relating to endocrine system, 277t
  relating to musculoskeletal system, 154–155
  relating to nervous system, 325
  relating to urinary system, 521–522
  on skin, 104
Suture lines, on newborn head, 140
Sweat glands, 81, 254
  temperature regulation and, 84
Sweet taste, 374, 374f
Swollen glands, 229
Sympathetic nervous system, 294
Symphysis pubis, 568
Synapse, 295
Synarthroses, 125
Syndactyly, 142
Synovial Cell Sarcoma, 147
Synovial fluid, 126
Synovial membrane, 125
Syphilis, 582
Sysphagia, 310
Systemic circulation, 430
Systemic lupus erythematosus, 514

pg 68 abbreviations

Photo Credits

Ch 2 — Page 58: Corbis; Page 59 (top): Corbis; Page 59 (bottom): Corbis • Ch 3 — Page 81: Image Vault; Page 90 (top): Medical-On-Line/Corbis; Page 90 (middle): Corbis; Page 90 (bottom): Medical-On-Line/Corbis; Page 91: Medical-On-Line/Corbis; Page 92 (top): Medical-On-Line/Corbis; Page 92 (bottom): Corbis; Page 95: Image Vault • Ch 4 — Page 122: © Custom Medical Stock Photo; Page 139 (left): Custom Medical Stock Photo; Page 139 (right) © Science Photo Library/Custom Medical Stock Photo; Page 140: Image Vault; Page 142: Corbis; Page 143 (upper left): © Dr P. Marazzi/Science Photo Library/Custom Medical Stock Photo; Page 143 (upper right): Custom Medical Stock Photo; Page 143 (bottom): Image Vault; Page 144: © NMSB/Custom Medical Stock Photo; Page 146: © NMSB/Custom Medical Stock Photo • Ch 5 — Page 170: Image Vault; Page 173: Image Vault • Ch 6 — Page 217: Image Vault; Page 220: American Mosaic • Ch 7 — Page 268: Superstock Portfolio of Images • Ch 8 — Page 292: FPG International; Page 316 (top): Medical-On-Line/Corbis; Page 316 (lower left): Medical-On-Line/Corbis; Page 316 (lower right): Medical-On-Line/Corbis; Page 317: Photo Researchers Science Source • Ch 9 — Page 339: Image Vault • Ch 11 — Page 419: Stock Market; Page 420: Stock Market • Ch 12 — Page 462: Image Vault; Page 478: Image Vault; Page 479: Image Vault • Ch 13 — Page 502: Image Vault; Page 521: Image Vault • Ch 16 — Page 603, Figure 16.1: Superstock Portfolio of Images; Page 604, Figure 16.2: Photo Researchers Science Source; Page 613: Picture Perfect